AGING AND THE KIDNEY

AGING AND THE KIDNEY

MECHANISMS, CONSEQUENCES, AND MANAGEMENT STRATEGIES

Edited by

STEPHEN Z. FADEM

Department of Medicine, Section of Nephrology, Baylor College of Medicine, Houston, TX, United States

AHMED ARSLAN YOUSUF AWAN

Department of Internal Medicine, Baylor College of Medicine, Houston, TX, United States

EMAAD M. ABDEL-RAHMAN

Division of Nephrology, University of Virginia, Charlottesville, VA, United States

ELSEVIER

ACADEMIC PRESS

An imprint of Elsevier

Academic Press is an imprint of Elsevier
125 London Wall, London EC2Y 5AS, United Kingdom
50 Hampshire Street, 5th Floor, Cambridge, MA 02139, United States

For accessibility purposes, images in electronic versions of this book are accompanied by alt text descriptions provided by Elsevier. For more information, see https://www.elsevier.com/about/accessibility.

Books and Journals published by Elsevier comply with applicable product safety requirements. For any product safety concerns or queries, please contact our authorised representative, Elsevier B.V., at productsafety@elsevier.com.

Publisher's note: Elsevier takes a neutral position with respect to territorial disputes or jurisdictional claims in its published content, including in maps and institutional affiliations.

Notices

Knowledge and best practice in this field are constantly changing. As new research and experience broaden our understanding, changes in research methods, professional practices, or medical treatment may become necessary.

Practitioners and researchers must always rely on their own experience and knowledge in evaluating and using any information, methods, compounds, or experiments described herein. In using such information or methods they should be mindful of their own safety and the safety of others, including parties for whom they have a professional responsibility.

To the fullest extent of the law, neither the Publisher nor the authors, contributors, or editors, assume any liability for any injury and/or damage to persons or property as a matter of products liability, negligence or otherwise, or from any use or operation of any methods, products, instructions, or ideas contained in the material herein.

ISBN: 978-0-443-34069-7

For information on all Elsevier publications visit our website at https://www.elsevier.com/books-and-journals

Publisher: Andre Wolff
Acquisitions Editor: Wendi Baker
Editorial Project Manager: Kshitij Jha
Production Project Manager: Sruthi Satheesh
Cover Designer: Raman Kumar

Typeset by Integra Software Services

About the cover

The cover of this book reflects its central theme: aging is a complex interplay of biological, physiological, and clinical factors. While these factors influence kidney health, the kidney itself plays an important role in the aging process.

The illuminated kidney symbolizes the organ at the center of this discussion and represents the intricate networks of cellular signaling, molecular pathways, and systemic interactions that contribute to both aging and age-related kidney disease. The interconnected digital pattern highlights the growing role of systems biology, translational science, artificial intelligence, and precision medicine in unraveling these mechanisms.

The images embedded within the kidney were selected to illustrate several key concepts. The older adult who maintains physical strength and independence represents successful aging, resilience, and functional longevity. The healthcare interaction emphasizes the importance of patient-centered care, prevention, and multidisciplinary management in optimizing outcomes for older adults.

The long-lived animal species depicted on the cover—the naked mole rat, Greenland shark, and Galápagos giant tortoise—have become important models for studying exceptional longevity, disease resistance, and biological mechanisms that may inform human aging research.

The naked mole-rat (*Heterocephalus glaber*) is the longest-lived rodent known, with a maximum lifespan exceeding 37 years, approximately 10 times that of a mouse. It is the only known thermoconforming mammal and behaves as if it were cold-blooded. Thus, the small animals bundle together in large huddles deep in burrowed tunnels. It resists hypoxia, exhibits negligible senescence, shows little or no age-related increase in mortality, shows remarkable resistance to cancer, and preserves reproductive capacity throughout life. Recent investigations have identified unique adaptations in naked mole rat DNA damage-sensing pathways, including modifications of cyclic GMP–AMP synthase (cGAS), that enhance recruitment of DNA repair machinery and promote genomic stability. These adaptations may contribute to the species' extraordinary longevity and resistance to age-related decline (Chen et al., 2025).

The Greenland shark (*Somniosus microcephalus*) is the longest-lived vertebrate known. Radiocarbon dating of eye lens proteins has estimated lifespans of at least 272 years and potentially approaching 400 years (Nielsen et al., 2016). The species does not reach sexual maturity until 150 to 170 years of age, thrives in cold deep waters, and has a slow metabolism. They have adapted to support DNA repair and cancer resistance and are apex predators.

The Galápagos giant tortoise (*Chelonoidis* spp.) can live well beyond 100 years, with some individuals documented to survive for more than 175 years. Their slow metabolism reduces cellular damage. Genome sequencing studies have identified lineage-specific variants and gene duplications involving DNA repair, tumor suppression, and inflammatory signaling pathways, providing a potential genomic basis for their reduced cancer risk and exceptional longevity. They have no predators (Quesada et al., 2019).

Collectively, these species illustrate several converging biological themes, enhanced DNA repair, cancer resistance, maintenance of genomic integrity, and resilience to cellular stress, that are directly relevant to understanding human aging. The aging kidney undergoes nephron loss, fibrosis, mitochondrial dysfunction, and declining regenerative capacity, processes closely linked to the pathways long-lived species have evolved to preserve.

The cover symbolizes the continuum from basic scientific discovery to clinical application. Insights gained from comparative biology and aging research inform our understanding of kidney disease and will ultimately lead to new strategies for preserving renal function throughout the lifespan.

This cover serves as a visual reminder that aging is both a biological journey and a clinical challenge, requiring the integration of fundamental science, compassionate care, and innovative research to improve outcomes for older adults with kidney disease.

References

Chen, Y., Chen, Z., Wang, H., et al., 2025. A cGAS-mediated mechanism in naked mole-rats potentiates DNA repair and delays aging. Science.

Nielsen, J., Hedeholm, R.B., Heinemeier, J., Bushnell, P.G., Christiansen, J.S., Olsen, J., Ramsey, C.B., Brill, R.W., Simon, M., Steffensen, K.F., Steffensen, J.F., 2016. Eye lens radiocarbon reveals centuries of longevity in the Greenland shark (*Somniosus microcephalus*). Science 353 (6300), 702–704.

Quesada, V., Freitas-rodríguez, S., Miller, J., Perez-Silva, J.G., Jiang, Z.F., Tapia, W., Santiago-Fernández, O., Campos-Iglesias, D., Kuderna, L.F.K., Quinzin, M., Álvarez, M.G., Carrero, D., Beheregaray, L.B., Gibbs, J.P., Chiari, Y., Glaberman, S., Ciofi, C., Araujo-Voces, M., Mayoral, P., Arango, J.R., Tamargo-Gómez, I., Roiz-Valle, D., Pascual-Torner, M., Evans, B.R., Edwards, D.L., Garrick, R.C., Russello, M.A., Poulakakis, N., Gaughran, S.J., Rueda, D.O., Bretones, G., Rodríguez, F., Muntané, G., Puente, X.S., López-Otín, C., 2019. Giant tortoise genomes provide insights into longevity and age-related disease. Nat. Ecol. Evol. 3 (1), 87–95.

Contents

6. The influence of acute kidney injury on aging

Gonzalo Ramírez-Guerrero and Mitchell Rosner

7. Nutritional considerations and aging

Yoko Narasaki, Connie M. Rhee, and Kamyar Kalantar-Zadeh

8. Proteomics

Stephen Z. Fadem and Emaad M. Abdel-Rahman

Part 2

Unique characteristics of kidney diseases in the elderly

9. Impaired quality of life in elderly CKD patients

Zara Ijaz and Angelina Edwards

10. Sleep

Seki A. Balogun and Emaad M. Abdel-Rahman

11. Falls

Stephen Z. Fadem

12. Fatigue and frailty in kidney disease

Totini Sagorika Chatterjee and Lucile Parker Gregg

13. Hospitalizations

Neha Siddiqui and Samaya Anumudu

14. Depression

Jessica Lowe and Angelina Edwards

15. Sarcopenia

Sheryl Cababat Caberto, Lynn Schlanger, and Stephen Z. Fadem

Part 3

Aging in specific diseases

16. Hypertension

Faruk Hilmi Turgut and Emaad M. Abdel-Rahman

17. Diabetes in kidney disease progression

Sheryl Cababat Caberto, Lynn Schlanger, and Stephen Z. Fadem

18. Glomerulonephritis

Akwe Nyabera and Gerald Appel

19. Peripheral vascular disease

Eric Peden, Omodele Durojaye, and Brianna Whithorn

Part 4

Management and prevention

20. Diagnosis of CKD in an elderly individual, due to a decline in GFR with normal healthy aging

Bryce M. Churilla, Jae Hun Son, Khan Shabtab, Sheryl Cababat Caberto, and Stephen Z. Fadem

21. Myths about chronic kidney disease in the elderly

Ahmed Awan and Sarwar Khan

22. The living donor and aging

Catherine Cecelia Vatsis and Sean Hebert

23. CNS limitations in elderly kidney patients

Stephen Z. Fadem and Totini Sagorika Chatterjee

24. Cancer and the kidney in an elderly individual

Raad Chowdhury and Si Yuan Khor

25. Cardiovascular disease in aging kidney

Ahmad Armoghan Yousuf Awan, Muhammad Rizwan, Rameesha Awan, and Carl Peter Walther

26. Benefits of renin angiotensin aldosterone system blockage

Faruk Hilmi Turgut and Emaad M. Abdel-Rahman

27. Active medical care without dialysis

Ojaswi Singh Tomar, Rebecca J. Schmidt, and Alvin Howard Moss

28. Drugs to avoid with geriatric kidney disease

Stephen Z. Fadem

29. Innovations in chronic kidney disease and aging

Stephen Z. Fadem

Contributors

Emaad M. Abdel-Rahman Division of Nephrology, University of Virginia, Charlottesville, VA, United States

Samaya Anumudu Baylor College of Medicine, Houston, TX, United States

Gerald Appel Nephrology, Columbia University Medical Center, New York, NY, United States

Ahmad Armoghan Yousuf Awan Memorial Heart and Vascular Center, Interventional and Endovascular Cardiologist, Lake Charles, LA, United States

Ahmed Awan Department of Internal Medicine, Baylor College of Medicine, Houston, TX, United States

Rameesha Awan Hull York Medical School, York, United Kingdom

Seki A. Balogun Geriatric Medicine Fellowship Program, University of Oklahoma, Norman, OK, United States

Brendan Bowman Division of Nephrology, University of Virginia, Charlottesville, VA, United States

Sheryl Cababat Caberto Division of Renal Medicine, Emory University School of Medicine, Atlanta, GA, United States

Sheryl Cababat Caberto Division of Renal Medicine, Emory University School of Medicine, Atlanta, GA, United States

Totini Sagorika Chatterjee Division of Geriatrics; Division of Nephrology, Department of Medicine, University of Texas Medical Branch, Galveston, TX, United States

Raad Chowdhury BWH-MGH Combined Renal Fellowship, Medical Director of Onconephrology, Dana-Farber Cancer Institute, Harvard Medical School, Brigham and Women's Hospital, Boston, MA, United States

Bryce M. Churilla Division of Renal Medicine, Emory University, Atlanta, GA, United States

Zheng Dong Department of Cellular Biology and Anatomy, Medical College of Georgia, Augusta University; Charlie Norwood VA Medical Center, Augusta, GA, United States

Omodele Durojaye Vascular Surgery; Department of Cardiovascular Surgery, Houston Methodist Hospital, Houston, TX, United States

Angelina Edwards Department of Medicine, Division of Nephrology, Houston Methodist Academic Institute, Houston Methodist Hospital, Weill Cornell Medical College, Houston, TX, United States

Stephen Z. Fadem Department of Medicine, Section of Nephrology, Baylor College of Medicine, Houston, TX, United States

Lucile Parker Gregg Medicine, Selzman Institute for Kidney Health, Baylor College of Medicine; Center for Innovations in Quality, Effectiveness and Safety, Michael E. DeBakey VA Medical Center, Houston, TX, United States

Sean Hebert MaineHealth Transplant Program, Maine Medical Center, Portland, ME, United States

Zara Ijaz Department of Internal Medicine, Houston Methodist Hospital, Houston, TX, United States

Shuta Ishibe Section of Nephrology, Yale University, New Haven, CT, United States

Kamyar Kalantar-Zadeh Division of Nephrology, Hypertension, and Kidney Transplantation, University of California Irvine, Orange; Division of Nephrology and Hypertension, The Lundquist Institute at Harbor-UCLA Medical Center, Torrance, CA, United States

Sarwar Khan Department of Internal Medicine, Baylor College of Medicine, Houston, TX, United States

Si Yuan Khor Renal Division, Department of Medicine, Brigham and Women's Hospital, Boston, MA, United States

Jessica Lowe Internal Medicine Resident, Department of Medicine, Houston Methodist Hospital, Houston, TX, United States

Alvin Howard Moss Department of Medicine, Division of Geriatrics, Palliative Medicine and Hospice, West Virginia University School of Medicine, Morgantown, WV, United States

Yoko Narasaki Department of Medicine, David Geffen School of Medicine at UCLA; Nephrology Section, Veterans Affairs Greater Los Angeles Healthcare System, Los Angeles, CA, United States

Akwe Nyabera Nephrology, Columbia University Medical Center, New York, NY, United States

Eric Peden Vascular Surgery, Houston Methodist Hospital, Houston, TX, United States

Jeffrey W. Pippin Division of Nephrology, University of Washington, Seattle, WA, United States

Gonzalo Ramírez-Guerrero International Renal Research Institute of Vicenza (IRRIV), Vicenza, Italy; Carlos Van Buren Hospital, Nephrology and Dialysis Unit; Department of Medicine, Universidad de Valparaíso, Valparaíso, Chile

Connie M. Rhee Department of Medicine, David Geffen School of Medicine at UCLA; Nephrology Section, Veterans Affairs Greater Los Angeles Healthcare System, Los Angeles; Division of Nephrology, Hypertension, and Kidney Transplantation, University of California Irvine, Orange, CA, United States

Muhammad Rizwan Medstar Washington Hospital Center, Washington, DC, United States

Mitchell Rosner Division of Nephrology, Department of Medicine, University of Virginia Health System, Charlottesville, VA, United States

Lynn Schlanger Division of Renal Medicine, Emory University School of Medicine, Atlanta, GA, United States

Rebecca J. Schmidt Department of Medicine, Division of Nephrology, West Virginia University School of Medicine, Morgantown, WV, United States

Khan Shabtab Renal Medicine, Atlanta VA Medical Center; Division of Renal Medicine, Emory University School of Medicine, Atlanta, GA, United States

Stuart J. Shankland Division of Nephrology; Institute for Stem Cell & Regenerative Medicine, University of Washington, Seattle, WA, United States

Neha Siddiqui Baylor College of Medicine, Houston, TX, United States

Jae Hun Son Division of Renal Medicine, Emory University, Atlanta, GA, United States

Ojaswi Singh Tomar Department of Medicine, Division of Nephrology, West Virginia University School of Medicine, Morgantown, WV, United States

Faruk Hilmi Turgut Department of Internal Medicine, Division of Nephrology, Hatay Mustafa Kemal University, Hatay, Turkey

Catherine Cecelia Vatsis Southwest Kidney Institute, Phoenix, AZ, United States

Carl Peter Walther Department of Nephrology, Baylor St. Luke's Medical Center, Houston, TX, United States

Qingqing Wei Department of Cellular Biology and Anatomy, Medical College of Georgia, Augusta University, Augusta, GA, United States

Oliver Wessely Cleveland Clinic Research, Cleveland Clinic, Cleveland, OH, United States

Brianna Whithorn Vascular Surgery, Houston Methodist Hospital, Houston, TX, United States

Foreword

The dream of eternal youth has been alive in our imagination since the dawn of human evolution. Myths and legends abound in searching for a magic antiaging potion, whether it be Ponce de Leon and the Fountain of Youth, Sir Galahad and the search for the Holy Grail, or the elixirs of nectar and ambrosia sought by the ancient Greeks. Yet, despite our dreams, aging seems undeniable and unavoidable.

Or is it? In the last few decades, there has been much interest in the fundamental mechanisms driving aging. Furthermore, we have all witnessed how some individuals age faster than others. And it is not just the duration of life, but the quality of life. Jeanne Calmet, who holds the record for being the longest-lived human by living to 122 years of age, remained active in tennis and roller-skating for many years, and even took up fencing at age 85. She quit smoking at age 117, not because she thought smoking was bad, but because she had trouble using the lighter. And if we look across species, we can see that some animals, like the Greenland shark, can live over 400 years. Even more impressive is Ming, the ocean quahog clam that was documented to have lived over 500 years. But the record may be a specific species of jellyfish (*Turritopsis*) that is so good at tissue regeneration that it can survive for a thousand years or more. Thus, nature has informed us that immortality is not an unachievable goal. But immortality is not a destination; rather an extension of maximal healthy life span, or longevity is the objective. The search for longevity has led to the discovery of the importance of mechanisms to protect the DNA, mitochondria, and other key aspects of cellular metabolism that can slowly deteriorate over time. Today, there are many investigators and pharmaceutical companies looking for the magical solutions to help people live longer (lifespan) and healthier (healthspan). It is very clear that the rate of aging differs between individuals, even if they are genetically identical. Furthermore, the organs and organ systems undergo aging (senescence) at variable rates even in a single individual.

One way to live longer and healthier is to understand what processes might be responsible for the rate of aging in organs or organ systems. In this regard, the kidney is a very metabolically active organ that works around the clock to help regulate body fluids and electrolyte concentrations, and as an organ, it is especially sensitive to aging. Indeed, most (but not all) people will show signs of an aging process in kidney function (and anatomy) after 40 years of age. Similarly, it is being increasingly recognized that chronic kidney disease itself has many features in common with the aging kidney. Indeed, it has been hypothesized that some forms of chronic kidney disease may represent an acceleration of normative aging. In this remarkable monograph, Dr. Stephen Z. Fadem and colleagues take a deep dive into the intricacies of aging and the relationship of the organ-specific aging process of the kidney and kidney diseases per se. By evaluating the science of these relationships (and differences), new insights have emerged that will likely be helpful to anyone who manages or has an interest in the patient with kidney disease. Fadem and colleagues do not just review the insights of how aging and kidney disease are similar (or different) but also use this information to provide valuable clinical approaches to aid in the management of older and elderly patients. This includes not only advice on lifestyle, diet, exercise, and sleep but also both nonpharmacological and pharmacological approaches to help the patients with the manifestation of kidney disease.

As older physicians with a deep interest in the kidneys, we both greatly enjoyed and profited from reading *Aging and the Kidney* by Fadem and colleagues. Practical means for improving healthy longevity might be of great interest to all, but especially to subjects with bona fide chronic kidney disease. This monograph tackles this key objective in a rigorous way and provides clinician's a rational approach to management. The pearls of wisdom it uncovers contained between the covers of this book are worth remembering.

Richard J. Johnson, MD
Richard J. Glassock, MD

Preface

People are living longer than ever before, reshaping medicine's core challenge: not just prolonging life but also preserving dignity and independence across decades. Nowhere is this more urgent than in the care of older adults with kidney disease. The aging kidney occupies a unique crossroads in science—vulnerable to molecular wear and tear, yet also deeply shaped by cumulative exposures, comorbidities, therapies, and social context. *Aging and the Kidney: Possible Mechanisms, Consequences, and Management Strategies* seeks to unpack these complexities.

This book moves purposefully between mechanism and bedside, building from biological foundations to clinical realities. The opening chapters in the first part outline the structural and functional changes in aging kidneys and review experimental models that make these shifts tractable. We delve into molecular mechanisms of aging and devote focused attention to podocyte function. Throughout, aging is positioned as a dynamic, partially modifiable process—explored through advances in epigenetics and the expanding lens of proteomics, with an eye toward signatures that may one day inform prognosis and therapy. We close the section with discussions on acute kidney injury and nutrition—two central modifiers of aging trajectories.

In the second part, the focus turns to the lived experience. Kidney disease in later life is not captured by laboratory values alone; it manifests as disrupted sleep, falls, frailty, muscle weakness, depression, and hospitalizations. These chapters highlight geriatric syndromes as outcomes unto themselves and as key mediators of survival, resilience, and, crucially, quality of life. What matters to patients—functional status, symptom burden, and life priorities—anchors our discussion of how living with chronic kidney disease can become more manageable.

The third part addresses clinical decision-making. We examine the major drivers of kidney and general health decline—hypertension, diabetes, glomerular, and vascular disease—and analyze diagnostic nuances that can complicate care in older adults. Common myths and misperceptions about kidney disease in elders are confronted to empower sound clinical judgment.

Patients age differently. For some, transplantation remains feasible; for others, even routine dialysis becomes burdensome, demanding nuanced, shared decisions. Cognitive decline, stroke, cardiovascular disease, and cancer often intersect in these timelines. In the final part, we discuss selecting therapies that maximize benefit while minimizing harm and trace innovations in diagnosis and treatment that are reshaping the field.

This book is written for nephrologists, geriatricians, internists, primary care clinicians, advanced practice providers, pharmacists, nurses, dietitians, trainees, and researchers. Health-system leaders and policymakers may find support here for integrated care models, investments in fall prevention and rehabilitation, and metrics that align with patient priorities.

Readers may engage with chapters nonlinearly—clinic preparation may benefit from sections on sleep, fatigue, frailty, and falls; inpatient teams might prioritize hospitalizations, delirium, and medication safety; researchers may gravitate toward early mechanistic and technology chapters. Nonetheless, we encourage starting with the foundational science, then the patient experience, and finally management strategies.

We thank our patients and their families, whose questions and lives shape these pages as much as any data or metric. Their lived experiences—struggles with sleep, balance, travel, and independence—frame our work. We are equally grateful to our contributors for their knowledge, dedication, and clarity. Finally, we extend heartfelt thanks to our families for steadfast support during the long hours of this project.

Our hope is that *Aging and the Kidney* enables you to think biologically, act pragmatically, and care wholeheartedly—to translate advances in research and discoveries into practical decisions that help older adults with kidney disease live the lives they choose.

Stephen Z. Fadem
Emaad M. Abdel-Rahman
Ahmed Arsian Yousuf Awan

PART 1

Mechanisms of aging in the kidney

CHAPTER

1

Structural and functional changes in aging

Emaad M. Abdel-Rahman[a], *Stephen Z. Fadem*[b], *and Brendan Bowman*[a]

[a]Division of Nephrology, University of Virginia, Charlottesville, VA, United States
[b]Department of Medicine, Section of Nephrology, Baylor College of Medicine, Houston, TX, United States

Introduction

We, as the human race, are aging. Epidemiological data are quite clear about this fact, showing an increase in both the average age and the number of older adults worldwide.

Aging has been defined as a physiological process coupled with a sequence of events involving the growth and development of living organisms. While aging remains an unavoidable process, longitudinal studies suggest that some older adults may experience minimal changes throughout their lives. "Older adults" is the term used to identify individuals aged 65 years or older.

Data from the US Census Bureau and Centers for Disease Control and Prevention (CDC) project that older adults will account for 20% of the population in the US (around 72 million), and 24.8% and 33% in China and Europe, respectively, by 2030, just a few years from now (Hoerger et al., 2015). The average age is now 76.5 years in economically developed countries and 65.4 years in economically developing countries (Kanasaki et al., 2012).

This increase in the number of older adults, while a positive indicator, is associated with enormous implications for various social and economic aspects worldwide and, more specifically, with significant challenges for health systems.

Kidneys are among the organs most affected by the aging process. Both structural and functional changes have been clearly documented in the aging kidney through imaging studies, autopsies, and renal biopsies from healthy older individuals.

In this chapter, we will highlight the changes that occur in the aging kidney.

Aging and the Kidney
https://doi.org/10.1016/B978-0-443-34069-7.00003-3

Structural and functional changes in the kidneys with aging

Changes noted in the aging kidney may vary according to an individual's health condition and kidney status. While kidney structural and functional changes in healthy older adults may be minimal, these changes can be significant in patients with kidney impairment and/or significant comorbidities.

Structural kidney changes with aging

The structural changes in the kidney may be both macroscopic and microscopic, affecting all parts of the kidney.

Macroscopic changes in the kidney with aging (Table 1.1)

Renal mass With aging, there is a significant decline in renal mass associated with fibrosis, which may replace the remaining functional cortical parenchyma. While initial renal mass increases from birth to the fourth decade of life, reaching about 400 g, autopsy and imaging

TABLE 1.1 Changes in the kidney with aging.

Macroscopic changes		Microscopic changes		Functional kidney changes	
Renal mass	• Decline	Number and size of nephrons	• Decrease in the number of nephrons • Decrease in the size of nephrons	Glomerular Filtration Rate	• Decline, but not in every aging individual.
Renal volume	• Decrease • Focal cortical thinning	Shape of nephrons	• Change in the shape of nephrons • GBM thickening, glomerular tuft collapse	Renal plasma flow filtration fraction	• Decrease • Increase
Renal cysts	• More frequent and larger • Increase number of benign tumors	Nephrosclerosis • Glomeruli • Tubulointerstitium • Renal vascular	• Glomerulosclerosis • GBM thickening • Accumulation of extracellular matrix • Mesangial widening • Glomerular capillary loop obliteration • Podocytes' hypertrophy • Foot process fusion • Tubular atrophy • Decrease the number and size of renal tubules • Increase the number of renal tubule diverticula • Interstitial fibrosis • Atrophy of renal arteries and arterioles • Intimal and medial hypertrophy of intrarenal arteries • Arterioles' lumen obliteration	Proteinuria	• Increased association with worsening kidney function

studies have estimated that over 3–4 decades after the age of 40, kidney mass decreases by 10%–30% to about 300 g (McLachlan and Wasserman, 1981). Loss of renal mass occurs primarily in the cortical region, with relative sparing of the medulla (Emamian et al., 1993; Tauchi et al., 1971).

Renal volume The decrease in renal mass is usually associated with a decrease in renal parenchymal volume, focal cortical thinning with unaltered medulla, and parenchymal calcification (Emamian et al., 1993; Glassock and Rule, 2012; Hommos et al., 2017; Wang et al., 2014; Foster et al., 2011; Denic et al., 2016; Dybiec et al., 2022). This decrease in renal parenchymal volume is noted as part of the aging process, regardless of the presence or absence of comorbidities.

Imaging studies of kidneys obtained from autopsies estimated a loss of around 16 cm^2/decade in the renal parenchymal volume (Hommos et al., 2017). Similar results were noted when assessing imaging studies of living kidney donors (Wang et al., 2014). A study using CT scans in 360 patients with no kidney disease showed that the parenchymal thickness of a kidney declined by 10% per decade of age (Gourtsoyiannis et al., 1990).

While Glodny and coworkers (Glodny et al., 2009) confirmed these findings in asymptomatic patients, Johnson and coworkers (Johnson et al., 2011) failed to show a correlation between aging and kidney parenchymal volume in healthy potential kidney transplant donors.

Renal cysts Renal cysts in the glomeruli have been demonstrated to be more frequent and larger in size in the aging population, particularly in hypertensive males and in patients with proteinuria (McNamara et al., 2010). A study of kidneys obtained from donors demonstrated a tenfold increase in the number of kidney parenchymal cysts ≥ 5 mm in men and a fourfold increase in women when comparing kidneys obtained from donors in their seventh decade to those obtained from patients in their third decade (Rule et al., 2012). Similarly, there is a noted increase in the incidence of some benign tumors with aging.

Microscopic changes in the kidney with aging (Table 1.1)

Several microscopic changes in the aging kidney have been well described in the literature. These changes affect all the microstructures of the kidney.

Number and size of nephrons Along with the decrease in renal mass, the number and size of the nephrons are also noted to decline (McNamara et al., 2010). The decline in the mean number of nephrons per kidney was observed to drop from close to a million nephrons for subjects in their twenties to almost half that number by the eighth decade.

Studies of kidney autopsy series (Hoy et al., 2003) and kidney biopsies of living kidney donors (Denic et al., 2017) have demonstrated a loss of kidney nephrons with aging. This decline in the number of nephrons is associated with changes in the shape of the nephrons (Mclachlan, 1978; Goyal, 1982), including progressive thickening and folding of the glomerular basement membrane (GBM), which later condenses into hyaline material with glomerular tuft collapse.

Nephrosclerosis Nephrosclerosis, defined as focal global glomerulosclerosis, arteriosclerosis, tubular atrophy, and interstitial fibrosis, is a common feature of an aging kidney (Glassock and Rule, 2012; Dybiec et al., 2022). The prevalence of nephrosclerosis was noted to increase markedly with aging, from only 2.7% for healthy adults in their third decade to 73% in the eighth decade (Rule et al., 2010).

Glomerular changes Several changes occur in the glomeruli of the aging kidney, including glomerulosclerosis, GBM thickening, accumulation of extracellular matrix, and mesangial widening (Nyengaard and Bendtsen, 1992).

The number of globally sclerosed glomeruli obtained from normotensive kidney donors was shown to increase by more than fivefold between the age of 20 and 70 (Kremers et al., 2015), and may account for as much as 30% of the glomeruli by that age (Kaplan and Shah, 1975). It is believed that the glomerulosclerosis noted with aging is secondary to ischemic injury to the glomeruli subsequent to age-associated arteriosclerosis.

The noted accumulation of extracellular matrix and the mesangial widening may further obliterate the glomerular capillary loops, with capillary tuft collapse and intra-capsular fibrosis, as shown in mice and rat models (Zheng et al., 2003; Bolton and Sturgill, 1980). While early in life both glomerular mesangial cells and endothelial cells increase in number, they both decline later in life. Podocytes are also affected by aging. The aging podocytes exhibit hypertrophy, foot process fusion, and may detach from the GBM (Bolton and Sturgill, 1980; Ortmann et al., 2004).

Furthermore, the shape of the glomeruli may change with aging. The spherical glomerulus in the fetal kidney develops lobular indentations as it matures, which tend to diminish with aging. In addition, the length of the glomerular tuft perimeter decreases relative to the total area with age (Mclachlan, 1978).

Tubulointerstitial changes Both tubular atrophy, characterized by a decline in the number and size of renal tubules, and interstitial fibrosis, marked by the accumulation of scar tissue in the kidney's interstitial space, are prevalent in the aging kidney. Tubular atrophy and interstitial fibrosis may be a function of aging or may occur due to chronic inflammation or vascular disease (Takazakura et al., 1972). This tubulointerstitial fibrosis, noted in aging, is an active process associated with interstitial inflammation and fibroblast activity. The distal renal tubules develop diverticula, which increase in number with advancing age (Zhou et al., 2008).

Renal vascular changes Renal arteries are also affected by the aging process. Several changes are noted upon examining the aging renal arteries and arterioles (Takazakura et al., 1972; Ljungqvist and Lagergren, 1962). While both the afferent and efferent arterioles show atrophic changes with global sclerosis, the renal arteries are observed to exhibit renal artery fibromuscular dysplasia and atherosclerotic narrowing. The presence of arteriosclerosis in the small arteries of the kidneys may potentially contribute to ischemic injury to the nephrons, which may further progress into global glomerulosclerosis and tubular atrophy (Denic et al., 2016).

Several studies have shown intimal and medial hypertrophy in the intrarenal arteries with aging, while the arterioles may exhibit hyaline deposits within the vessel walls, leading to vessel lumen obliteration (Kubo et al., 2003; McLachlan et al., 1977).

Functional kidney changes with aging (Table 1.1)

With aging and the accompanying changes in the macro- and microscopic structure of the kidneys, several physiological changes also occur in the aging kidney.

As kidneys age, the balance between several mediators is altered, thus playing a major role in the kidney's response to acute injury.

There is reduced renin production, aldosterone levels (Thomas et al., 2005), and nitric oxide (NO) (Sverdlov et al., 2014), as well as decreased sensitivity to the vasodilatory response. On the contrary, there is a propensity toward increased sensitivity to vasoconstrictor stimuli and heightened oxidative stress, resulting in endothelial cell dysfunction and changes in vasoactive mediators.

Glomerular filtration rate (GFR)

Several functional changes occur in kidney function with aging. Assessing these functional changes is challenging, as there is no way to directly assess the single nephron GFR in human subjects. The most common practical method to evaluate kidney function is by measuring serum creatinine. However, assessing serum creatinine remains relatively unreliable because creatinine generation reflects muscle mass, which usually decreases with aging.

Clear evidence is available regarding a reduction in kidney function with aging. Earlier studies among apparently healthy adults demonstrated a linear decline in GFR beyond the fourth decade, such that by age 90 years, GFR was reduced by an average of 46% compared to levels found in youth (Davies and Shock, 1950).

That was confirmed two decades later by a study showing a decline in creatinine clearance from 140 ml/min/1.73 m^2 at the age of 25 years to 34 to 97 ml/min/1.73 m^2 at the age of 75–84 years (Rowe et al., 1976). In a longitudinal study of normal subjects (n = 254) over 23 years, GFR, approximated by urinary creatinine clearance, declined at about 0.75 ml/min per year (Lindeman et al., 1985). This decline was not uniform for all subjects, with one-third of these 254 individuals experiencing an increase rather than a decrease in creatinine clearance with aging, which suggests that the decline in renal function over time might not be due solely to the aging process itself. Instead, comorbidities that are more prevalent in older adults, such as high blood pressure and diabetes mellitus, play a major role in this decline.

Renal plasma flow

Renal blood flow (RBF) is maintained at 600 mL/min until approximately the age of 30, and then begins declining by about 10% per decade (Davies and Shock, 1950). This decrease in RBF represents a progressive decline per unit of kidney mass and is most profound in the renal cortex.

It is also greater than the decrease in GFR, resulting in an increased filtration fraction in elderly persons (Davies and Shock, 1950). A possible explanation for the decreased renal blood flow may be that it is caused by an imbalance and alterations in the responsiveness of vasoactive substances.

Proteinuria

Proteinuria is usually not a function of normal aging but more likely represents an underlying kidney disease process. In a study that compared proteinuria in younger individuals aged 38 ± 2 years (n = 45) with older individuals aged 69 ± 1 year (n = 24), while the degree of proteinuria in both age groups was similar, the proteinuria in the older group was associated with CKD, as shown by a high serum creatinine, a low creatinine clearance, and a higher systolic blood pressure (Sureshkumar et al., 2003). The presence of albuminuria in older adults may also increase cardiovascular mortality when eGFR is ≤ 45 ml/min/1.73 m^2 (Glassock and Rule, 2012).

Several kidney pathologies were noted in these patients on renal biopsies, including focal segmental glomerulosclerosis (FSGS), membranous nephropathy, minimal change disease, and diabetic nephropathy (Davison and Johnston, 1996) (Table 1.1).

Effects of the kidney's structural and pathological changes on kidney disease

The changes observed in the kidney as we age may have no significant effects on kidney function, as demonstrated in the Baltimore Longitudinal Study (Lindeman et al., 1985) where one-third of the population studied showed improvement in GFR. However, these changes may, on the other hand, contribute to various renal pathologies. Elderly individuals are more susceptible to experiencing a decrease in their kidney reserve capacity and are more prone to developing CKD and AKI.

Several primary glomerular diseases were noted in the elderly population, including membranous nephropathy, FSGS, and minimal change disease. Secondary glomerular diseases included diabetic glomerulosclerosis, systemic amyloidosis, systemic necrotizing and crescentic glomerulonephritis, and malignancy-associated glomerulopathy (Davison and Johnston, 1996). The tubular changes noted with aging may contribute to abnormal osmoregulation and impaired water handling, resulting in hyponatremia or hypernatremia. Hyponatremia in the elderly was estimated to affect around 8% of healthy older adults and increase with aging (Liamis et al., 2013) while hypernatremia was prevalent in 1% of nursing home residents (Beck and Lavizzo-Mourey, 1987), increasing to over 30% in these nursing home patients requiring acute hospitalization (Lavizzo-Mourey et al., 1988).

The changes in the renal vasculature, along with a decrease in nitric oxide production with aging, may contribute to high blood pressure, which is prevalent in the elderly population.

Summary

In summary, numerous changes affect the structure as well as the function of the aging kidney. These changes may contribute to the development of further kidney diseases. It is crucial to highlight that, while these changes may make the kidney more vulnerable to diseases, excellent care of older adults and minimizing or mitigating comorbid conditions may help preserve kidney function.

References

Beck, L.H., Lavizzo-Mourey, R., 1987. Geriatric hypernatremia [Editorial]. Ann. Intern. Med. 107, 768–769.

Bolton, W.K., Sturgill, B.C., 1980. Spontaneous glomerular sclerosis in aging Sprague-Dawley rats. II. Ultrastructural studies. Am. J. Pathol. 98 (2), 339–356.

Davies, D.F., Shock, N.W., 1950. Age changes in glomerular filtration rate, effective renal plasma flow, and tubular excretory capacity in adult males. J. Clin. Invest. 00219738. 29 (5), 496–507. doi:10.1172/JCI102286.

Davison, A.M., Johnston, P.A., 1996. Glomerulonephritis in the elderly. Nephrol. Dial. Transplant. 09310509. 9 (11), 34–37. http://ndt.oxfordjournals.org/. doi:10.1093/ndt/11.supp9.34.

Denic, A., Glassock, R.J., Rule, A.D., 2016. Structural and functional changes with the aging kidney. Adv. Chronic Kidney Dis. 15485609. 23 (1), 19–28. Available from: http://www.elsevier.com/wps/find/journaldescription.cws_home/703170/description#description. doi:10.1053/j.ackd.2015.08.004.

Denic, A., Lieske, J.C., Chakkera, H.A., Poggio, E.D., Alexander, M.P., Singh, P., Kremers, W.K., Lerman, L.O., Rule, A.D., 2017. The substantial loss of nephrons in healthy human kidneys with aging. J. Am. Soc. Nephrol. 15333450. 28 (1), 313–320. Available from: http://jasn.asnjournals.org/content/28/1/313.full.pdf+html. doi:10.1681/ASN.2016020154.

Dybiec, J., Szlagor, M., Młynarska, E., Rysz, J., Franczyk, B., 2022. Structural and functional changes in aging kidneys. Int. J. Mol. Sci. 1422-0067. 23 (23), 15435. doi:10.3390/ijms232315435.

Emamian, S.A., Nielsen, M.B., Pedersen, J.F., Ytte, L., 1993. Kidney dimensions at sonography: correlation with age, sex, and habitus in 665 adult volunteers. Am. J. Roentgenol. 0361803X. 160 (1), 83–86. doi:10.2214/ajr.160.1.8416654.

Foster, M.C., Hwang, S.-J., Porter, S.A., Massaro, J.M., Hoffmann, U., Fox, C.S., 2011. Fatty kidney, hypertension, and chronic kidney disease. Hypertension. 0194-911X. 58 (5), 784–790. doi:10.1161/hypertensionaha.111.175315.

Glassock, R.J., Rule, A.D., 2012. The implications of anatomical and functional changes of the aging kidney: with an emphasis on the glomeruli. Kidney Int. 15231755. 82 (3), 270–277. Available from: https://www.journals.elsevier.com/kidney-international. doi:10.1038/ki.2012.65.

Glodny, B., Unterholzner, V., Taferner, B., Hofmann, K.J., Rehder, P., Strasak, A., Petersen, J., 2009. Normal kidney size and its influencing factors - a 64-slice MDCT study of 1.040 asymptomatic patients. BMC Urol. 1471-2490. 9 (1). doi:10.1186/1471-2490-9-19.

Gourtsoyiannis, N., Prassopoulos, P., Cavouras, D., Pantelidis, N., 1990. The thickness of the renal parenchyma decreases with age: a CT study of 360 patients. Am. J. Roentgenol. 0361-803X. 155 (3), 541–544. doi:10.2214/ajr.155.3.2117353.

Goyal, V.K., 1982. Changes with age in the human kidney. Exp. Gerontol. 05315565. 17 (5), 321–331. doi:10.1016/0531-5565(82)90032-8.

Hoerger, T.J., Simpson, S.A., Yarnoff, B.O., Pavkov, M.E., Ríos Burrows, N., Saydah, S.H., Williams, D.E., Zhuo, X., 2015. The future burden of CKD in the United States: a simulation model for the CDC CKD initiative. Am. J. Kidney Dis. 0272-6386. 65 (3), 403–411. Available from: https://www.sciencedirect.com/science/article/pii/S0272638614013638. doi:10.1053/j.ajkd.2014.09.023.

Hommos, M.S., Glassock, R.J., Rule, A.D., 2017. Structural and functional changes in human kidneys with healthy aging. J. Am. Soc. Nephrol. 15333450. 28 (10), 2838–2844. Available from: http://jasn.asnjournals.org/content/28/10/2838.full.pdf+html. doi:10.1681/ASN.2017040421.

Hoy, W.E., Douglas-Denton, R.N., Hughson, M.D., Cass, A., Johnson, K., Bertram, J.F., 2003. A stereological study of glomerular number and volume: preliminary findings in a multiracial study of kidneys at autopsy. Kidney Int. 00986577. 83 (Suppl. 63), S31–S37. http://www.nature.com/ki/about_supplements.html. doi:10.1046/j.1523-1755.63.s83.8.x.

Johnson, S., Rishi, R., Andone, A., Khawandi, W., Al-Said, J., Gletsu-Miller, N., Lin, E., Baumgarten, D.A., O'Neill, W.C., 2011. Determinants and functional significance of renal parenchymal volume in adults. Clin. J. Am. Soc. Nephrol. 1555905X. 6 (1), 70–76. Available from: http://cjasn.asnjournals.org/content/6/1/70.full.pdf+html. doi:10.2215/CJN.00030110.

Kanasaki, K., Kitada, M., Koya, D., 2012. Pathophysiology of the aging kidney and therapeutic interventions. Hypertens. Res. 13484214. 35 (12), 1121–1128. doi:10.1038/hr.2012.159.

Kaplan, B.P., Shah, G., 1975. Age-related incidence of sclerotic glomeruli in human kidneys. Am. J. Pathol. 80 (2), 227–234.

Kremers, W.K., Denic, A., Lieske, J.C., Alexander, M.P., Kaushik, V., Elsherbiny, H.E., Chakkera, H.A., Poggio, E.D., Rule, A.D., 2015. Distinguishing age-related from disease-related glomerulosclerosis on kidney biopsy: the Aging Kidney Anatomy study. Nephrol. Dial. Transplant. 14602385. 30 (12), 2034–2039. Available from: http://ndt.oxfordjournals.org/. doi:10.1093/ndt/gfv072.

Kubo, M., Kiyohara, Y., Kato, I., Tanizaki, Y., Katafuchi, R., Hirakata, H., Okuda, S., Tsuneyoshi, M., Sueishi, K., Fujishima, M., Iida, M., 2003. Risk factors for renal glomerular and vascular changes in an autopsy-based population survey: the Hisayama study. Kidney Int. 00852538. 63 (4), 1508–1515. Available from: https://www.journals.elsevier.com/kidney-international. doi:10.1046/j.1523-1755.2003.00886.x.

Lavizzo-Mourey, R., Johnson, J., Stolley, P., 1988. Risk factors for dehydration among elderly nursing home residents. J. Am. Geriatr. Soc. 00028614. 36 (3), 213–218. doi:10.1111/j.1532-5415.1988.tb01803.x.

Liamis, G., Rodenburg, E.M., Hofman, A., Zietse, R., Stricker, B.H., Hoorn, E.J., 2013. Electrolyte disorders in community subjects: prevalence and risk factors. Am. J. Med. 15557162. 126 (3), 256–263. doi:10.1016/j.amjmed.2012.06.037.

Lindeman, R.D., Tobin, J., Shock, N.W., 1985. Longitudinal studies on the rate of decline in renal function with age. J. Am. Geriatr. Soc. 15325415. 33 (4), 278–285. doi:10.1111/j.1532-5415.1985.tb07117.x.

Ljungqvist, A., Lagergren, C., 1962. Normal intrarenal arterial pattern in adult and ageing human kidney. A microangiographical and histological study. J. Anat. 00218782. 96, 285–300.

Mclachlan, M.S.F., 1978. The ageing kidney. Lancet. 01406736. 312 (8081), 143–146. doi:10.1016/S0140-6736(78)91522-2.

McLachlan, M.S.F., Guthrie, J.C., Anderson, C.K., Fulker, M.J., 1977. Vascular and glomerular changes in the ageing kidney. J. Pathol. 10969896. 121 (2), 65–78. doi:10.1002/path.1711210202.

McLachlan, M., Wasserman, P., 1981. Changes in sizes and distensibility of the aging kidney. Br. J. Radiol. 00071285. 54 (642), 488–491. doi:10.1259/0007-1285-54-642-488.

McNamara, B.J., Diouf, B., Douglas-Denton, R.N., Hughson, M.D., Hoy, W.E., Bertram, J.F., 2010. A comparison of nephron number, glomerular volume and kidney weight in Senegalese Africans and African Americans. Nephrol. Dial. Transplant. 14602385. 25 (5), 1514–1520. doi:10.1093/ndt/gfq030.

Nyengaard, J.R., Bendtsen, T.F., 1992. Glomerular number and size in relation to age, kidney weight, and body surface in normal man. Anat. Rec. 10970185. 232 (2), 194–201. doi:10.1002/ar.1092320205.

Ortmann, J., Amann, K., Brandes, R.P., Kretzler, M., Münter, K., Parekh, N., Traupe, T., Lange, M., Lattmann, T., Barton, M., 2004. Role of podocytes for reversal of glomerulosclerosis and proteinuria in the aging kidney after endothelin inhibition. Hypertension 44 (6), 974–981. doi:10.1161/01.HYP.0000149249.09147.b4.

Rowe, J.W., Andres, R., Tobin, J.D., Norris, A.H., Shock, N.W., 1976. The effect of age on creatinine clearance in men: a cross sectional and longitudinal study. J. Gerontol. 00221422. 31 (2), 155–163. doi:10.1093/geronj/31.2.155.

Rule, A.D., Amer, H., Cornell, L.D., Taler, S.J., Cosio, F.G., Kremers, W.K., Textor, S.C., Stegall, M.D., 2010. The association between age and nephrosclerosis on renal biopsy among healthy adults. Ann. Intern. Med. 15393704. 152 (9), 561–567. Available from: http://www.annals.org/contents-by-date.2008.shtml. doi:10.7326/0003-4819-152-9-201005040-00006.

Rule, A.D., Sasiwimonphan, K., Lieske, J.C., Keddis, M.T., Torres, V.E., Vrtiska, T.J., 2012. Characteristics of renal cystic and solid lesions based on contrast-enhanced computed tomography of potential kidney donors. Am. J. Kidney Dis. 15236838. 59 (5), 611–618. doi:10.1053/j.ajkd.2011.12.022.

Sureshkumar, K.K., Ray, T., Clark, B.A., 2003. Evaluation and outcome of proteinuria in older and younger adults. J. Gerontol. A Biol. Sci. Med. Sci. 1079-5006. 58 (4), M378. doi:10.1093/gerona/58.4.m378.

Sverdlov, A.L., Ngo, D.T.M., Chan, W.P.A., Chirkov, Y.Y., Horowitz, J.D., 2014. Aging of the nitric oxide system: are we as old as our NO? J. Am. Heart Assoc. 20479980. 3 (4). Available from: http://jaha.ahajournals.org/content/by/year. doi:10.1161/JAHA.114.000973.

Takazakura, E., Sawabu, N., Handa, A., Takada, A., Shinoda, A., Takeuchi, J., 1972. Intrarenal vascular changes with age and disease. Kidney Int. 00852538. 2 (4), 224–230. doi:10.1038/ki.1972.98.

Tauchi, H., Tsuboi, K., Okutomi, J., 1971. Age changes in the human kidney of the different races. Gerontologia. 0016898X. 17 (2), 87–97. doi:10.1159/000211811.

Thomas, M.C., Tikellis, C., Burns, W.M., Bialkowski, K., Cao, Z., Coughlan, M.T., Jandeleit-Dahm, K., Cooper, M.E., Forbes, J.M., 2005. Interactions between renin angiotensin system and advanced glycation in the kidney. J. Am. Soc. Nephrol. 10466673. 16 (10), 2976–2984. Available from: https://journals.lww.com/jasn/pages/default.aspx. doi:10.1681/ASN.2005010013.

Wang, X., Vrtiska, T.J., Avula, R.T., Walters, L.R., Chakkera, H.A., Kremers, W.K., Lerman, L.O., Rule, A.D., 2014. Age, kidney function, and risk factors associate differently with cortical and medullary volumes of the kidney. Kidney Int. 15231755. 85 (3), 677–685. Available from: https://www.journals.elsevier.com/kidney-international. doi:10.1038/ki.2013.359.

Zheng, F., Plati, A.R., Potier, M., Schulman, Y., Berho, M., Banerjee, A., Leclercq, B., Zisman, A., Striker, L.J., Striker, G.E., 2003. Resistance to glomerulosclerosis in B6 mice disappears after menopause. Am. J. Pathol. 00029440. 162 (4), 1339–1348. Available from: http://ajp.amjpathol.org/. doi:10.1016/S0002-9440(10)63929-6.

Zhou, X.J., Rakheja, D., Yu, X., Saxena, R., Vaziri, N.D., Silva, F.G., 2008. The aging kidney. Kidney Int. 15231755. 74 (6), 710–720. Available from: https://www.sciencedirect.com/science/journal/00852538. doi:10.1038/ki.2008.319.

CHAPTER

2

Models of kidney aging

Emaad M. Abdel-Rahman[a], Stephen Z. Fadem[b], and Brendan Bowman[c]

[a]Division of Nephrology, University of Virginia, Charlottesville, VA, United States
[b]Department of Medicine, Section of Nephrology, Baylor College of Medicine, Houston, TX, United States
[c]Division of Nephrology, University of Virginia, Charlottesville, VA, United States

Introduction

It is a fact that we, as individuals and communities, are getting older. Increasing in age, or aging, is complicated as it involves multiple processes affecting different aspects of an organism over time, which, in turn, increases the susceptibility of these organisms to diseases and makes them more vulnerable to death. The search for the "fountain of youth" has been a dream for mankind for centuries. This dream has driven continuous research aimed at understanding the mechanism(s) of aging.

Multiple mechanisms have been suggested to contribute to aging, as discussed in Chapter 3. These diverse mechanisms make studying aging in humans a challenging and cumbersome task. Thus the search for models of aging was proposed as an alternative method for researching different aspects of aging, including mechanisms of aging, with a focus on species models that range from short-lived to long-lived ones. Consequently, aging research has utilized lower organisms with short lifespans, such as *Caenorhabditis* elegans (*C. elegans*) and *Drosophila melanogaster* (fruit fly), to study gene expression, while relatively longer-lived species, such as the naked mole-rat (NMR), have been used to study antiaging defenses.

Mice were suggested as reasonable models to study aging, being easy to breed and having the potential to obtain large amounts of data that can be detected from their various phenotypic and genetic variability. Other models of aging used in research include fish, rats, canines, and whales.

Kidney diseases are highly prevalent, particularly in the aging population. Kidney diseases in humans, including their more advanced and severe form, end-stage kidney disease (ESKD), are on the rise, especially among older adult individuals; the fastest-growing group

Aging and the Kidney
https://doi.org/10.1016/B978-0-443-34069-7.00009-4

of ESKD patients consists of older adults. Given the irreversible nature of nephron loss, aging models are very important alternatives for aging kidney research.

As kidney diseases are a heterogeneous group encompassing different pathologies, the number and specificity of research models have grown exponentially. Several organisms have been utilized as research models for kidney diseases associated with aging. While the nematode *C. elegans* has been used in studying ciliary diseases such as autosomal dominant and recessive polycystic kidney disease, its use has been expanded to include longevity research, as it has a short lifespan. The rat model "Heymann Nephritis" has been used for membranous nephropathy research. Aged canine kidneys share some characteristics with human kidneys, with different aged canine breeds demonstrating age-related glomerular and tubulointerstitial changes and declining kidney function. There are animal models for acute kidney injury (AKI), chronic kidney disease (CKD), diabetes, hypertension, and glomerular diseases.

Similar to kidney disease research models, there are models used for normal aging research aimed at understanding the mechanisms of aging and exploring antiaging drugs. Human kidneys change both their structure and function with aging. Macroscopic studies of the kidney, though variable, show that their size, weight, number of glomeruli, and amount of cortex decrease with age, while microscopic examination demonstrates glomerulosclerosis, glomerular basement membrane (GBM) thickening, tubular atrophy, interstitial fibrosis, and vascular sclerosis. Functional changes with aging include a decline in glomerular filtration rate (GFR) and renal plasma flow (RPF) in the majority of aging individuals. Thus advancing research on the aging kidney is of crucial importance, and animal models of the aging kidney are indispensable in shedding further light on the mechanisms of aging and the search for antiaging drugs.

We will divide the models of kidney aging into premature aging, nonmammalian, and mammalian models (Table 2.1).

Premature models for kidney aging

The relatively recent discovery of the Klotho family has contributed significantly to aging research. Decreased levels of the Klotho protein have been shown to be associated with increased mortality in humans (John et al., 2011). Several Klotho-deficient animal models have been used in aging research. Klotho-deficient mice exhibited a phenotype similar to premature aging, including a shortened lifespan (Kuro-o et al., 1997). Conversely, mice with overexpressed Klotho genes demonstrated an increased lifespan of around 20–30% (Kurosu et al., 2005). Due to the interplay between Klotho, fibroblast growth factor-23 (FGF-23), serum phosphorus, and vitamin D, a low-phosphorus and vitamin D diet was shown to attenuate the changes observed in Klotho and FGF-23 knockout mice (Kuro-o, 2010). A possible explanation for the accelerated kidney failure noted with low Klotho levels is that Klotho deficiency triggers and increases calcium flux, thereby reducing the cytoskeletal spectrin, which leads to cellular damage and kidney injury (Akasaka-Manya et al., 2016).

Telomeres are nucleoproteins consisting of repetitive DNA sequences and specific proteins that are located at the ends of eukaryotic chromosomes. Telomeres and telomerase enzymes are believed to play a role in the irreversible growth arrest of the cell cycle. Although the cells remain viable, they lack mitogenic stimuli and cannot divide. This phenomenon is known as senescence.

When telomeres are damaged or very short, their protective function is impaired, and cells stop dividing. The enzyme telomerase counteracts the shortening of telomeres.

TABLE 2.1 Characteristics of animal models used in aging research.

Animal model	Lifespan	Renal aging features	Key advantages	Limitations
Fish (Zebrafish, Killifish)	Zebrafish: 3 years; Killifish: 6 to 12 months	Capable of tubular regeneration Model for AKI and PCKD Model telomerase defects	Genetic manipulability, regeneration capacity, and rapid aging in killifish make them suitable for drug testing	Anatomical differences from mammals and limited lifespan data for all species
Mouse (C57BL/6)	2 to 3 yrs	Age-associated glomerulosclerosis, mesangial expansion, GBM thickening, albuminuria, and tubular atrophy	Well-characterized genetics, short lifespan, and availability of inbred strains	High tumor incidence in old age (lymphomas, amyloidosis) is not fully representative of human aging
Rat (Sprague-Dawley, Wistar, F344)	2 to 3 years	Age-related nephropathy, GBM thickening, glomerulosclerosis, proteinuria, and tubulointerstitial fibrosis	Various disease models (CPN, GN, hypertension) and a large body of research	Obesity in outbred stocks, high spontaneous disease in inbred lines
Naked mole-rat	30 years	Long lifespan with resistance to age-related diseases; a model for antiaging studies	Exceptional longevity and cancer resistance Overexpression of a-Klotho	Historically not used in renal research, but this is changing
Canine	10 to 15 years	Glomerulosclerosis, GBM thickening, tubular atrophy, interstitial fibrosis, and a decline in GFR (small breeds)	Close structural and functional similarity to human kidneys, spontaneous disease	Scarcity of healthy aged tissue and postnatal nephron development complicate analysis
Whale (Bowhead)	Around 200 years	Reticulated kidneys—individual lobules are adapted to a hyperosmolar environment	Extreme longevity, natural resistance to renal degeneration, and the ability to repair double-strand DNA breaks more efficiently	Limited availability, logistical, and ethical research constraints

In the kidneys, it was shown that shortened telomeres or a lack of telomere repair may impair cellular regeneration capacity, leading to an impaired response to AKI (Westhoff et al., 2010). Schildhorn demonstrated changes in kidney structure and function consistent with aging in telomerase-deficient mice, regardless of their age (Schildhorn et al., 2015). These changes in the kidney included lower body and kidney weight, GBM thickening, increased glomerulosclerosis, proteinuria, and lower creatinine clearance compared to a control group.

Nonmammalian models for kidney aging

Fish

Fish are the largest class of vertebrates. Several fish models have been utilized to study normal kidney development as well as diseased kidneys. The kidneys of fish share both differences and similarities with mammalian kidneys. While the kidney of fish is less organized than that of mammals, with a flattened structure located along the dorsal inner body wall, the specific segments—including glomeruli, tubules, interstitium, and vascular supply—are preserved. There are even structural differences in the kidneys among various fish species. For instance, the zebra fish's kidneys have morphologically separable head, trunk, and tail regions, with nephrons being detected, whereas the African killifish's kidneys consist only of the head region (Sander and Davidson, 2014; McCampbell et al., 2015). Despite these differences, there are similarities in life span nephron composition. The lifespan of the African killifish (*Nothobranchius furzeri*) is very short (Valdesalici and Cellerino, 2003) while it is relatively long in the zebrafish (*Danio rerio*). Thus these fish species serve as ideal models for studying human kidneys (Bates et al., 2018).

Fish may exhibit both age-related senescence with increased mortality and a definite lifespan, as well as serve as a model for human kidney disease, making them a valuable subject for study. The guppy fish (*Poecilia reticulata*) and the killifish have been studied from the perspectives of senescence and aging, while the zebrafish has been demonstrated to be an excellent model for kidney diseases. Several studies have shown that zebrafish embryos, larvae, and adults can model human kidney diseases, including acute kidney injury (AKI) and polycystic kidney disease (Woodhead, 1978; Woodhead et al., 1983; Liu and Walford, 1970).

Adult fish kidneys are able to maintain and restore their regenerative abilities following AKI. The regeneration starts with tubular regeneration and re-population of the basement membrane with epithelial cells, followed by compensation for the lost nephrons (Reimschuessel, 2001)

Another area that captured the interest of researchers studying aging was the effect of certain drugs acting as antiaging agents. The very short life span of the killifish allowed for the study of antiaging drugs in this species (Valenzano and Cellerino, 2006). Fish have also been used to study organ regeneration. The effects of aging and temperature on fin regeneration were studied in the guppy (Comfort, 1969). Furthermore, the effects of telomerase defects as a mechanism of aging, causing a premature aging phenotype, were evaluated in the zebrafish.

Mammalian models for renal aginghave also been explored.

Mammalian models for kidney aging

Mice

The laboratory mouse has been identified as an excellent model of human aging (Ackert-Bicknell et al., 2015). The reason for this stems from its relatively short lifespan, the ease of controlling its environment, the availability of tools to examine it, and the availability of over 500 different inbred mouse strains to choose from as a model for aging (Masoro, 1991).

Cai and colleagues reviewed the common mouse models of aging, focusing on senescence models and models of specific diseases, such as the aging brain, the aging muscle, the aging heart, the aging liver, and the aging kidney (Cai et al., 2022). Among the kidney diseases that utilized mouse models were models of CKD, diabetic nephropathy, and AKI.

There are similarities between mice and humans in terms of genetic background and the structure and function of various organs or systems. As a result, mice have become one of the most important animal models for studying various aging-related human diseases, for researching the mechanisms of aging and studying the pathogenesis of various chronic diseases. Mice have functioned as a target for many therapeutic trials for such chronic diseases (Cai et al., 2022). An example of a model examined is the C57BL/6. The C57BL/6 mouse model has a short lifespan of two to three years, while naked mole-rats can live up to 30 years. This short lifespan of the C57BL/6 mouse model allows for maximum lifespan studies. Unfortunately, almost half of the C57BL mice and three-quarters of both sexes had lymphoreticular tumors and amyloidosis, respectively, at death, a finding hindering the use of this strain as a model for normal aging (Cai et al., 2022; Masoro, 1991; Weindruch and Masoro, 1991).

Despite this, Lim and colleagues conducted a study aiming to show the effect of aging on kidney structure and function in C57/BL mice. Male C57BL/BL6 mice of 2-, 12-, and 24-month-old were used in this study. The researchers observed an increase in mesangial volume and tubulointerstitial fibrosis in the older mice (24-month-old mice). These histological changes in the 24-month-old mice were associated with increased albuminuria and decreased creatinine clearance (Lim et al., 2012). Another mouse strain, the B10C3F hybrid mouse, despite being long-lived, shares the same concern as the C57BL mice; close to half of the male mice suffered from hepatoma and/or lymphoma at death (Weindruch and Walford, 1982).

To study lupus nephritis, several mouse models of lupus nephritis were identified, including mice of the NZB strain, the (NZB × NZW) F1 hybrid (termed NZB/W), and the MRL/*lpr* and BXSB strains. The MRL/*lpr* and NZB/W mice spontaneously develop lupus nephritis that closely resembles human histological findings (Morel and Wakeland, 1998). Another mouse model used for kidney disease was the Alport mouse, which genetically lacked alpha3 (IV) collagen, making it a good model to study Alport syndrome. Anti-GBM was induced in these mice and used for Goodpasture's syndrome studies (Reynolds et al., 1998).

In conclusion, while mouse models seem like excellent tools for research, especially in age-related studies, researchers in this field must acknowledge their limitations, as they may not portray aging in humans accurately.

Rats

As in mouse models, rats have been used as models for normal and diseased aging kidney research. The most common rat strains used are outbred stocks, such as Sprague-Dawley and Wistar rats. These outbred stocks are not genetically uniform, with the additional limitation of becoming obese as they age (Masoro, 1991).

On the other hand, inbred rats, such as the Fischer 344 (F344) rat, are genetically homogeneous and do not become obese with aging. The limitation observed in this rat strain is evident when studying normal aging due to the high prevalence of diseases such as nephropathy and leukemia/lymphoma (Maeda et al., 1985).

Changes noted in aging kidney rats are influenced by their gender and genetic background. Sprague-Dawley rats are more susceptible than other strains to developing age-related kidney scarring. Other morphologic changes noted within the aging rat model include early mesangial expansion and GBM thickening. These morphological changes may later show an increase in both GBM thickness and mesangial matrix by 2–3 fold compared to young adults. As rats continue to age, glomerulosclerosis and tubulointerstitial fibrosis develop (Yang et al., 2010).

Associated with kidney morphological changes due to aging, Goldstein and colleagues demonstrated worsening proteinuria with aging, showing that 25% of male Sprague-Dawley rats became proteinuric with urinary protein excretion > 10 mg/day by 3 months of age, 38% by 6 months, 56% at 12 months, and 94% at 24 months (Goldstein et al., 1988).

One of the earliest proposed models for renal senescence is the chronic progressive nephropathy (CPN) found commonly among various rat strains. CPN is an age-related renal disease, particularly affecting male rats, characterized by a spectrum of distinct histological changes. In certain rat strains, it begins early in the animal's life and progresses to ESKD. CPN is generally regarded as a degenerative-to-atrophic disease with compensatory regenerative hyperplasia.

Owen and colleagues accumulated data from 500 male and 500 female Sprague-Dawley rats. Data were sampled at 17, 30, 56, 82, or 108 weeks of age. The researchers showed that aging was associated with increased proteinuria and decreased urinary concentrating ability, in addition to increased size, weight, and degree of cortical scarring of the kidneys. These changes were secondary to age-associated CPN, noted more in male rats (Owen and Heywood, 1986).

Yang and colleagues reviewed various models of CKD depending on the type of injury contributing to CKD. Spontaneous hypertensive rats (SHR) proved to be an excellent model for hypertension (Yang et al., 2010). Several rat models were used to study glomerulonephritis (GN); Thy-1 nephritis was used to study mesangioproliferative GN (Ishizaki et al., 1986) while the Wistar Kyoto (WKY) rat was used in crescentic glomerulonephritis studies (Reynolds et al., 2006).

Another kidney disease associated with aging in rats was examined by Bolton and colleagues, who studied the pathogenesis of focal glomerulosclerosis. They noted that as the animals aged, there was an increase in GBM permeability with a loss of selectivity associated with increasing proteinuria (Bolton et al., 1976).

Studies of the naked mole-rat (NMR; *Heterocephalus glaber*) offer a unique perspective in the study of aging, as these animals age at a slower rate and have a life span 9–10 times that of a laboratory mouse. NMRs possess characteristic features, including a low adult weight of up to 35 g, and they live in subterranean burrows primarily in eastern Africa. Several renal histological changes and renal diseases have been observed in NMRs. Delaney et al., more than a decade ago, conducted a retrospective study in which they analyzed necropsy and histological data from 138 adult NMRs (Delaney et al., 2013). They noted that 57% of the NMRs studied had chronic progressive nephropathy (CPN). In a subsequent study by the same group (Delaney et al., 2016), the authors provided more detailed descriptions of the renal lesions in the same 138 NMRs and compared these findings to changes observed in the kidneys of mice and rats. While histological changes were noted in 92% of the NMRs' kidneys studied, renal diseases were reported in only 16.7% of cases. Diseased kidneys appeared diffusely pale tan, exhibited abnormal sizes (either enlarged or shrunken), and contained microcysts. Both CPN and thickened basement membranes were the most common histological kidney changes, observed in 57.5% and 30.7% of NMRs, respectively. Both similarities and discrepancies were identified in renal diseases among NMRs, rats, and mice.

In an effort to explain the longevity of NMRs, Morevati et al. studied the expression of Klotho in the kidneys of NMRs and compared it with that of another species, *Rattus norvegicus* (RN) (Morevati et al., 2021). The researchers showed that while Klotho levels were similar in the kidneys of both species, they were highly expressed in the liver of NMRs but not in the liver of RN. These results suggest that Klotho, a longevity-related gene, is expressed extra-renally in NMRs and might have a specific function in expanding the life span of NMRs.

Canines

While mouse and rat models are the most familiar small animal models for aging, many similarities exist among histological lesions in aged human and canine kidneys. Dogs are frequently used in aging research as they are a desirable size and are tractable in a research environment. Their renal morphology and function are similar to those of humans in many respects. Aging in canines affects all components of the nephron.

The study of dogs as models of aging has its limitations due to the scarcity of renal tissues from aged healthy dogs, limited kidney biopsies, and a lack of adequate clinical data. Canine kidneys, contrary to human kidneys, continue to develop postnatally. Until approximately 8 days of age, there is a distinct subcapsular zone in which new nephrons are formed (Cianciolo et al., 2016).

The glomeruli of aged dogs show changes similar to those in humans, with an increased frequency of glomerulosclerosis (GS) and obsolescent glomeruli. These kidney changes were noted in autopsy studies of pet dogs older than 7 years, purpose-bred laboratory Beagles older than 2 years, and Portuguese Water Dogs (McCarthy et al., 2001). Furthermore, microscopic kidney changes in dogs were similar to those observed in humans; aged dogs exhibited age-related GBM thickening (34). Tubular atrophy and interstitial fibrosis were also found in the aging kidney (Cowgill and Spangler, 1981).

In addition to the structural changes noted in the kidneys of aging dogs, functional changes also occur. eGFR, examined by iohexol clearance in 699 dogs, demonstrated an age-associated decline in GFR in small dogs (<15 kg) but not in larger ones (Miyagawa et al., 2010).

Besides using dogs as models for normal aging, dogs have been used to study kidney-related diseases. Kidney disease is a significant cause of morbidity and mortality in dogs, with more than half of dogs over five years old experiencing decreased kidney function due to spontaneous diseases, including acute and chronic glomerulonephritis, pyelonephritis, acute and chronic tubulointerstitial nephritis, renal amyloidosis, neoplasms of the kidney, congenital and acquired polycystic disease, and kidney stone disease (Robertson, 1986). In addition to changes associated with aging in dogs, they may serve as good models for certain kidney diseases, such as focal segmental glomerulosclerosis (FSGS) (Cowgill and Spangler, 1981).

Whales

Whales, dolphins, and porpoises belong to the Cetacea order. Cetaceans are generally long-lived (Seim et al., 2014). The bowhead whale (*Balaena mysticetus*) is the longest-lived mammal known, with a lifespan of over 200 years (George et al., 1999). Its longevity makes the bowhead whale an excellent model for aging research.

The kidneys of all Cetacea are composed of many small, relatively independent kidney lobules known as renicules. Whales may also be utilized as a model for aging organs, particularly kidneys. Aging-induced changes in the kidney include reduced repair and/or regeneration of cells, which is concomitant with decreases in GFR and RBF (Weinstein and Anderson, 2010).

The long life span of the bowhead whale, along with its huge mass exceeding 80,000 kg, predisposes it to a large number of DNA mutations throughout its life. The longevity of the bowhead whale, despite the increased risks of DNA mutations, suggests a protective genetic mechanism for efficient DNA repair, preventing age-related diseases. Firsanov et al. showed that the bowhead whale relies on an efficient double-strand break repair mechanism prompted by the protein CIRBP and its downstream protein RPA2 which are found in high levels in bowhead whales (Firsanov et al., 2024). The study suggests that an efficient DNA repair system could lead to increased longevity.

More research on this model is needed, as it offers researchers a golden opportunity to understand the factors affecting their long lifespan.

Effects of caloric intake on aging and expression of renal diseases

The role of caloric intake and caloric restriction (CR) on aging and the expression of age-related kidney disease in rodents has been well studied. The lifespan-prolonging effects of CR have been demonstrated in various species. CR acts by reducing body temperature, thereby increasing longevity. This was shown in mice (Duffy et al., 1990), rats (Keenan et al., 2000), and nonhuman primates (Lane et al., 1996).

The effect of CR on renal diseases was demonstrated in Sprague-Dawley rats fed low-calorie/low-protein diets, where CPN was attenuated, indicating that control of body and renal growth through CR may be essential to prevent the development and progression of kidney disease in laboratory rats (Keenan et al., 2000).

Conclusion and future directions

Studies of aging may be rewarding to mankind. Models of aging are excellent tools to facilitate such studies. Though the models discussed offer many advantages, there are numerous challenges and limitations in relying on them to establish accurate data that may eventually help humans in their quest to live longer and healthier lives.

Kidneys are affected by aging, and kidney diseases are on the rise, especially in the elderly population. Conducting studies that may delay or even reverse the processes of kidney aging and kidney disease will be a significant step forward for humanity.

Developing more models that mimic human aging without the current limitations will prove to be of great value.

References

Ackert-Bicknell, C.L., Anderson, L.C., Sheehan, S., Hill, W.G., Chang, B., Churchill, G.A., Chesler, E.J., Korstanje, R., Peters, L.L., 2015. Aging research using mouse models. Curr. Protoc. Mouse Biol. 21612617. 5 (2), 95–133. doi:10.1002/9780470942390.mo140195.

Akasaka-Manya, K., Manya, H., Endo, T., 2016. Function and change with aging of α-klotho in the kidney. Vitam. Horm. 101, 239–256. Available from: http://www.elsevier.com/wps/find/bookdescription.cws_home/704835/description#description. doi:10.1016/bs.vh.2016.02.006.

Bates, T., Naumann, U., Hoppe, B., Englert, C., 2018. Kidney regeneration in fish. Int. J. Dev. Biol. 0214-6282. 62 (6-7-8), 419–429. doi:10.1387/ijdb.170335ce.

Bolton, W.K., Benton, F.R., Maclay, J.G.B.C., 1976. Spontaneous glomerular sclerosis in aging Sprague Dawley rats. I. Lesions associated with mesangial IgM deposits. Am. J. Pathol. 85 (2), 277–300.

Cai, N., Yifan, W., Huang, Y., 2022. Induction of accelerated aging in a mouse model. Cells. 2073-4409. 11 (9), 1418. doi:10.3390/cells11091418.

Cianciolo, R.E., Benali, S.L., Aresu, L., 2016. Aging in the canine kidney. Vet. Pathol. 15442217. 53 (2), 299–308. Available from: http://vet.sagepub.com/content/by/year. doi:10.1177/0300985815612153.

Comfort, A., 1969. Effect of temperature on tail regeneration in lebistes. Gerontology. 14230003. 15 (4-5), 248–251. doi:10.1159/000211692.

Cowgill, L.D., Spangler, W.L., 1981. Renal insufficiency in geriatric dogs. Vet. Clin. North Am. Small Anim. Pract. 01955616. 11 (4), 727–748. doi:10.1016/S0195-5616(81)50083-0.

Delaney, M.A., Kinsel, M.J. and Treuting, P.M., 2016. Renal Pathology in a Nontraditional Aging Model. The Naked Mole-Rat (Heterocephalus glaber). Vet. Pathol. 53(2), 493–503. doi:10.1177/0300985815612557.

Delaney, M.A., Nagy, L., Kinsel, M.J., Treuting, P.M., 2013. Spontaneous histological lesions of the adult naked mole rat (Heterocephalus glaber): a retrospective survey of lesions in a zoo population. Vet. Pathol. 50(4), 607–621. doi:10.1177/0300985812471543.

Duffy, P.H., Feuers, R.J., Hart, R.W., 1990. Effect of chronic caloric restriction on the circadian regulation of physiological and behavioral variables in old Male b6c3f1 mice. Chronobiol. Int. 07420528. 7 (4), 291–303. doi:10.1080/07420529009064635.

Firsanov, D., Zacher, M., Tian, X., Sformo, T.L., Zhao, Y., Tombline, G., 2024. DNA repair and anti-cancer mechanisms in the long-lived bowhead whale. bioRxiv. doi:10.1101/2023.05.07.539748

George, J.C., Bada, J., Zeh, J., Scott, L., Brown, S.E., O'Hara, T., Suydam, R., 1999. Age and growth estimates of bowhead whales (*Balaena mysticetus*) via aspartic acid racemization. Can. J. Zool. 00084301. 77 (4), 571–580. Available from: http://pubs.nrc-cnrc.gc.ca/rp-ps/journalDetail.jsp?jcode=cjz&lang=eng. doi:10.1139/cjz-77-4-571.

Goldstein, R.S., Tarloff, J.B., Hook, J.B., 1988. Age-related nephropathy in laboratory rats. FASEB J. 08926638. 2 (7), 2241–2251. doi:10.1096/fasebj.2.7.3280378.

Ishizaki, M., Masuda, Y., Fukuda, Y., Sugisaki, Y., Yamanaka, N., Masugi, Y., 1986. Experimental mesangioproliferative glomerulonephritis in rats induced by intravenous administration of anti-thymocyte serum. Acta Pathol. Jpn. 0001-6632. 36 (8), 1191–1203. doi:10.1111/j.1440-1827.1986.tb02839.x.

John, G.B., Cheng, C.Y., Kuro-O, M., 2011. Role of klotho in aging, phosphate metabolism, and CKD. Am. J. Kidney Dis. 15236838. 58 (1), 127–134. doi:10.1053/j.ajkd.2010.12.027.

Keenan, K.P., Coleman, J.B., McCoy, C.L., Hoe, C.M., Soper, K.A., Laroque, P., 2000. Chronic nephropathy in ad libitum overfed Sprague-Dawley rats and its early attenuation by increasing degrees of dietary (caloric) restriction to control growth. Toxicol. Pathol. 01926233. 28 (6), 788–798. Available from: http://tpx.sagepub.com/archive/. doi:10.1177/019262330002800604.

Kuro-o, M., 2010. A potential link between phosphate and aging-Lessons from Klotho-deficient mice. Mech. Ageing Dev. 00476374. 131 (4), 270–275. doi:10.1016/j.mad.2010.02.008.

Kuro-o, M., Matsumura, Y., Aizawa, H., Kawaguchi, H., Suga, T., Utsugi, T., Ohyama, Y., Kurabayashi, M., Kaname, T., Kume, E., Iwasaki, H., Iida, A., Shiraki-Iida, T., Nishikawa, S., Nagai, R., Nabeshima, Y.I., 1997. Mutation of the mouse klotho gene leads to a syndrome resembling ageing. Nature 00280836. 390 (6655), 45–51. Available from: http://www.nature.com/nature/index.html. doi:10.1038/36285.

Kurosu, H., Yamamoto, M., Clark, J.D., Pastor, J.V., Nandi, A., Gurnani, P., McGuinness, O.P., Chikuda, H., Yamaguchi, M., Kawaguchi, H., Shimomura, I., Takayama, Y., Joachim Herz, C.R.K., Rosenblatt, K.P., Kuro-o, M., 2005. Suppression of aging in mice by the hormone Klotho. Science. 0036-8075. 309 (5742), 1829–1833. doi:10.1126/science.1112766.

Lane, M.A., Baer, D.J., Rumpler, W.V., Weindruch, R., Ingram, D.K., Tilmont, E.M., Cutler, R.G., Roth, G.S., 1996. Calorie restriction lowers body temperature in rhesus monkeys, consistent with a postulated anti-aging mechanism in rodents. Proc. Natl. Acad. Sci. U.S.A. 00278424. 93 (9), 4159–4164. doi:10.1073/pnas.93.9.4159.

Lim, J.H., Kim, E.N., Kim, M.Y., Chung, S., Shin, S.J., Kim, H.W., Yang, C.W., Kim, Y.S., Chang, Y.S., Park, C.W., Choi, B.S., 2012. Age-associated molecular changes in the kidney in aged mice. Oxid. Med. Cell. Longev. 19420994. doi:10.1155/2012/171383.

Liu, R.K., Walford, R.L., 1970. Observations on the lifespans of several species of annual fishes and of the world's smallest fishes. Exp. Gerontol. 05315565. 5 (3), 241–246. doi:10.1016/0531-5565(70)90044-6.

Maeda, H., Gleiser, C.A., Masoro, E.J., Murata, I., McMahan, C.A., Yu, B.P., 1985. Nutritional influences on aging of Fischer 344 rats: II. Pathology. J. Gerontol. 00221422. 40 (6), 671–688. doi:10.1093/geronj/40.6.671.

Masoro, E.J., 1991. Use of rodents as models for the study of "normal aging": conceptual and practical issues. Neurobiol. Aging. 01974580. 12 (6), 639–643. doi:10.1016/0197-4580(91)90114-Y.

McCampbell, K.K., Springer, K.N., Wingert, R.A., 2015. In: Atlas of cellular dynamics during zebrafish adult kidney regeneration. Stem Cells Int. Hindawi Publishing Corporation, 2015, pp. 16879678. Available from: http://www.hindawi.com/journals/sci/contents/. doi: 10.1155/2015/547636.

McCarthy, R.A., Steffens, W.L., Brown, C.A., Brown, S.A., Ard, M., Finco, D.R., 2001. Effects of dietary protein on glomerular mesangial area and basement membrane thickness in aged uninephrectomized dogs. Can. J. Vet. Res. 08309000. 65 (2), 125–130.

Miyagawa, Y., Takemura, N., Hirose, H., 2010. Assessments of factors that affect glomerular filtration rate and indirect markers of renal function in dogs and cats. J. Vet. Med. Sci. 0916-7250. 72 (9), 1129–1136. doi:10.1292/jvms.09-0443.

Morel, L., Wakeland, E.K., 1998. Susceptibility to lupus nephritis in the NZB/W model system. Curr. Opin. Immunol. 09527915. 10 (6), 718–725. Available from: http://www.journals.elsevier.com/current-opinion-in-immunology/. doi:10.1016/S0952-7915(98)80094-0.

Morevati, M., Mace, M.L., Egstrand, S., Nordholm, A., Doganli, C. and Strand, J., 2021. Extrarenal expression of α-klotho, the kidney related longevity gene, in Heterocephalus glaber, the long living Naked Mole Rat. Sci. Rep. 11(1), 15375. doi:10.1038/s41598-021-94972-1.

Owen, R.A., Heywood, R., 1986. Age-related variations in renal structure and function in sprague-dawley rats. Toxicol. Pathol. 0192-6233. 14 (2), 158–167. doi:10.1177/019262338601400203.

Reimschuessel, R., 2001. A fish model of renal regeneration and development. ILAR J. 1084-2020. 42 (4), 285–291. doi:10.1093/ilar.42.4.285.

Reynolds, J., Albouainain, A., Duda, M.A., Evans, D.J., Pusey, C.D., 2006. Strain susceptibility to active induction and passive transfer of experimental autoimmune glomerulonephritis in the rat. Nephrol. Dial. Transplant. 14602385. 21 (12), 3398–3408. doi:10.1093/ndt/gfl523.

Reynolds, J., Mavromatidis, K., Cashman, S.J., Evans, D.J., Pusey, C.D., 1998. Experimental autoimmune glomerulonephritis (EAG) induced by homologous and heterologous glomerular basement membrane in two substrains of Wistar-Kyoto rat. Nephrol. Dial. Transplant. 09310509. 13 (1), 44–52. doi:10.1093/ndt/13.1.44.

Robertson, J.L., 1986. Spontaneous renal disease in dogs. Toxicol. Pathol. 01926233. 14 (1), 101–108. doi:10.1177/019262338601400112.

Sander, V., Davidson, A.J., 2014. Kidney injury and regeneration in zebrafish. Semin. Nephrol. 15584488. 34 (4), 437–444. Available from: http://www.elsevier.com/inca/publications/store/6/2/3/3/3/5/index.htt. doi:10.1016/j.semnephrol.2014.06.010.

Schildhorn, C., Jacobi, C., Weißbrodt, A., Hermstedt, C., Westhoff, J.H., Hömme, M., Bhayadia, R., Gretz, N., Falk, C.S., Schmitt, R., Bröcker, V., Kränzlin, B., Melk, A., 2015. Renal phenotype of young and old telomerase-deficient mice. Mech. Ageing Dev. 18726216. 150, 65–73. Available from: https://www.elsevier.com/locate/mechagedev. doi:10.1016/j.mad.2015.08.004.

Seim, I., Ma, S., Zhou, X., Gerashchenko, M.V., Lee, S.G., Suydam, R., George, J.C., Bickham, J.W., Gladyshev, V.N., 2014. The transcriptome of the bowhead whale *Balaena mysticetus* reveals adaptations of the longest-lived mammal. Aging 19454589. 6 (10), 879–899. Available from: http://www.impactaging.com/papers/v6/n10/pdf/100699.pdf. doi:10.18632/aging.100699.

Valdesalici, S., Cellerino, A., 2003. Extremely short lifespan in the annual fish Nothobranchius furzeri. Proc. R. Soc. B Biol. Sci. 14712970. 270 (2), s189. Available from: http://rspb.royalsocietypublishing.org/. doi:10.1098/rsbl.2003.0048.

Valenzano, D.R., Cellerino, A., 2006. Resveratrol and the pharmacology of aging: a new vertebrate model to validate an old molecule. Cell Cycle 15514005. 5 (10), 1027–1032. Available from: http://www.landesbioscience.com/journals/cc/ccpdf/a11820916767671121y00gf30471010/valenzanoCC5-10.pdf?PHPSESSID=c93a1574f77c570e538535051f300121. doi:10.4161/cc.5.10.2739.

Weindruch, R., Masoro, E.J., 1991. Concerns about rodent models for aging research. J. Gerontol. 0022-1422. 46 (3), B87. doi:10.1093/geronj/46.3.B87.

Weindruch, R., Walford, R.L., 1982. Dietary restriction in mice beginning at 1 year of age: effect on life-span and spontaneous cancer incidence. Science. 00368075. 215 (4538), 1415–1418. doi:10.1126/science.7063854.

Weinstein, J.R., Anderson, S., 2010. The aging kidney: physiological changes. Adv. Chronic Kidney Dis. 15485595. 17 (4), 302–307. doi:10.1053/j.ackd.2010.05.002.

Westhoff, J.H., Schildhorn, C., Jacobi, C., Hömme, M., Hartner, A., Braun, H., Kryzer, C., Wang, C., von Zglinicki, T., Kränzlin, B., Gretz, N., Melk, A., 2010. Telomere shortening reduces regenerative capacity after acute kidney injury. J. Am. Soc. Nephrol. 1046-6673. 21 (2), 327–336. doi:10.1681/asn.2009010072.

Woodhead, A.D., 1978. Fish in studies of aging. Exp. Gerontol. 05315565. 13 (3-4), 125–140. doi:10.1016/0531-5565(78)90005-0.

Woodhead, A.D., Pond, V., Dailey, K., 1983. Aging changes in the kidneys of two poeciliid fishes, the guppy *Poecilia reticulatus* and the Amazon molly *P. formosa*. Exp. Gerontol. 05315565. 18 (3), 211–221. doi:10.1016/0531-5565(83)90033-5.

Yang, H.C., Zuo, Y., Fogo, A.B., 2010. Models of chronic kidney disease. Drug Discov. Today Dis. Model. 17406757. 7 (1-2), 13–19. Available from: http://www.elsevier.com/wps/find/journaldescription.cws_home/702727/description#description. doi:10.1016/j.ddmod.2010.08.002.

CHAPTER

3

Molecular mechanisms of aging

Stephen Z. Fadem[a], Brendan Bowman[b], and Emaad M. Abdel-Rahman[b]

[a]Department of Medicine, Section of Nephrology, Baylor College of Medicine, Houston, TX, United States

[b]Division of Nephrology, University of Virginia, Charlottesville, VA, United States

Introduction

While aging is a pathway of life, it occurs at varying speeds and with different consequences on an individual level. Studies of how aging occurs have given scientists insight into therapeutic approaches that can delay it or at least preserve a high quality of life. Mechanisms of aging in the kidney have been extensively studied and parallel systemic aging. Aging stimuli have been divided by López-Otín et al. (2023) into twelve well-recognized hallmarks, which the authors highlight as being highly integrated and mutually influential: (1) genomic instability, (2) telomere attrition, (3) epigenetic alterations, 4) loss of proteostasis, (5) impaired macroautophagy, (6) deregulated nutrient sensing, (7) mitochondrial dysfunction, (8) cellular senescence, (9) (stem cell exhaustion, (10) altered intercellular communication, (11) chronic inflammation, and (12) dysbiosis (Fig. 3.1).

These hallmarks contribute to both systemic aging and aging in the kidney. A discussion of each hallmark follows, aiming to integrate them and improve our understanding of the sequelae of the aging process in the kidney. We will also explore what is available regarding therapeutic interventions.

Genomic instability

The genome is susceptible to damage from oxidative stress and other factors. Many of these factors are environmental, but others, such as DNA errors, are endogenous. DNA is highly susceptible to oxidative stress. An intricate repair system is integrated into its survival mechanism. This system must ensure that DNA functions properly, replicates, and divides when necessary. Over millions of years, the DNA damage response (DDR) has evolved and can effectively determine when DNA can be repaired or when it must be replaced. As organs

https://doi.org/10.1016/B978-0-443-34069-7.00005-7

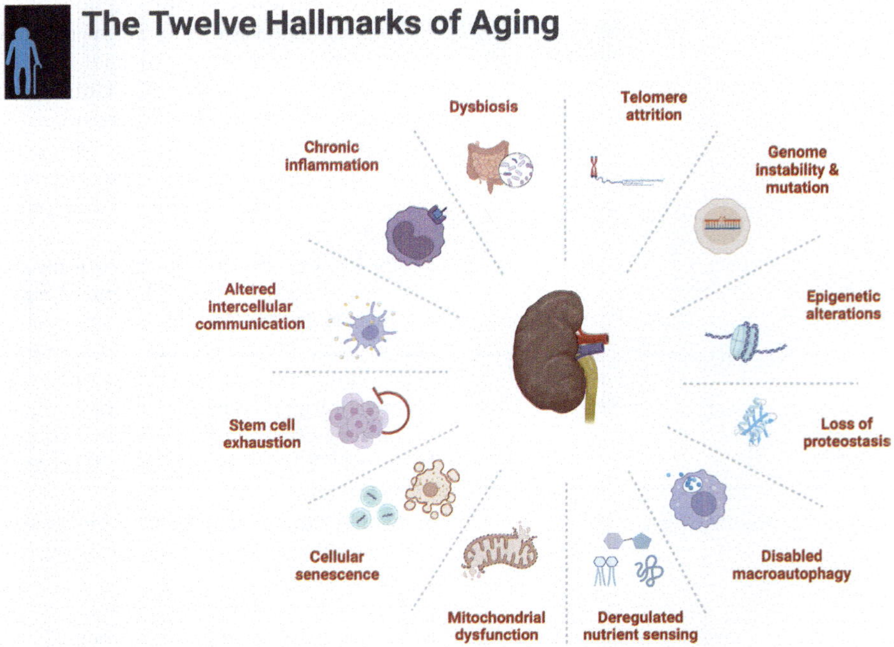

FIG. 3.1 The twelve hallmarks of aging. Hallmarks of aging modified for kidney disease. *Created in BioRender. Fadem, S., 2025. https://BioRender.com/ap91cqy; From López-Otín, C., Blasco, M.A., Partridge, L., Serrano, M., Kroemer, G., 2023. Hallmarks of aging: an expanding universe. Cell. 10974172. 186 (2), 243–278. Available from: https://www.sciencedirect.com/journal/cell. doi:10.1016/j.cell.2022.11.001.*

and organisms age, the DNA repair mechanisms lose their effectiveness while stress factors continue to accumulate.

In health, DNA is tightly wound around an octamer of eight histones and is repressive to signal transduction. This nucleosome serves as a subunit of chromatin.

When transcription factors like NF-κB and STAT are needed in response to stress or growth, they work in concert with an activator protein. Both can enter the nucleus, although STAT must first be phosphorylated into a dimer by Janus Kinase (JAK). The activators may either acetylate or methylate sections of the histone tail, loosening the histone and enabling the transcription factor to interface with the DNA. This allows RNA polymerase to generate a ribonucleotide chain that corresponds with the DNA. The RNA can then move to a ribosome, where it assembles amino acids in a specific sequence. This assembly is known as translation. These peptides are subsequently refined and folded (Kornberg, 1999). In the case of NF-κB, the proteins generated are the cytokines and chemokines that further potentiate the inflammatory response.

Aging is associated with longstanding environmental exposure. The toxic agents that the body is exposed to on a daily basis include oxidative radiation, environmental chemical substances, lifestyle abuses such as cigarette use, and food breakdown products. These factors damage DNA, leading to lesions that several pathways repair. This also requires chromatin remodeling, as the DNA-histone section must be taken offline for the repair to happen. Transcription must be temporarily halted. The repair must be synchronized to the cell cycle stage. After repair, other factors may be required, such as nucleotide substitution, ubiquitination, phosphorylation, methylation, and acetylation. For instance, ultraviolet damage requires nucleotide excision. Hemodialysis is associated with oxidative stress and results in DNA damage, including double-stranded breaks (DSBs). It was shown that DNA repair significantly increases after dialysis and reduces DSBs (Herman et al., 2008).

Double-stranded breaks

DSBs can be quite damaging to DNA and may lead to cell death. They can occur during natural processes such as DNA replication, meiosis, or mitosis. The nonhomologous end joining (NHEJ) repair mechanism used in mammals is faster and tends to be more error-prone compared to homologous recombination. This mechanism rejoins the broken ends of DNA; however, since it does not match the original sequence, it may result in small insertions or deletions that could cause frameshifts, thereby altering protein production. DSBs trigger an enzymatic reaction that results in the phosphorylation of downstream substrates. These can inhibit cell cycle progression and lead to apoptosis. This phosphorylation cascade can activate p53, a tumor suppressor gene that leads to cell cycle arrest. If the DSB is repaired, the phosphorylation cascade is inactivated. While DNA damage and methylation are associated with proteinuria, DSBs and glomerular DNA methylation are associated with a decline in eGFR in diabetic nephropathy patients (Yoshimoto et al., 2023).

Cyclic guanosine monophosphate–adenosine monophosphate synthase (cGAS) impairs homologous recombination DNA repair. The naked mole-rat cGAS differs from its human homologs by four amino acids, and these substitutions abolish its suppressive effect, allowing naked mole-rat cGAS to remain on chromatin longer after DNA damage, enhancing DNA repair factors FANCI and RAD50. When the naked mole-rat cGAS variant was introduced into Drosophila and mice, it antagonized cellular and tissue aging and extended lifespan, raising the prospect that pharmacological or genetic manipulation of cGAS could one day be harnessed to enhance DNA repair and delay aging in humans (Chen et al., 2025).

Sirtuins and DNA repair

Silent information regulators (SIRTs) are transcription regulators that help defend against mitochondrial dysfunction, endoplasmic reticulum stress, and the increased p16 expression that causes cell cycle arrest. They are also involved in genome stability. When recruited to DSBs, they deacetylate histones and promote the DDR factor. They also assist in chromatin remodeling (Vazquez et al., 2017).

Telomere attrition

Telomeres are repeating nucleotides, TTAGGG tags, that shorten with each cell division. They are also shortened by oxidative stress. Thus, after multiple cell divisions, the DNA attracts the DDR and is degraded, decreasing cell functionality. Telomerase is an enzyme complex that codes new telomeres and, in health, can balance stressors that shorten telomeres. The telomeres shorten in the renal cortex with aging (Melk et al., 2000) and they are sensitive to oxidative stress (von Zglinicki, 2000). Chronic systemic diseases that have a kidney component further aggravate shortening and may accelerate glomerulosclerosis.

In mouse models of kidney fibrosis, short telomeres in response to folic acid become fibrotic. They exacerbate an epithelial-to-mesenchymal transition (EMT). During this transition, epithelial cells lose their adhesion properties and become capable of migrating. They are able to change their phenotype to mesenchymal cells. Telomeric repeat-binding factor 1 (Trf1) is a protein that binds to telomeres and maintains their stability. Mice with Trf1 deletions develop fibrosis and EMT activation (Saraswati et al., 2021).

Epigenetic alterations

Epigenetic modifications can occur based on the following: (1) DNA methylation, (2) posttranslational nucleosome modifications of histones, including acetylation, methylation, and phosphorylation, or (3) chromatin-level epigenesis. Muscle protein loss is a characteristic of CKD. There are several causes, including the activation of caspase-3, ubiquitin-proteasomal degradation, inflammation, insulin resistance, and metabolic acidosis. NO66, a JmjC domain-containing protein, demethylates histones and can repress transcription. It is expressed in CKD muscle stimulated by NF-κB. It demethylates and silences ribosomal DNA transcription at two domains, suppressing muscle synthesis (Zhang et al., 2020).

MicroRNAs (miRNAs) are small strands of noncoding single-stranded RNA, approximately 18–14 nucleotides in length. They block mRNA posttranscriptionally and cause its degradation. Their repression is associated with disease, and they are often decreased in CKD. In one study, their downregulation was associated with vascular smooth muscle changes linked to the transcription factor runt-related transcription factor-2 (RUNX2), which converts smooth muscle cells to a bone phenotype. When stimulated by indoxyl sulfate, their upregulation has been implicated in endothelial dysfunction in CKD. Other diseases they have been associated with include inflammation, vascular calcification, AKI, podocyte injury, and angiotensin II renal injury (Piko et al., 2023).

Loss of proteostasis

The accumulation of intracellular damaged fragments can occur with aging as the control processes for regulating protein functionality degrade. Proteins that are misfolded or unfolded must be chaperoned. Unfolded proteins lead to endoplasmic reticulum stress, activating the unfolded protein response-endoplasmic reticulum (UPR^{ER}). The UPR^{ER} detects improperly folded proteins in the endoplasmic reticulum and initiates a chaperone response. ER stress also initiates a hypoxia-inducible factor (HIF-1) response. Chaperone molecules are heat shock protein molecules that maintain proteostasis. They ensure proper folding, unfolding, and remodeling, attempting to initiate repair when misfolding occurs. If the misfolding is severe or if protein aggregates have formed, the proteins are degraded by either the ubiquitin-proteasome system or undergo autophagy. Protein stability is essential for enzymes, protein structure, and most other functions (Kaushik and Cuervo, 2015).

Ubiquitin protease

Ubiquitin-conjugation tags misfolded or nonfunctioning proteins and transfer them to a 26S proteasome. The proteasome catalyzes proteins into smaller peptides or amino acids. The ubiquitin complex also destroys short-lived proteins and is involved in several cell regulation processes, including hemostasis, iron turnover, immune responses, metabolism, cell cycle progression, and cell death. It is also involved in signal transduction. Misfolded proteins that aggregate are eliminated by autophagy (see below), as are organelle fragments, ubiquitinated aggregate proteins, and mitochondrial fragments.

Dysregulated macroautophagy

When aggregation is excessive, it can overburden autophagy. Autophagy is responsive to cellular stress and is regulated by adenosine monophosphate-activated protein kinase (AMPK), which also activates forkhead box O (FoxO). Sirt1 activates nuclear factor erythroid-2-related factor 2 (Nrf2). Nrf1, AMPK, and Klotho inhibit the mechanistic target of rapamycin (mTOR) pathway, which stimulates autophagosome biogenesis, the first step in developing an autophagosome carrying cargo to be degraded by the lysosome. Increased mTOR, AMPK, and Klotho have the opposite effect of decreasing mTOR. While mTOR is critical for protein synthesis, its abundance can severely decrease autophagy. Autophagy impairment has been linked to a decline in kidney function with aging. Mice fed a high-fat diet exhibited dysfunctional autophagy and accelerated aging.

An additional duty of the proteins is maintaining DNA repair. As protein function deteriorates in CKD, so does its ability to repair DNA, resulting in further genomic instability (Yamamoto and Isaka, 2024).

Deregulated nutrient sensing

Any organism's ability to utilize nutrients is essential, and the mechanisms for nutrient sensing that were developed millions of years ago still exist today. The major nutrients are glucose, amino acids, and lipids. Nutrient sensing must also detect the availability of nutrients. Adaptation swings between growth and conservation are well-devised plans that work together to optimize homeostasis. The two systems that control nutrient sensing are AMPK and mTOR.

AMPK

The AMPK complex has three subunits, each being activated by phosphorylation at a threonine site. The α subunit has kinase properties. The β subunit binds to glycogen during times of plenty, while the γ subunits bind to nucleotides like AMP or ADP under stress. AMPK may respond to calcium and osmotic stress. Metformin, exercise, caloric restriction, glycogen depletion, and AMP or ADP binding are known to activate AMPK to act on specific downstream catabolic processes that help regenerate ATP and recycle components that can be sourced for energy. In the kidney, it is activated by ischemia and inhibited by hypertension. It upregulates the GLUT1 receptor to increase glucose entry into cells, whether in the gut, muscle, or kidney. It also inhibits energy-dependent SGLT1. It can stimulate glycolysis by activating phosphofructokinase-2. It increases fatty acid metabolism and shuts off mTOR. It can decrease cell growth and protein synthesis but also suppress inflammation. The inhibition of AMPK blocks the protective effect of adiponectin on podocyte permeability (Huynh et al., 2023). In the tubule, AMPK activation may modulate ion transport in sodium, potassium, and chloride channels. AMPK inhibits the cystic fibrosis transmembrane conductance regulator (CFTR), a chloride transporter channel, and mTOR, thereby inhibiting cyst formation (Pastor-Soler and Hallows, 2012).

When activated, AMPK inhibits caspase-6. AMPK inhibition leads to reduced AMPK-dependent phosphorylation of caspase-6 activation, increasing nonphosphorylated caspase and inducing the release of cytochrome C from mitochondria, which leads to hepatocyte apoptosis, resulting in nonalcoholic steatohepatitis.

Mechanistic target of rapamycin (mTOR)

Easter Island (Rapa Nui) was discovered on Easter Sunday, April 5, 1722. The Mataveri Airport on Easter Island is over 3500 km from the nearest continent. It lies at the base of Rano Kau, a dormant volcano. When NASA made plans to extend the airport's runway, scientists wanted to first thoroughly study multiple soil samples on the island, fearing that if the island became a popular tourist attraction, the uniqueness of this remote environment would be lost. In 1975, a soil sample from Rano Kau was discovered to contain a Streptomyces species that exhibited both antifungal and immunosuppressive properties. They named it Rapamycin. Since 1999, it has been extensively used in clinical practice as an immunosuppressant in kidney transplantation. The targets of rapamycin, TORC1 and TORC2 are serine/threonine-protein kinases and have been extensively studied since 1994. The mTORC1 complex is a regulator built on scaffolding proteins known as Raptor. It receives nutrient signals from the insulin growth factor pathway, an amino acid signaling pathway, and indirectly from the stress pathway, AMPK. mTOR can be blocked by rapamycin through complexing with the adjacent FK506-binding protein 12 and binding to the FRB domain, restricting its activation. With mTORC2, Rictor hinders FRB binding, but mORC2 blocking is nonspecific. Although mTORC1-dependent S6-kinase1 (S6K1) can be completely blocked, rapamycin does not totally block other substrates.

Amino acids, particularly leucine and arginine, through sensing proteins, lead to the activation of GATOR1, localizing the Rag heterodimer anchored by the Ragulator complex to the lysosomal surface to recruit mTORC1. mTORC1 promotes the activation of ribosomal protein S6 and the translation initiation factor eIF-4E to initiate protein synthesis. The lysosomes can excrete amino acids that are stimulated by the juxtaposed mTORC1 to also enter mRNA protein translation pathways.

Growth factors like insulin growth factor stimulate PI3 kinase to activate mTORC2 and AKT. AKT phosphorylates and inhibits the tuberous sclerosis complex (TSC). TSC normally inactivates RHEB; thus when inhibited, RHEB is able to activate MTORC1. Lipids, fructose, glucose, and pyruvate work through pathways that activate dihydroxyacetone phosphate (DHAP) to activate mTORC1 through phosphatidic acid. These factors activate anabolic mechanisms that enable growth, while autophagy is suppressed. Inhibition of mTORC1 induces factors that activate mTORC1. mTOR hyperactivation inhibits necessary repair processes such as autophagy, blocking key recycling systems that help rid the cell of harmful wastes, which can release inflammasomes. The overactivation of mTORC1 results in podocyte hypertrophy and dysfunction. In the proximal tubule, excessive mTORC1 activity causes tubular cell hypertrophy and dysfunction (Huynh et al., 2023).

Mitochondrial dysfunction

The mitochondria are organelles that have been derived from ancient oxygen-using bacteria. They are capable of respiration. Glucose or fatty acids cross the cell membrane and go through a series of metabolic steps that release electrons while degrading the molecule to a single carbon. The electrons drive the production of adenosine triphosphate from adenosine diphosphate. At the end of the cycle, they are passed along cofactors and taken up by oxygen, which reacts to form carbon dioxide and water. If there is any breach in the system, there is an electron mismatch, and a free radical is created. Mitochondrial membrane disruption results in a leakage of mtDNA, which activates interferon and the inflammatory cascade. Powerful oxidants can be scavenged or can produce oxidative stress. Oxidative stress drives a host of adaptive responses that may lead to the release of proinflammatory cytokines, apoptosis, cell senescence, or fibrosis. In either event, it is associated with both the progression of kidney disease and aging. Mitochondrial dysfunction mediates oxidative stress and inflammation, and when mitophagy is impaired, the repair mechanisms are overburdened. This results in increased senescence and fibrosis and reduced kidney function (Yang et al., 2024b).

Disrupted mitochondria—reactive oxygen species

Reactive species at normal levels are not particularly harmful. However, with aging and chronic kidney disease (CKD), the balance between antioxidants and oxidants is disturbed, and the oxidative burden increases, damaging cells. Since the kidney requires a large amount of energy, it is loaded with mitochondria, the major source of reactive oxygen species production. The NADPH oxidases (NOX) move electrons, and NOX isoforms are located in the kidney. Cytokines and glucose can trigger NOX to produce reactive oxygen species. Nitric oxide in blood vessels stabilizes the endothelium. In disease, uncoupling results in the production of ROS at the vascular level. In inflammation, the oxidation of cysteine residues converts xanthine dehydrogenase to xanthine oxidase, which produces uric acid and reactive oxygen as a byproduct. When reactive oxygen species overburden antioxidants, they interfere with cellular pathways and cause disease or turn on cell degradation processes that constitute aging or chronic disease progression (Daenen et al., 2019). Diabetes mellitus is an example of a disease that causes oxidative stress in the kidneys. The high glucose associated with diabetes impairs electron chain transport to oxygen. The lack of proper delivery of electrons to oxygen leads to free oxygen radicals that further damage mitochondria (Zhang et al., 2023). The high blood sugars associated with diabetes also cause advanced glycation endproducts (AGEs), the formation of insoluble complexes between proteins and sugars. They also can lead to oxidative stress. Additional mechanisms besides elevated glucose that are responsible for oxidative stress in CKD, with and without diabetes, are renal ischemia, inflammation, and uremic toxins.

Stem cell exhaustion

Stem cells decrease as one ages. Since they play key roles in the upkeep of cells, the disrepair and reduced function of cellular organelles drive inflammation and senescence. Stem cells have been demonstrated to renew intracellular mechanisms and reduce fibrosis.

Altered intercellular communication

In the kidney, extracellular vesicles (EVs) are able to transfer proteins and RNA back and forth to cells. They play a role in the homeostasis and progression of glomerular, tubular, and interstitial disease. In hyperglycemia, EV release transfers factors that cause podocyte dysfunction. Mesangial cells can release EVs that stimulate the p-AKT pathway as well as the TGF-β1 pathway. It has been shown that injured podocytes release the microRNA miR-221, and that it may be a useful marker for diabetic nephropathy (Carney, 2016). In the collecting duct, the EVs are regulated by vasopressin (Oosthuyzen et al., 2016).

Molecular mechanisms of inflammation

The causes of inflammation associated with CKD are multifactorial. It can occur early in kidney disease, as evidenced by the presentation and persistence of C-reactive protein (CRP). CRP is produced by the liver as a response to inflammation and is recognized as a risk factor for CKD, cardiovascular events, and mortality when elevated in Stages 3 and 4 of CKD. It is not just a biomarker but can also stimulate the transcription factor NF-κB and, hence, macrophages that contribute to inflammation. CRP has been implicated in the upregulation of FGF-23, an NF-κB transcription stimulator. NF-κB transcribes proteins that are chemotactic to macrophages, which recruit another potent cytokine, tumor necrosis factor α (TNF-α). TNF-α regulates the release of other inflammatory pathways, including caspase, NF-κB, and MAPK (mitogen-activated protein kinase). It enhances tissue damage and the regulation of immunity, especially in infection and sepsis. It is also released by chronically diseased organs.

CD40

The CD40/CD40 ligand dyad is a member of the TNF superfamily and is important in adaptive immunity. It induces adhesion molecules and proinflammatory cytokines. In the kidney, it is present in mesangial, glomerular epithelial, and tubular cells, leading to chronic inflammation. In glomerular epithelial cells, it causes nephrin loss and reorganizes the podocyte cytoskeleton, modifying permselectivity and causing albuminuria. It also leads to F-actin accumulation and cell retraction. In vivo experiments demonstrate that inactivating CD40 blocks the permeability effect (Doublier et al., 2017).

C-reactive protein

CRP can also promote the release of transforming growth factor β1 (TGF-β1), leading to fibrosis. Decreased clearance of uremic toxins, like indoxyl sulfate, potentiates inflammation by activating the environmental sensing receptor aryl hydrocarbon receptor (AHR), enabling its translocation to the nucleus, where it forms a dimer with a nuclear receptor, Arnt. This binds to the DNA sequence xenobiotic response element, which is important in detoxification.

Interleukin-6

Interleukin-6 (IL-6) is a complex protein with a molecular weight between 21 and 28 kDa. It is a uremic toxin poorly cleared by the kidney. It is released by macrophages into the bloodstream and is a proinflammatory cytokine, inciting the hepatic release of phase reactants such as CRP, hepcidin, and fibrinogen. It also decreases albumin synthesis. IL-6 can appear as early as stage 2 CKD, and its levels rise as the disease progresses (Barreto et al., 2010). In the kidney, it is associated with oxidative stress, vascular damage, and fibrosis that lead to nephrosclerosis.

The delicate balance between oxidants and antioxidants tips toward oxidants in CKD, leading to oxidative stress, which further potentiates mitochondrial dysfunction. Oxidative stress is proinflammatory, recruiting cells to release IL-6 and TNFα. IL-6 is released by several cells, including podocytes, tubular epithelial cells, endothelial cells, mesangial cells, adipose tissue, and lymphocytes. It induces lymphocyte proliferation, B-cell differentiation, and the release of additional cytokines. It also decreases endothelial nitric oxide synthase, leading to blood vessel damage. In addition, IL-6 reduces adiponectin.

IL-6 and NF-κB

IL-6 triggers a further inflammatory response by binding to its receptor, IL-6R, promoting the phosphorylation and degradation of inhibitor kappa B (Kβ), freeing the proinflammatory transcription factor NF-κB to translocate to the nucleus and bind DNA. The IL-6/IL-6R complex triggers the dimerization of Janus kinase (JAK), which activates the phosphorylation of "signal transducer and activator of transcription-3" (STAT3) to form a dimer that translocates to the nucleus, where it binds histone tails, loosening histones and enabling the transcription machinery. Along with NF-κB and RNA polymerase, mRNA transcribes proteins like the monocyte chemotactic protein – 1 (MCP-1) and the adhesion molecule (ICAM-1), recruiting macrophages that release IL-1β and more TNF-α (Anders et al., 2002; Attiq et al., 2024).

While CKD is inexorably progressive as a consequence of inflammatory and oxidative stress, it can be further aggravated by hemodynamic changes, infections, medications/toxins, and acute kidney injury (AKI). Patients who develop AKI are at a disadvantage in eventually developing CKD because macrophages stimulated during an acute inflammatory event stimulate CRP release and its binding to CD32, an immune cell receptor. CD32 orchestrates the signaling cascades that activate NF-κB transcription to generate proteins that attract the cells that will elicit further inflammation and more oxidative stress.

Transforming growth factor β1 (TGF-β1)

TGF-β1 is a cytokine and one of three TGF-β isomers. It is implicated in both aging and uremia. TGF-β is latent until activated by factors such as oxidative stress. Once active, it combines with its receptor and phosphorylates Smad2 and Smad3 to form a complex with Smad 4, which then translocates to the nucleus, where it transcribes proteins such as actin and collagen. It also activates Smad 7, a competitive inhibitor that potentiates the ubiquitination of TGF-β1. This blocks TGF-β1's role by acting as an antifibrotic feedback loop. Smad7 also suppresses NF-κB activation. Wnt9a induces TGF-β1 in senescent tubular cells, leading to collagen production and fibroblast activation. The result is renal fibrosis (Luo et al., 2018).

Other pathways that can activate TGF-β1 include angiotensin II, ERK/MAP kinase/p38, epidermal growth factor (EGF), p53, and advanced AGE. Bone morphogenetic protein (BMP) can counter the fibrosis pathways. Kidney Toll-like receptors, IL-6, and TNF stimulate the IKK complex to phosphorylate IκB, the inhibitor of NF-κB. Activation of NF-κB occurs when its repressor is phosphorylated and degraded by the proteasome.

αKlotho (Klotho)

Klotho is highly expressed in the kidney, and knockout mice with the Klotho gene deleted exhibit a CKD phenotype. It serves as a co-receptor to fibroblast growth factor (FGF) 23 and blocks phosphorus reabsorption as a protective mechanism in CKD. The large Klotho hormone may have a beneficial effect on CKD. It can regulate p53/p21 signaling, which suppresses the phosphorylation cascade resulting from checkpoint activation and blocks the DNA cell cycle. Hence, it is a key factor in cellular senescence. Soluble Klotho blocks Wnt signaling and decreases βcatenin. By blocking the insulin growth factor-protein kinase C pathway, it can increase FOXO (Oskuye et al., 2025). It also activates NRF2 and can modulate TGF-β. A key Klotho mechanism of action may be to stabilize the IKK/NF-κB complex and prevent the NF-κB transcription factor from entering the cell (Buendía et al., 2015) Through these mechanisms, it creates antioxidant activity that helps stabilize mitochondrial dysfunction, reduce inflammation, and oxidative stress.

When bound to its receptor, the FGF23/klotho complex decreases 1α hydroxylase, thereby reducing active vitamin D. Since active vitamin D is necessary for klotho production, a high dietary phosphate intake and the resultant FGF23 production decrease both.

SDS-PAGE, or sodium dodecyl sulfate-polyacrylamide gel electrophoresis, is a method used to separate different protein types and study posttranslational modifications. A single N-linked site mutant of Klotho may modulate its folding properties. Other Klotho modifications can affect its function as an FGF-23 cofactor (Hong et al., 2020). The ability to modify the Klotho molecule may be useful therapeutically. Klotho expression may be increased with PPAR-γ antagonism, ARB, vitamin D and vitamin D analogs, exercise, phosphorus restriction, ketoanalogs, a low-fat diet, soluble fiber, a plant-dominant diet, and prebiotics (Buchanan et al., 2020). In its circulating form, it may have multiple beneficial effects on the neurological system and is being considered as a treatment to decrease dementia. It plays a role in cognitive processes and in remyelination.

Patients with CKD not on dialysis have a high risk of hypomagnesemia. Hypomagnesemia is also a predictor of mortality in this CKD population. In an analysis of 11,387 subjects aged 40–79 participating in the National Health and Nutrition Examination Survey (NHANES), it was demonstrated that the magnesium depletion score (MDS) was inversely related to Klotho levels. The MDS indicates a risk of magnesium depletion secondary to diuretic use, proton pump inhibitors, alcohol use, and kidney function. The higher the MDS, the lower the serum magnesium. The serum Klotho means were 864.5 pg/mL in the low-risk group, 755.01 pg/mL in the middle group, and 755.032 pg/mL in the high-risk group ($p < 0.0001$) (Zhuang et al., 2025). It is not clear whether the Klotho changes were related to magnesium levels or to underlying diseases. In another NHANES data study of 9958 participants aged

40–79 years, body roundness index, an approximation of central obesity, was inversely associated with serum Klotho levels ($p < 0.001$) (Zhuang et al., 2025; Zhong et al., 2020).

Uremic toxins play a role in oxidative stress and inflammation

Uremic toxins are the residues of organic compounds ordinarily removed by the kidney. When kidney function is diminished, these substances accumulate. Since they are biologically active, they trigger pathways that lead to lost cellular functionality and death, senescence, fibrosis, and inexorable organ failure. They also have systemic consequences and are a cause of premature aging. A systematic review published in 2003 (Vanholder et al., 2003) advanced the concept of uremic toxins. Falconi et al. (2021) also reviewed uremic toxins and their role in cardiovascular disease.

Some uremic toxins are bound to proteins and are not removed during dialysis. Examples include indoxyl sulfate, phenyl sulfate, indole-3 acetic acid, uric acid, p-cresyl sulfate, and homocysteine. Parathyroid hormone, FGF-23, IL-6, and β-microglobulin are also uremic toxins. Trimethylamine N-oxide (TMAO) is a low molecular weight toxin that accumulates in CKD and is associated with atherosclerosis (Yachun et al., 2023). Serum phosphorus is also considered a uremic toxin because of its role in vascular calcification. Phosphorus increases the transcription factor RUNX2 to modify the vascular smooth muscle cell, causing it to express a bone-forming phenotype, which leads to vascular calcification. The osteopenia associated with CKD mineral-bone disease increases the risk of fractures related to falls.

Indoxyl sulfate can be taken up by macrophages to activate the inflammatory process through the activation of the TGF-β Smad complex transcription. Indoxyl sulfate can cause fibrosis in the heart and kidney, increase cell senescence, and induce oxidative stress in the kidney.

Dysbiosis

The gastrointestinal tract (gut) of humans contains trillions of commensal bacteria that live in a stable symbiosis with their host organism. The two enterotypes most frequently encountered are *Bacteroides* and *Prevotella*. Among the *Bacteroides* are *Lactobacillus* and *Bifidobacteria*. As long as the gut microbiome is balanced, the barrier that restricts bacteria and toxins from entering the gut remains intact. With aging and kidney disease, this barrier may leak. Both the diet and intrinsic chronic diseases have an impact on the host's physiological response. In CKD, the gut flora changes. Also, bacterial DNA is more commonly found in the circulation. In addition, in CKD, bacteria in the *Lactobacillus* genus are decreased, while those in the Enterobacteriaceae family are increased. The gut epithelial cells rely on fermentable or soluble fiber. When amino acid loads are not excessive, the amino acids can be incorporated into the fecal biomass. However, an imbalance occurs when the amino acid load is higher than the fiber load, as when the diet high in excessive animal proteins break down to amino acids such as phenylalanine, tyrosine, and tryptophan. The first two can metabolize to a cresol that is conjugated in the liver to p-cresyl sulfate. Tryptophan is broken down to an indole that is conjugated in the liver to indoxyl sulfate. These toxins can be traced to indigenous gut bacteria, helping to account for the negative effects that coronary artery disease has on the heart and the brain. They impair cognitive hippocampal function and promote atherosclerosis. They also activate macrophages and promote systemic inflammation. In the kidney, they cause tubulointerstitial damage, glomerulosclerosis, and endothelial dysfunction. When the diet is high in soluble fiber, the bacterial fermentation leads to short-chain fatty acids that nourish gut bacteria.

CKD shifts an increase in nitrogen to the intestines, deranging gut homeostasis and leading to an increase in toxins. As urea losses shift from the kidney to the colon, the delicate epithelial barrier in the colon is disrupted.

Cellular senescence (Fang et al., 2020)

The arrest of cell cycle progression is a consequence of increased ROS damage to DNA, mitochondria, and proteins, extending beyond the capability of autophagy and ubiquitin-proteasome mechanisms. While apoptosis causes programmed cell death in cells, senescent cells remain metabolically active even though they have stopped dividing. They are resistant to apoptosis and release proteases, growth factors, proinflammatory cytokines, and chemokines collectively known as the senescence-associated secretory phenotype (SASP).

Increased ROS damages DNA, proteins, and mitochondria, overwhelming cell recovery mechanisms and triggering senescence. Senescent load builds up when repair mechanisms such as autophagy, chaperones, and ubiquitin-proteasome systems are impaired. SASP contains inflammatory cytokines that further amplify the inflammatory response. Senescence is characterized by increased lysosomal mass and the expression of cyclin-dependent kinases. The lysosomal mass is marked by the presence of senescence-associated β-galactosidase (SA-β-gal), which is detectable at a pH of 6.0. When elevated, SA-β-gal and p16 are indicators of cellular senescence used to identify aging cells.

Checkpoints recognize DNA damage and trigger a series of kinases like ATM (Ataxia-telangiectasia mutated) and ATR (Ataxia-telangiectasia-Rad3). This phosphorylation cascade also activates the tumor suppressor gene p53. These activate p21, p16, and the retinoblastoma protein (Rb), suppressing phosphorylation and the E2 transcription factor (E2F), which is essential for cell cycle progression. Klotho and Sirt1 can block this mechanism.

Acute senescence is a programmed event that transiently releases SASPs. These are antifibrotic and facilitate wound healing, and they can increase renal recovery. Chronic aging is the consequence of oxidative stress, genomic instability, and mitochondrial dysfunction. Chronic stress and senescence are associated with the abnormal accumulation of senescent cells, each contributing to SASP release. The overexpression of Wnt9a produces TGF-β1, leading to increased fibroblast activation and collagen production. In contrast to the acute form of senescence, fibrosis is increased. In addition, with chronic senescence, renal recovery and allograft survival are compromised. Renal function declines, and renal aging results.

Management interventions

Renal acid secretion declines with age. In 2020, Frassetto et al. (2020) emphasized the role of acidosis in accelerating aging. William Mitch and his team, in 1995, demonstrated that acidosis in rats caused a 2.5 to 4-fold increase in ubiquitin, which normalized when acidosis was treated (Mitch et al., 1994). They later demonstrated several other mechanisms for decreased muscle synthesis, including protein proteasomal degradation related to increased myostatin levels and metabolic acidosis. Longitudinal studies demonstrate that the decline in kidney function, although frequent, does not occur in everyone. Since acidosis occurs early in CKD, dietary choices could have made a difference in GFR over many years. Meats are high in acid content, while vegetables and fruits are high in bicarbonate. Wesson's team has demonstrated that management of metabolic acidosis with either oral bicarbonate tablets or a diet high in fruits and vegetables helps delay CKD regardless (Goraya and Wesson, 2019; Goraya and Wesson, 2025; Silva et al., 2023).

Multivitamins may increase telomere length

In a self-reporting assessment of 586 women in the Sister Study, leukocyte DNA was assessed for telomere length and compared with a 146-item questionnaire. Vitamin use extended telomere length by 5.1% ($P = 0.002$). The most beneficial foods were those containing vitamins E and C (Qun et al., 2009). Vitamins may modulate oxidative stress and help reduce chronic inflammation.

Calorie restriction, AMPK, mTOR inactivation—CR, exercise, metformin, berberine.

Caloric restriction studies in rats demonstrate increased autophagy. Metformin stimulates AMPK, opposes aging in rats, and reduces transcription of genes through transcription factors like Zeb1 that drive the transition from the epithelial to mesenchymal phenotype (EMT). Metformin has also been shown to decrease TGFβ. Metformin and caloric restriction have also been shown to decrease the transcription factor Zeb1 and markers of fibroblasts, alleviating cell senescence. High glucose downregulated AMPK/mTOR and induced senescence in rats (Dong et al., 2017). The Comprehensive Assessment of Long-term Effects of Reducing Intake of Energy (CALERIE) 2 trial randomized 199 participants to a 25% calorie-restricted diet for 2 years. The HOMA-IR was identified as a robust predictor, as were IL6, GDF15, ICAM1, RAGE, and MDC. The earlier CALERIE study also demonstrated quantifiable longitudinal reductions in biomarkers of aging. Combined, these markers showed a decreased level of senescence in healthy, young, middle-aged, overweight, but not obese subjects (Aversa et al., 2024).

Skeletal muscle mass decreases naturally with aging but is accelerated in individuals with CKD. Branched-chain amino acids, in concert with resistance exercises, activate mTOR to promote muscle synthesis.

Fat restriction and adiponectin

Central adiposity can be measured by the body roundness index (Du et al., 2025). It is inversely associated with serum klotho. Adiponectin naturally decreases with aging and plays a role in preserving kidney function. It decreases with dietary excess, and this decline worsens lipid and glucose metabolism, leading to further damage in the kidneys and liver. In animal studies, adiponectin knockout mice have a shortened lifespan. Although there are currently no medications that increase adiponectin, it can be improved through dietary control and exercise.

ACE/ARB therapy

Renin synthesis from the juxtaglomerular apparatus decreases with age in rat models, but locally, angiotensin II is increased. This contributes to inflammation, oxidative stress, mitochondrial dysfunction, efferent arteriolar constriction, glomerular hyperfiltration, and glomerulosclerosis. The glomerulosclerosis may be activated by angiotensin II starting around age 30. The elderly are predisposed to hypovolemia, hyponatremia, acidosis, and hyperkalemia. Many patients carry a genotype that decreases sodium excretion. Renin-angiotensin system inhibition with angiotensin-converting enzyme (ACE) inhibition or angiotensin receptor blockade (ARB) therapy is established to protect the kidney from aging. It works by decreasing the mitochondrial damage associated with aging in the kidney as well as several diseases. These therapies can also preserve Klotho expression and Sirtuins (Musso and Jauregui, 2014; Yoon and Choi, 2014).

SGLT1, semaglutides and nonsteroidal mineralocorticoid inhibitors

Innovative medications targeting specific pathophysiological mechanisms have advanced the ability to manage CKD.

Sodium-glucose cotransporter-2 inhibition (SGLT2i)

These drugs have been shown to reduce CKD progression by 30%–40% and are recommended with GFR levels as low as 20 mL/min/1.73 m^2. In the CREDENCE trial, using canagliflozin 100 mg daily vs. placebo, the HR was 0.70 (95% CI 0.59–0.82) (n = 4,401). The DAPA-CKD trial used dapagliflozin 10 mg daily vs. placebo in 4304 patients. Here, the HR was 0.61 (95% CI 0.51–0.72). In the EMPA-Kidney trial, using empagliflozin in 6609 patients and with GFR levels as low as 20 mL/min/1.73 m^2, the HR was 0.72 (95% CI 0.64–0.82). The majority of subjects were on ACE or ARB therapy. The CREDENCE trial excluded eGFR < 30 mL/min/1.73 m^2 and DAPA-CKD excluded CKD < 25 mL/min/1.73 m^2 (Perkovic et al., 2019; Herrington et al., 2023; Heerspink et al., 2020).

In addition, SGLT2 inhibitors improve cardiovascular outcomes (Spiazzi et al., 2024). The co-transporter blocks both glucose and sodium reentry. The increased tubular load is delivered to the macula densa, where it decreases glomerular capillary pressure through arteriolar vasoconstriction. This decreases the GFR and protects the kidney. In animal studies, it has been shown to increase AMPK, which would inhibit mTORC1 and promote autophagy. It may have other mechanisms of action: blocking the microbiome conversion of tryptophan and phenylalanine to indole and p-cresol, reducing proximal tubule oxygen consumption, and having a mild diuretic effect, to name a few (Vallon, 2024).

Nonsteroidal mineralocorticoid antagonist (NS-MRA)

Finerenone was shown to reduce albuminuria in CKD and type 2 diabetic patients by decreasing the mineralocorticoid receptor (MR). Overactivation of the MR contributes to the pathophysiology of CKD through increased inflammation and fibrosis. The primary outcome was a sustained decrease in GFR of at least 40% from baseline over a four-week period. A total of 5734 patients from 48 countries were randomized, and 5674 were included for statistical analysis. The patients were followed for a median of 2.6 years, with a hazard ratio of 0.82 (95% CI, 0.73–0.93) (Bakris et al., 2020).

Glucagon-like peptide-1 receptor agonist (GLP-RA)

The indication for using semaglutide to reduce the risk of worsening kidney disease has been approved by the US FDA. It is available as an injectable in 0.5 mg, 1 mg, and 2 mg doses. This approval was based on the FLOW Phase 3b Kidney Outcomes Trial, which investigated the once-weekly injection of semaglutide. The drug demonstrated a 24% relative risk reduction in the worsening of kidney disease (HR 0.76; 95% CI, 0.66 to 0.88; P = 0.0003). FLOW was an international, randomized, double-blind, placebo-controlled trial that studied 3533 adult participants for 3.4 years (Perkovic et al., 2024). GLP-1 is secreted from the gut when eating and is insulinotropic. Aside from controlling weight and blood pressure, the agonist may directly affect the kidney by reducing inflammation and oxidative stress. Its mechanism of action in the kidney is still not clearly understood. It inhibits the sodium-hydrogen ion exchanger isoform 3 in the proximal tubule. GLP1-R is a G-protein. It stimulates protein kinase A and adenylate cyclase in the renal vasculature and proximal tubule. It may affect tubuloglomerular feedback and reduce hyperfiltration (Skov, 2014).

Mediterranean diet

The Mediterranean diet includes healthy portions of vegetables, nuts, monounsaturated oleic acid fat (olive oil), and fish. It is considered antiinflammatory and has been studied in CKD patients. It has been associated with better kidney graft survival after kidney transplantation (Gomes-Neto et al., 2020). However, neither the Mediterranean nor DASH diets impact mortality in the dialysis population (Saglimbene et al., 2018). Starting earlier may be beneficial. A Swedish study of 1110 men found medium and high adherents were 23% and 42% less likely to develop CKD, with an odds ratio of 0.77 (95% CI 0.57–1.05) and 0.58 (95% CI 0.38–0.87), respectively. The study also predicted survival (Huang et al., 2013). Epigenetic modifications of histones are usually related to either environmental or metabolic causes. These include the Western diet and cigarette smoking and are reversed with exercise. NF-κB induces NO66, a nucleolar enzyme that demethylates the epigenetic histone sites, H3Kme3 and H3Kme6 in the ribosome, blocking transcription of muscle proteins (Zhang et al., 2020).

Other drugs in the pipeline

The pipeline has several medications on the horizon that promise novel therapeutic approaches to kidney disease. Aldosterone synthase inhibitors may be useful as an adjunct to ACE/ARB therapy for CKD. Vicadrostat is being studied in combination with an SGLT2 inhibitor in the EASi-KIDNEY trial, a multicenter, randomized, double-blind, placebo-controlled trial that aims to include 11,000 people with CKD (https://www.easikidney.org/health-professionals).

Endothelin receptor antagonists (ERA)

Endothelin A is a smooth muscle receptor found on vascular endothelial cells. It can increase intercellular calcium, causing vasoconstriction and increased blood pressure. Zibotentan blocks the endothelin receptor and was investigated for cancer. It did not achieve primary outcomes in a clinical trial for cardiovascular disease but did lower blood pressure (Morrow et al., 2024). A side effect was fluid retention. It is being investigated in a Phase III trial along with dapagliflozin for CKD (Heerspink et al., 2023).

Soluble guanylate cyclase (sGC) agonist

sGC agonists target the sGC receptor to enhance nitric oxide bioavailability in endothelial cells, leading to vasodilation. It exhibits antiinflammatory and antithrombotic properties. Nitric oxide is synthesized by nitric oxide synthase and activates sGC. sGC facilitates the conversion of guanosine triphosphate to guanosine 3′5′-monophosphate, forming cyclic GMP (cGMP), which subsequently causes a downstream decrease in intracellular calcium and smooth muscle relaxation (Nossaman et al., 2012). Runcaciguat is an sGC stimulator that has been studied for CKD. A total of 229 patients were randomized. Among those receiving the sGC stimulator, the urine albumin-to-creatinine ratio dropped by 45.2% without SGLT2i and 48.1% with SGLT2i; however, the changes were not significant when compared with the group receiving SGLT2i alone (Gansevoort et al., 2024).

Interleukin-6 inhibitors

The inhibition of IL-6 or its receptor is being studied in CKD prevention and to minimize negative outcomes in the dialysis population. It is not indicated for individuals with active infections such as tuberculosis or thrombocytopenia. Tocilizumab is directed against the receptor, while siltuximab is directed against the cytokine. Both have been in use and are approved by the US FDA. In the phase 2b randomized trial, Clazakizumab was studied in dialysis patients with chronic inflammation and was found to significantly reduce CRP levels by 86% to 92%, depending on the dose. Further studies are under investigation (Chertow et al., 2024).

Sirtuins activation and DNA

Sirtuins can decrease aging in the kidney and change the expression of several biomarkers, including PPARα, HIF-1α, and Klotho. Since a reduction in SIRT1 causes podocyte damage, it follows that its preservation with aging would be beneficial. Caloric restriction promotes SIRT1 and FOXO expression. Angiotensin II blocks sirtuins in the tubules, and this effect can be inhibited with angiotensin blockade. Sirtuin deficiency also causes renal fibrosis (Hong et al., 2020).

Prebiotics (Kemp et al., 2025)

The gut contains trillions of bacteria that work in symbiosis with organ systems. A multicenter randomized, placebo-controlled 12-week intervention trial with 200 subjects evaluated elderly individuals, classifying them according to frailty status and treating them with prebiotics or placebo. In those randomized to prebiotics, frailty and kidney function improved. Body fat percentage, walking speed, and grip strength—all indices of frailty—also improved with changes in the microbiome (Yang et al., 2024a).

The use of probiotics containing the Lactobacillus and Bifidobacterium genera was reviewed. In the three studies that examined inflammatory markers, C-reactive protein (CRP), TNF-α, interleukin-5 (IL-5), and interleukin-6 (IL-6) decreased, while IL-10 levels rose (Fagundes et al., 2018).

In hemodialysis patients, prebiotics, probiotics, and synbiotics decreased circulating levels of p-cresyl sulfate, CRP, and IL-6 compared to placebos (Nguyen et al., 2021; Nossaman et al., 2012; Vazquez et al., 2017). Trimethylamine is derived from the gut by the bacterial breakdown of betaine, choline, and carnitine. The liver converts trimethylamine to trimethylamine N-oxide (TMAO), a risk factor for cardiac events. This TMAO risk was observed in patients without CKD and patients with CKD but not on dialysis. It is not worsened by dialysis (Li et al., 2023). Shifting the diet away from eggs and meat products toward a plant-dominant diet high in fiber can decrease TMAO. Probiotic supplements have not been associated with serious adverse events in immunocompetent individuals, but bacteria-derived probiotics are not recommended for immunocompromised patients.

Supplements such as coenzyme Q10 and nicotinamide riboside have been evaluated in a placebo-controlled, double-blind, randomized, crossover trial in CKD (Clinical trial NCT03579693). There was no improvement in GFR VO2 peak, but they did improve markers of systemic mitochondrial metabolism and lipid levels (Ahmadi et al., 2023).

Berberine can inhibit g_*Clostridium_sensu_stricto-1* and reduce the metabolite p-cresol. It may also increase butyrate production by increasing *Butyricimonas* and *Akkermansia* levels in the gut. This can improve epithelial barrier function. It reduces TMAO levels by 35% and has been shown in animals to decrease renal fibrosis (Pan et al., 2023). As an antioxidant, it blocks NF-κB's transcription of proinflammatory cytokines, protecting the release of cytochrome-C from the mitochondria and thus canceling the effect of Caspase 3 on apoptosis. Meanwhile, it activates NRF2 and PPARγ (Hassanein et al., 2022).

Conclusion

The molecular mechanisms of kidney aging parallel those associated with systemic aging, and both are worsened by CKD. Through a review of well-grounded hallmarks of aging, this chapter explores features that are present in both, namely inflammation and oxidative stress. The kidney's response to inflammation depends on its ability to sustain stresses through repair mechanisms that deteriorate with age, with the end results being the deposition of senescent cells, cell death, or fibrosis. Understanding the molecular basis of kidney aging provides the reader with insights into how therapeutic interventions may delay the process. Lifestyle, dietary, and pharmacological strategies offer promise by focusing on ways to mitigate the inflammatory and oxidative stress response.

AI disclosure

During the preparation of this work, the author(s) used Grammarly to assist with punctuation and readability. After using this tool/service, the author(s) reviewed and edited the content as needed and take(s) full responsibility for the content of the publication.

References

Ahmadi, A., Begue, G., Valencia, A.P., Norman, J.E., Lidgard, B., Bennett, B.J., Van Doren, M.P., Marcinek, D.J., Fan, S., Prince, D.K., Gamboa, J., Himmelfarb, J., de Boer, I.H., Kestenbaum, B.R., Roshanravan, B., 2023. Randomized crossover clinical trial of coenzyme Q10 and nicotinamide riboside in chronic kidney disease. JCI Insight. 23793708. 8 (11). Available from: https://insight.jci.org/articles/view/167274/version/3/pdf/render.pdf. doi:10.1172/jci.insight.167274.

Anders, H.-J., Vielhauer, V., Frink, M., Linde, Y., Cohen, C.D., Blattner, S.M., Kretzler, M., Strutz, F., Mack, M., 2002. A chemokine receptor CCR1 antagonist reduces renal fibrosis after unilateral ureter ligation. J. Clin. Invest. 109 (2), 251–259. doi:10.1172/JCI200214092.

Attiq, A., Afzal, S., Ahmad, W., Kandeel, M., 2024. Hegemony of inflammation in atherosclerosis and coronary artery disease. Eur. J. Pharmacol. 966, 176338. doi:10.1016/j.ejphar.2024.176338.

Aversa, Z., White, T.A., Heeren, A.A., Hulshizer, C.A., Saul, D., Zhang, X., Molina, A.J.A., Redman, L.M., Martin, C.K., Racette, S.B., Huffman, K.M., Bhapkar, M., Khosla, S., Das, S.K., Fielding, R.A., Atkinson, E.J., LeBrasseur, N.K., 2024. Calorie restriction reduces biomarkers of cellular senescence in humans. Aging Cell. 14749726. 23 (2). Available from: http://onlinelibrary.wiley.com/journal/10.1111/(ISSN)1474-9726. doi:10.1111/acel.14038.

Bakris, G.L., Agarwal, R., Anker, S.D., Pitt, B., Ruilope, L.M., Rossing, P., Kolkhof, P., Nowack, C., Schloemer, P., Joseph, A., Filippatos, G., 2020. Effect of finerenone on chronic kidney disease outcomes in type 2 diabetes. N. Engl. J. Med. 15334406. 383 (23), 2219–2229. Available from: http://www.nejm.org/medical-index. doi:10.1056/NEJMoa2025845.

Barreto, D.V., Barreto, F.C., Liabeuf, S., Temmar, M., Lemke, H.D., Tribouilloy, C., Choukroun, G., Vanholder, R., Massy, Z.A., 2010. Plasma interleukin-6 is independently associated with mortality in both hemodialysis and pre-dialysis patients with chronic kidney disease. Kidney Int. 15231755. 77 (6), 550–556. Available from: https://www.sciencedirect.com/science/journal/00852538. doi:10.1038/ki.2009.503.

Buchanan, S., Combet, E., Stenvinkel, P., Shiels, P.G., 2020. Klotho, aging, and the failing kidney. Front. Endocrinol. 16642392. 11. Available from: https://www.frontiersin.org/journals/endocrinology#. doi:10.3389/fendo.2020.00560.

Buendía, P., Carracedo, J., Soriano, S., Madueño, J.A., Ortiz, A., Martín-Malo, A., Aljama, P., Ramírez, R., 2015. Klotho prevents NFκB translocation and protects endothelial cells from senescence induced by uremia. J. Gerontol. A Biol. Sci. Med. Sci. 1079-5006. 70 (10), 1198–1209. doi:10.1093/gerona/glu170.

Carney, E.F., 2016. Intercellular communication in the kidney. Nat. Rev. Nephrol. 1759-5061. 12 (6), 314–314. doi:10.1038/nrneph.2016.50.

Chen, Y., Chen, Z., Wang, H., et al., 2025. A cGAS-mediated mechanism in naked mole-rats potentiates DNA repair and delays aging. Science 390 (6769). doi:10.1126/science.adq0782.

Chertow, G.M., Chang, A.M., Felker, G.M., Heise, M., Velkoska, E., Fellström, B., Charytan, D.M., Clementi, R., Gibson, C.M., Goodman, S.G., Jardine, M., Levin, A., Lokhnygina, Y., Mears, J., Mehran, R., Stenvinkel, P., Wang, A.Y.M., Wheeler, D.C., Zoccali, C., Ridker, P.M., Mahaffey, K.W., Tricoci, P., Wolf, M., 2024. IL-6 inhibition with clazakizumab in patients receiving maintenance dialysis: a randomized phase 2b trial. Nat. Med. 1546170X. 30 (8), 2328–2336. Available from: https://www.nature.com/nm/. doi:10.1038/s41591-024-03043-1.

Daenen, K., Andries, A., Mekahli, D., Van Schepdael, A., Jouret, F., Bammens, B., 2019. Oxidative stress in chronic kidney disease. Pediatr. Nephrol. 0931-041X. 34 (6), 975–991. doi:10.1007/s00467-018-4005-4.

Dong, D., Cai, G.Y., Ning, Y.C., Wang, J.C., Lv, Y., Hong, Q., Cui, S.Y., Fu, B., Guo, Y.N., Chen, X.M., 2017. Alleviation of senescence and epithelial-mesenchymal transition in aging kidney by short-term caloric restriction and caloric restriction mimetics via modulation of AMPK/mTOR signaling. Oncotarget. 19492553. 8 (10), 16109–16121. Available from: http://www.impactjournals.com/oncotarget/index.php?journal=oncotarget&page=article&op=download&path%5B%5D=14884&path%5B%5D=47556. doi:10.18632/oncotarget.14884.

Doublier, S., Zennaro, C., Musante, L., Spatola, T., Candiano, G., Bruschi, M., Besso, L., Cedrino, M., Carraro, M., Ghiggeri, G.M., Camussi, G., Lupia, E., Dryer, S.E., 2017. Soluble CD40 ligand directly alters glomerular permeability and may act as a circulating permeability factor in FSGS. PLoS One. 1932-6203. 12 (11), e0188045. doi:10.1371/journal.pone.0188045.

Du, R., Tang, X., Guan, L., Lai, Y., Xiang, H., Huang, W., 2025. Central adiposity and α-klotho: inflammatory mechanisms underlying aging biomarkers related to body roundness index. Lipids Health Dis. 1476-511X. 24 (1). doi:10.1186/s12944-025-02541-6.

Fagundes, R.A.B., Soder, T.F., Grokoski, K.C., Benetti, F., Mendes, R.H., 2018. Probiotics in the treatment of chronic kidney disease: a systematic review. J. Bras. Nefrol. 21758239. 40 (3), 278–286. doi:10.1590/2175-8239-JBN-3931.

Falconi, C.A., Junho, C.V.D.C., Fogaça-Ruiz, F., Vernier, I.C.S., da Cunha, R.S., Stinghen, A.E.M., Carneiro-Ramos, M.S., 2021. Uremic toxins: an alarming danger concerning the cardiovascular system. Front. Physiol. 1664042X. 12. Available from: http://www.frontiersin.org/Physiology/archive/. doi:10.3389/fphys.2021.686249.

Fang, Y., Gong, A.Y., Haller, S.T., Dworkin, L.D., Liu, Z., Gong, R., 2020. The ageing kidney: molecular mechanisms and clinical implications. Ageing Res. Rev. 18729649. 63. Available from: http://www.elsevier.com/locate/arr. doi:10.1016/j.arr.2020.101151.

Frassetto, L.A., Sebastian, A., DuBose, T.D., 2020. How metabolic acidosis and kidney disease may accelerate the aging process. Eur. J. Clin. Nutr. 14765640. 74, 27–32. Available from: https://www.nature.com/ejcn/. doi:10.1038/s41430-020-0693-5.

Gansevoort, R.T., Wheeler, D.C., Martínez Debén, F., Speeckaert, M., Thomas, D., Berger, M., Klein, S., Friedrichs, F., Paraschin, K., Schmieder, R.E., 2024. The soluble guanylate cyclase activator runcaciguat significantly improves albuminuria in patients with chronic kidney disease: a randomized placebo-controlled clinical trial. Nephrol. Dial. Transplant. 0931-0509. doi:10.1093/ndt/gfae261.

Gomes-Neto, A.W., Osté, M.C.J., Sotomayor, C.G., van den Berg, E., Geleijnse, J.M., Berger, S.P., Gans, R.O.B., Bakker, S.J.L., Navis, G.J., 2020. Mediterranean style diet and kidney function loss in kidney transplant recipients. Clin. J. Am. Soc. Nephrol. 1555905X. 15 (2), 238–246. Available from: https://cjasn.asnjournals.org/content/clinjasn/15/2/238.full.pdf. doi:10.2215/CJN.06710619.

Goraya, N., Wesson, D.E., 2019. Clinical evidence that treatment of metabolic acidosis slows the progression of chronic kidney disease. Curr. Opin. Nephrol. Hypertens. 14736543. 28 (3), 267–277. Available from: http://journals.lww.com/co-nephrolhypertens/pages/default.aspx. doi:10.1097/MNH.0000000000000491.

Goraya, N., Wesson, D.E., 2025. Plant-based diets across the spectrum of kidney disease. Clin. J. Am. Soc. Nephrol. 1555905X. Available from: https://journals.lww.com/CJASN/Pages/default.aspx. doi:10.2215/CJN.0000000706.

Hassanein, E.H.M., Ibrahim, I.M., Abd-alhameed, E.K., Mohamed, N.M., Ross, S.A., 2022. Protective effects of berberine on various kidney diseases: emphasis on the promising effects and the underlined molecular mechanisms. Life Sci. 18790631. 306. Available from: https://www.elsevier.com/locate/lifescie. doi:10.1016/j.lfs.2022.120697.

Heerspink, H.J.L., Kiyosue, A., Wheeler, D.C., Lin, M., Wijkmark, E., Carlson, G., Mercier, A.K., Åstrand, M., Ueckert, S., Greasley, P.J., Ambery, P., 2023. Zibotentan in combination with dapagliflozin compared with dapagliflozin in patients with chronic kidney disease (ZENITH-CKD): a multicentre, randomised, active-controlled, phase 2b, clinical trial. Lancet 1474547X. 402 (10416), 2004–2017. Available from: https://www.sciencedirect.com/science/journal/01406736. doi:10.1016/S0140-6736(23)02230-4.

Heerspink, H.J.L., Stefánsson, B.V., Correa-Rotter, R., Chertow, G.M., Greene, T., Hou, F.F., Mann, J.F.E., McMurray, J.J.V., Lindberg, M., Rossing, P., Sjöström, C.D., Toto, R.D., Langkilde, A.M., Wheeler, D.C., 2020. Dapagliflozin in patients with chronic kidney disease. N. Engl. J. Med. 15334406. 383 (15), 1436–1446. Available from: http://www.nejm.org/medical-index. doi:10.1056/NEJMoa2024816.

Herman, M., Ori, Y., Chagnac, A., Korzets, A., Weinstein, T., Malachi, T., Gafter, U., 2008. Spontaneous DNA repair increases during hemodialysis. Nephron Clin. Pract. 1660-2110. 108 (3), c188. doi:10.1159/000118941.

Herrington, W.G., Staplin, N., Wanner, C., Green, J.B., Hauske, S.J., Emberson, J.R., Preiss, D., Judge, P., Mayne, K.J., Ng, S.Y.A., Sammons, E., Zhu, D., Hill, M., Stevens, W., Wallendszus, K., Brenner, S., Cheung, A.K., Liu, Z.H., Li, J., Hooi, L.S., Liu, W., Kadowaki, T., Nangaku, M., Levin, A., Cherney, D., Maggioni, A.P., Pontremoli, R., Deo, R., Goto, S., Rossello, X., Tuttle, K.R., Steubl, D., Petrini, M., Massey, D., Eilbracht, J., Brueckmann, M., Landray, M.J., Baigent, C., Haynes, R., 2023. Empagliflozin in patients with chronic kidney disease. N. Engl. J. Med. 15334406. 388 (2), 117–127. Available from: http://www.nejm.org/medical-index. doi:10.1056/NEJMoa2204233.

Hong, Y.A., Kim, J.E., Jo, M., Ko, G.J., 2020. The role of sirtuins in kidney diseases. Int. J. Mol. Sci. 14220067. 21 (18), 1–21. Available from: https://www.mdpi.com/1422-0067/21/18/6686/pdf. doi:10.3390/ijms21186686.

Huang, X., Juan Jiménez-Moleón, J., Lindholm, B., Cederholm, T., Ärnlöv, J., Risérus, U., Sjögren, P., Jesús Carrero, J., Diet, M., 2013. Kidney function, and mortality in men with CKD. Clin. J. Am. Soc. Nephrol. 1555-9041. 8 (9), 1548–1555. doi:10.2215/cjn.01780213.

Huynh, C., Ryu, J., Lee, J., Inoki, A., Inoki, K., 2023. Nutrient-sensing mTORC1 and AMPK pathways in chronic kidney diseases. Nat. Rev. Nephrol. 1759-5061. 19 (2), 102–122. doi:10.1038/s41581-022-00648-y.

Kaushik, S., Cuervo, A.M., 2015. Proteostasis and aging. Nat. Med. 1546170X. 21 (12), 1406–1415. Available from: http://www.nature.com/nm/index.html. doi:10.1038/nm.4001.

Kemp, J.A., Ribeiro, M., Borges, N.A., Cardozo, L.F.M.F., Fouque, D., Mafra, D., 2025. Dietary intake and gut microbiome in CKD. Clin. J. Am. Soc. Nephrol. 1555905X. 20 (7), 1003–1013. Available from: https://journals.lww.com/CJASN/Pages/default.aspx. doi:10.2215/CJN.0000000705.

Kornberg, R.D., 1999. Eukaryotic transcriptional control. Trends Cell Biol. 9, M46-9.

Li, Y., Lu, H., Guo, J., Zhang, M., Zheng, H., Liu, Y., Liu, W., 2023. Gut microbiota-derived trimethylamine N-oxide is associated with the risk of all-cause and cardiovascular mortality in patients with chronic kidney disease: a systematic review and dose-response meta-analysis. Ann. Med. 55, 2215542.

López-Otín, C., Blasco, M.A., Partridge, L., Serrano, M., Kroemer, G., 2023. Hallmarks of aging: an expanding universe. Cell. 10974172. 186 (2), 243–278. Available from: https://www.sciencedirect.com/journal/cell. doi:10.1016/j.cell.2022.11.001.

Luo, C., Zhou, S., Zhou, Z., Liu, Y., Yang, L., Liu, J., Zhang, Y., Li, H., Liu, Y., Hou, F.F., Zhou, L., 2018. Wnt9a promotes renal fibrosis by accelerating cellular senescence in tubular epithelial cells. J. Am. Soc. Nephrol. 15333450. 29 (4), 1238–1256. Available from: http://jasn.asnjournals.org/content/29/4/1238.full.pdf+html. doi:10.1681/ASN.2017050574.

Melk, A., Ramassar, V., Helms, L.M.H., Moore, R., Rayner, D., Solez, K., Halloran, P.F., 2000. Telomere shortening in kidneys with age. J. Am. Soc. Nephrol. 10466673. 11 (3), 444–453. Available from: https://journals.lww.com/jasn/pages/default.aspx. doi:10.1681/asn.v113444.

Mitch, W.E., Medina, R., Grieber, S., May, R.C., England, B.K., Price, S.R., Bailey, J.L., Goldberg, A.L., 1994. Metabolic acidosis stimulates muscle protein degradation by activating the adenosine triphosphate-dependent pathway involving ubiquitin and proteasomes. J. Clin. Invest. 0021-9738. 93 (5), 2127–2133. doi:10.1172/JCI117208.

Morrow, A., Young, R., Abraham, G.R., Hoole, S., Greenwood, J.P., Arnold, J.R., Shibly, M.E., Shanmuganathan, M., Ferreira, V., Rakhit, R., Galasko, G., Sinha, A., Perera, D., Al-Lamee, R., Spyridopoulos, I., Kotecha, A., Clesham, G., Ford, T.J., Davenport, A., Padmanabhan, S., Jolly, L., Kellman, P., Kaski, J.C., Weir, R.A., Sattar, N., Kennedy, J., Macfarlane, P.W., Welsh, P., McConnachie, A., Berry, C., 2024. Zibotentan in microvascular angina: a randomized, placebo-controlled, crossover trial. Circulation. 15244539. 150 (21), 1671–1683. Available from: http://circ.ahajournals.org. doi:10.1161/CIRCULATIONAHA.124.069901.

Musso, C.G., Jauregui, J.R., 2014. Renin-angiotensin-aldosterone system and the aging kidney. Expert Rev. Endocrinol. Metab. 17448417. 9 (6), 543–546. Available from: http://www.tandfonline.com/loi/iere20#.V6Qca01f1Fo. doi:10.1586/17446651.2014.956723.

Nguyen, T.T.U., Kim, H.W., Kim, W., 2021. Effects of probiotics, prebiotics, and synbiotics on uremic toxins, inflammation, and oxidative stress in hemodialysis patients: a systematic review and meta-analysis of randomized controlled trials. J. Clin. Med. 20770383. 10 (19). Available from: https://www.mdpi.com/2077-0383/10/19/4456/pdf. doi:10.3390/jcm10194456.

Nossaman, B., Pankey, E., Kadowitz, P., 2012. Stimulators and activators of soluble guanylate cyclase: review and potential therapeutic indications. Crit. Care Res. Pract. 2090-1305. 2012, 1–12. doi:10.1155/2012/290805.

Oosthuyzen, W., Scullion, K.M., Ivy, J.R., Morrison, E.E., Hunter, R.W., Lewis, P.J.S., O'Duibhir, E., Street, J.M., Caporali, A., Gregory, C.D., Forbes, S.J., Webb, D.J., Bailey, M.A., Dear, J.W., 2016. Vasopressin regulates extracellular vesicle uptake by kidney collecting duct cells. J. Am. Soc. Nephrol. 15333450. 27 (11), 3345–3355. Available from: http://jasn.asnjournals.org/content/27/11/3345.full.pdf+html. doi:10.1681/ASN.2015050568.

Oskuye, Z.Z., Mehri, K., Khalilpour, J., Nemati, S., Hosseini, L., Bafadam, S., Abdollahzade, N., Badalzadeh, R., 2025. Klotho in age-related cardiovascular diseases: insights into mitochondrial dysfunction and cell death. IJC Heart Vasculature. 23529067. 57, 101629. doi:10.1016/j.ijcha.2025.101629.

Pan, L., Hang, Y., Jie, F., Jiachun, H., Hui, X., Zhang, Z., Mengmeng, B., Yang, X., Zhang, H., Jinyue, L., Jiang, J., Wang, Y., 2023. Berberine ameliorates chronic kidney disease through inhibiting the production of gut-derived uremic toxins in the gut microbiota. Acta Pharm. Sin. B. 22113835. 13 (4), 1537–1553. doi:10.1016/j.apsb.2022.12.010.

Pastor-Soler, N.M., Hallows, K.R., 2012. AMP-activated protein kinase regulation of kidney tubular transport. Curr. Opin. Nephrol. Hypertens. 14736543. 21 (5), 523–533. doi:10.1097/MNH.0b013e3283562390.

Perkovic, V., Jardine, M.J., Neal, B., Bompoint, S., Heerspink, H.J.L., Charytan, D.M., Edwards, R., Agarwal, R., Bakris, G., Bull, S., Cannon, C.P., Capuano, G., Chu, P.L., De Zeeuw, D., Greene, T., Levin, A., Pollock, C., Wheeler, D.C., Yavin, Y., Zhang, H., Zinman, B., Meininger, G., Brenner, B.M., Mahaffey, K.W., 2019. Canagliflozin and renal outcomes in type 2 diabetes and nephropathy. N. Engl. J. Med. 15334406. 380 (24), 2295–2306. Available from: http://www.nejm.org/medical-index. doi:10.1056/NEJMoa1811744.

Perkovic, V., Tuttle, K.R., Rossing, P., Mahaffey, K.W., Mann, J.F.E., Bakris, G., Baeres, F.M.M., Idorn, T., Bosch-Traberg, H., Lausvig, N.L., Pratley, R., 2024. Effects of semaglutide on chronic kidney disease in patients with type 2 diabetes. N. Engl. J. Med. 15334406. 391 (2), 109–121. Available from: http://www.nejm.org/medical-index. doi:10.1056/NEJMoa2403347.

Piko, N., Bevc, S., Hojs, R., Ekart, R., 2023. Atherosclerosis and epigenetic modifications in chronic kidney disease. Nephron. 1660-8151. 147 (11), 655–659. doi:10.1159/000531292.

Qun, X., Parks, C.G., DeRoo, L.A., Cawthon, R.M., Sandler, D.P., Chen, H., 2009. Multivitamin use and telomere length in women. Am. J. Clin. Nutr. 00029165. 89 (6), 1857–1863. Available from: http://www.ajcn.org/cgi/reprint/89/6/1857. doi:10.3945/ajcn.2008.26986.

Saglimbene, V.M., Wong, G., Craig, J.C., Ruospo, M., Palmer, S.C., Campbell, K., Garcia-Larsen, V., Natale, P., Teixeira-Pinto, A., Carrero, J.J., Stenvinkel, P., Gargano, L., Murgo, A.M., Johnson, D.W., Tonelli, M., Gelfman, R., Celia, E., Ecder, T., Bernat, A.G., Castillo, D.D., Timofte, D., Török, M., Bednarek-Skublewska, A., Duława, J., Stroumza, P., Hoischen, S., Hansis, M., Fabricius, E., Felaco, P., Wollheim, C., Hegbrant, J., Strippoli, G.F.M., 2018. The association of Mediterranean and DASH diets with mortality in adults on hemodialysis: the DIET-HD multinational cohort study. J. Am. Soc. Nephrol. 15333450. 29 (6), 1741–1751. Available from: https://journals.lww.com/jasn/pages/default.aspx. doi:10.1681/asn.2018010008.

Saraswati, S., Martínez, P., Graña-Castro, O., Blasco, M.A., 2021. Short and dysfunctional telomeres sensitize the kidneys to develop fibrosis. Nat. Aging 26628465. 1 (3), 269–283. Available from: https://www.nature.com/nataging/. doi:10.1038/s43587-021-00040-8.

Silva, P.H.I., Wesson, D.E., Wagner, C.A., 2023. The mechanisms of alkali therapy in targeting renal diseases. Portland Press Ltd. Switz. Biochem. Soc. Trans. 14708752. 51 (1), 223–232. Available from: https://portlandpress.com/biochemsoctrans/article/51/1/223/232534/The-mechanisms-of-alkali-therapy-in-targeting. doi:10.1042/BST20220690.

Skov, J., 2014. Effects of GLP-1 in the Kidney. Rev. Endocr. Metab. Disord. 1389-9155. 15 (3), 197–207. doi:10.1007/s11154-014-9287-7.

Spiazzi, P., Wayerbacher, L., Scalco, S., Fraga, C., Gerchman, 2024. SGLT2 inhibitors and kidney outcomes across the spectrum of kidney disease: a systematic review and meta-analysis. Clin. J. Am. Soc. Nephrol. 20, 39–49.

Thomas von Zglinicki, 2000. Role of oxidative stress in telomere length regulation and replicative senescence. Ann. N. Y. Acad. Sci. 0077-8923. 908 (1), 99–110. doi:10.1111/j.1749-6632.2000.tb06639.x.

Vallon, V., 2024. State-of-the-Art-Review: mechanisms of Action of SGLT2 Inhibitors and Clinical Implications. Am. J. Hypertens. 0895-7061. 37 (11), 841–852. doi:10.1093/ajh/hpae092.

Vanholder, R., De Smet, R., Glorieux, G., Argilés, A., Baurmeister, U., Brunet, P., Clark, W., Cohen, G., De Deyn, P.P., Deppisch, R., Descamps-Latscha, B., Henle, T., Jörres, A., Lemke, H.D., Massy, Z.A., Passlick-Deetjen, J., Rodriguez, M., Stegmayr, B., Stenvinkel, P., Tetta, C., Wanner, C., Zidek, W., 2003. Review on uremic toxins: classification, concentration, and interindividual variability. Kidney Int. 00852538. 63 (5), 1934–1943. Available from: https://www.journals.elsevier.com/kidney-international. doi:10.1046/j.1523-1755.2003.00924.x.

Vazquez, B.N., Thackray, J.K., Serrano, L., 2017. Sirtuins and DNA damage repair: SIRT7 comes to play. Nucleus. 19491042. 8 (2), 107–115. Available from: http://www.tandfonline.com/loi/kncl20. doi:10.1080/19491034.2016.1264552.

Yachun, L., Hongmei, L., Guo, J., Zhang, M., Zheng, H., Liu, Y., Liu, W., 2023. Gut microbiota-derived trimethylamine N-oxide is associated with the risk of all-cause and cardiovascular mortality in patients with chronic kidney disease: a systematic review and dose-response meta-analysis. Ann. Med. 0785-3890. 55 (1). doi:10.1080/07853890.2023.2215542.

Yamamoto, T., Isaka, Y., 2024. Pathological mechanisms of kidney disease in ageing. Nat. Rev. Nephrol. 1759-5061. 20 (9), 603–615. doi:10.1038/s41581-024-00868-4.

Yang, J., Hou, L., Wang, A., Shang, L., Jia, X., Xu, R., Wang, 2024a. Prebiotics improve frailty status in community-dwelling older individuals in a double-blind, randomized, controlled trial. J. Clin. Invest. 134 (18), e176507.

Yang, S., Hou, F.F., Qin, X., 2024b. Pure healthy diet score, genetic susceptibility, and new-onset CKD. J. Am. Soc. Nephrol. 1046-6673. 35 (10S). doi:10.1681/asn.2024a9qaecmn.

Yoon, H.E., Choi, B.S., 2014. The renin-angiotensin system and aging in the kidney. Korean J. Intern. Med. 20056648. 29 (3), 291–295. Available from: http://www.ncbi.nlm.nih.gov/pmc/articles/PMC4028516/pdf/kjim-29-291.pdf. doi:10.3904/kjim.2014.29.3.291.

Yoshimoto, N., Hayashi, K., Hishikawa, A., Hashiguchi, A., Nakamichi, R., Sugita-Nishimura, E., Yoshida-Hama, E., Azegami, T., Nakayama, T., Itoh, H., 2023. Significance of podocyte DNA damage and glomerular DNA methylation in CKD patients with proteinuria. Hypertens. Res. 0916-9636. 46 (4), 1000–1008. doi:10.1038/s41440-023-01169-2.

Zhang, L., Chen, Q., Chen, Z., Wang, Y., Gamboa, J.L., Ikizler, T.A., Garibotto, G., Mitch, W.E., 2020. Mechanisms regulating muscle protein synthesis in CKD. J. Am. Soc. Nephrol. 15333450. 31 (11), 2573–2587. Available from: https://jasn.asnjournals.org/content/jnephrol/31/11/2573.full.pdf?with-ds=yes. doi:10.1681/ASN.2019121277.

Zhang, Z., Huang, Q., Zhao, D., Lian, F., Xiangyan, L., Wenxiu, Q., 2023. The impact of oxidative stress-induced mitochondrial dysfunction on diabetic microvascular complications. Front. Endocrinol. 1664-2392. 14. doi:10.3389/fendo.2023.1112363.

Zhong, X., Jagarlapudi, S., Weng, Y., Ly, M., Rouse, J.C., McClure, K., Ishino, T., Zhang, Y., Sousa, E., Cohen, J., Tzvetkova, B., Cote, K., Scarcelli, J.J., Johnson, K., Palandra, J., Apgar, J.R., Yaddanapudi, S., Gonzalez-Villalobos, R.A., Opsahl, A.C., Lam, K., Yao, Q., Duan, W., Sievers, A., Zhou, J., Ferguson, D., D'Antona, A., Zollner, R., Zhu, H.L., Kriz, R., Lin, L., Clerin, V., 2020. Structure-function relationships of the soluble form of the antiaging protein Klotho have therapeutic implications for managing kidney disease. J. Biol. Chem. 1083351X. 295 (10), 3115–3133. Available from: https://www.jbc.org/content/295/10/3115.full.pdf. doi:10.1074/jbc.RA119.012144.

Zhuang, Z., Huang, S., Xiong, Y., Peng, Y., Cai, S., 2025. Association of magnesium depletion score with serum anti-aging protein Klotho in the middle-aged and older populations. Front. Nutr. 2296-861X. (12). doi:10.3389/fnut.2025.1518268.

CHAPTER

4

A review of podocyte senescence and aging

Stuart J. Shankland[a,b], *Shuta Ishibe*[c], *Jeffrey W. Pippin*[a], *and Oliver Wessely*[d]

[a]Division of Nephrology, University of Washington, Seattle, WA, United States
[b]Institute for Stem Cell & Regenerative Medicine, University of Washington, Seattle, WA, United States
[c]Section of Nephrology, Yale University, New Haven, CT, United States
[d]Cleveland Clinic Research, Cleveland Clinic, Cleveland, OH, United States

Learning objectives

- Glomerular aging is a risk factor for chronic kidney disease.
- Aging affects all glomerular cell types, with podocytes being the central cell type.
- Aging podocytes exhibit signs of cellular senescence characteristic of nondividing cells.
- The senescence-associated secretory phenotype mediates autocrine and paracrine effects in the glomerulus.
- Podocyte injury causes a senescent phenotype that intertwines with aging, leading to augmented disease in the elderly.

Scope of the problem

Glomerular and tubulointerstitial diseases are disproportionately more common in people over 65 and have worse outcomes compared to younger individuals with the same disease (Reichert et al., 1998; Cui et al., 2011; Ge et al., 2016; Gerstoft et al., 1986). Progressive glomerular diseases are the leading causes of chronic kidney disease (CKD) and end-stage kidney disease (ESKD). Diabetic glomerulopathy is the leading cause of CKD and ESKD, and about 50% of patients with primary focal segmental glomerulosclerosis (FSGS) progress to ESKD. Proteinuric glomerular diseases share a key common pathological theme—injury

https://doi.org/10.1016/B978-0-443-34069-7.00006-9

to podocytes. Terminally differentiated glomerular epithelial cells are a central driver of proteinuria, glomerular scarring, and ultimately the decline in glomerular filtration rate (GFR). The progression of glomerular disease to CKD typically occurs over many years. Even in healthy people, nephron numbers and GFR decline predictably after age 40 by 0.8%–1.0% per year (Levy and Douglas, 1989). Thus, it is of little surprise that the risk, incidence, and prevalence of CKD are strongly linked to advancing age. As a result, elderly patients are now the largest group of patients undergoing chronic dialysis for the first time (Kurella et al., 2007).

Clinical relevance of aged podocytes

Each glomerulus is a microcosm within the kidney, where its different cell types interact and communicate extensively. Aging causes glomerulosclerosis through changes in the number, structure, and function of all four resident glomerular cell types, resulting in a decline in GFR (Wiggins, 2012; Iwamoto et al., 2015; Sweetwyne et al., 2017; Denic et al., 2016; Regan, 1986; Anderson and Brenner, 1986). Of these four cell types, compelling evidence points toward podocytes as the most critical in aging. In 1997, Floege et al. (1997) first described age-related glomerulosclerosis as a podocyte disorder. This was subsequently confirmed by others (Hodgin et al., 2015; Wiggins, 2012). Clinically, the development of age-associated glomerulosclerosis is accompanied by a predictable decrease in podocyte number and density with advancing age (Hodgin et al., 2015; Puelles et al., 2016; Wiggins et al., 2005). This contributes to the higher likelihood of a poorer outcome of glomerular diseases in older compared to younger patients (Schneider et al., 2017; Cui et al., 2011), as well as the reduced life expectancy of transplanted kidneys (Naik et al., 2016). Age also negatively affects the normal function of podocytes in their role as important conductors for the health of other glomerular cell types, including making survival factors for glomerular endothelial cells (Dimke et al., 2015), regulating parietal epithelial cell differentiation (Romoli et al., 2018) and mesangial cell recruitment (Ebefors et al., 2021).

In this chapter, we will not review the normal structure or function of podocytes but will focus specifically on what is known about podocyte aging. As expected, podocyte aging is a synthesis of pathways involved in the general aging process and additional cell type-specific aspects (da Costa et al., 2016). However, we will limit our discussion to published data and refrain from extrapolating general aging studies of other cells to podocytes.

Podocyte senescence

It is important to note that molecular signatures for aging and senescence are still only partially established for any cell type or organ. There are ongoing efforts to deepen our understanding, such as the Common Fund's Cellular Senescence Network (SenNet) (Suryadevara et al., 2024; Lee et al., 2022). In podocytes, their healthy physiological state is characterized by terminal differentiation, replicative quiescence, and cell cycle exit. As such, cell cycle arrest, a classical hallmark of senescence in proliferating cell types, does not serve

TABLE 4.1 Characteristics of the podocyte senescence phenotype.

Process	Endpoint	Measurement
Senescence	↑Senescence	↑SA-ßGal, Lipofuscin staining ↓Telomere length
	↑Senescence mediators	↑p16, p19, p53, p21
	↑Senescent associated secretory phenotype (SASPs)	↑*Il1a, Mmp12, Ccl5, Osm, Areg, Il1b, Mmp13, Hgf, Cxcl3, Il6, Mmp3, Ccl8, Il13, Csf2, Icam1, Mmp14, Cxcl1, Tnsf11b*
	↑DNA damage	↑p-H2ax, comet assay
	Polyploidy	Flow cytometry, PAS staining

as a qualifying criterion in podocytes. Instead, podocyte senescence is based on several other markers detected in podocytes of human and mouse kidneys with advancing age (Table 4.1). These include markers such as senescence-associated β-Galactosidase staining (SA-β-Gal) and lipofuscin staining, as well as markers of DNA damage such as γH2AX and polyploidy (Inoue et al., 2019). Importantly, they are characterized by an increase in the senescent-inducing cell cycle-associated proteins p16/CDKN2A, p19/CDKN2D, p21/CDKN1A, and p53 (Zhang et al., 2019; Chuang et al., 2017; Sweetwyne et al., 2017; Hamatani et al., 2018; Sis et al., 2007; Melk et al., 2005; Verzola et al., 2008). These activate the two hallmark senescence pathways: the age-associated p16/pRB signaling and the stress-associated p53/p21 pathway (Kumari and Jat, 2021). These are thought to explain the similarities between aged and injured podocytes and the clinical phenomenon of more severe kidney injury in the aged population. They are also responsible for the podocyte senescence-associated secretory phenotype (SASP), typified by the increased production and secretion of numerous cytokines, growth factors, and chemokines (Table 4.1), creating a senescent environment within each affected glomerulus. The relevance of podocyte senescence was demonstrated in a recent study where the combination of two senolytics, dasatinib and quercetin, enhanced autophagy and reduced podocyte dedifferentiation through the Notch pathway in diabetic mice (Zhu et al., 2024).

Podocyte aging phenotype

In addition to senescence, the aged podocyte is characterized by several other hallmarks, including foot process and ultrastructural changes, hypertrophy, endoplasmic reticulum stress, cellular and oxidative stress, and reduced autophagy (Table 4.2). One compelling interpretation of podocyte aging is the concept of a podocyte life- and health span (Shankland et al., 2021). The lifespan of an individual podocyte corresponds to how long a podocyte is alive and, as such, is binary (Fig. 4.1). The lifespan translates to the total number of podocytes comprising the glomerular filtration barrier of individual glomeruli. The health span, on the other hand, is the part of an individual podocyte's life spent in good health and able to

TABLE 4.2 Characteristics of the podocyte aging phenotype.

Process	Endpoint	Measurement
Aging Classical hallmarks observed in podocytes	↓Foot process length and ↑slit diaphragm width	Podocyte exact morphology measurement procedure and filtration slit density
	Hypertrophy	↑podocyte nuclear area/podocyte volume
	↓Ultrastructure	Expansion microscopy, actin cytoskeleton
	↓Autophagy	mTOR, ATG/MAP1LC3, p62
	Cell stress	↑Desmin
	Endoplasmic reticulum stress	↑GRP94/Hsp90b1
	Oxidative stress	↑Reactive oxygen species, Ncx4, Ncf1, Ncf2, Prkcd ↓Ndufa5, Ndufs2, Ndufs4, Sdha, Cox5b,6c,7b
	↑Aging genes	↑*Gpnmb, Ighm, Igkc, J Chain, Ms4a7, Rplp2, Ccr1, Emp3, Fn1, Vcam1, Selplg*
Lifespan Length of time a podocyte lives corresponds to the total number of podocytes comprising the glomerular filtration barrier	↓Podocyte number/density	↓p57 and ↓p57/glomerular size
	↑Apoptosis	↑Cleaved caspase-3, TUNEL
	↑Pyroptosis	↑Caspase-1, NLRP3, GasderminD
	↑Detachment	Podocyturia
	Cell cycle arrest	BrdU, DNA content by flow cytometry
	Polyploidy	Flow cytometry, PAS staining
	Mitotic catastrophe	Flow cytometry, PAS staining
Health span Part of a podocyte's life that is spent in good health to perform normal cellular and molecular functions that maintain physiology, structure, and function	↓Canonical genes/proteins	↓Actn4, Cdkn1, Col4a, Fat1, Lamb2, Nphs1, Nphs2, Podxl, Synpo
	↓Canonical transcription factors	↓Wt1, Lmx1b, Foxc2, MafB
	↓Function	↓VEGFa, Angiopoietin-1
	↑Inflammation	↑PD1, PD-L1, PD-L2, *Naip6, Nlrp3, Aim2, Naip5, Nlrp1b, Nlrc4, Naip2, Casp1, Gsdmd, Casp4, Nlrp1a, Pycard, TLR 8,3,4,2*

perform the cellular and molecular functions necessary to maintain its physiology, structure, and function (Fig. 4.1). In contrast to the lifespan, the health span is not definitive but is best considered a continuous variable, changing dynamically throughout the cell's life. There are many molecular pathways associated with the podocyte health span (Shankland et al., 2021). Many are intrinsic to the podocytes and change with age, while others are extrinsic confounders and include known podocyte stressors such as obesity, hypertension, premature birth, and glomerular disease.

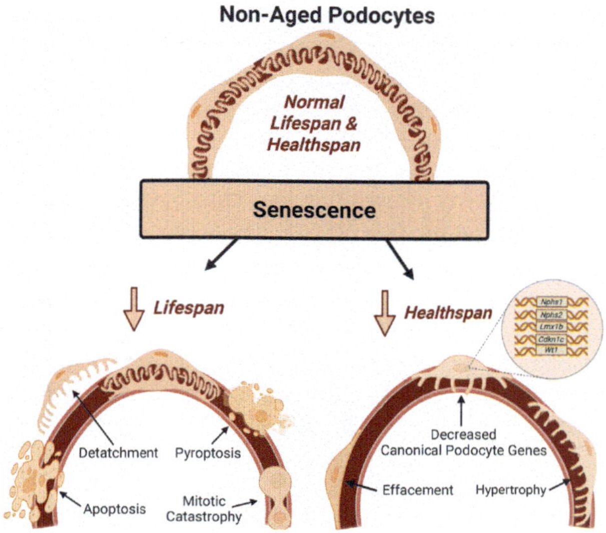

FIG. 4.1 Podocyte life- and health span. Illustration of how senescence affects healthy podocyte biology via two aspects. The podocyte lifespan is a binary outcome, caused by the loss of podocytes from the glomerulus via apoptosis, detachment, pyroptosis, or mitotic catastrophe (left panel). Conversely, the podocyte health span is a gradual change in the ability of a podocyte to perform its function, which is manifested by decreased expression of canonical podocyte genes, podocyte effacement, and hypertrophy (right panel). *Generated in Biorender.com.*

Podocyte lifespan - characterization

It is generally accepted that terminally differentiated podocytes are unable to self-renew (Griffin et al., 2003). However, some studies have demonstrated postnatal podocyte gain (Puelles and Moeller, 2019). Moreover, animal model studies have shown a direct correlation between podocyte depletion and glomerulosclerosis (Kim et al., 2001; Wharram et al., 2005; Fukuda et al., 2012b). Similarly, increasing age is associated with glomerulosclerosis (Kaplan et al., 1975; McLachlan, 1978; Rule et al., 2010; Glassock and Rule, 2012), which is paralleled by a decrease in absolute podocyte numbers and density (Kaverina et al., 2020; Wiggins et al., 2005; Zhang et al., 2012; Sweetwyne et al., 2017; Roeder et al., 2015; Schneider et al., 2017; McNicholas et al., 2016; Pippin et al., 2014; Wanner et al., 2014). It is important to note that this absolute loss of podocytes is accompanied by hypertrophy, i.e., an increase in podocyte size. This mechanism partially compensates for the decreased podocyte numbers yet is ultimately insufficient to match the overall reduction of podocyte density (Puelles et al., 2015; Goyal, 1982; Puelles et al., 2016). In fact, podocyte density decreases in both aged rats (Zhang et al., 2012) and mice (Schneider et al., 2017; Kaverina et al., 2020; Sweetwyne et al., 2017; Roeder et al., 2015; McNicholas et al., 2016; Pippin et al., 2014). In addition, the decrease in podocyte numbers with age differs between the glomeruli present in the cortical and juxtamedullary compartments of the kidney. Compared to young mice, podocyte density is 45.6% and 39% lower in the cortex and juxta-medulla of aged mice, respectively (Schneider et al., 2017).

Similar conclusions have been drawn regarding changes in podocyte number and density in humans. Kikuchi et al. (2017) reported that podocyte number per glomerulus increased from 326 ± 154 per glomerulus at the pre-capillary loop stage to 589 ± 166 podocytes per glomerulus in adults. Similarly, Puelles et al. (2015) reported that in children, the median podocyte count was 452, which increased to 558 podocytes per glomerulus in adults. With aging, podocyte number, as determined by nuclear density, was 300 podocytes per 10^6 μm^3 in young kidneys, which decreased to <100 per 10^6 μm^3 by 70–80 years of age. This equates to an annual podocyte loss of approximately 0.9% per year (Hodgin et al., 2015). Clinically, this decrease in podocyte number and density ultimately results in glomerulosclerosis (Wiggins, 2009; Camici et al., 2011) and therefore remains the best predictor for glomerulosclerosis risk in healthy aged kidneys (Naik et al., 2016; Hodgin et al., 2015; Puelles et al., 2015). Moreover, podocyte number and integrity are also critical in transplanted kidneys (Pippin et al., 2009), as kidney transplants with low podocyte endowment develop transplant glomerulopathy at a higher rate compared to those with normal podocyte density (Naik et al., 2019).

Podocyte lifespan - mechanisms of podocyte depletion

Several mechanisms ultimately cause podocyte depletion in aged kidneys, which are not mutually exclusive and likely occur in parallel or situation-dependently. Each will be briefly discussed below.

Apoptosis

This form of controlled cell death has been detected in aging podocytes (Lee et al., 2004; Tower, 2015). Yet, its overall contribution to podocyte depletion is technically difficult to quantify over the course of a lifespan because established assays, such as TUNEL, can only capture a short time period in the apoptotic program (Braun et al., 2016). Transcriptomic data from aged podocytes show a decrease in survival factors and an increase in pro-apoptotic pathways (Wang et al., 2020). However, their mechanistic contributions have not been experimentally tested. Other candidates can be extrapolated from published studies in nonaged podocytes (reviewed in Braun et al., 2016). These include: (1) the age-dependent decrease in nephrin and podocin, which likely reduces podocyte survival (Li et al., 2015); (2) the age-dependent decrease in WT1 resulting in increased WNT/ß-catenin signaling, which in turn can induce podocyte death (Wang et al., 2018); (3) the age-dependent increase of TGFß, which directly induces apoptosis (Schiffer et al., 2001); (4) the balance in autophagy, as an age-dependent decrease in autophagy induces apoptosis, while restoring it attenuates apoptosis (Yuan et al., 2025); and (5) increased levels of programmed cell death protein 1 in podocytes (Pippin et al., 2022).

Pyroptosis

This highly inflammatory form of lytic programmed cell death is characterized by the activation of caspase-1, with cells undergoing lysis, swelling, pore formation, blebbing, and DNA fragmentation (Bergsbaken et al., 2009). Pyroptosis is typically initiated by the inflammasome and generates an inflammatory response through the activation and release of IL-1ß and IL-18, followed by IFN-γ production. Pyroptosis has been implicated in several podocyte injury studies in nonaged kidneys, such as those associated with diabetes and APOL1 nephropathy (Shahzad et al., 2022; Wu et al., 2021). Moreover, genes causing pyroptosis are markedly increased in middle-aged and aged podocytes (Kaverina et al., 2023).

Podocyte detachment

The detection of podocytes in the urine is considered a sensitive marker of ongoing glomerular damage (Yu et al., 2005). Viable podocytes can be detected in the urine (Petermann et al., 2004). Moreover, the detachment of one podocyte can result in the subsequent detachment of neighboring healthy podocytes (Cho et al., 1993; Fukuda et al., 2012a; Ichikawa et al., 2005). Unfortunately, determining the actual number of podocytes lost due to detachment has been challenging, as detached podocytes can undergo secondary apoptosis in the urine via anoikis (Tharaux and Huber, 2012). Humans over the age of 60 exhibit a 3.3-fold increase in podocytes present in the urine compared to younger individuals (Hodgin et al., 2015). Transcriptomic data have identified several candidates for podocyte detachment, such as the downregulation of several cell-cell junction genes and the weakening of integrin-collagen interactions. Yet, validation of a causal relationship is still missing.

Mitotic catastrophe

As mentioned above, terminally differentiated podocytes cannot proliferate and self-renew, in part due to the expression of cell cycle inhibitors (Shankland et al., 2017). During aging, several inhibitory cell cycle regulatory genes are further upregulated (Wang et al., 2020), further limiting any possibility for cell cycle reentry and self-renewal. Injury studies have shown that if podocytes do manage to enter the cell cycle, they are unable to assemble an efficient mitotic spindle, which leads to aberrant chromosome segregation and ultimately cell death (Pippin et al., 2003; Tian et al., 2023; Mulay et al., 2013). This process is generally referred to as mitotic catastrophe (Lasagni et al., 2013; Shankland et al., 2024). Recent studies also implicate the loss of Profilin1, an actin-binding protein critical for cytoskeletal dynamics, in driving mitotic catastrophe through chromatin instability and failed cytokinesis (Tian et al., 2023). While not directly shown for aging, it is likely that changes in genes associated with cell cycle regulation in aged podocytes cause mitotic catastrophe and represent an additional mechanism that limits proliferation and increases podocyte loss.

Podocyte health span - age-dependent podocyte structural and synthetic changes

In contrast to the podocyte lifespan, the decline in the podocyte health span is accompanied by a range of major changes with advancing age (Table 4.2). Examples are discussed as follows.

Podocyte hypertrophy

Normal glomerular function requires that podocytes cover the underlying glomerular basement membrane (GBM). Glomerular volume increases by up to 700% between childhood and adulthood at a rate of 2.7% per year (Puelles et al., 2016). This is accompanied by an increase in total podocyte cell mass at a rate of 1.8% per year. However, as podocyte numbers decrease with age and glomerular volume increases, podocyte density is reduced as well (Hodgin et al., 2015). Due to the inability of podocytes to proliferate, this creates a mismatch between the number of podocytes and the increasing glomerular volume (Shankland et al., 2017). Thus, to continue to cover the GBM during aging, podocytes rely on compensatory hypertrophy (Wiggins et al., 2005). The average human podocyte volume at a young age (~38 weeks) is 335 ± 136 um^3(Kikuchi et al., 2017), but it then increases by 3.2% per year thereafter (Hodgin et al., 2015). In rats, five stages of podocyte hypertrophy have been described (Wiggins et al., 2005). Over time, the compensatory hypertrophy becomes maladaptive, leading to glomerulosclerosis (Wiggins et al., 2005; Hodgin et al., 2015; Wiggins, 2012). In particular, a denuded GBM lacking podocytes has been critically linked to the scarring process (Kriz, 2002). At the molecular level, the mechanisms of podocyte hypertrophy in the context of aging are not well understood. However, using cues from nonaged podocytes, candidate mechanisms include increased p21, p27, TGF-β, mTOR, and IL-6 (Wang et al., 2020). It is also noteworthy that, in contrast to the podocytes, increased glomerular size results in a proliferative and not a hypertrophic response in the two other glomerular cell types, the glomerular endothelial and mesangial cells (Hodgin et al., 2015).

Foot process effacement and podocyte stress

A characteristic feature of podocyte injury is a flattening of podocyte shape, generally referred to as effacement. It is a dynamic, ATP-consuming, signaling-based process that involves the rearrangement of the actin cytoskeleton and integrin-focal adhesion dynamics (Lennon et al., 2014). Effacement is accompanied by the loss of the interdigitating pattern of the foot processes between neighboring podocytes, decreased filtration slit density (Pippin et al., 2022), the loss of adherence to the GBM, and the loss of the sub-podocyte space between the podocyte cell body and the GBM (Garg, 2018; Shirato, 2002; Kriz et al., 2013). These changes are associated with reduced GFR due to their impact on the ultrafiltration coefficient Kf (Shankland, 2006) and proteinuria occurs due to the inability to compress the capillary wall (Butt et al., 2020; Benzing and Salant, 2021). In aging, podocytes in sclerosed glomeruli tend to be effaced in a highly similar process, likely contributing to a decrease in kidney function (Ali et al., 2025). The causes of age-associated podocyte effacement are not fully elucidated but clearly involve the remodeling of the cytoskeleton. In fact, many proteins involved in podocyte effacement in different clinical settings are also altered upon aging (Sweetwyne et al., 2017; Wang et al., 2020; Liu et al., 2017; Kakinuma et al., 2009). One major player is desmin, a type III intermediate filament protein that connects the nuclear and cell membrane with actin filaments and microtubules, thereby contributing to podocyte morphology and mechanics. While desmin is constitutively expressed in healthy podocytes, it is increased upon podocyte stress as well as aging (Wiggins et al., 2005; Floege et al., 1997). More importantly, increased desmin expression in aged podocytes in rats and mice precedes glomerulosclerosis, supporting that its dysregulation is a critical prerequisite for podocyte dysfunction (Floege et al., 1997; Wiggins et al., 2005).

Canonical podocyte gene expression

In podocytes, canonical genes are defined as proteins that are constitutively active and are required for their unique shape and function. Podocytes contain numerous canonical genes, many of which are unique to them. The function of the slit diaphragm as a size and charge barrier requires constitutive expression of a set of unique membrane proteins such as nephrin and podocin, typical adherens junction proteins such as cadherins and catenins, and scaffold proteins such as ZO-1, CD2AP, and MAGI-2 (Fukasawa et al., 2009; Garg, 2018). Decreased levels of these proteins lead to impaired signaling to the actin cytoskeleton, resulting in weakening of the foot processes, proteinuria, and, at times, glomerulosclerosis (Itoh et al., 2014). The expression of several of these proteins is significantly reduced in aged podocytes. For example, (Wiggins et al., 2005) reported that in 24-month-old rats, there was strongly reduced expression of *Tcf21*, *Nphs1*, *Col4a5*, *Glepp1*, and *Wt1*. Similarly, in aged mice, podocytes have decreased mRNA and protein expression of many critical slit diaphragm, tight junction, and other canonical podocyte genes (Wiggins et al., 2005; Wang et al., 2020; Kaverina et al., 2020; Sweetwyne et al., 2017; Pippin et al., 2022).

Reduced synthetic function and decreased crosstalk with other glomerular cell types

Podocytes do not act in isolation but extensively communicate with neighboring resident glomerular cells—the glomerular endothelial cells (GEnCs), parietal epithelial cells (PECs), and mesangial cells—to maintain glomerular integrity and function (Fig. 4.2). For example,

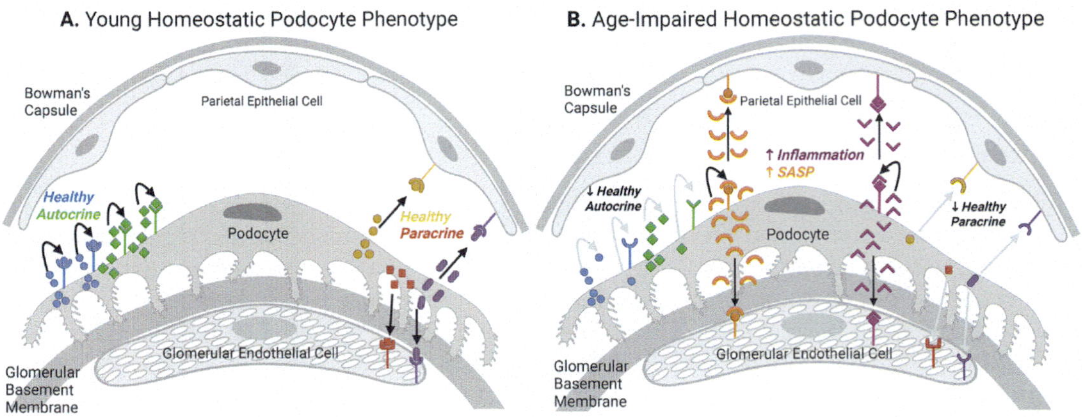

FIG. 4.2 Autocrine and paracrine signaling in the glomerulus. A schematic of a glomerulus with three of its four resident cells,the podocytes, the glomerular endothelial cells, and the parietal epithelial cells,depicts the young homeostatic podocyte phenotype (A) and the age-impaired homeostatic phenotype (B). The ligand-receptor interactions emanating from the podocytes and signaling to podocytes in an autocrine manner, as well as to glomerular endothelial cells and parietal epithelial cells in a paracrine manner, are illustrated. Note that the healthy autocrine and paracrine signaling in (A) is reduced upon aging, and a new set of ligands and receptors consisting of inflammatory markers and SASPs (senescence-associated secretory phenotypes), emerges in (B). *Generated in Biorender.com.*

a critical podocyte synthetic function is the production of angiopoietic factors required for the survival and health of neighboring GEnCs (Eremina et al., 2007). This crosstalk is best exemplified by a metaanalysis of recent transcriptomic data, which identified 55 ligand-receptor interactions specifically present in healthy podocytes, with 26 of them significantly reduced in aged podocytes (Wang et al., 2020). While the individual contributions of these to podocyte health and aging are still largely unexplored, these data show that aging podocytes are characterized by the lack or reduced activity of autocrine and perhaps paracrine signaling networks. This may explain why, for example, GEnC numbers are reduced in aged rats (Kang et al., 2001).

Mechanisms contributing to podocyte aging

Considering the multiple cellular and molecular manifestations of podocyte aging, it is not surprising that this requires an intricate interplay of cellular responses. There are at least four themes: *First*, the podocyte aging process involves aging mechanisms shared with many other cell types, such as senescence, loss of autophagy, or p53 signaling, as well as podocyte-specific aspects. *Second*, podocyte aging is a multifactorial process and not simply linear. Yet, the interactions between the pathways, their hierarchy, and chronology are mostly unexplored. *Third*, although not firmly established, podocyte aging is almost certainly accelerated by age-related comorbid stressors acting on podocytes, such as obesity (McKinzie et al., 2024), diabetes (Li and Liu, 2025), and hypertension (McKinzie et al., 2024), as well as environmental factors. These might involve pathways shared between aging and the stressors, such as senescence or mTORC1 signaling, or they could be distinct from each other. *Fourth*, as we outlined above, there exists a reciprocal crosstalk between the different glomerular cell types. In the following, we will discuss several of the published candidate mechanisms and their contribution to podocyte aging.

Senescence-associated secretory phenotypes

One of the hallmarks of senescence is the development of a hypersecretory state known as the senescence-associated secretory phenotype (SASP), which has both beneficial and detrimental effects (Wang et al., 2024; Ritschka et al., 2017). Short-term exposure to SASPs aids in cellular regeneration, while chronic exposure can induce tissue damage and promote senescence of neighboring cells. Our transcriptomic study of aged podocytes identified age-induced upregulation of classic inflammation-associated genes, components of the inflammasome pathway, and many SASP genes (Wang et al., 2020; Kaverina et al., 2023; Pippin et al., 2022). For example, *Nfkb1* and *Nfkb2* have been shown to be involved in glomerular aging (Wiggins et al., 2010) and are thus likely transcriptional drivers of this inflammatory phenotype. However, as there is little recruitment of immune cells into aging glomeruli (Kaneko et al., 2018), aging podocytes are likely in a state of sterile inflammation, i.e., inflammation not caused by infection (Shen et al., 2013; Zindel and Kubes, 2020). Yet, the precise role of individual SASPs, either alone or in combination, still needs to be addressed.

Mitochondrial dysfunction, oxidative stress, and changes in metabolism

Mitochondria generate most of the chemical energy needed for cellular homeostasis, and their dysfunction is often coupled with an increase in reactive oxygen species (ROS), a hallmark of aging in many cell types (Miwa et al., 2022). We reported that in 24-month-old mice, podocytes exhibited extensive mitochondrial damage, including disruption of the inner mitochondrial membranes, loss of cristae, changes to the mitochondrial matrix density, outer mitochondrial rupture, and increased expression of the ROS marker Nox4 (Sweetwyne et al., 2017). These changes were progressive, as mitochondria of 26-month-old mice were even more severely impacted. This was supported by transcriptomic data that showed global downregulation of genes involved in mitochondrial oxidative phosphorylation and upregulation of genes activated by ROS, supporting a concomitant increase in ROS production (Wang et al., 2020).

In addition, this study revealed that key metabolic pathways, including oxidative phosphorylation, the citric acid cycle, fatty acid oxidation, and amino acid catabolism, were reduced in aged podocytes (Wang et al., 2020). Such changes in metabolism have been described for most aged cells. Yet, in podocytes, the focus has largely been on oxidative phosphorylation (OXPHOS) (Balaban et al., 2005). Indeed, aged podocytes show dramatically reduced expression of enzymes involved in energy production via OXPHOS, such as peroxisome proliferator-activated receptor gamma coactivator 1 Alpha (*PGC1a*), a central regulator of mitochondrial biogenesis and OXPHOS (Ventura-Clapier et al., 2008; LeBleu et al., 2014). A similar situation applies to fatty acid oxidation. Podocytes primarily oxidize fatty acids instead of glutamine or pyruvate (Brinkkoetter et al., 2019) and the genes involved in fatty acid oxidation are downregulated in aged podocytes (Wang et al., 2020).

Anaerobic glycolysis has been identified as the predominant energy source for podocytes (Brinkkoetter et al., 2019), yet no significant age-dependent changes in the expression of glycolysis pathway genes have been observed (Sweetwyne et al., 2017). One hypothesis for this conundrum is that the age-dependent reduction in OXPHOS and fatty acid oxidation renders aged podocytes even more reliant on glycolysis for energy production.

Transcriptional changes

Transcriptional regulation is critical for normal podocyte development and homeostasis (Chugh, 2007). Yet, a transcriptional regulon analysis showed that many canonical transcription factors, their regulators, and their downstream targets were significantly downregulated in the aging podocyte, while injury-dependent transcription factors such as p53 were upregulated (Wang et al., 2020). One example is the transcription factor Cebpa, a member of the basic-region leucine zipper family of proteins. It is highly expressed in young podocytes (Zhong et al., 2016) but decreases in 20-month-old mice (Zhang et al., 2019). Moreover, podocyte-specific deletion of *Cebpa* induces podocyte senescence, reduces podocyte numbers, and decreases the expression of several canonical podocyte markers (Zhang et al., 2019). Similarly, in vitro studies of immortalized mouse podocytes show that Adriamycin-induced aging reduces *Cebpa* levels, and *Cebpa* overexpression reverses these changes (Zhang et al., 2019).

Sirtuins

The Sirtuins (Sirt) are a family of nicotinamide adenine dinucleotide-dependent deacetylases involved in several cellular processes, such as autophagy, and act largely through transcriptional repression by deacetylation (Salminen and Kaarniranta, 2009). Sirtuins have been implicated in the beneficial effects of calorie restriction via the regulation of autophagy (Madeo et al., 2019). Sirt1 and Sirt6 have been associated with normal podocyte function (Chuang et al., 2017). A decrease in Sirt1 expression augments podocyte aging, and knockdown of Sirt1 in mouse podocytes resulted in reduced levels of key podocyte proteins, an overall reduction in podocyte number, increased glomerulosclerosis, and albuminuria. This was accompanied by elevated expression of the senescent markers p16/Cdkn2a and p19/Cdkn2d, as well as increased levels of the cellular oxidative stress marker 8-OHdG in the urine (Chuang et al., 2017). This suggests that reduced Sirt1 levels in podocytes cause premature aging, increased oxidative stress, and mitochondrial injury, as has been observed in other cell types (Gomes et al., 2015).

Reduced autophagy

Autophagy is a healthy biological "cleaning" process that helps cells maintain homeostatic balance between the synthesis, degradation, and recycling of cellular proteins and organelles, with the ultimate purpose of supplying nutrients for survival (Lenoir et al., 2016). Podocytes, like other post-mitotic cells, have very high basal autophagic activity, which is essential for their energy homeostasis (Hartleben et al., 2010). When podocytes are unable to perform autophagy, damage occurs, resembling an aging phenotype. This notion is supported by the podocyte-specific deletion of autophagy-related 5 (*Atg5*), one of the key regulatory genes in the autophagy process in mice. These mice exhibit reduced autophagy and characteristics of enhanced aging, i.e., a decline in podocyte numbers and the accumulation of damaged organelles and protein aggregates (Hartleben et al., 2010) Surprisingly, the autophagy phenotype appears to be independent of one of its major known regulators, the mammalian target of rapamycin (mTOR) complex, which inhibits autophagy. As expected, mTOR activity is higher in the podocytes of aged mice (McNicholas et al., 2016). Two known inhibitors of mTOR activity are reduced: *Prkaa2*, which is part of the AMPK complex, and *Pkhd1*, while *Card11*, an activator of mTOR signaling, is upregulated 6.9-fold in aged podocytes (Wang et al., 2020). Yet, administering the mTOR inhibitor rapamycin to 26.5-month-old mice reduced mTOR activity but did not impact podocyte density (McNicholas et al., 2016). Thus further studies are needed to understand the mTOR-independent regulation of autophagy in aged podocytes and whether this can be harnessed toward antiaging approaches.

Epigenetic changes

Epigenetic changes play a critical role in influencing the senescence of kidney cells, including podocytes (Zheng et al., 2021; Yang et al., 2023). In podocytes, these changes include DNA methylation, DNA methyltransferases, and histone modifications. The latter was, for example, demonstrated in Hdac1/2 deletion, which induces loss of podocyte quiescence, leading to cell cycle entry, G1 arrest, and the onset of podocyte senescence, both in vivo and in vitro (Medina Rangel et al., 2023).

Additional mechanisms

In addition to these well-established mechanistic pathways, there are also several molecules that have clear aging-dependent phenotypes but are not yet incorporated into more generalizable schemes, as the following examples show: (1) Overexpression of retinoic acid receptor responder protein-1 (RARRES1) in podocytes increased albuminuria, blood urea nitrogen, and glomerulosclerosis in middle-aged mice compared to age-matched control mice (Feng et al., 2024). (2) Knocking down Rheb1, a member of the Ras superfamily of small GTPases, in cultured podocytes and in podocytes of diabetic mice decreased hyperglycemia-induced senescence (Lu et al., 2024). (3) Exposure of cultured podocytes or mice with STZ-induced diabetic kidney disease to ß-hydroxybutyrate, which inhibits GSK3ß, reduced podocyte senescence and activated Nrf2 (Fang et al., 2021). (4) NAT10, an enzyme that catalyzes the acetylation of cytidine in RNA, is increased in podocytes of mice with Adriamycin-induced podocyte injury, and its inhibitor, Remodelin, or small interfering RNAs targeting NAT10 reduced senescence through its interaction with TLR2 (Hu et al., 2025). (5) The expression of the RE1-silencing transcription factor REST increases in human and mouse podocytes with age and translocates from the cytoplasm in young podocytes to the nucleus with age (Magassa et al., 2021). Overexpression of REST improves the survival of podocytes, while a podocyte-specific deletion results in a reduced podocyte number. (6) Podocyte-specific deletion of G-protein-coupled receptor 124 (Gpr124) exacerbates senescence in mice with diabetic kidney disease, while overexpressing Gpr124 in cultured podocytes induces senescence (Li et al., 2025). (7) Estrogen-related receptor (ERR) alpha, which regulates the transcription of genes involved in many metabolic pathways and mitochondrial biogenesis, is decreased in aged mouse podocytes (Wang et al., 2023). Treating aged mice with the pan-ERR agonist SLU-PP-332 limited podocyte loss and increased the expression of podocin compared to age-matched untreated mice, which was accompanied by reduced albuminuria. (8) Arginase II is an enzyme that metabolizes L-arginine to urea and L-ornithine, is expressed in many kidney cell types, including podocytes, and increases with advancing age (Ajalbert et al., 2023). Interestingly, male but not female global Arginase II null mice at 20–22 months of age exhibited lower albuminuria and a higher number of podocytes compared to age-matched wildtype mice.

The intersection of kidney disease and aging

A critical clinical question that requires a mechanistic understanding is how podocyte aging and disease intersect. Glomerular diseases are more common in older patients (Reichert et al., 1998; Gerstoft et al., 1986) and their outcomes with the same disease are, on average, more severe than in a younger population (Reichert et al., 1998; Gerstoft et al., 1986; Cui et al., 2011). Healthy aging of podocytes and injury to young podocytes share many histological and molecular changes (Table 4.3). For example, in both settings, podocytes undergo effacement, experience changes to their slit diaphragms, and exhibit decreased canonical gene expression, resulting in an overall reduction in function. This phenomenon is also recapitulated in animal models. Induction of experimental podocyte injury compounds the preexisting age-dependent podocyte depletion, triggering increased glomerulosclerosis

TABLE 4.3 Comparison between podocyte aging and disease phenotypes.

Podocyte pathways/genes/proteins	Aging	Disease
Senescence genes (e.g., p16, p21, p53)	↑	↑
Polyploidy	↑	↑
DNA damage	↑	↑
Canonical podocyte proteins (e.g., nephrin, podocin)	↓	↓
Cell cycle arrest	↑	↑
Hypertrophy	↑	↑
Inflammatory phenotype (e.g., NLRP3, PD-1, IL-1β, IL-18)	↑	↑
Growth factors/cytokines (e.g., TGFß, bFGF, INF)	↑	↑
Chemokines (e.g., CXCR4, TLR4)	↑	↑
Podocyte function (e.g., VEGF secretion)	↓	↓
Proteases (e.g., MMP1, MMP9)	↑	↑
Mitochondrial dysfunction	↓	↓
Oxidative stress	↑	↑

(Schneider et al., 2017). As such, from a clinical treatment standpoint, it is important to determine whether changes in gene expression during podocyte aging overlap with or are distinct from those in common podocyte diseases. Indeed, several changes observed in nonaged podocytes injured by glomerular disease overlap with those seen in podocytes from healthy-aged kidneys, including a decrease in podocyte health and lifespan (Shankland et al., 2021, 2023). However, another study comparing published data concluded that pathways perturbed in diabetic kidney disease and FSGS were largely distinct from each other (Wang et al., 2020). Thus more studies are needed to identify distinct and common pathways between aging and disease. Intriguingly, from a therapeutic perspective, changes to podocytes in both disease and aging can be halted or even partially reversed by improving mitochondrial health (Sweetwyne et al., 2017; Gujarati et al., 2020), PD1 blockade (Pippin et al., 2022) and inhibiting the NLRP3-inflammasome (Kaverina et al., 2023; Wu et al., 2021; Shahzad et al., 2022; Wu et al., 2021).

In animal models of experimental FSGS induced by both Adriamycin and anti-podocyte antibody, the glomerular expression of p16/Cdkn2a, p21/Cdkn1a, and senescence-associated beta-galactosidase (SA-β-gal) is increased in young mice (Pereira et al., 2024). However, when long-term effects were assessed, these markers of senescence were no longer consistently upregulated. Yet, podocyte density and expression of canonical podocyte proteins were reduced, accompanied by increased glomerular scarring. Thus this study supports the clinical observations that injury during youth accelerates podocyte aging, contributing to more severe disease progression.

Future directions - antiaging therapies

There is a substantial effort to identify treatments and drugs that mitigate the effects of aging in humans. To date, several different approaches or compounds have shown promise in reducing podocyte aging or are at least conceptually advanced.

Calorie restriction

This approach is the oldest and most robust way to extend rodent life span systemically. In the kidney, Wiggins et al. showed that calorie restriction in rats prevented age-associated podocyte hypertrophy, upregulated podocyte function genes, and reduced podocyte stress markers (Wiggins et al., 2005). Similarly, we reported that calorie restriction in male F344 rats during aging limited their podocyte loss compared to their counterparts on an ad libitum diet (Zhang et al., 2012). The precise mechanism(s) whereby calorie restriction alters aging podocyte biology, and whether they differ from what is described for other aging cell types, is unknown. One possible link between the effect of calorie restriction in podocytes is the sirtuins discussed above, as these have been implicated as effectors of calorie restriction (Zullo et al., 2018).

Senotherapy

This therapeutic approach aims to reverse aging-related processes by directly targeting senescent cells. Among these, senolytics are a class of drugs designed to selectively eliminate senescent cells (Lelarge et al., 2024). While not yet tested extensively in the kidney, one example includes the cancer drugs quercetin and dasatinib, which have been shown to reduce markers of aging (O'Hare et al., 2005; Russo et al., 2012; Zhu et al., 2015) and also improve podocyte function (Palmer et al., 2019). One possibility is that if senescent podocytes are secreting SASPs and this is damaging neighboring podocytes, senolytics may have a positive effect. Conversely, senolytics, by removing terminally differentiated podocytes, could exacerbate podocytopathies in vivo by causing the remaining podocytes to undergo hypertrophy and/or trigger scarring. Thus, further studies are needed. The second group of senotherapy drugs is senomorphics, a class of drugs that target senescent cells and aim to revert them to resemble younger cells again (Zhang et al., 2023). They are thought to act primarily by attenuating the pathological function of SASPs. The best-studied example is the inhibition of the mTOR pathway, which induces autophagy, thereby sustaining cell survival under conditions of nutrient deprivation. In podocytes, it has been shown that increased mTOR signaling causes disease and augments injury, while reducing it limits injury (reviewed in Lenoir et al., 2016). However, while rapamycin treatment can revert podocyte hypertrophy (Puelles et al., 2019), it did not impact podocyte density in aged mice (McNicholas et al., 2016). Thus its antiaging activity in podocytes is still unresolved. Another example is the well-studied senomorphic metformin, one of the most prescribed drugs for treating type 2 diabetes mellitus. Similar to rapamycin, metformin has been shown to remediate diabetes-induced podocyte injury (Lehtonen, 2020), but its antiaging activities have not been investigated.

Novel targets

Besides these conceptual approaches, several studies have identified potential targets to reverse the aged podocyte phenotype. Three examples include: (1) The endothelin receptor antagonist Darusentan, which was clinically evaluated for congestive heart failure and hypertension treatment. It induces substantial recovery of podocyte structure in 23-month-old male Wistar rats treated for 28 days (Ortmann et al., 2004). (2) The mitochondrial antioxidant SS-31/Elamipretide, a small cell-permeable synthetic peptide that is in clinical trials for heart failure, primary mitochondrial myopathy, and other mitochondrial diseases (Szeto, 2014). SS-31 improves mitochondrial function by enhancing electron transfer through cytochrome c, improving oxidative phosphorylation coupling, increasing ATP synthesis, and reducing ROS production (Fouron, 1985; Cornel et al., 1986). In podocytes of aged 24-month-old mice, SS-31 preserved podocyte mitochondrial integrity, reduced podocyte hypertrophy, foot process effacement, the injury marker desmin, and preserved the expression of synaptopodin (Sweetwyne et al., 2017). (3) Glycogen synthase kinase 3β (GSK3β) is overexpressed and hyperactive in aged podocytes, targeting key mediators of senescence signaling, such as p16/Cdkn2A and p53 (Fang et al., 2022). Therapeutic targeting of GSK3β by lithium in aged mice reduced senescence and kidney aging. While this has not yet been translated to humans, the FDA-approved use of lithium in schizophrenia establishes feasibility (Shankland and Wessely, 2022; Fang et al., 2022).

Future directions - podocyte replacement

As podocyte depletion is a critical pathophysiological process in the aged kidney, one might ask if replacement can be augmented from the putative adult podocyte progenitors, namely glomerular parietal epithelial cells (Kaverina et al., 2020; Romoli et al., 2018; Lasagni et al., 2015; Appel et al., 2009) and renin-producing cells (Pippin et al., 2014). Both progenitors are detected in individual aged glomeruli in which podocytes are depleted, albeit in low numbers (Kaverina et al., 2020; Romoli et al., 2018; Lasagni et al., 2015; Appel et al., 2009; Pippin et al., 2014). Notably, these aged glomeruli have a normal morphology with no scarring. However, the numbers of both types of podocyte progenitors decrease with advancing age. They also acquire additional adverse changes, such as mesenchymal transformation, that limit their progenitor function (Roeder et al., 2015; Hamatani et al., 2018). Thus, while corrective, podocyte progenitor augmentation is not fully capable of countering the age-associated decrease in podocyte numbers. Based on this observation, boosting adult podocyte progenitors should be considered a target for future therapies to improve podocyte numbers.

Conclusion

This chapter focuses on published studies of podocyte aging under nonstressed conditions, where p16/CDKN2A and p19/CDKN2D are the predominant senescence-inducing genes, and under stressed conditions, where the senescence-inducing genes include p16/CDKN2A, p21/CDKN1A, and p53. The podocyte aging responses include a shorter lifespan and a reduced health span. Moreover, the resultant senescence-associated secretory phenotype causes deleterious autocrine and paracrine signaling effects on podocytes and neighboring glomerular cells, respectively. Future studies will be needed to better understand the intersection of podocyte aging and disease-induced injury and whether limiting podocyte senescence can impact clinical outcomes.

Acknowledgments

Grants Supporting Work: 5R01DK056799, 1R01DK097598-01A1, 5R01AG079935, 5R01DK083294, 5R01DK093629, DOD HT9425-23-10440.

References

Ajalbert, G., Brenna, A., Ming, X.F., Yang, Z., Potenza, D.M., 2023. Elevation of arginase-II in podocytes contributes to age-associated albuminuria in male mice. Int. J. Mol. Sci. 14220067. 24 (13). Available from: http://www.mdpi.com/journal/ijms. doi:10.3390/ijms241311228.

Ali, A., Liu, Z., Kenan, Y., Guan, Y., Chen, S., Liu, T., Guo, Z., Wong, M.K., Vasquez, P., Poudel, C., Mustonen, B.C., Eng, D.G., Pippin, J.W., Shankland, S.J., Wang, S., Vaughan, J.C., 2025. Super-resolved optical imaging, reconstruction, and spatial analysis of whole mouse glomeruli via the Glomerulus Mapping and Analysis Pipeline. Kidney Int. doi:10.1016/j.kint.2025.07.024.

Anderson, S., Brenner, B.M., 1986. Effects of aging on the renal glomerulus. Am. J. Med. 00029343. 80 (3), 435–442. doi:10.1016/0002-9343(86)90718-7.

Appel, D., Kershaw, D.B., Smeets, B., Yuan, G., Fuss, A., Frye, B., Elger, M., Kriz, W., Floege, J., Moeller, M.J., 2009. Recruitment of podocytes from glomerular parietal epithelial cells. J. Am. Soc. Nephrol. 15333450. 20 (2), 333–343. Available from: http://jasn.asnjournals.org/cgi/reprint/20/2/333. doi:10.1681/ASN.2008070795.

Balaban, R.S., Nemoto, S., Finkel, T., 2005. Mitochondria, oxidants, and aging. Cell. 00928674. 120 (4), 483–495. Available from: https://www.cell.com. doi:10.1016/j.cell.2005.02.001.

Benzing, T., Salant, D., 2021. Insights into glomerular filtration and albuminuria. N. Engl. J. Med. 384, 1437–1446.

Bergsbaken, T., Fink, S.L., Cookson, B.T., 2009. Pyroptosis: host cell death and inflammation. Nat. Rev. Microbiol. 17401526. 7 (2), 99–109. doi:10.1038/nrmicro2070.

Braun, F., Becker, J.U., Brinkkoetter, P.T., 2016. Live or let die: is there any cell death in podocytes? Semin. Nephrol. 15584488. 36 (3), 208–219. Available from: http://www.elsevier.com/inca/publications/store/6/2/3/3/3/5/index.htt. doi:10.1016/j.semnephrol.2016.03.008.

Brinkkoetter, P.T., Bork, T., Salou, S., Liang, W., Mizi, A., Özel, C., Koehler, S., Hagmann, H.H., Ising, C., Kuczkowski, A., Schnyder, S., Abed, A., Schermer, B., Benzing, T., Kretz, O., Puelles, V.G., Lagies, S., Schlimpert, M., Kammerer, B., Handschin, C., Schell, C., Huber, T.B., 2019. Anaerobic glycolysis maintains the glomerular filtration barrier independent of mitochondrial metabolism and dynamics. Cell Rep. 22111247. 27 (5), 1551. Available from: http://www.sciencedirect.com/science/journal/22111247. doi:10.1016/j.celrep.2019.04.012.

Butt, L., Unnersjö-Jess, D., Höhne, M., Edwards, A., Binz-Lotter, J., Reilly, D., Hahnfeldt, R., Ziegler, V., Fremter, K., Rinschen, M.M., Helmstädter, M., Ebert, L.K., Castrop, H., Hackl, M.J., Walz, G., Brinkkoetter, P.T., Liebau, M.C., Tory, K., Hoyer, P.F., Beck, B.B., Brismar, H., Blom, H., Schermer, B., Benzing, T., 2020. A molecular mechanism explaining albuminuria in kidney disease. Nat. Metab. 25225812. 2 (5), 461–474. Available from: https://www.nature.com/natmetab/. doi:10.1038/s42255-020-0204-y.

Camici, M., Carpi, A., Cini, G., Galetta, F., Abraham, N., 2011. Podocyte dysfunction in aging - Related glomerulosclerosis. Front. Biosci. Scholar. 19450524. 3 (3), 995–1006. Available from: http://www.bioscience.org/fbs/getfile.php?FileName=/2011/v3s/af/204/204.pdf.

Cho, C.R., Lumsden, C.J., Whiteside, C.I., 1993. Epithelial cell detachment in the nephrotic glomerulus: a receptor co-operativity model. J. Theor. Biol. 00225193. 160 (4), 407–426. doi:10.1006/jtbi.1993.1027.

Chuang, P.Y., Cai, W., Li, X., Fang, L., Xu, J., Yacoub, R., He, J.C., Lee, K., 2017. Reduction in podocyte SIRT1 accelerates kidney injury in aging mice. Am. J. Physiol. Renal Physiol. 15221466. 313 (3), F621. Available from: http://ajprenal.physiology.org/content/313/3/F621.full.pdf. doi:10.1152/ajprenal.00255.2017.

Chugh, S.S., 2007. Transcriptional regulation of podocyte disease. Transl. Res. 19315244. 149 (5), 237–242. Available from: http://www.sciencedirect.com/science/journal/19315244. doi:10.1016/j.trsl.2007.01.002.

Cornel, M.C., Swagemakers, M.L., te Meerman, G.J., Haayer, E.J., ten Kate, L.P., 1986. EUROCAT registration of congenital abnormalities and multiple births; aims, methods and results of the Dutch share of the project 1981–1983. Ned. Tijdschr. Geneeskd. 130 (27), 1233–1237.

Cui, Z., Zhao, J., Jia, X.Y., Zhu, S.N., Zhao, M.H., 2011. Clinical features and outcomes of anti-glomerular basement membrane disease in older patients. Am. J. Kidney Dis. 02726386. 57 (4), 575–582. doi:10.1053/j.ajkd.2010.09.022.

da Costa, J.P., Vitorino, R., Silva, G.M., Vogel, C., Duarte, A.C., Rocha-Santos, T., 2016. A synopsis on aging—Theories, mechanisms and future prospects. Ageing Res. Rev. 18729649. 29, 90–112. Available from: http://www.elsevier.com/locate/arr. doi:10.1016/j.arr.2016.06.005.

Denic, A., Glassock, R.J., Rule, A.D., 2016. Structural and functional changes with the aging kidney. Adv. Chronic Kidney Dis. 15485609. 23 (1), 19–28. Available from: http://www.elsevier.com/wps/find/journaldescription.cws_home/703170/description#description. doi:10.1053/j.ackd.2015.08.004.

Dimke, H., Maezawa, Y., Quaggin, S.E., 2015. Crosstalk in glomerular injury and repair. Curr. Opin. Nephrol. Hypertens. 14736543. 24 (3), 231–238. Available from: http://journals.lww.com/co-nephrolhypertens/pages/default.aspx. doi:10.1097/MNH.0000000000000117.

Ebefors, K., Bergwall, L., Nystrom, J., 2021. The glomerulus according to the mesangium. Front. Med. (Lausanne) 8, 740527.

Eremina, V., Baelde, H.J., Quaggin, S.E., 2007. Role of the VEGF-A signaling pathway in the glomerulus: evidence for crosstalk between components of the glomerular filtration barrier. Nephron Physiol. 16602137. 106 (2), 32. doi:10.1159/000101798.

Fang, Y., Chen, B., Gong, A.Y., Malhotra, D.K., Gupta, R., Dworkin, L.D., Gong, R., 2021. The ketone body β-hydroxybutyrate mitigates the senescence response of glomerular podocytes to diabetic insults. Kidney Int. 15231755. 100 (5), 1037–1053. Available from: https://www.journals.elsevier.com/kidney-international. doi:10.1016/j.kint.2021.06.031.

Fang, Y., Chen, B., Liu, Z., Gong, A.Y., Gunning, W.T., Yan, G., Malhotra, D., Gohara, A.F., Dworkin, L.D., Gong, R., 2022. Age-related GSK3β overexpression drives podocyte senescence and glomerular aging. J. Clin. Invest. 132 (4). doi:10.1172/JCI141848.

Feng, Y., Sun, Z., Fu, J., Zhong, F., Zhang, W., Wei, C., Chen, A., Liu, B.C., He, J.C., Lee, K., 2024. Podocyte-derived soluble RARRES1 drives kidney disease progression through direct podocyte and proximal tubular injury. Kidney Int. 15231755. 106 (1), 50–66. Available from: https://www.sciencedirect.com/science/journal/00852538. doi:10.1016/j.kint.2024.04.011.

Floege, J., Hackmann, B., Kliem, V., Kriz, W., Alpers, C.E., Johnson, R.J., Kühn, K.W., Koch, K.M., Brunkhorst, R., 1997. Age-related glomerulosclerosis and interstitial fibrosis in Milan normotensive rats: a podocyte disease. Kidney Int. 00852538. 51 (1), 230–243. Available from: https://www.journals.elsevier.com/kidney-international. doi:10.1038/ki.1997.28.

Fouron, J.C., 1985. Pulmonary edema with upper airway obstruction. Am. J. Dis. Child. 23742976. 139 (4), 331. doi:10.1001/archpedi.1985.02140060013005.

Fukasawa, H., Bornheimer, S., Kudlicka, K., Farquhar, M.G., 2009. Slit diaphragms contain tight junction proteins. J. Am. Soc. Nephrol. 15333450. 20 (7), 1491–1503. Available from: http://jasn.asnjournals.org/cgi/reprint/20/7/1491. doi:10.1681/ASN.2008101117.

Fukuda, A., Chowdhury, M.A., Venkatareddy, M.P., Wang, S.Q., Nishizono, R., Suzuki, T., Wickman, L.T., Wiggins, J.E., Muchayi, T., Fingar, D., Shedden, K.A., Inoki, K., Wigg, R.C., 2012b. Growth-dependent podocyte failure causes glomerulosclerosis. J. Am. Soc. Nephrol. 15333450. 23 (8), 1351–1363. Available from: http://jasn.asnjournals.org/content/23/8/1351.full.pdf+html. doi:10.1681/ASN.2012030271.

Fukuda, A., Wickman, L.T., Venkatareddy, M.P., Sato, Y., Chowdhury, M.A., Wang, S.Q., Shedden, K.A., Dysko, R.C., Wiggins, J.E., Wiggins, R.C., 2012a. Angiotensin II-dependent persistent podocyte loss from destabilized glomeruli causes progression of end stage kidney disease. Kidney Int. 15231755. 81 (1), 40–55. Available from: https://www.journals.elsevier.com/kidney-international. doi:10.1038/ki.2011.306.

Garg, P., 2018. A review of podocyte biology. Am. J. Nephrol. 0250-8095. 47 (Suppl. 1), 3–13. doi:10.1159/000481633.

Ge, S., Nie, S., Liu, Z., Chen, C., Zha, Y., Qian, J., Liu, B., Teng, S., Xu, A., Bin, W., Xu, X., Xu, G., 2016. Epidemiology and outcomes of acute kidney injury in elderly chinese patients: a subgroup analysis from the EACH study. BMC Nephrol. 17 (1), 136. doi:10.1186/s12882-016-0351-2. PMID: 27682843; PMCID: PMC5041437.

Gerstoft, J., Balsløv, J.T., Brahm, M., Brun, C., Jørgensen, F., Jørgensen, H.E., Larsen, M., Larsen, S., Lorenzen, I., Løber, M., 1986. Prognosis in glomerulonephritis. II. Regression analyses of prognostic factors affecting the course of renal function and the mortality in 395 patients. Calculation of a prognostic model. Report from a Copenhagen study group of renal diseases. Acta Med. Scand. 219 (2), 179–187.

Glassock, R.J., Rule, A.D., 2012. The implications of anatomical and functional changes of the aging kidney: with an emphasis on the glomeruli. Kidney Int. 15231755. 82 (3), 270–277. Available from: https://www.journals.elsevier.com/kidney-international. doi:10.1038/ki.2012.65.

Gomes, P., Outeiro, T.F., Cavadas, C., 2015. Emerging role of Sirtuin 2 in the regulation of mammalian metabolism. Trends Pharmacol. Sci. 01656147. 36 (11), 756–768. doi:10.1016/j.tips.2015.08.001.

Goyal, V.K., 1982. Changes with age in the human kidney. Exp. Gerontol. 05315565. 17 (5), 321–331. doi:10.1016/0531-5565(82)90032-8.

Griffin, S.V., Petermann, A.T., Durvasula, R.V., Shankland, S.J., 2003. Podocyte proliferation and differentiation in glomerular disease: role of cell-cycle regulatory proteins. Nephrol. Dial. Transplant. 09310509. 18, vi8.

Gujarati, N.A., Vasquez, J.M., Bogenhagen, D.F., Mallipattu, S.K., 2020. The complicated role of mitochondria in the podocyte. Am. J. Physiol. Renal Physiol. 15221466. 319 (6), F955. Available from: https://journals.physiology.org/doi/10.1152/ajprenal.00393.2020. doi:10.1152/AJPRENAL.00393.2020.

Hamatani, H., Eng, D.G., Kaverina, N.V., Gross, K.W., Freedman, B.S., Pippin, J.W., Shankland, S.J., 2018. Lineage tracing aged mouse kidneys shows lower number of cells of renin lineage and reduced responsiveness to RAAS inhibition. Am. J. Physiol. Renal Physiol. 15221466. 315 (1), F97. Available from: https://www.physiology.org/doi/pdf/10.1152/ajprenal.00570.2017. doi:10.1152/ajprenal.00570.2017.

Hartleben, B., Gödel, M., Meyer-Schwesinger, C., Liu, S., Ulrich, T., Köbler, S., Wiech, T., Grahammer, F., Arnold, S.J., Lindenmeyer, M.T., Cohen, C.D., Pavenstädt, H., Kerjaschki, D., Mizushima, N., Shaw, A.S., Walz, G., Huber, T.B., 2010. Autophagy influences glomerular disease susceptibility and maintains podocyte homeostasis in aging mice. J. Clin. Invest. 15588238. 120 (4), 1084–1096. Available from: http://www.jci.org/articles/view/39492/pdf. doi:10.1172/JCI39492Germany.

Hodgin, J.B., Bitzer, M., Wickman, L., Afshinnia, F., Wang, S.Q., O'Connor, C., Yang, Y., Meadowbrooke, C., Chowdhury, M., Kikuchi, M., Wiggins, J.E., Wiggins, R.C., 2015. Glomerular aging and focal global glomerulosclerosis: a podometric perspective. J. Am. Soc. Nephrol. 15333450. 26 (12), 3162–3178. Available from: http://jasn.asnjournals.org/content/26/12/3162.full.pdf+html. doi:10.1681/ASN.2014080752.

Hu, M., Lv, L., Lei, Y., Chen, M., Zhou, S., Liu, Z., 2025. NAT10 mediates TLR2 to promote podocyte senescence in Adriamycin-induced nephropathy. Cell Death Dis. 20414889. 16 (1). Available from: https://www.nature.com/cddis/. doi:10.1038/s41419-025-07515-1.

Ichikawa, I., Ma, J., Motojima, M., Matsusaka, T., 2005. Podocyte damage damages podocytes: autonomous vicious cycle that drives local spread of glomerular sclerosis. Curr. Opin. Nephrol. Hypertens. 1062-4821. 14 (3), 205–210. doi:10.1097/01.mnh.0000165884.85803.e1.

Inoue, K., Gan, G., Ciarleglio, M., Zhang, Y., Tian, X., Pedigo, C.E., Cavanaugh, C., Tate, J., Wang, Y., Cross, E., Groener, M., Chai, N., Wang, Z., Justice, A., Zhang, Z., Parikh, C.R., Wilson, F.P., Ishibe, S., 2019. Podocyte histone deacetylase activity regulates murine and human glomerular diseases. J. Clin. Invest. 15588238. 129 (3), 1295–1313. Available from: https://www.jci.org/articles/view/124030/pdf. doi:10.1172/JCI124030.

Itoh, M., Nakadate, K., Horibata, Y., Matsusaka, T., Jianliang, X., Hunziker, W., Sugimoto, H., Fanning, A.S., 2014. The structural and functional organization of the podocyte filtration slits is regulated by Tjp1/ZO-1. PLoS One. 1932-6203. 9 (9), e106621. doi:10.1371/journal.pone.0106621.

Iwamoto, M., Nakahira, Y., Kimpara, H., 2015. Development and validation of the total human model for safety (THUMS) toward further understanding of occupant injury mechanisms in precrash and during crash. Traffic Inj. Prev. 1538-9588. 16 (sup1), S36. doi:10.1080/15389588.2015.1015000.

Kakinuma, N., Zhu, Y., Wang, Y., Roy, B.C., Kiyama, R., 2009. Kank proteins: structure, functions and diseases. Cell. Mol. Life Sci. 1420-682X. 66 (16), 2651–2659. doi:10.1007/s00018-009-0038-y.

Kaneko, Y., Cho, T., Sato, Y., Goto, K., Yamamoto, S., Goto, S., Madaio, M.P., Narita, I., 2018. Attenuated macrophage infiltration in glomeruli of aged miceresultinginamelioratedkidneyinjuryinnephrotoxic serum nephritis. J. Gerontol. A Biol. Sci. Med. Sci. 1758535X. 73 (9), 1178–1186. Available from: http://biomedgerontology.oxfordjournals.org/. doi:10.1093/gerona/gly019.

Kang, D.H., Anderson, S., Kim, Y.G., Mazzalli, M., Suga, S.I., Jefferson, J.A., Gordon, K.L., Oyama, T.T., Hughes, J., Hugo, C., Kerjaschki, D., Schreiner, G.F., Johnson, R.J., 2001. Impaired angiogenesis in the aging kidney: vascular endothelial growth factor and thrombospondin-1 in renal disease. Am. J. Kidney Dis. 02726386. 37 (3), 601–611. Available from: http://www.elsevier.com/inca/publications/store/6/2/3/2/7/6/index.htt. doi:10.1053/ajkd.2001.22087.

Kaplan, C., Pasternack, B., Shah, H., Gallo, G., 1975. Age-related incidence of sclerotic glomeruli in human kidneys. Am. J. Pathol. 80 (2), 227–234.

Kaverina, N., Schweickart, R.A., Chan, G.C., Maggiore, J.C., Eng, D.G., Zeng, Y., McKinzie, S.R., Perry, H.S., Ali, A., O'Connor, C., Pereira, B.M.V., Theberge, A.B., Vaughan, J.C., Loretz, C.J., Chang, A., Hukriede, N.A., Bitzer, M., Pippin, J.W., Wessely, O., Shankland, S.J., 2023. Inhibiting NLRP3 signaling in aging podocytes improves their lifeand health-span. Aging. 19454589. 15 (14). Available from: http://www.aging-us.com/. doi:10.18632/aging.204897.

Kaverina, N.V., Eng, D.G., Miner, J.H., Pippin, J.W., Shankland, S.J., 2020. Parietal epithelial cell differentiation to a podocyte fate in the aged mouse kidney. Aging. 19454589. 12 (17), 1–24. Available from: https://paperchase-aging.s3-us-west-1.amazonaws.com/pdf/uWaLgY9hv34g9NCvw.pdf. doi:10.18632/AGING.103788.

Kikuchi, M., Wickman, L., Rabah, R., Wiggins, R.C., 2017. Podocyte number and density changes during early human life. Pediatr. Nephrol. 1432198X. 32 (5), 823–834. Available from: https://link.springer.de/link/service/journals/00467/index.htm. doi:10.1007/s00467-016-3564-5.

Kim, Y.H., Goyal, M., Kurnit, D., Wharram, B., Wiggins, J., Holzman, L., Kershaw, D., Wiggins, R., 2001. Podocyte depletion and glomerulosclerosis have a direct relationship in the PAN-treated rat. Kidney Int. 00852538. 60 (3), 957–968. doi:10.1046/j.1523-1755.2001.060003957.x.

Kriz, W., 2002. Podocyte is the major culprit accounting for the progression of chronic renal disease. Microsc. Res. Tech. 1059-910X. 57 (4), 189–195. doi:10.1002/jemt.10072.

Kriz, W., Shirato, I., Nagata, M., LeHir, M., Lemley, K.V., 2013. The podocyte's response to stress: the enigma of foot process effacement. Am. J. Physiol. Renal Physiol. 15221466. 304 (4), F333. Available from: http://ajprenal.physiology.org/content/304/4/F333.full.pdf+html. doi:10.1152/ajprenal.00478.2012.

Kumari, R., Jat, P., 2021. Mechanisms of cellular senescence: cell cycle arrest and senescence associated secretory phenotype. Front. Cell Dev. Biol. 9. doi:10.3389/fcell.2021.645593.

Kurella, M., Covinsky, K.E., Collins, A.J., Chertow, G.M., 2007. Octogenarians and nonagenarians starting dialysis in the United States. Ann. Intern. Med. 00034819. 146 (3), 177–183. Available from: http://www.annals.org/cgi/reprint/146/3/177.pdf. doi:10.7326/0003-4819-146-3-200702060-00006.

Lasagni, L., Angelotti, M.L., Ronconi, E., Lombardi, D., Nardi, S., Peired, A., Becherucci, F., Mazzinghi, B., Sisti, A., Romoli, S., Burger, A., Schaefer, B., Buccoliero, A., Lazzeri, E., Romagnani, P., 2015. Podocyte regeneration driven by renal progenitors determines glomerular disease remission and can be pharmacologically enhanced. Stem Cell Rep. 22136711. 5 (2), 248–263. Available from: http://www.elsevier.com/journals/stem-cell-reports/2213-6711. doi:10.1016/j.stemcr.2015.07.003.

Lasagni, L., Lazzeri, E., Shankland, S.J., Anders, H.-J., Romagnani, P., 2013. Podocyte mitosis - a catastrophe. Curr. Mol. Med. 15665240. 13 (1), 13–23. doi:10.2174/156652413804486250.

LeBleu, V.S., O'Connell, J.T., Herrera, K.N.G., Wikman, H., Pantel, K., Haigis, M.C., de Carvalho, F.M., Damascena, A., Chinen, L.T.D., Rocha, R.M., Asara, J.M., Kalluri, R., 2014. PGC-1α mediates mitochondrial biogenesis and oxidative phosphorylation in cancer cells to promote metastasis. Nat. Cell Biol. 16 (10). doi:10.1038/ncb3039.

Lee, J.H., Jung, K.J., Kim, J.W., Kim, H.J., Yu, B.P., Chung, H.Y., 2004. Suppression of apoptosis by calorie restriction in aged kidney. Exp. Gerontol. 05315565. 39 (9), 1361–1368. doi:10.1016/j.exger.2004.06.015.

Lee, P.J., Benz, C.C., Blood, P., Börner, K., Campisi, J., Chen, F., Daldrup-Link, H., De Jager, P., Ding, L., Duncan, F.E., Eickelberg, O., Fan, R., Finkel, T., Furman, D., Garovic, V., Gehlenborg, N., Glass, C., Heckenbach, I., Joseph, Z.-B., Katiyar, P., Kim, S.-J., Königshoff, M., Kuchel, G.A., Lee, H., Lee, J.H., Jian, M., Qin, M., Melov, S., Metis, K., Mora, A.L., Musi, N., Neretti, N., Passos, J.F., Rahman, I., Rivera-Mulia, J.C., Robson, P., Rojas, M., Roy, A.L., Scheibye-Knudsen, M., Schilling, B., Shi, P., Silverstein, J.C., Suryadevara, V., Xie, J., Wang, J., Wong, A.I., Niedernhofer, L.J., Wang, S., Anvari, H., Balough, J., Benz, C., Bons, J., Brenerman, B., Evans, W., Gerencser, A., Gregory, H., Hansen, M., Justice, J., Kapahi, P., Murad, N., O'Broin, A., Pavone, M.E., Powell, M., Scott, G., Shanes, E., Shankaran, M., Verdin, E., Winer, D., Fei, W., Adams, A., Blood, P.D., Bueckle, A., Cao-Berg, I., Chen, H., Davis, M., Filus, S., Hao, Y., Hartman, A., Hasanaj, E., Helfer, J., Herr, B., Joseph, Z.B., Molla, G., Mou, G., Puerto, J., Quardokus, E.M., Ropelewski, A.J., Ruffalo, M., Satija, R., Schwenk, M., Scibek, R., Shirey, W., Sibilla, M., Welling, J., Yuan, Z., Bonneau, R., Christiano, A., Izar, B., Menon, V., Owens, D.M., Phatnani, H., Smith, C., Suh, Y., Teich, A.F., Bekker, V., Chan, C., Coutavas, E., Hartwig, M.G., Zhicheng, J., Nixon, A.B., Dou, Z., Rajagopal, J., Slavov, N., Holmes, D., Jurk, D., Kirkland, J.L., Lagnado, A., Tchkonia, T., Abraham, K., Dibattista, A., Yih-Woei Fridell, T.K.H., Jhappan, C., Montes, V.P., Prabhudas, M., Resat, H., Taylor, V., Kumar, M., Suryadevara, V., Cigarroa, F., Cohn, R., Cortes, T.M., Courtois, E., Chuang, J., Davé, M., Domanskyi, S., Enninga, E.A.L., Eryilmaz, G.N., Espinoza, S.E., Gelfond, J., Kirkland, J., Kuchel, G.A., Kuo, C.-L., Lehman, J.S., Aguayo-Mazzucato, C.,

Meves, A., Rani, M., Sanders, S., Thibodeau, A., Tullius, S.G., Ucar, D., White, B., Qian, W., Ming, X., Yamaguchi, S., Assarzadegan, N., Cho, C.-S., Hwang, I., Hwang, Y., Jingyue, X., Adeyi, O.A., Aliferis, C.F., Bartolomucci, A., Dong, X., DuFresne-To, M.J., Ikramuddin, S., Johnson, S.G., Nelson, A.C., Niedernhofer, L.J., Revelo, X.S., Trevilla-Garcia, C., Sedivy, J.M., Thompson, E.L., Robbins, P.D., Wang, J., Aird, K.M., Alder, J.K., Beaulieu, D., Bueno, M., Calyeca, J., Chamucero-Millaris, J.A., Chan, S.Y., Chung, D., Corbett, A., Gorbunova, V., Gowdy, K.M., Gurkar, A., Horowitz, J.C., Qianjiang, H., Kaur, G., Khaliullin, T.O., Lafyatis, R., Lanna, S., Dongmei, L., Anjun, M., Morris, A., Muthumalage, T.M., Peters, V., Pryhuber, G.S., Reader, B.F., Rosas, L., Sembrat, J.C., Shaikh, S., Shi, H., Stacey, S.D., Croix, C.S., Wang, C., Wang, Q., Watts, A., Liangcai, G., Lin, Y., Rabinovitch, P.S., Sweetwyne, M.T., Artyomov, M.N., Ballentine, S.J., Chheda, M.G., Davies, S.R., DiPersio, J.F., Fields, R.C., Fitzpatrick, J.A.J., Fulton, R.S., Imai, S.-I., Jain, S., Tao, J., Kushnir, V.M., Link, D.C., Major, M.B., Oh, S.T., Rapp, D., Rettig, M.P., Stewart, S.A., Veis, D.J., Vij, K.R., Wendl, M.C., Wyczalkowski, M.A., Craft, J.E., Enninful, A., Farzad, N., Gershkovich, P., Halene, S., Kluger, Y., VanOudenhove, J., Mina, X., Yang, J., Yang, M., 2022. NIH SenNet Consortium to map senescent cells throughout the human lifespan to understand physiological health. Nat. Aging. 2662-8465. 2 (12), 1090–1100. doi:10.1038/s43587-022-00326-5.

Lehtonen, S., 2020. Metformin protects against podocyte injury in diabetic kidney disease. Pharmaceuticals. 1424-8247. 13 (12), 452. doi:10.3390/ph13120452.

Lelarge, V., Capelle, R., Oger, F., Mathieu, T., Calvé, B.L., 2024. Senolytics: from pharmacological inhibitors to immunotherapies, a promising future for patients' treatment. Npj Aging. 2731-6068. 10 (1). doi:10.1038/s41514-024-00138-4.

Lennon, R., Randles, M.J., Humphries, M.J., 2014. The importance of podocyte adhesion for a healthy glomerulus. Front. Endocrinol. 16642392. 5. Available from: http://journal.frontiersin.org/Journal/10.3389/fendo.2014.00160/full. doi:10.3389/fendo.2014.00160.

Lenoir, O., Tharaux, P.L., Huber, T.B., 2016. Autophagy in kidney disease and aging: lessons from rodent models. Kidney Int. 15231755. 90 (5), 950–964. Available from: https://www.journals.elsevier.com/kidney-international. doi:10.1016/j.kint.2016.04.014.

Levy, J., Douglas, S.D., 1989. Role of acid proteinases in inflammatory processes. Harefuah 117 (10), 310–312.

Li, L., Liu, Y., 2025. Podocyte aging and diabetic kidney disease. Kidney Int. 15231755. 107 (4), 596–598. Available from: https://www.sciencedirect.com/science/journal/00852538. doi:10.1016/j.kint.2025.01.011.

Li, X., Chuang, P.Y., D'Agati, V.D., Dai, Y., Yacoub, R., Fu, J., Xu, J., Taku, O., Premsrirut, P.K., Holzman, L.B., He, J.C., 2015. Nephrin preserves podocyte viability and glomerular structure and function in adult kidneys. J. Am. Soc. Nephrol. 15333450. 26 (10), 2361–2377. Available from: http://jasn.asnjournals.org/content/26/10/2361.full.pdf. doi:10.1681/ASN.2014040405.

Li, Y., Duan, Y., Chu, Q., Lv, H., Li, J., Guo, X., Gao, Y., Liu, M., Tang, W., Hu, H., Liu, H., Sun, J., Wang, X., Yi, F., 2025. G-protein coupled receptor GPR124 protects against podocyte senescence and injury in diabetic kidney disease. Kidney Int. 107, 652–665.

Liu, M., Liang, K., Zhen, J., Zhou, M., Wang, X., Wang, Z., Wei, X., Zhang, Y., Sun, Y., Zhou, Z., Hua, S., Zhang, C., Ningjun, L., Gao, C., Peng, J., Fan, Y., 2017. Sirt6 deficiency exacerbates podocyte injury and proteinuria through targeting Notch signaling. Nat. Commun. 2041-1723. 8 (1). doi:10.1038/s41467-017-00498-4.

Lu, Q., Hu, X., Hou, Q., Yu, L., Cao, K., Ding, D., Lu, Y., Dai, C., 2024. Rheb1 deficiency elicits mitochondrial dysfunction and accelerates podocyte senescence through promoting Atp5f1c acetylation. Cell. Signal. 124, 111451.

Madeo, F., Carmona-Gutierrez, D., Hofer, S.J., Kroemer, G., 2019. Caloric restriction mimetics against age-associated disease: targets, mechanisms, and therapeutic potential. Cell Metab. 19327420. 29 (3), 592–610. Available from: http://www.cellmetabolism.org/. doi:10.1016/j.cmet.2019.01.018.

Magassa, S., Aron, L., Hoguin, C., Isnard, P., Terzi, F., Legendre, C., Yankner, B.A., Canaud, G., 2021. Rest and stress resistance in the aging kidney. J. Am. Soc. Nephrol. 15333450. 32 (8), 1974–1986. Available from: https://jasn.asnjournals.org/content/32/8/1974. doi:10.1681/ASN.2021020231.

McKinzie, S.R., Kaverina, N., Schweickart, R.A., Chaney, C.P., Eng, D.G., Pereira, B.M.V., Kestenbaum, B., Pippin, J.W., Wessely, O., Shankland, S.J., 2024. Podocytes from hypertensive and obese mice acquire an inflammatory, senescent, and aged phenotype. Am. J. Physiol. Renal Physiol. 15221466. 326 (4), F644. Available from: https://journals.physiology.org/doi/full/10.1152/ajprenal.00417.2023. doi:10.1152/ajprenal.00417.2023.

McLachlan, M.S., 1978. The ageing kidney. Lancet. 01406736. 2 (8081), 143–145.

McNicholas, B.A., Eng, D.G., Lichtnekert, J., Rabinowitz, P.S., Pippin, J.W., Shankland, S.J., 2016. Reducing mTOR augments parietal epithelial cell density in a model of acute podocyte depletion and in aged kidneys. Am. J. Physiol. Renal Physiol. 15221466. 311 (3), F626. Available from: http://ajprenal.physiology.org/content/311/3/F626.full.pdf. doi:10.1152/ajprenal.00196.2016.

Melk, A., Schmidt, B.M.W., Vongwiwatana, A., Rayner, D.C., Halloran, P.F., 2005. Increased expression of senescence-associated cell cycle inhibitor p16/INK4a in deteriorating renal transplants and diseased native kidney. Am. J. Transplant. 5 (6), 1375–1382. doi:10.1111/j.1600-6143.2005.00846.x.

Miwa, S., Kashyap, S., Chini, E., von Zglinicki, T., 2022. Mitochondrial dysfunction in cell senescence and aging. J. Clin. Invest. 1558-8238. 132 (13). doi:10.1172/jci158447.

Mulay, S.R., Thomasova, D., Ryu, M., Kulkarni, O.P., Migliorini, A., Bruns, H., Gröbmayr, R., Lazzeri, E., Lasagni, L., Liapis, H., Romagnani, P., Anders, H.J., 2013. Podocyte loss involves MDM2-driven mitotic catastrophe. J. Pathol. 10969896. 230 (3), 322–335. doi:10.1002/path.4193.

Naik, A.S., Afshinnia, F., Aqeel, J., Cibrik, D.M., Samaniego, M., Wickman, L., Wang, S.Q., Chowdhury, M., Wiggins, R.C., 2019. Accelerated podocyte detachment early after kidney transplantation is related to long-term allograft loss of function. Nephrol. Dial. Transplant. 14602385. 34 (7), 1232–1239. Available from: http://ndt.oxfordjournals.org/. doi:10.1093/ndt/gfy350.

Naik, A.S., Afshinnia, F., Cibrik, D., Hodgin, J.B., Wu, F., Zhang, M., Kikuchi, M., Wickman, L., Samaniego, M., Bitzer, M., Wiggins, J.E., Ojo, A., Li, Y., Wiggins, R.C., 2016. Quantitative podocyte parameters predict human native kidney and allograft half-lives. JCI Insight 23793708. 1 (7). Available from: https://insight.jci.org/articles/view/86943/pdf. doi:10.1172/jci.insight.86943.

O'Hare, T., Walters, D.K., Stoffregen, E.P., Jia, T., Manley, P.W., Mestan, J., Cowan-Jacob, S.W., Lee, F.Y., Heinrich, M.C., Deininger, M.W., Druker, B.J., 2005. In vitro activity of Bcr-Abl inhibitors AMN107 and BMS-354825 against clinically relevant imatinib-resistant Abl kinase domain mutants. Cancer Res. 65, 4500–4505.

Ortmann, J., Amann, K., Brandes, R.P., Kretzler, M., Münter, K., Parekh, N., Traupe, T., Lange, M., Lattmann, T., Barton, M., 2004. Role of podocytes for reversal of glomerulosclerosis and proteinuria in the aging kidney after endothelin inhibition. Hypertension 44 (6), 974–981. doi:10.1161/01.HYP.0000149249.09147.b4.

Palmer, A.K., Xu, M., Zhu, Y., Pirtskhalava, T., Weivoda, M.M., Hachfeld, C.M., Prata, L.G., van Dijk, T.H., Verkade, E., Casaclang-Verzosa, G., Johnson, K.O., Cubro, H., Doornebal, E.J., Ogrodnik, M., Jurk, D., Jensen, M.D., Chini, E.N., Miller, J.D., Matveyenko, A., Stout, M.B., Schafer, M.J., White, T.A., Hickson, L.T.J., Demaria, M., Garovic, V., Grande, J., Arriaga, E.A., Kuipers, F., von Zglinicki, T., LeBrasseur, N.K., Campisi, J., Tchkonia, T., Kirkland, J.L., 2019. Targeting senescent cells alleviates obesity-induced metabolic dysfunction. Aging Cell 14749726. 18 (3). Available from: http://onlinelibrary.wiley.com/journal/10.1111/(ISSN)1474-9726. doi:10.1111/acel.12950.

Pereira, B.M.V., Zeng, Y., Maggiore, J.C., Schweickart, R.A., Eng, D.G., Kaverina, N., McKinzie, S.R., Chang, A., Loretz, C.J., Thieme, K., Hukriede, N.A., Pippin, J.W., Wessely, O., Shankland, S.J., 2024. Podocyte injury at young age causes premature senescence and worsens glomerular aging. Am. J. Physiol. Renal Physiol. 15221466. 326 (1), F120. Available from: https://journals.physiology.org/doi/epdf/10.1152/ajprenal.00261.2023. doi:10.1152/ajprenal.00261.2023.

Petermann, A.T., Pippin, J., Krofft, R., Blonski, M., Griffin, S., Durvasula, R., Shankland, S.J., 2004. Viable podocytes detach in experimental diabetic nephropathy: potential mechanism underlying glomerulosclerosis. Nephron Exp. Nephrol. 16602129. 98 (4), e114. doi:10.1159/000081555.

Pippin, J., Kumar, V., Stein, A., Jablonski, P., Shankland, S.J., Davis, C.L., 2009. The contribution of podocytes to chronic allograft nephropathy. Nephron Exp. Nephrol. 16602129. 111 (1), e1. doi:10.1159/000178762.

Pippin, J.W., Durvasula, R., Petermann, A., Hiromura, K., Couser, W.G., Shankland, S.J., 2003. DNA damage is a novel response to sublytic complement C5b-9-induced injury in podocytes. J. Clin. Invest. 111 (6), 877–885. doi:10.1172/JCI200315645.

Pippin, J.W., Glenn, S.T., Krofft, R.D., Rusiniak, M.E., Alpers, C.E., Hudkins, K., Duffield, J.S., Gross, K.W., Shankland, S.J., 2014. Cells of renin lineage take on a podocyte phenotype in aging nephropathy. Am. J. Physiol. Renal Physiol. 15221466. 306 (10), F1198. Available from: http://ajprenal.physiology.org/content/306/10/F1198.full.pdf. doi:10.1152/ajprenal.00699.2013.

Pippin, J.W., Kaverina, N., Wang, Y., Eng, D.G., Zeng, Y., Tran, U., Loretz, C.J., Chang, A., Akilesh, S., Poudel, C., Perry, H.S., O'Connor, C., Vaughan, J.C., Bitzer, M., Wessely, O., Shankland, S.J., 2022. Upregulated PD-1 signaling antagonizes glomerular health in aged kidneys and disease. J. Clin. Invest. 15588238. 132 (16). Available from: https://www.jci.org/articles/view/156250/pdf. doi:10.1172/JCI156250.

Puelles, V.G., Cullen-McEwen, L.A., Taylor, G.E., Li, J., Hughson, M.D., Kerr, P.G., Hoy, W.E., Bertram, J.F., 2016. Human podocyte depletion in association with older age and hypertension. Am. J. Physiol. Renal Physiol. 15221466. 310 (7), F656. Available from: http://ajprenal.physiology.org/content/310/7/F656.full.pdf. doi:10.1152/ajprenal.00497.2015.

Puelles, V.G., Douglas-Denton, R.N., Cullen-McEwen, L.A., Li, J., Hughson, M.D., Hoy, W.E., Kerr, P.G., Bertram, J.F., 2015. Podocyte number in children and adults: associations with glomerular size and numbers of other glomerular resident cells. J. Am. Soc. Nephrol. 15333450. 26 (9), 2277–2288. Available from: http://jasn.asnjournals.org/content/26/9/2277.full.pdf+html. doi:10.1681/ASN.2014070641.

Puelles, V.G., Moeller, M.J., 2019. Postnatal podocyte gain: is the jury still out? Semin. Cell Dev. Biol. 10963634. 91, 147–152. Available from: http://www.elsevier.com/inca/publications/store/6/2/2/9/4/4/index.htt. doi:10.1016/j.semcdb.2018.07.007.

Puelles, V.G., Wolde, J.W.V.D., Wanner, N., Scheppach, M.W., Cullen-McEwen, L.A., Bork, T., Lindenmeyer, M.T., Gernhold, L., Wong, M.N., Braun, F., Cohen, C.D., Kett, M.M., Kuppe, C., Kramann, R., Saritas, T., Van Roeyen, C.R., Moeller, M.J., Tribolet, L., Rebello, R., Sun, B.Y.Y., Li, J., Müller-Newen, G., Hughson, M.D., Hoy, W.E., Person, F., Wiech, T., Ricardo, S.D., Kerr, P.G., Denton, K.M., Furic, L., Huber, T.B., Nikolic-Paterson, D.J., Bertram, J.F., 2019. MTOR-mediated podocyte hypertrophy regulates glomerular integrity in mice and humans. JCI Insight 23793708. 4 (18). Available from: https://insight.jci.org/articles/view/99271/pdf. doi:10.1172/jci.insight.99271.

Rangel, P.X.M., Cross, E., Liu, C., Pedigo, C.E., Tian, X., Gutiérrez-Calabrés, E., Nagata, S., Priyadarshini, A., Lerner, G., Bunda, P., Perincheri, S., Gu, J., Zhao, H., Wang, Y., Inoue, K., Ishibe, S., 2023. Cell cycle and senescence regulation by podocyte histone deacetylase 1 and 2. J. Am. Soc. Nephrol. 15333450. 34 (3), 433–450. Available from: https://journals.lww.com/jasn/pages/default.aspx. doi:10.1681/ASN.2022050598.

Regan, C.M., 1986. Rapid drug haptenization procedure: application to gentamicin and quinidine. J. Pharm. Pharmacol. 20427158. 38 (11), 834–836. doi:10.1111/j.2042-7158.1986.tb04504.x.

Reichert, L.J., Koene, R.A., Wetzels, J.F., 1998. Prognostic factors in idiopathic membranous nephropathy. Am. J. Kidney Dis. 02726386. 31 (1), 1–11. doi:10.1053/ajkd.1998.v31.pm9428445.

Ritschka, B., Storer, M., Mas, A., Heinzmann, F., Ortells, M.C., Morton, J.P., Sansom, O.J., Zender, L., Keyes, W.M., 2017. The senescence-associated secretory phenotype induces cellular plasticity and tissue regeneration. Genes Dev. 15495477. 31 (2), 172–183. Available from: http://genesdev.cshlp.org/content/31/2/172.full.pdf. doi:10.1101/gad.290635.116.

Roeder, S.S., Stefanska, A., Eng, D.G., Kaverina, N., Sunseri, M.W., McNicholas, B.A., Rabinovitch, P., Enge, F.B., Danie, C., Amann, K., Lichtnekert, J., Pippin, J.W., Shankland, S.J., 2015. Changes in glomerular parietal epithelial cells in mouse kidneys with advanced age. Am. J. Physiol. Renal Physiol. 15221466. 309 (2), F164. Available from: http://ajprenal.physiology.org/content/309/2/F164.full-text.pdf. doi:10.1152/ajprenal.00144.2015.

Romoli, S., Angelotti, M.L., Antonelli, G., VR, S.K., Mulay, S.R., Desai, J., Gomez, L.A., Thomasova, D., Eulberg, D., Klussmann, S., Melica, M.E., Conte, C., Lombardi, D., Lasagni, L., Anders, H.J., Romagnani, P., 2018. CXCL12 blockade preferentially regenerates lost podocytes in cortical nephrons by targeting an intrinsic podocyte-progenitor feedback mechanism. Kidney Int. 15231755. 94 (6), 1111–1126. Available from: https://www.journals.elsevier.com/kidney-international. doi:10.1016/j.kint.2018.08.013.

Rule, A.D., Amer, H., Cornell, L.D., Taler, S.J., Cosio, F.G., Kremers, W.K., Textor, S.C., Stegall, M.D., 2010. The association between age and nephrosclerosis on renal biopsy among healthy adults. Ann. Intern. Med. 15393704. 152 (9), 561–567. Available from: http://www.annals.org/contents-by-date.2008.shtml. doi:10.7326/0003-4819-152-9-201005040-00006.

Russo, M., Spagnuolo, C., Tedesco, I., Bilotto, S., Russo, G.L., 2012. The flavonoid quercetin in disease prevention and therapy: facts and fancies. Biochem. Pharmacol. 18732968. 83 (1), 6–15. Available from: https://www.elsevier.com/locate/biochempharm. doi:10.1016/j.bcp.2011.08.010.

Salminen, A., Kaarniranta, K., 2009. SIRT1: regulation of longevity via autophagy. Cell. Signal. 08986568. 21 (9), 1356–1360. doi:10.1016/j.cellsig.2009.02.014.

Schiffer, M., Bitzer, M., Roberts, I.S.D., Kopp, J.B., Dijke, P., Mundel, P., Böttinger, E.P., 2001. Apoptosis in podocytes induced by TGF-β and Smad7. J. Clin. Invest. 108 (6), 807–816. doi:10.1172/JCI200112367.

Schneider, R.R.S., Eng, D.G., Kutz, J.N., Sweetwyne, M.T., Pippin, J.W., Shankland, S.J., 2017. Compound effects of aging and experimental FSGS on glomerular epithelial cells. Aging 19454589. 9 (2), 524–546. Available from: https://s3-us-west-1.amazonaws.com/paperchase-aging/pdf/ikgK4CGaTSpaTB3DY.pdf. doi:10.18632/aging.101176.

Shahzad, K., Fatima, S., Khawaja, H., Elwakiel, A., Gadi, I., Ambreen, S., Zimmermann, S., Mertens, P.R., Biemann, R., Isermann, B., 2022. Podocyte-specific Nlrp3 inflammasome activation promotes diabetic kidney disease. Kidney Int. 15231755. 102 (4), 766–779. Available from: https://www.journals.elsevier.com/kidney-international. doi:10.1016/j.kint.2022.06.010.

Shankland, S.J., 2006. The podocyte's response to injury: role in proteinuria and glomerulosclerosis. Kidney Int. 00852538. 69 (12), 2131–2147. doi:10.1038/sj.ki.5000410.

Shankland, S.J., Freedman, B.S., Pippin, J.W., 2017. Can podocytes be regenerated in adults? Curr. Opin. Nephrol. Hypertens. 14736543. 26 (3), 154–164. Available from: http://journals.lww.com/co-nephrolhypertens/pages/default.aspx. doi:10.1097/MNH.0000000000000311.

Shankland, S.J., Najafian, B., Wessely, O., 2024. The tragedy of mitotic catastrophe in podocytes. Kidney Int. 15231755. 105 (6), 1153–1156. Available from: https://www.sciencedirect.com/science/journal/00852538. doi:10.1016/j.kint.2024.01.015.

Shankland, S.J., Rule, A.D., Kutz, J.N., Pippin, J.W., Wessely, O., 2023. Podocyte senescence and aging. Kidney360 26417650. 4 (12), 1784–1793. Available from: https://kidney360.asnjournals.org/. doi:10.34067/KID.0000000000000284.

Shankland, S.J., Wang, Y., Shaw, A.S., Vaughan, J.C., Pippin, J.W., Wessely, O., 2021. Podocyte aging: why and how getting old matters. J. Am. Soc. Nephrol. 15333450. 32 (11), 2697–2713. Available from: https://jasn.asnjournals.org/content/jnephrol/32/11/2697.full.pdf?with-ds=yes. doi:10.1681/ASN.2021050614.

Shankland, S.J., Wessely, O., 2022. GSKβ as a target in podocyte aging. Kidney Int. 15231755. 102 (3), 463–465. Available from: https://www.journals.elsevier.com/kidney-international. doi:10.1016/j.kint.2022.04.041.

Shen, H., Kreisel, D., Goldstein, D.R., 2013. Processes of sterile inflammation. J. Immunol. 15506606. 191 (6), 2857–2863. Available from: http://www.jimmunol.org/content/191/6/2857.full.pdf+html. doi:10.4049/jimmunol.1301539.

Shirato, I., 2002. Podocyte process effacement in vivo. Microsc. Res. Tech. 1059-910X. 57 (4), 241–246. doi:10.1002/jemt.10082.

Sis, B., Tasanarong, A., Khoshjou, F., Dadras, F., Solez, K., Halloran, P.F., 2007. Accelerated expression of senescence associated cell cycle inhibitor p16INK4A in kidneys with glomerular disease. Kidney Int. 00852538. 71 (3), 218–226. doi:10.1038/sj.ki.5002039.

Suryadevara, V., Hudgins, A.D., Rajesh, A., Pappalardo, A., Karpova, A., Dey, A.K., Hertzel, A., Agudelo, A., Rocha, A., Soygur, B., Schilling, B., Carver, C.M., Aguayo-Mazzucato, C., Baker, D.J., Bernlohr, D.A., Jurk, D., Mangarova, D.B., Quardokus, E.M., Enninga, E.A.L., Schmidt, E.L., Chen, F., Duncan, F.E., Cambuli, F., Kaur, G., Kuchel, G.A., Lee, G., Daldrup-Link, H.E., Martini, H., Phatnani, H., Al-Naggar, I.M., Rahman, I., Nie, J., Passos, J.F., Silverstein, J.C., Campisi, J., Wang, J., Iwasaki, K., Barbosa, K., Metis, K., Nernekli, K., Niedernhofer, L.J., Ding, L., Wang, L., Adams, L.C., Ruiyang, L., Doolittle, M.L., Teneche, M.G., Schafer, M.J., Xu, M., Hajipour, M., Boroumand, M., Basisty, N., Sloan, N., Slavov, N., Kuksenko, O., Robson, P., Gomez, P.T., Vasilikos, P., Adams, P.D., Carapeto, P., Zhu, Q., Ramasamy, R., Perez-Lorenzo, R., Fan, R., Dong, R., Montgomery, R.R., Shaikh, S., Vickovic, S., Yin, S., Kang, S., Suvakov, S., Khosla, S., Garovic, V.D., Menon, V., Xu, Y., Song, Y., Suh, Y., Dou, Z., Neretti, N., 2024. SenNet recommendations for detecting senescent cells in different tissues. Nat. Rev. Mol. Cell Biol. 14710080. 25 (12), 1001–1023. Available from: https://www.nature.com/molcellbio. doi:10.1038/s41580-024-00738-8.

Sweetwyne, M.T., Pippin, J.W., Eng, D.G., Hudkins, K.L., Chiao, Y.A., Campbell, M.D., Marcinek, D.J., Alpers, C.E., Szeto, H.H., Rabinovitch, P.S., Shankland, S.J., 2017. The mitochondrial-targeted peptide, SS-31, improves glomerular architecture in mice of advanced age. Kidney Int. 15231755. 91 (5), 1126–1145. Available from: https://www.journals.elsevier.com/kidney-international. doi:10.1016/j.kint.2016.10.036.

Szeto, H.H., 2014. First-in-class cardiolipin-protective compound as a therapeutic agent to restore mitochondrial bioenergetics. Br. J. Pharmacol. 14765381. 171 (8), 2029–2050. Available from: http://onlinelibrary.wiley.com/journal/10.1111/%28ISSN%291476-5381. doi:10.1111/bph.12461.

Tharaux, P.L., Huber, T.B., 2012. How many ways can a podocyte die? Semin. Nephrol. 15584488. 32 (4), 394–404. doi:10.1016/j.semnephrol.2012.06.011.

Tian, X., Pedigo, C.E., Li, K., Ma, X., Bunda, P., Pell, J., Lek, A., Gu, J., Zhang, Y., Rangel, P.X.M., Li, W., Schwartze, E., Nagata, S., Lerner, G., Perincheri, S., Priyadarshini, A., Zhao, H., Lek, M., Menon, M.C., Fu, R., Ishibe, S., 2023. Profilin1 is required for prevention of mitotic catastrophe in murine and human glomerular diseases. J. Clin. Invest. 15588238. 133 (24). Available from: https://www.jci.org/articles/view/171237/pdf. doi:10.1172/JCI171237.

Tower, J., 2015. Programmed cell death in aging. Ageing Res. Rev. 15681637. 23 (Pt A), 90–100. doi:10.1016/j.arr.2015.04.002.

Ventura-Clapier, R., Garnier, A., Veksler, V., 2008. Transcriptional control of mitochondrial biogenesis: the central role of PGC-1. Cardiovasc. Res. 0008-6363. 79 (2), 208–217. doi:10.1093/cvr/cvn098.

Verzola, D., Gandolfo, M.T., Gaetani, G., Ferraris, A., Mangerini, R., Ferrario, F., Villaggio, B., Gianiorio, F., Tosetti, F., Weiss, U., Traverso, P., Mji, M., Deferrari, G., Garibotto, G., 2008. Accelerated senescence in the kidneys of patients with type 2 diabetic nephropathy. Am. J. Physiol. Renal Physiol. 15221466. 295 (5), F1563. Available from: http://ajprenal.physiology.org/cgi/reprint/295/5/F1563. doi:10.1152/ajprenal.90302.2008.

Wang, B., Han, J., Elisseeff, J.H., Demaria, M., 2024. The senescence-associated secretory phenotype and its physiological and pathological implications. Nat. Rev. Mol. Cell Biol. 14710080. 25 (12), 958–978. Available from: https://www.nature.com/molcellbio. doi:10.1038/s41580-024-00727-x.

Wang, X.X., Myakala, K., Libby, A.E., Krawczyk, E., Panov, J., Jones, B.A., Bhasin, K., Shults, N., Qi, Y., Krausz, K.W., Zerfas, P.M., Takahashi, S., Daneshpajouhnejad, P., Titievsky, A., Taranenko, E., Billon, C., Chatterjee, A., Elgendy, B., Walker, J.K., Albanese, C., Kopp, J.B., Rosenberg, A.Z., Gonzalez, F.J., Guha, U., Brodsky, L., Burris, T.P., Levi, M., 2023. Estrogen-related receptor agonism reverses mitochondrial dysfunction and inflammation in the aging kidney. Am. J. Pathol. 15252191. 193 (12), 1969–1987. Available from: http://ajp.amjpathol.org/. doi:10.1016/j.ajpath.2023.07.008.

Wang, Y., Eng, D.G., Kaverina, N.V., Loretz, C.J., Koirala, A., Akilesh, S., Pippin, J.W., Shankland, S.J., 2020. Global transcriptomic changes occur in aged mouse podocytes. Kidney Int. 15231755. 98 (5), 1160–1173. Available from: https://www.journals.elsevier.com/kidney-international. doi:10.1016/j.kint.2020.05.052.

Wang, Y., Li, H., Song, S.P., 2018. β-arrestin 1/2 aggravates podocyte apoptosis of diabetic nephropathy via wnt/β-catenin pathway. Med. Sci. Monit. 16433750. 24, 1724–1732. Available from: https://www.medscimonit.com/download/index/idArt/905642. doi:10.12659/MSM.905642.

Wanner, N., Hartleben, B., Herbach, N., Goedel, M., Stickel, N., Zeiser, R., Walz, G., Moeller, M.J., Grahammer, F., Huber, T.B., 2014. Unraveling the role of podocyte turnover in glomerular aging and injury. J. Am. Soc. Nephrol. 15333450. 25 (4), 707–716. Available from: http://jasn.asnjournals.org/content/25/4/707.full.pdf+html. doi:10.1681/ASN.2013050452.

Wharram, B.L., Goyal, M., Wiggins, J.E., Sanden, S.K., Hussain, S., Filipiak, W.E., Saunders, T.L., Dysko, R.C., Kohno, K., Holzman, L.B., Wiggins, R.C., 2005. Podocyte depletion causes glomerulosclerosis: diphtheria toxin-induced podocyte depletion in rats expressing human diphtheria toxin receptor transgene. J. Am. Soc. Nephrol. 10466673. 16 (10), 2941–2952. Available from: https://journals.lww.com/jasn/pages/default.aspx. doi:10.1681/ASN.2005010055.

Wiggins, J., 2009. Podocytes and glomerular function with aging. Semin. Nephrol. 02709295. 29 (6), 587–593. doi:10.1016/j.semnephrol.2009.07.012.

Wiggins, J.E., 2012. Aging in the glomerulus. J. Gerontol. A Biol. Sci. Med. Sci. 1079-5006. 67 (12), 1358–1364. doi:10.1093/gerona/gls157.

Wiggins, J.E., Goyal, M., Sanden, S.K., Wharram, B.L., Shedden, K.A., Misek, D.E., Kuick, R.D., Wiggins, R.C., 2005. Podocyte hypertrophy, "adaptation," and "decompensation" associated with glomerular enlargement and glomerulosclerosis in the aging rat: prevention by calorie restriction. J. Am. Soc. Nephrol. 16 (10), 2953–2966.

Wiggins, J.E., Patel, S.R., Shedden, K.A., Goyal, M., Wharram, B.L., Martini, S., Kretzler, M., Wiggins, R.C., 2010. NFkappaB promotes inflammation, coagulation, and fibrosis in the aging glomerulus. J. Am. Soc. Nephrol. 21 (4), 587–597. doi:10.1681/ASN.2009060663.

Wu, J., Raman, A., Coffey, N.J., Sheng, X., Wahba, J., Seasock, M.J., Ma, Z., Beckerman, P., Laczkó, D., Palmer, M.B., Kopp, J.B., Kuo, J.J., Pullen, S.S., Boustany-Kari, C.M., Linkermann, A., Susztak, K., 2021. The key role of NLRP3 and STING in APOL1-associated podocytopathy. J. Clin. Invest. 15588238. 131 (20). Available from: https://www.jci.org/articles/view/136329/pdf. doi:10.1172/JCI136329.

Yang, J.H., Hayano, M., Griffin, P.T., Amorim, J.A., Bonkowski, M.S., Apostolides, J.K., Salfati, E.L., Blanchette, M., Munding, E.M., Bhakta, M., Chew, Y.C., Guo, W., Yang, X., Maybury-Lewis, S., Tian, X., Ross, J.M., Coppotelli, G., Meer, M.V., Rogers-Hammond, R., Vera, D.L., Lu, Y.R., Pippin, J.W., Creswell, M.L., Dou, Z., Xu, C., Mitchell, S.J., Das, A., O'Connell, B.L., Thakur, S., Kane, A.E., Su, Q., Mohri, Y., Nishimura, E.K., Schaevitz, L., Garg, N., Balta, A.M., Rego, M.A., Gregory-Ksander, M., Jakobs, T.C., Zhong, L., Wakimoto, H., Andari, J.E., Grimm, D., Mostoslavsky, R., Wagers, A.J., Tsubota, K., Bonasera, S.J., Palmeira, C.M., Seidman, J.G., Seidman, C.E., Wolf, N.S., Kreiling, J.A., Sedivy, J.M., Murphy, G.F., Green, R.E., Garcia, B.A., Berger, S.L., Oberdoerffer, P., Shankland, S.J., Gladyshev, V.N., Ksander, B.R., Pfenning, A.R., Rajman, L.A., Sinclair, D.A., 2023. Loss of epigenetic information as a cause of mammalian aging. Cell 10974172. 186 (2), 305. Available from: https://www.sciencedirect.com/science/journal/00928674. doi:10.1016/j.cell.2022.12.027.

Yu, D., Petermann, A., Kunter, U., Rong, S., Shankland, S.J., Floege, J., 2005. Urinary podocyte loss is a more specific marker of ongoing glomerular damage than proteinuria. J. Am. Soc. Nephrol. 10466673. 16 (6), 1733–1741. Available from: https://journals.lww.com/jasn/pages/default.aspx. doi:10.1681/ASN.2005020159.

Yuan, Q., Tang, B., Xie, Y., Xie, Y., Zhu, Y., Hua, S., Liu, Y., Zhang, C., 2025. PRDM16 deficiency promotes podocyte injury by impairing insulin receptor signaling. Cell Death Differ. 1350–9047. doi:10.1038/s41418-025-01477-9.

Zhang, J., Hansen, K.M., Pippin, J.W., Chang, A.M., Taniguchi, Y., Krofft, R.D., Pickering, S.G., Liu, Z.H., Abrass, C.K., Shankland, S.J., 2012. De novo expression of podocyte proteins in parietal epithelial cells in experimental aging nephropathy. Am. J. Physiol. Renal Physiol. 15221466. 302 (5), F571. Available from: http://ajprenal.physiology.org/content/302/5/F571.full.pdf#page=1&view=FitH. doi:10.1152/ajprenal.00516.2011.

Zhang, L., Pitcher, L.E., Prahalad, V., Niedernhofer, L.J., Robbins, P.D., 2023. Targeting cellular senescence with senotherapeutics: senolytics and senomorphics. FEBS J. 17424658. 290 (5), 1362–1383. Available from: http://onlinelibrary.wiley.com/journal/10.1111/(ISSN)1742-4658. doi:10.1111/febs.16350.

Zhang, L., Zhou, F., Xialian, Y., Zhu, Y., Zhou, Y., Liu, J., Liu, Y., Qingyang, M., Zhang, Y., Wang, W., Chen. N., 2019. C/EBPα deficiency in podocytes aggravates podocyte senescence and kidney injury in aging mice. Cell Death Dis. 10 (10). doi:10.1038/s41419-019-1933-2.

Zheng, W., Guo, J., Liu, Z.S., 2021. Effects of metabolic memory on inflammation and fibrosis associated with diabetic kidney disease: an epigenetic perspective. Clin. Epigenetics 18687083. 13 (1). Available from: http://www.springer.com/biomed/human+genetics/journal/13148. doi:10.1186/s13148-021-01079-5.

Zhong, F., Wang, W., Lee, K., John Cijiang, H., Chen, N., 2016. Role of C/EBP-α in Adriamycin-induced podocyte injury. Sci. Rep. 6. doi:10.1038/srep33520.

Zhu, X., Zhang, C., Liu, L., Xu, L., Yao, L., 2024. Senolytic combination of dasatinib and quercetin protects against diabetic kidney disease by activating autophagy to alleviate podocyte dedifferentiation via the Notch pathway. Int. J. Mol. Med. 1107-3756. 53 (3). doi:10.3892/ijmm.2024.5350.

Zhu, Y., Tchkonia, T., Pirtskhalava, T., Gower, A.C., Ding, H., Giorgadze, N., Palmer, A.K., Ikeno, Y., Hubbard, G.B., Lenburg, M., O'Hara, S.P., LaRusso, N.F., Miller, J.D., Roos, C.M., Verzosa, G.C., LeBrasseur, N.K., Wren, J.D., Farr, J.N., Khosla, S., Stout, M.B., McGowan, S.J., Fuhrmann-Stroissnigg, H., Gurkar, A.U., Zhao, J., Colangelo, D., Dorronsoro, A., Ling, Y.Y., Barghouthy, A.S., Navarro, D.C., Sano, T., Robbins, P.D., Niedernhofer, L.J., Kirkland, J.L., 2015. The Achilles' heel of senescent cells: from transcriptome to senolytic drugs. Aging Cell 14 (4), 644–658. doi:10.1111/acel.12344.

Zindel, J., Kubes, P., 2020. DAMPs, PAMPs, and LAMPs in immunity and sterile inflammation. Annu. Rev. Pathol. 1553-4006. 15 (1), 493–518. doi:10.1146/annurev-pathmechdis-012419-032847.

Zullo, A., Simone, E., Grimaldi, M., Musto, V., Mancini, F.P., 2018. Sirtuins as mediator of the anti-ageing effects of calorie restriction in skeletal and cardiac muscle. Int. J. Mol. Sci. 14220067. 19 (4). Available from: http://www.mdpi.com/1422-0067/19/4/928/pdf. doi:10.3390/ijms19040928.

CHAPTER

5

Epigenetics and the kidney

Qingqing Wei[a] *and Zheng Dong*[a,b]

[a]Department of Cellular Biology and Anatomy, Medical College of Georgia, Augusta University, Augusta, GA, United States

[b]Charlie Norwood VA Medical Center, Augusta, GA, United States

Epigenetic dysregulation in aging

Epigenetic regulations

In addition to transmitting hereditary characteristics through DNA sequence information (genetic regulation), cells can also control gene expression through epigenetic regulation, a heritable mechanism that does not alter the DNA sequence. Eukaryotic cells, in contrast to prokaryotic cells, exhibit much more complex epigenetic mechanisms, including histone modifications, DNA methylation, chromatin remodeling, noncoding RNA regulation, and RNA modifications. Unlike genetic regulation, epigenetic regulation is relatively reversible and undergoes dynamic changes in response to environmental factors, such as aging (Pal and Tyler, 2016; Zhang et al., 2020; Ma et al., 2022).

Histone modifications

Histones are positively charged proteins that bind to genomic DNA to form nucleosomes, the fundamental units of chromatin structure. Each nucleosome contains eight core histones (two copies of H2A, H2B, H3, and H4) wrapped by 147 base pairs (BP) of genomic DNA, and one linker histone (H1) binds to the linker DNA between nucleosomes. Their amino acid residues, especially the lysine in core histone tails, can undergo modifications by various chemical groups or small proteins, such as acetyl, phosphate, methyl, small ubiquitin-like modifier (SUMO), or ubiquitin. These post-translational modifications change the binding affinity between histones and genomic DNA, modulate the accessibility of specific DNA sequences, and play a crucial role in gene transcription regulation (Fig. 5.1).

- *Histone acetylation* (Fig. 5.1A): Lysine is one of the primary contributors to maintaining the positive charge of histones. During histone acetylation, an acetyl group is added to the ε-amino group of lysine by histone acetyltransferases (HATs) (Yang and Seto, 2007).

Aging and the Kidney
https://doi.org/10.1016/B978-0-443-34069-7.00008-2

This modification neutralizes the positive charge of histones and weakens their interaction with genomic DNA. This reduction in binding affinity relaxes the chromatin structure, transitioning it from condensed heterochromatin to open euchromatin, thereby facilitating gene transcription (Grunstein, 1997; Eberharter and Becker, 2002). While the lysine on the N-terminal tails of histones is the primary site of acetylation, this modification can also occur on the globular domains (Morales and Richard-Foy, 2000; Pradeepa et al., 2016). Conversely, histone deacetylases (HDACs) remove acetyl groups from lysine residues, leading to chromatin condensation and transcriptional repression. Multiple HDACs, including HDAC1, HDAC2, HDAC3, HDAC4, HDAC5, HDAC8, HDAC9, SIRT1, SIRT3, and SIRT6, have been reported to play important roles in histone deacetylation in the kidney (Hong et al., 2020; Hyndman, 2020). Notably, the availability of the acetyl group for histone acetylation is directly linked to the levels of acetyl-CoA, which are closely influenced by metabolic changes during aging (Peleg et al., 2016; Bradshaw, 2021).

- *Histone methylation* (Fig. 5.1B): In this posttranslational modification of histones, histone methyltransferases (HMTs) mediate the addition of one to three methyl groups from S-adenosylmethionine (SAM) to basic residues (lysine, arginine, or histidine) in histones (Greer and Shi, 2012). Different from histone acetylation, histone methylation does not neutralize the positive charge of lysine and can either activate or repress gene transcription by promoting chromatin compaction or relaxation, depending on the specific site of methylation. In addition, histone methylation at specific sites can recruit nonhistone proteins to facilitate other cellular functions (Greer and Shi, 2012). For example, certain methylation marks, such as H4K20me2 and H3K9me3, are crucial for recruiting DNA repair proteins during the DNA damage response (DDR) (Gong and Miller, 2019). While some histone methylation marks are stable and inheritable through cell division, they are reversible by demethylation catalyzed by histone demethylases (Greer and Shi, 2012; Kooistra and Helin, 2012). Furthermore, specific histone methylation marks, including H3K4me3, H3K27me3, H3K36me3, and H3K9me3, have been reported to play significant roles in the processes of senescence and aging (Michalak et al., 2019; Wang et al., 2022).
- *Histone phosphorylation* (Fig. 5.1C): Similar to other proteins, the serine, threonine, or tyrosine residues in histones undergo phosphorylation and dephosphorylation, catalyzed by protein kinases (e.g., ATM/ATR and AMPK) and phosphatases (e.g., PP1 and PP2A), respectively (Rossetto et al., 2012). Among all histone phosphorylation events, histone H3 phosphorylation is highly conserved and plays a key role in regulating chromatin condensation and segregation, as well as gene transcription. One important mark is H3S10ph, which is critical for regulating the transcription of cell proliferation-related genes and influences the post-translational modifications of adjacent sites, such as H3K9 methylation (Komar and Juszczynski, 2020). Another pivotal function of histone phosphorylation is its involvement in the DDR. In addition to H3S10ph, an important phosphorylation mark is H2AX (an H2A variant) phosphorylation (γH2AX), which serves as a well-established marker of DNA double-strand breaks, initiating and signaling DNA repair pathways (Kinner et al., 2008; Collins et al., 2020).

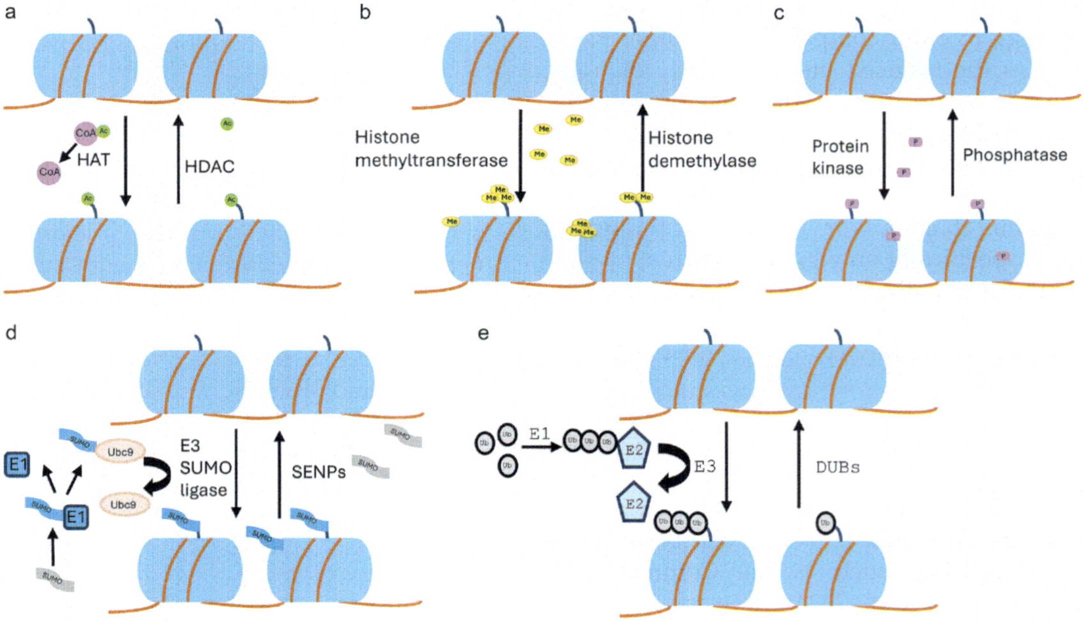

FIG. 5.1 The illustration of histone modifications. (A) Histone acetylation. Histone acetylation is catalyzed by histone acetyltransferase (HAT), which transfers an acetyl group from acetyl-CoA to lysine residues in histones. Histone deacetylation is mediated by histone deacetylase (HDAC), which removes acetyl groups from lysine residues, reversing the acetylation process. (B) Histone methylation. Histone methylation is catalyzed by methyltransferases, which add one to three methyl groups to lysine, arginine, or histidine residues. This process can be reversed by histone demethylases. (C) Histone phosphorylation. Histone phosphorylation is catalyzed by protein kinases, which add phosphate groups to serine, threonine, or tyrosine residues on histones. These phosphate groups can be removed by phosphatases. (D) Histone SUMOylation. Histone SUMOylation involves the covalent attachment of a small ubiquitin-like modifier (SUMO) protein to specific lysine residues on histones by a serial of enzymes: activated by SUMO-activating enzymes (E1), conjugated to Ubc9 (a major E2 enzyme), and ligated to histone by SUMO ligases (E3). SUMO modifications can be removed by SUMO-specific proteases (SENPs). (E) Histone ubiquitination. Histone ubiquitination involves the covalent attachment of one or multiple ubiquitins to specific lysine residues on histone proteins This process is mediated by a cascade of enzymatic reactions involving ubiquitin-activating enzyme E1, ubiquitin-conjugating enzymes E2, and ubiquitin ligases E3. Histone ubiquitination can be removed by deubiquitinating enzymes (DUBs).

- *Histone SUMOylation* (Fig. 5.1D): SUMO is a small protein of approximately 12 kDa. It is primarily covalently attached to lysine residues within a conserved SUMOylation consensus motif, ΨKxE, where Ψ represents a hydrophobic amino acid, K is lysine, x is any amino acid, and E is glutamate. The conjugation of SUMO to histones involves a cascade of reactions catalyzed by the SUMOylation machinery: E1 activating enzymes, E2 conjugating enzymes, and E3 ligases. SUMO is first activated by an E1 enzyme complex (e.g., SAE1/SAE2), which uses ATP hydrolysis to form a thioester bond with SUMO. The activated SUMO is then transferred to an E2 enzyme, primarily Ubc9, which facilitates its attachment to target proteins. Finally, E3 ligases enhance the specificity and efficiency of SUMO ligation to the target lysine residue. SUMOylation is reversible and can be removed by SUMO-specific proteases (SENPs) (Wilkinson and Henley, 2010; Celen and Sahin, 2020). SUMOylation often interacts with other histone modifications, contributing to the complexity of chromatin regulation.

- *Histone ubiquitination* (Fig. 5.1E): Ubiquitin (a 76-amino acid, ~8.6 kDa protein) is covalently attached to specific lysine residues on histone proteins. This process is mediated by a cascade of enzymatic reactions involving E1 ubiquitin-activating enzymes, E2 ubiquitin-conjugating enzymes, and E3 ubiquitin ligases (Wilkinson, 2000). Unlike the classical role of ubiquitination in targeting proteins for degradation, histone ubiquitination primarily regulates chromatin structure and gene expression, frequently crosstalking with other histone modifications such as methylation and acetylation, as well as with other epigenetic processes like chromatin remodeling or m^6A RNA methylation (Vaughan et al., 2021; Yadav et al., 2022; Mandal et al., 2024). While polyubiquitination may occasionally result in histone degradation, monoubiquitination of histones, particularly H2A and H2B, has been extensively studied for its role in gene transcription regulation and DDR regulation (Uckelmann and Sixma, 2017; Mandal et al., 2024). In addition, deubiquitinases (DUBs) are responsible for removing ubiquitin from histones and other proteins and are critical for maintaining the proper balance of the histone ubiquitin pattern (Snyder and Silva, 2021; Mandal et al., 2024).

DNA methylation

In mammalian DNA, there are a large number of CpG sites (sites where a cytosine [C] nucleotide is followed immediately by a guanine [G] nucleotide in the 5′ to 3′ direction) that are subject to methylation regulation. Many of these CpG sites are enriched in certain areas, forming CpG islands. DNA methylation is catalyzed by DNA methyltransferases (DNMTs), primarily including DNMT1, DNMT3a, DNMT3b, and DNMT3c, which convert cytosine into 5-methylcytosine (5mC) (Fig. 5.2). During cell division, the DNA methylation pattern in daughter cells is restored by DNMT1, which copies the methylation marks from the parental DNA strand to the newly synthesized strand. DNMT3a, DNMT3b, and DNMT3c are classified as de novo DNMTs, which establish new DNA methylation patterns based on the physiological status of the cell or in response to stress. On the contrary, DNA demethylation can occur via ten-eleven translocation enzymes (TETs) or activation-induced cytidine deaminases (AIDs) (Fig. 5.2). The TETs are dioxygenases that catalyze the oxidation of 5mC and ultimately cause demethylation after a series of intermediate reactions. AIDs deaminate 5mC to thymine (T) to create a T:G mismatch, which can be corrected by the base excision repair mechanism, leading to demethylation (Guo et al., 2019; Greenberg and Bourc'his, 2019).

The function of DNA methylation depends on the location of the methylated CpG sites (Greenberg and Bourc'his, 2019). The methylation of CpG islands in the promoter region of a gene usually suppresses transcription by preventing the binding of specific transcription factors, leading to gene silencing. DNA methylation also plays critical roles in X-chromosome inactivation and the suppression of transposon activity, helping to maintain genomic stability. Although highly conserved DNA methylation is also found in gene bodies, its precise function is not well understood yet. A balanced DNA methylation pattern, regulated by DNMTs, TETs, and AIDs, is essential for normal cellular function. This balance can be disrupted by aging, leading to either hypermethylation or hypomethylation, which are associated with various pathological changes (Unnikrishnan et al., 2019).

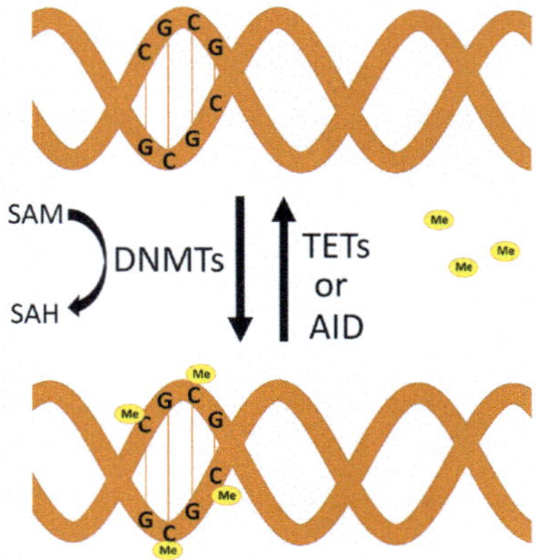

FIG. 5.2 The illustration of DNA methylation regulation. DNA Methyltransferases (DNMTs) catalyze the addition of a methyl group to cytosine in a CpG site, forming 5-methylcytosine (5mC). During this reaction, S-adenosyl-L-methionine (SAM) serves as the methyl group donor and is converted to S-adenosyl-L-homocysteine (SAH). DNA methylation can be reversed by ten-eleven translocation (TET) enzymes or activation-induced cytidine deaminase (AID).

Chromatin remodeling

Chromatin is a highly compact structure composed of genomic DNA and associated binding proteins, such as histones. This complex structure undergoes dynamic changes to become loose (euchromatin, more accessible) or tight (heterochromatin, less accessible), thereby modulating gene transcription activity. Chromatin structure is regulated by various factors, including histone modifications, DNA methylation, and noncoding RNAs. In the past decade, another critical mechanism, ATP-dependent chromatin remodeling, has been extensively explored (Clapier et al., 2017; Giles et al., 2019; Eustermann et al., 2024). This process is mediated by remodeler complexes—enzymes that use energy derived from ATP hydrolysis to alter the interactions between genomic DNA and histones. Based on their specific ATPase domains and functions, remodeler complexes are categorized into four subfamilies: SWItch/Sucrose Non-Fermentable (SWI/SNF), Imitation SWItch (ISWI), Chromodomain Helicase DNA-binding (CHD), and Inositol-requiring 80 (INO80). These remodeler complexes are directed to specific genomic DNA regions by transcription factors or noncoding RNAs. Functionally, they regulate chromatin dynamics by establishing and repositioning nucleosomes, ejecting histones to disassemble nucleosomes, or restructuring nucleosomes by incorporating histone variants or modified histones (Fig. 5.3). Therefore they activate or silence gene expression by exposing specific genomic sequence regions and facilitate DDR by providing access for DNA repair complexes. Though the role of ATP-dependent chromatin remodeling in aging is unclear, emerging evidence has elucidated the involvement of some remodelers in life span and senescence regulation (Watanabe et al., 2017; Li et al., 2019; Schoberleitner et al., 2021).

Noncoding RNAs

Noncoding RNAs (ncRNAs) are RNA molecules that do not encode proteins. Various types of ncRNAs are expressed in mammalian cells, including long noncoding RNAs

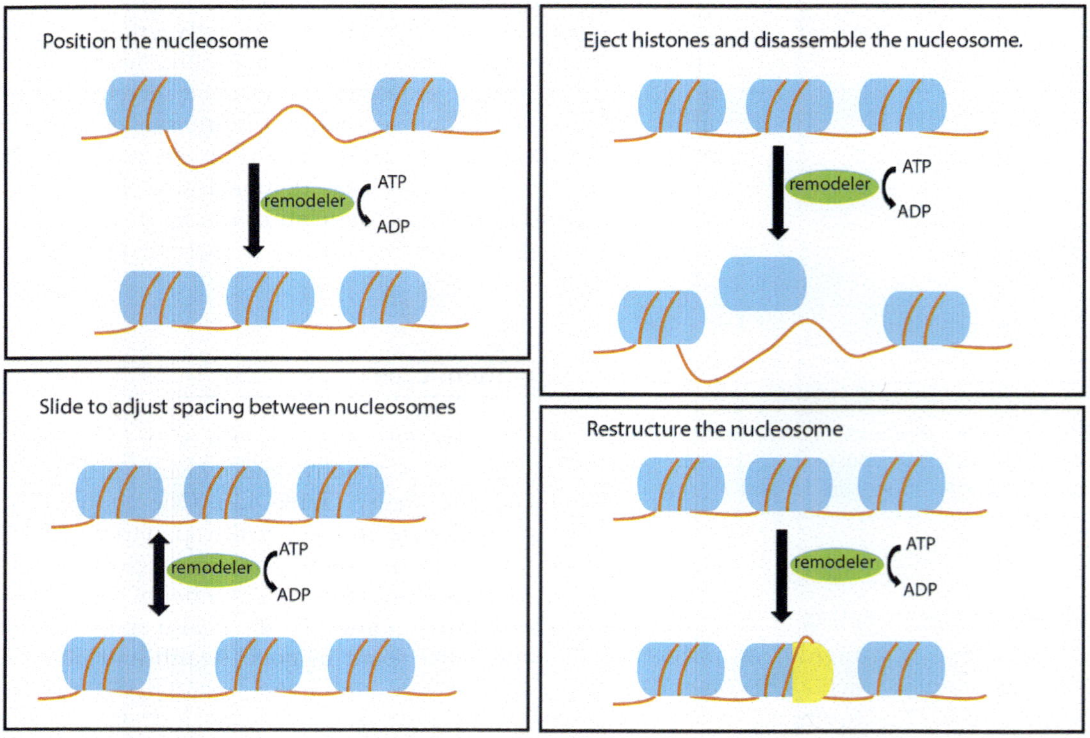

FIG. 5.3 ATP-dependent Chromatin remodeling. The remodeler complex contains an ATPase domain that hydrolyzes ATP into ADP. This enzymatic activity enables the complex to modulate chromatin structure through various mechanisms, including positioning new nucleosomes on genomic DNA, sliding nucleosomes along DNA to adjust the spacing between them, ejecting histones from DNA, or restructuring nucleosomes by incorporating different histone variants or modified histones.

(lncRNAs), microRNAs (miRNAs), small interfering RNAs (siRNAs), circular RNAs (circRNAs), Piwi-interacting RNAs (piRNAs), ribosomal RNAs (rRNAs), transfer RNAs (tRNAs), small nuclear RNAs (snRNAs), small nucleolar RNAs (snoRNAs), and enhancer RNAs (eRNAs). Among them, rRNAs and tRNAs serve as structural and functional RNAs for ribosomes and protein synthesis, respectively, and snRNAs are primary components in spliceosomes for RNA splicing. The other ncRNAs perform diverse roles in epigenetic regulation.

- *MiRNAs* are small ncRNAs of 21–25 nucleotides in length. Thousands of miRNAs have now been identified, and many of them are highly conserved between species. They are transcribed from miRNA genes as primary miRNAs and processed in the nucleus by the Drosha-DGCR8 complex into precursor miRNAs (pre-miRNAs), which have a hairpin structure. The pre-miRNAs are then exported to the cytoplasm, where they are cleaved by Dicer to form miRNA duplexes, generating two mature miRNAs (the functional form of miRNA): one from the 3′-arm (−3p) and the other from the 5′-arm (−5p) (Shang et al., 2023). Typically, one of these strands acts as the major strand, while the other one (the passenger strand) is degraded. However, recent studies have revealed that both strands can function as mature miRNAs, mediating distinct biological functions (Mitra et al., 2015; Yurikova et al., 2019). Canonically, miRNAs regulate gene expression by binding to the 3′-untranslated region (3′-UTR) of target mRNAs in the RNA-induced silencing complex (RISC), thereby suppressing protein translation. The miRNA-mRNA interaction typically involves partial base pairing, primarily within the miRNA seed sequence (nucleotides 2–8) (Guo et al., 2019). This partial complementarity allows a single miRNA to target multiple mRNAs, enabling it to fine-tune biological pathways by suppressing related proteins. In addition, recent studies have identified lncRNAs as targets of miRNAs. The interaction between miRNAs and lncRNAs often results in antagonistic effects on each other, adding complexity to the regulatory networks involving miRNAs (Li et al., 2024a). Two mechanisms have been reported for miRNA turnover (Shang et al., 2023; Wei et al., 2024b). During miRNA biogenesis, the passenger strand miRNA undergoes degradation without protection from RISC proteins. Another mechanism is target-directed miRNA degradation (TDMD), which can be triggered by a long RNA (such as mRNA or lncRNA) with a complementary seed sequence binding to the miRNA in the TDMD complex.

- *SiRNAs* are a class of small ncRNAs similar to miRNAs (Piatek and Werner, 2014). However, unlike miRNAs, siRNAs are not directly transcribed from siRNA genes. Instead, they are derived from double-stranded or hairpin-structured precursor RNAs, which are processed by Dicer into 21–25 nucleotide siRNAs. Like miRNAs, the major strands of siRNAs are incorporated into the RISC to guide target recognition, while the passenger strands are degraded. Unlike miRNAs, siRNAs typically exhibit full complementarity to their target sequences, leading to the degradation of one specific target RNA and silencing of its expression. SiRNAs are widely used in biomedical research and therapeutic applications as a tool to knock down specific gene expression (Hu et al., 2020). Endogenous siRNAs have also been identified in a variety of species, including plants, *Caenorhabditis elegans* (*C. elegans*), fruit flies, and vertebrates. In *C. elegans*, one study has shown that endogenous siRNAs play critical roles in lifespan regulation (Cohen-Berkman et al., 2020). In human cells, endogenous siRNAs have been found to regulate LINE-1 retrotransposons, highlighting their importance in maintaining genomic stability (Chen et al., 2012).
- *PiRNAs* are another class of small ncRNAs ranging from 21 to 35 nucleotides in length, expressed exclusively in animal cells (Ozata et al., 2019). They are primarily derived from long precursor RNAs transcribed from genomic loci called piRNA clusters. The process of piRNA biogenesis is independent of Dicer. Processed intermediate piRNAs are loaded onto Piwi proteins (a subclass of Argonaute proteins) for final trimming and modification (Watanabe and Lin, 2014). PiRNAs are highly abundant in germ cells, where they play a critical role in suppressing transposon activity during gametogenesis and are essential for maintaining genome integrity. PiRNA-Piwi protein complexes bind to transposon genomic loci, regulating DNA methylation or histone methylation to suppress transposon transcription (Watanabe and Lin, 2014; Ozata et al., 2019; Wang et al., 2023). These complexes can also bind to complementary sequences in transposon RNA in the cytosol, leading to RNA degradation. In addition, some piRNAs have been identified in somatic cells. Emerging evidence indicates that piRNAs are not only

important in embryonic development but also involved in disease development, such as age-related cancer and Alzheimer's disease (Wang et al., 2023). However, more evidence is needed to fully understand the role of piRNAs in aging.

- *CircRNAs* are a class of noncoding RNAs characterized by their closed-loop structure (Kristensen et al., 2019; Zhou et al., 2020). They are typically derived from pre-mRNAs through a unique RNA splicing mechanism called backsplicing, which covalently links the 5′-splice site to the 3′-splice site. Without free 5′ and 3′ ends, circRNAs are resistant to exonucleases and are more stable than other linear RNA molecules. CircRNAs are classified into three categories based on their origin: exonic circRNA (only derived from exon sequences), intronic circRNA (only derived from intron sequences), and exon-intron circRNA (containing both exon and intron sequence regions). After biogenesis, the intron-containing circRNAs are predominantly retained in the nucleus, while the exonic circRNAs are exported to the cytoplasm. The understanding of circRNA biological function is limited. They are commonly recognized for their role as sponges for miRNAs or proteins, antagonizing or modulating their function, respectively. In addition, nuclear circRNAs can regulate the transcription of their parent genes by interacting with transcriptional machinery. Although circRNAs are mainly considered as ncRNAs, some of them may be translatable (Zhou et al., 2020). Notably, circRNAs have been reported to accumulate during aging, suggesting a potential role in age-related patho-physiology (Kristensen et al., 2019).
- *LncRNAs* are ncRNAs longer than 200 nucleotides that do not fall into other ncRNA categories. They can be transcribed from lncRNA-specific genes or processed from precursors, such as intronic RNAs (Statello et al., 2021). The functions of lncRNAs are highly diverse and depend on their specific sequences and structures (Guo et al., 2019; Statello et al., 2021; Mattick et al., 2023; Wei et al., 2024b). In the nucleus, some lncRNAs interact with DNA, chromatin, or chromatin-binding proteins, such as transcription factors, to remodel chromatin and regulate gene transcription by recruiting or inhibiting other transcriptional regulators. LncRNAs can also guide RNA splicing in the nucleus. In the cytoplasm, lncRNAs can bind to other RNA molecules, including mRNAs and ncRNAs, to modulate mRNA translation, neutralize the activity of miRNAs or siRNAs, or promote miRNA degradation. In addition, lncRNAs can bind to RNA-binding proteins as structural RNAs to influence other cellular functions, such as maintaining telomere integrity and participating in stress responses in stress granules. Due to their length, lncRNAs may contain multiple functional domains within a single sequence, enabling them to perform diverse roles. Although over 100,000 lncRNAs have been identified, most of them are not conserved across species, which has hindered the exploration of their detailed functions (Mattick et al., 2023).
- *eRNAs* are ncRNAs transcribed from active enhancer regions of the genome, discovered in the last decade (Kim et al., 2015; Sartorelli and Lauberth, 2020; Harrison and Bose, 2022). They vary in length, often ranging from ~200 BP to 2 kb, overlapping partially with the size of lncRNAs. Unlike canonical lncRNAs, eRNAs are typically transcribed bidirectionally from enhancers. Most eRNAs lack maturation processes such as splicing or polyadenylation but are 5′-capped. They are short-lived and exhibit a high turnover rate. Functionally, eRNAs facilitate gene transcription by being recruited to the promoter regions of target genes, where they recruit chromatin remodelers, promote

active enhancer-specific histone modifications and DNA methylation patterns, interact with transcription factors, or directly modulate transcription machinery activity (Harrison and Bose, 2022). The secondary structure of eRNAs is critical for their function, making their activity sensitive to mutations. Emerging evidence suggests that eRNAs may play roles in cancer and age-related diseases (Wijesinghe et al., 2021; Xiao et al., 2021; Ahmed et al., 2023).

- *snoRNAs* are small ncRNAs ranging in length from 60 to 300 nucleotides, originating from the intronic regions of coding or noncoding genes. They are mainly localized in the nucleolus, with some found in Cajal bodies, where they assemble into small nucleolar ribonucleoproteins (snoRNPs) by binding to specific proteins. The primary responsibility of snoRNAs involves guiding 2′-O–Methylation and pseudouridylation of rRNAs or tRNAs (Bratkovič et al., 2020; Huang et al., 2022c). Emerging evidence supports additional functions, such as acetylation of rRNAs, regulation of mRNA 3′-end processing, regulation of host gene splicing, and the generation of even smaller RNAs to silence gene expression, similar to miRNAs (Bratkovič et al., 2020; Bergeron et al., 2023). Furthermore, a recent report has revealed some noncanonical functions of SNORA13 in promoting cellular senescence (Cheng et al., 2024).

RNA modifications

Similar to DNA, all RNA molecules undergo certain types of epitranscriptomic modifications, which significantly impact their structure, stability, and function. To date, over 150 types of RNA modifications have been identified. Some major RNA modifications will be introduced below, which include: N6-methyladenosine (m^6A); 5-methylcytosine (m^5C); pseudouridine (Ψ); N1-methyladenosine (m^1A); adenosine-to-inosine editing (A-to-I editing); 2′-O–methylation (2′-O–Me); N7-methylguanosine (m^7G); and N^4-acetylcytosine (Ac^4C).

- *m^6A:* m^6A is one of the most prevalent RNA modifications for all types of RNAs and is abundant in mRNAs. This modification involves the addition of a methyl group to the sixth nitrogen of adenine and is catalyzed by writer enzymes such as METTL3, METTL5, and METTL14. The m^6A signal is recognized by reader proteins, e.g., YTH domain-containing m^6A-binding proteins, which further regulate processes including RNA biogenesis, maturation, protein translation or ncRNA functions, and degradation of RNAs. Importantly, the m6A modification is reversible and can be removed by eraser proteins such as ALKBH5 and FTO. Overall, m^6A modification plays a critical role in regulating diverse biological processes and is implicated in the development and progression of various diseases (Sendinc and Shi, 2023; Petri and Klinge, 2023).
- *m^1A:* m^1A is the second most abundant RNA methylation, involving the addition of a methyl group to the first nitrogen of adenine. It is most prevalent in tRNA and rRNA, although it has also been identified in other types of RNAs such as mRNAs, lncRNAs, circRNAs, and miRNAs (Konno et al., 2019; Zhang et al., 2023). The characterized writer enzymes for m^1A include TRMT6/TRMT61A (for m^1A in tRNAs), TRMT10C (for m^1A in mitochondrial tRNAs), and Nucleomethylin (NML) (for m^1A in rRNAs). However, the writers for mRNAs, lncRNAs, microRNAs, and circRNAs are not well characterized yet. The m^1A signals are detected by reader proteins, mainly from the YTH domain-containing family. m^1A modification is also reversible and can be removed by AlkB

family demethylases. Different from m^6A, m^1A introduces a positive charge to RNA, which significantly impacts RNA structure and RNA-protein binding, ultimately affecting protein translation efficiency (Xiong et al., 2023).

- *m^5C:* Similar to DNA methylation, RNAs can be modified by m^5C which adds a methyl group to the fifth carbon of cytosine. It is another abundant RNA modification affecting all types of RNAs. This modification is catalyzed by NSUN family proteins or DNMT2, and the signal is recognized by reader proteins such as ALYREF YBX1 (Gao and Fang, 2021). Generally, m^5C modification enhances RNA stability, which further impacts key cellular functions such as protein translation efficiency and fidelity, microRNA maturation, or ncRNA-protein bindings (Cui et al., 2022). The removal of m^5C modification in RNA is not yet fully understood, possibly involving enzymes such as TETs and ALKBH1. m^5C modifications of RNA have diverse biological functions, including roles in stress response and senescence (Gao and Fang, 2021).
- *Ψ:* Pseudouridylation, the isomerization of a uridine base to Ψ, is the first identified and most abundant RNA modification in all types of RNAs. This reaction is catalyzed by pseudouridine synthases (PUS). Most PUS independently recognize their targets for modification, while pseudouridylation in rRNAs and snRNAs is guided by snoRNAs within snoRNPs (Borchardt et al., 2020). Compared to uridine, Ψ forms stronger base-pairing with adenine. Overall, Ψ stabilizes both the single-strand RNA conformation and the secondary structure, impacting RNA biogenesis, function, and decay (Borchardt et al., 2020; Zhao et al., 2023; Rodell et al., 2024). The profiling of Ψ landscapes in different types of RNAs has revealed cellular and tissue-specific distributions, suggesting potential developmental and pathological roles (Borchardt et al., 2020; Rodell et al., 2024; Herridge et al., 2024). However, the biological function of Ψ has not been fully understood yet.
- *A-to-I editing:* A-to-I editing is a process in which adenosine is deaminated to inosine in a double-stranded RNA, catalyzed by adenosine deaminase acting on RNA (ADAR) proteins (Nishikura, 2016). This modification can occur in any RNA with a double-stranded secondary structure, including mRNAs, miRNAs, lncRNAs, and circRNAs. Since inosine is recognized as guanine during protein translation, A-to-I editing in coding regions can alter the protein sequence by changing the codon in mRNA. In the noncoding region of mRNA, A-to-I editing can influence RNA splicing (Goncharov et al., 2022). Similarly, A-to-I editing may impact ncRNA processing and splicing. Notably, A-to-I editing is enriched in the seed sequence of microRNAs, which can potentially change their target specificity (Paul et al., 2017). The understanding of this A-to-I editing mechanism has also driven the development of RNA editing therapeutic techniques by introducing guide RNAs to directly edit and modify the sequence of target RNAs, offering promising approaches for precision medicine (Booth et al., 2023).
- *2′-O–Me:* 2′-O–Me, also called Nm, is a common and highly conserved RNA modification that adds a methyl group to the 2′-hydroxyl group of the ribose sugar. This modification is abundant in rRNAs, tRNAs, and snRNAs, and has also been reported in mRNAs and other ncRNAs. The 2′-O–Me modifications in regular rRNAs, snRNAs, lncRNAs, and the internal regions (coding region and UTRs) of mRNAs are typically guided by snoRNPs. In contrast, independent writer enzymes, such as the Trm family proteins or Hen1, can introduce 2′-O–Me to mitochondrial rRNAs, tRNAs,

miRNAs, piRNAs, and the 5′-cap of mRNAs. It is believed that 2′-O–Me is an irreversible modification, as no eraser protein has been detected (Zhou et al., 2024). However, 2′-O–Me modification undergoes dynamic changes in a cell-specific manner, possibly due to RNA turnover or writer enzyme level regulation (Khoshnevis et al., 2022; Drazkowska et al., 2022; Zhou et al., 2024). While 2′-O–Me does not directly affect base pairing, it does stabilize RNA duplex structures and alter RNA-protein binding. It has been reported to affect protein translation by promoting mRNA stability, ribosome assembly, and tRNA decoding, thereby further modulating diverse cellular functions (Erales et al., 2017; Choi et al., 2018b; Yelland et al., 2023; Li et al., 2024c). Despite these insights, the roles of 2′-O–Me in development and disease remain poorly understood and require further exploration.

- *m^7G:* m^7G is another type of broadly distributed RNA methylation that adds a methyl group to the seventh nitrogen of guanosine. Initially discovered in the 5′-cap of mRNAs, it has now been reported in internal mRNAs, tRNAs, rRNAs, and miRNAs (Pandolfini et al., 2019; Zhang et al., 2019; Xia et al., 2023). m^7G modification has gained significant attention in recent years (Xia et al., 2023). The METTL1/WDR4 complex has been shown to catalyze this modification, though not all responsible writer enzymes have been identified (Li et al., 2023a). It has been reported that IGF2BP family proteins can read the m^7G signal in cancer cells (Liu et al., 2024a). While many m^7G modification sites have been revealed, information about their precise locations, dynamic changes, and functions remains largely unknown.
- *Ac^4C:* Ac^4C is the acetylation modification of RNA at the N4 position of cytidine. It is predominantly studied in mRNAs, tRNAs, and rRNAs, with recent studies identifying its presence in primary miRNAs and lncRNAs (Jin et al., 2020; Zhang et al., 2024c; Gong et al., 2024). This modification is catalyzed by N-acetyltransferase 10 (NAT10) (Xie et al., 2023). Although the full scope of the function of Ac^4C remains unclear, it has been shown to influence RNA stability, biogenesis, and mRNA translation efficiency (Jin et al., 2020). Notably, a recent study suggested that Ac^4C may promote the recruitment of mRNAs into stress granules, indicating a potential role in the oxidative stress response (Kudrin et al., 2024).

The crosstalk between epigenetic regulations

The epigenetic regulation layers introduced above actively collaborate at different levels to regulate gene expression. The 3D organization and spatial arrangement of chromatin are influenced by various factors, including histone modifications, DNA methylation patterns, ATP-dependent chromatin remodeling, and ncRNAs such as lncRNAs, piRNAs, circRNAs, and eRNAs. These elements collectively determine chromatin accessibility, which in turn governs gene transcription. At the translational level, the inhibitory effects of miRNAs and siRNAs can be counteracted by interactions with other ncRNAs. The regulatory effects of ncRNAs are further altered by various RNA modifications. The crosstalk between RNAs and distinct RNA modification patterns ultimately dictates mRNA translation efficiency.

- *The interplay between histone modifications*: Different histone modifications exert divergent effects on chromatin conformation regulation, and they either facilitate or antagonize each other. For instance, recent studies have reported that histone SUMOylation can be stimulated by histone acetylation, further enhancing chromatin condensation and gene repression (Ryu and Hochstrasser, 2021). In addition, the accumulation of γH2AX after DNA damage is accompanied by H3 acetylation to facilitate DNA repair (Lee et al., 2010). In contrast, histone methylation and acetylation can compete for the same residue, H3K9 to counteract the function of each other (Park et al., 2011). While acetylation of H3K9 promotes an open chromatin structure and active transcription, methylation of H3K9 supports chromatin compaction and transcriptional repression.

- *Histone modification and DNA methylation feedback*: Histone modifications can guide DNA methylation by recruiting or rejecting DNMTs, depending on H3K9 or H3K4 methylation, respectively. On the other hand, DNA methylation is critical for maintaining histone modification patterns during cell division. MBD proteins recognize methylated DNA and recruit HDACs or HMTs to promote histone deacetylation or methylation. In addition, enzymes such as HMTs and DNMTs can interact with each other to establish the connection between these two epigenetic mechanisms (Cedar and Bergman, 2009).
- *Crosstalk between histone modification and chromatin remodeling*: Both histone modifications and ATP-dependent chromatin remodeling play critical roles in modulating chromatin conformation changes. Their interplay ensures dynamic regulation of chromatin accessibility and precise control of genomic processes, such as gene transcription (Petty and Pillus, 2013). Histone modifications can act as recruiters of chromatin remodelers. For example, acetylated H3 and H4 can recruit the Swi2/Snf2-ADCR complex, facilitating local chromatin remodeling (Yamada et al., 2004). On the contrary, ATP-dependent chromatin remodelers influence histone modification patterns by exposing histone tails or facilitating the recruitment of histone-modifying enzymes. For instance, the ISWI family remodeler BAZ1B-SMARCA5 mediates the recruitment of H3K36 methyltransferases NSD2 and induces H3K36Me2 modification in some mouse cell lines (Goto et al., 2024).
- *The interplay between chromatin conformation modulation and ncRNA expression and function*: The levels of ncRNAs are regulated at multiple stages, including gene transcription, biogenesis, and degradation. Changes in chromatin conformation, governed by DNA methylation, histone modifications, and ATP-dependent chromatin remodeling, can profoundly influence their transcriptional activity. For example, the hypermethylation of the mir-219-2 gene in renal fibrosis significantly suppressed mir-219a-5p expression (Wei et al., 2024a). Conversely, ncRNAs can directly or indirectly modulate chromatin conformation. In the nucleus, certain lncRNAs, piRNAs, and eRNAs can bind directly to genomic DNA, facilitating the recruitment of chromatin remodelers or other chromatin regulatory enzymes. PiRNAs can suppress transposon expression by guiding DNA methylation and histone modification patterns (Wang et al., 2023). In the cytoplasm, miRNAs and siRNAs inhibit mRNA translation, which can indirectly influence the expression of enzymes involved in chromatin conformation regulation (Wang et al., 2017). This dynamic interplay between ncRNAs and chromatin conformation cooperatively controls genomic stability and cellular homeostasis.
- *The interaction between ncRNAs*: In addition to the gene transcription regulation function exerted by some lncRNAs or eRNAs, ncRNAs interact with each other by base pairing (Han et al., 2022). LncRNAs and circRNAs can bind to miRNAs, acting as sponges to

block their interaction with target mRNAs. Depending on the degree of sequence complementarity, these interactions can even lead to miRNA degradation through TDMD (Wei et al., 2024b). In fact, such miRNA/lncRNA or miRNA/circRNA interactions effectively neutralize each other's function, with the more prevalent ncRNA exerting a stronger influence on the regulatory network. Although not well characterized, it is possible that siRNAs may have similar interactions with lncRNAs or circRNAs.

- *ncRNA modifications*: Although most RNA modifications were initially identified in mRNAs, tRNAs, or rRNAs, emerging evidence highlights the widespread presence of these modifications in other ncRNAs. These modifications influence the splicing, processing, function, and degradation of ncRNAs, thereby modulating their epigenetic roles. Multiple RNA modifications, including m^6A, m^1A, m^5C, m^7G, and Ψ, have been detected in lncRNAs, regulating their processing, localization, and stability (Yang et al., 2024a). Mature miRNAs have been reported to undergo modifications such as m^1A, m^5C and 2′-O-Me, although the detailed cellular functions of these modifications remain unclear (Xiong and Zhang, 2023; Su et al., 2025). In contrast, some primary miRNAs can be modified by m^6A and A-to-I editing, potentially influencing miRNA biogenesis (Xiong and Zhang, 2023). For circRNAs, m^6A and m^1A are prevalent, while A-to-I editing can alter circRNA sequences, enabling their translation (Shen et al., 2022; Huang et al., 2022b; Zhang et al., 2023). Despite these discoveries, much of the ncRNA modification landscape remains unexplored, largely due to the limitations of current techniques.

Epigenetic hallmarks in aging

The gradual loss of physiological function during aging is characterized by the accumulation of cellular oxidative stress and metabolic waste, increased molecular, cellular, and organismal damage, and alterations in epigenetic modification patterns. As aging progresses, chromatin conformation undergoes significant changes, including a general loss of heterochromatin, leading to a more open chromatin structure (Lee et al., 2020). This shift is accompanied by changes in histone modifications and DNA methylation patterns. These alterations contribute to substantial changes in gene expression, including the dysregulation of ncRNAs.

- *Histone modification changes*: Although global histone acetylation tends to decrease with age, some specific regions show increased acetylation to activate stress response or proinflammatory genes. Reduced acetylation of H4K16 is linked to genomic instability and impaired DNA repair and is considered a hallmark of cellular aging (Krishnan et al., 2011). Histone methylation changes are context-specific, and some markers also undergo significant changes during aging, such as H3K4me3, H3K27me3, H3K36me3, and H3K9me3 (Wang et al., 2022). γH2AX, a histone phosphorylation marker of DNA damage, reflects accumulating genomic instability and is a key hallmark of cellular senescence and aging (Mah et al., 2010).
- *DNA methylation*. DNA methylation change is also context-specific (Michalak et al., 2019). While overall DNA methylation levels may not change significantly with age, recent studies have revealed decreased methylation in heterochromatin regions and

increased methylation in CpG islands within specific gene promoters. In addition, hypomethylation of transposon promoter regions has been reported, leading to higher transposon activity and reduced genomic stability. With advances in DNA methylation profiling techniques and machine learning-based data analysis, age-related changes in DNA methylation have been characterized across various tissue types and species. These studies have led to the concept of **epigenetic clocks**, which utilize a set of conserved methylation sites identified through genome-wide DNA methylation analysis to estimate biological or chronological age (Field et al., 2018). Multiple laboratories have proposed a variety of epigenetic clocks (such as Horvath Clock, 2013; Hannum Clock, 2013, GrimAge, PhenoAge) to assess universal aging across species, species-specific aging (such as in humans and mice), and tissue-specific aging (Hannum et al., 2013; Horvath, 2013; Field et al., 2018; Horvath et al., 2018; Bernabeu et al., 2023; Lu et al., 2023).

- *Dysregulation of ncRNAs* Due to the high conservation of miRNAs, they are considered excellent biomarker candidates for diseases and pathological conditions. Changes in miRNA expression levels have been examined across different species and tissues. Multiple miRNAs have been identified to be closely associated with aging and lifespan in a tissue-specific manner (Kinser and Pincus, 2020). In a recent study by Wagner et al., aging-related miRNA changes were systematically examined across various tissue types (Wagner et al., 2024). They identified several common miRNA markers of aging, with miR-29c-3p showing the strongest correlation with aging. Aging is also associated with the dysregulation of other ncRNAs, including lncRNAs and circRNAs. Some of these ncRNAs are evolutionarily conserved and show differential expression patterns linked to aging, such as NFKBMARL-1, NEAT1, circFOXO3, and circEP300 (Kim et al., 2021; Cai and Han, 2021). However, further mechanistic studies are needed to determine whether their expression changes are tissue-specific or if they can be considered universal aging markers.

Cellular stresses and repair during aging

Oxidative stress is a major contributing factor to aging, driven by excessive production of reactive oxygen species (ROS) resulting from mitochondrial dysfunction and declined efficiency of antioxidant defense mechanisms. The accumulation of ROS leads to widespread cellular damage and disrupts the balance between damage and repair in various organelles, including the mitochondria, endoplasmic reticulum (ER), and DNA. Mitochondrial function and DNA repair are highly regulated by epigenetic mechanisms. In addition, autophagy plays a critical role in the repair process by removing dysfunctional organelles and mitigating cellular senescence, a process that is also epigenetically regulated.

Oxidative stress in aging

ROS, such as hydroxyl radicals, superoxide anions, and hydrogen peroxide, induce the oxidation of key cellular components, including nucleic acids, proteins, and lipids. The early free radical theory proposed a strong link between ROS and lifespan (Harman, 1956). While it is now understood that ROS play a complex role in cellular processes and are not the sole determinant of lifespan, uncontrolled ROS remains a significant contributor to aging (Giorgi et al., 2018). ROS originate from endogenous sources like NADPH oxidases, peroxisomes, and mitochondria, as well as environmental factors such as UV light, toxins, and radiation. Mitochondria are the primary producers of ROS, generating superoxides along the respiratory chain during oxidative phosphorylation (Balaban et al., 2005). Cells counteract oxidative stress through antioxidant defense mechanisms, including superoxide dismutases (SODs), glutathione peroxidases, and peroxiredoxins, which protect cellular components from oxidative damage (Balaban et al., 2005). However, aging is associated with a decline in mitochondrial function, characterized by reduced mitochondrial abundance, accumulation of impaired mitochondria, decreased respiratory chain enzyme activity, and lower SOD2 levels. These age-related changes result in increased ROS production due to electron leakage and diminished ROS clearance, contributing to overall ROS accumulation (Jastroch et al., 2010; Bratic and Larsson, 2013).

The accumulation of oxidative stress during aging disrupts normal cellular functions and damages critical biomolecules at multiple levels. It induces DNA damage through base modifications and strand breaks, triggering the DNA damage response (DDR). Oxidative stress also harms mitochondrial DNA (mtDNA) and essential proteins involved in energy production, further exacerbating ROS generation. Protein oxidation leads to misfolding and ER stress, activating the unfolded protein response. These cellular insults stimulate autophagy and various cellular repair mechanisms. However, when the damage is severe, these defense systems can be overwhelmed, resulting in cell death or senescence.

ROS production, detoxification, and oxidative stress-induced injury are tightly regulated by various epigenetic pathways. MiRNAs play an extensive role in this regulation by targeting key pathways such as the Nrf2/KEAP1 axis and mitochondrial proteins to control ROS production, as well as the SOD/catalase pathway to enhance detoxification. In addition, miRNAs respond to oxidative stress by modulating downstream signaling pathways (Ghafouri-Fard et al., 2020; Lu et al., 2020). lncRNAs are another group of critical regulators. Some well-characterized lncRNAs, such as HOTAIR, NEAT1, XIST, TUG1, and MALAT1, have been shown to influence ROS production and detoxification, by either interacting with chromatin to regulate protein transcription or sponging miRNAs to affect protein translation (Gast et al., 2019; Liu et al., 2019; Cai et al., 2020; Su et al., 2020; Ghafouri-Fard et al., 2020; You et al., 2023). Notably, RNA can also be oxidized by ROS. Although the downstream effects are not fully understood, emerging evidence suggests that RNA oxidation may influence RNA modifications (Yan et al., 2024). In addition, some RNA modification enzymes have been shown to directly sense ROS levels, potentially linking oxidative stress to RNA regulatory processes (Lee et al., 2023).

DNA damage and repair in aging

A major consequence of uncontrolled ROS is DNA damage. ROS can directly attack DNA, causing oxidative lesions such as 8-oxo-7,8-dihydroguanine, along with single-strand or double-strand breaks (Srinivas et al., 2019). These damages can be detected by some sensor proteins in DDR, such as ATM, ATR, and PARP1, to activate different DNA repair pathways.

Depending on the type of damage, different repair mechanisms are employed (Hakem, 2008). The direct reversal of the DNA damage pathway can reverse the modification of nucleotides such as O^6-alkylguanine. The mismatch repair system can fix mismatches. Nucleotide excision repair corrects bulky lesions that distort the DNA helix, while base excision repair fixes small, nonhelix-distorted base lesions. Double-strand breaks are repaired by nonhomologous end joining through ligating the broken ends or homologous recombination using a sister chromatid as a template to achieve error-free repair. However, excessive DNA damage can overwhelm repair systems, resulting in aberrant DNA repair (Qian et al., 2023). MtDNA is especially vulnerable to oxidative damage due to its proximity to ROS production sites and the limited availability of robust repair mechanisms within mitochondria (Druzhyna et al., 2008). Oxidative damage to mtDNA impairs mitochondrial function, creating a feedback loop that promotes further ROS generation and exacerbates cellular dysfunction (Rowe et al., 2008).

In addition to oxidative stress-induced DNA damage, telomere shortening is another aging hallmark closely related to DNA damage. Telomeres are repetitive DNA-protein structures that cap chromosome ends, protecting them from degradation, fusion, and recognition as DNA damage. With each cell division, telomeres progressively shorten due to the inability of DNA polymerase to fully replicate the lagging strand. When telomeres become critically short, they lose their protective function, exposing chromosome ends, triggering a persistent DNA damage response, and leading to cellular senescence (Hewitt et al., 2012; Rossiello et al., 2022).

DNA damage and genomic instability drive significant changes in epigenetic regulation, including alterations in chromatin conformation, to enhance DNA repair system accessibility. The chromatin conformation change involves alterations in DNA methylation, histone modifications, and chromatin remodeling. In addition to the dynamic DNA methylation changes that expose damaged DNA and promote gene expression for DNA repair, DNMT1 is recruited to the damaged site to modulate the DNA repair machinery (Sriraman et al., 2020; Soto-Palma et al., 2022). One of the most well-characterized histone modifications associated with DNA damage is the phosphorylation of histone H2AX (γ-H2AX), a hallmark of double-strand breaks. Additional histone modifications induced by DNA damage include H2AX acetylation and ubiquitination, H3K79 methylation, H4K20 methylation, and acetylation of histones H3 and H4 (Ikura et al., 2007; Pei et al., 2011; Lenart et al., 2018; Ljungman et al., 2019). In addition, PARP family protein-mediated poly-ADT-ribosylation (PARylation) of histones and other chromatin-associated proteins is essential to recruit DNA repair proteins such as ATM to the damage sites (Ray Chaudhuri and Nussenzweig, 2017). Chromatin remodelers also respond by modulating chromatin conformation, sliding or ejecting nucleosomes near DNA breaks, incorporating histone variants, spreading γ-H2AX along double-strand breaks, and recruiting DNA repair enzymes (Dabin et al., 2016; Qian et al., 2023).

NcRNAs, particularly lncRNAs, play critical roles in initiating and regulating the DDR and repair processes. Some lncRNAs, known as damage-induced long noncoding RNAs (dilncRNAs), can be transcribed from the sequences flanking double-strand breaks. DilncRNAs are cleaved to generate small DNA damage response RNAs (ddRNAs), which form RNA-RNA pairing complexes with dilncRNAs to recruit DNA repair machinery (Michelini et al., 2017). HMGB1, a chromatin-associated protein essential for DNA repair, requires binding to the lncRNA BS-DRL1 to function effectively (Lou et al., 2021). In addition, the lncRNA TERRA binds to telomeric DNA to control telomere-shortening-induced DNA damage response (Silva et al., 2021). LncRNA NORAD is significantly induced after DNA damage, sequestering PUMILIO proteins to reverse their suppression of DDR-related gene expression (Lee et al., 2016). Furthermore, the p53 pathway, a central regulator of DDR, controls the expression of DDR-associated lncRNAs and is itself regulated by numerous lncRNAs and eRNAs. Multiple lncRNAs, including GUARDIN, MEG3, PANDA, and DINO, are activated by p53 during DDR, reinforcing downstream signaling and facilitating genomic stability (Hung et al., 2011; Schmitt et al., 2016; Hu et al., 2018; Li et al., 2019). On the other hand, the transcriptional activity of p53 is influenced by a specific set of eRNAs (Melo et al., 2013).

MiRNAs play crucial regulatory roles in DDR and aging, particularly in modulating the p53 pathway. Several miRNAs, including miR-125b, miR-25, miR-30d, miR-380-5p, miR-504, and miR-1285, directly target the 3′-UTR of p53, suppressing its expression and influencing cell fate decisions (Le et al., 2009; Hu et al., 2010; Swarbrick et al., 2010; Tian et al., 2010; Kumar et al., 2011). MiR-29 is transcriptionally induced by p53 during aging and promotes the development of aging phenotypes. This occurs through a positive feedback loop, as miR-29 activates p53 by targeting Ppmd1, a negative regulator of p53 (Ugalde et al., 2011; Swahari et al., 2024). In addition, numerous miRNAs regulate downstream effectors of the p53 pathway, modulating cell cycle arrest and DNA repair to maintain genomic stability and influence cellular longevity (Majidinia et al., 2020; Potter et al., 2021).

Mitochondrial repair in aging

Mitochondria are the powerhouses of cells, highly efficient in ATP generation through oxidative phosphorylation. In addition, they play essential roles in maintaining calcium homeostasis, regulating ROS production and detoxification. Mitochondrial function is crucial in determining cell fate, influencing survival, senescence, or cell death. Mitochondrial function is influenced by several processes, including mitochondrial biogenesis, mitochondrial dynamics, mitochondrial damage and repair, and the selective removal of damaged mitochondria through mitophagy.

The decline of mitochondrial biogenesis

Mitochondrial biogenesis is the process of creating new mitochondria, coordinated by the master regulator PGC-1α (Palikaras et al., 2015; Guo et al., 2023). This process involves the synthesis of mitochondrial proteins from both nuclear and mitochondrial genes, assembling them with other mitochondrial components to form functional mitochondria. During aging, the expression of PGC-1α declines through the regulation of multiple pathways. Chronic inflammation and elevated cytokine levels activate the NF-κB pathway, which can suppress PGC-1α expression (Alvarez-Guardia et al., 2010; Tilstra et al., 2011). Overactivation of the mTOR pathway further reduces PGC-1α activation during aging (Summer et al., 2019). In addition, aging lowers NAD + levels, decreasing the activity of Sirt1, an NAD +-dependent deacetylase (Imai and Guarente, 2016; Chini et al., 2024), while Sirt1 can activate PGC-1α by direct deacetylation (Nemoto et al., 2005). Epigenetic mechanisms also modulate PGC-1α expression during aging and in age-related diseases. In type II diabetic conditions, hypermethylation of the PGC-1α promoter mediated by DNMT3b suppresses its transcription in muscle (Barrès et al., 2009). HDAC4-mediated histone deacetylation downregulates PGC-1α expression, contributing to muscle atrophy (Luo et al., 2019). Mir-696 directly suppresses PGC-1α, while mir-149 targets PARP2 to enhance Sirt1 and PGC-1α activation in response to metabolic stresses in muscle (Mohamed et al., 2014; Queiroz et al., 2021). Overall, suppression of the PGC-1α pathway results in impaired mitochondrial biogenesis, contributing to mitochondrial dysfunction during aging.

Mitochondrial unfolded protein response (UPR^{mt})

During aging, mitochondrial dysfunction leads to the accumulation of misfolded or damaged proteins, triggering UPR^{mt}—a protective stress response within mitochondria. ATFS-1 (in worms) or ATF5 (in mammals) plays a crucial role by translocating from the mitochondria to the nucleus upon mitochondrial stress, initiating UPR^{mt}. Activation of UPR^{mt} affects mitochondrial protein import, activates proteases to degrade misfolded proteins, and stimulates mitophagy to remove irreparable mitochondria. In addition, UPR^{mt} enhances communication between mitochondria and the nucleus, promoting chromatin remodeling and histone acetylation to induce gene expression to support mitochondrial recovery (e.g., increased chaperone production for protein folding). While UPR^{mt} is essential for mitochondrial repair and recovery, prolonged activation can be detrimental. Interestingly, UPR^{mt} activity declines with age, but it remains unclear whether this decline represents a self-protective mechanism or an age-related impairment (Shpilka and Haynes, 2018).

MtDNA damage

MtDNA is more vulnerable to ROS-induced damage due to its lack of histone protection and proximity to the electron transport chain, where ROS is produced. During aging, mtDNA accumulates various types of damage, including point mutations, deletions, strand breaks, oxidative lesions, and large-scale rearrangements (Chocron et al., 2019). Similar to nuclear DNA, mtDNA can be repaired through multiple mechanisms, including base excision repair (BER), DNA break repair, and mismatch repair (Kazak et al., 2012). While BER is well characterized and considered the primary repair pathway in mitochondria, the robustness of other repair mechanisms, such as double-strand break repair and mismatch repair, remains less clear. When mtDNA damage is irreparable, damaged mtDNA may be degraded, or dysfunctional mitochondria may be removed through mitophagy. If these processes fail, damaged mitochondria can release mtDNA into the cytosol, which is associated with cellular senescence and aging (Victorelli et al., 2023).

The epigenetic regulation of mtDNA involves DNA methylation, modifications of mtDNA-binding proteins, and ncRNA regulation (Stoccoro and Coppedè, 2021; Mongelli et al., 2023). Enzymes responsible for genomic DNA methylation, including DNMT1, DNMT3a, DNMT3b, and TETs, are also present in mitochondria. De novo methylation is thought to play a critical role in protecting mtDNA from oxidative stress-induced damage (Yue et al., 2022). However, the impact of aging on mtDNA methylation remains unclear. In addition, mtDNA associates with mitochondrial transcription factor A (TFAM) to form nucleoids, which are essential for maintaining mtDNA stability and regulating mitochondrial gene expression. Posttranslational modifications of TFAM, such as acetylation and phosphorylation, influence its binding affinity to mtDNA, thereby modulating mitochondrial function

(Mongelli et al., 2023). Furthermore, ncRNAs, including lncRNA MALAT1 and a couple of miRNAs, have been identified in mitochondria (Mongelli et al., 2023). MALAT1 directly interacts with mtDNA to regulate gene expression, while mitochondrial miRNAs primarily target mitochondrial mRNAs, suppressing protein translation.

Mitochondrial dynamic dysregulation and mitophagy

Mitochondrial quality is tightly regulated to maintain proper cellular function. Mitochondria form dynamic networks within cells, and the balance of their dynamic morphology is controlled by mitochondrial fusion and fission to match the cellular metabolic status. Fusion-generated elongated mitochondria enhance ATP production efficiency and reduce ROS generation, while fission-induced fragmentation is often associated with increased glycolysis and elevated ROS levels. Notably, fission also plays a crucial role in mitochondrial quality control by enabling the selective removal of damaged mitochondrial parts through mitophagy. Aging disrupts this balance, leading to species- or tissue-specific alterations, such as excessive mitochondrial fragmentation or hyper-elongation. Furthermore, key fusion and fission proteins, including MFN2, OPA1, and Drp1, have been reported to decline with age, contributing to mitochondrial dysfunction (Wu et al., 2019; Lima et al., 2022).

When parts of mitochondria become damaged and cannot be repaired, they are separated from the healthy mitochondrial network by fission and subsequently removed through mitophagy (Burman et al., 2017). Mitophagy is a selective form of autophagy that degrades damaged mitochondria within autophagosomes (Picca et al., 2023). The canonical mitophagy pathway is mediated by PINK1 and Parkin. When mitochondria are damaged, the degradation of PINK1 is disrupted, causing it to accumulate on the outer mitochondrial membrane. This accumulation recruits Parkin, an E3 ubiquitin ligase, which ubiquitinates outer membrane proteins. Ubiquitinated proteins then attract autophagy adaptors (e.g., p62/SQSTM1, NBR1), facilitating the encapsulation of damaged mitochondria by autophagosomes. In addition to the PINK1/Parkin pathway, several PINK1/Parkin-independent mitophagy pathways have been identified. These are regulated by proteins such as Bnip3, NIX, and FUNDC1. Mitophagy levels are crucial for the aging process, and suppression of basal mitophagy levels can lead to cellular senescence (Kelly et al., 2024). While mitophagy generally declines with aging in short-lived model organisms, a recent study in mouse brains reveals tissue- and cell-type-specific changes. In certain neurons, mitophagy remains active even during aging, suggesting that the regulation of mitochondrial quality control may differ across tissues and cell populations (Rappe et al., 2024).

Currently, only a few epigenetic mechanisms have been identified in the modulation of mitochondrial dynamics and mitophagy in aging. Among them, ncRNAs play important regulatory functions (Giordani et al., 2021; Gallo Cantafio et al., 2023). One example is lncRNA H19, which disrupts the interaction between PINK1 mRNA and eIF4A2, thereby suppressing PINK1 expression and reducing mitophagy in obesity (Wang et al., 2021a). During aging, TET1-mediated demethylation of the GSNOR promoter is impaired. This leads to a reduction in GSNOR, a denitrosylase, resulting in increased S-nitrosylation and functional inactivation of Parkin, ultimately inhibiting mitophagy (Rizza et al., 2018). In addition, during epidermal aging, the overexpression of miR-30a targets Bnip3L, suppressing Bnip3L/NIX-dependent mitophagy (Chevalier et al., 2022).

Mitonuclear signaling

Mitochondria and the nucleus closely communicate with each other, a process known as mitonuclear signaling, to maintain cellular homeostasis, energy production, and stress responses (English et al., 2020; Kim and Lee, 2024). The nucleus encodes most mitochondrial proteins, such as PGC-1α to regulate mitochondrial biogenesis, TFAM for mtDNA structure and expression, and Drp1/PINK1/PARKIN for mitochondrial dynamics and mitophagy. On the other hand, mitochondria send signals to the nucleus, such as ROS, calcium, ATP/AMP ratio, and UPR^{mt}, in response to stress, damage, or changes in energy demand. This feedback regulates nuclear gene expression to adapt to mitochondrial dysfunction.

Mitonuclear signaling is closely linked to epigenetic regulation. For example, mtDNA gene expression is modulated by DNA methylation/demethylation enzymes, TFAM, lncRNAs, and miRNAs encoded by nuclear genes (Yue et al., 2022; Mongelli et al., 2023). Conversely, mitochondria produce ncRNAs, which can influence nuclear gene expression (Rackham et al., 2011; Ren et al., 2023). With aging, mitochondrial production of acetyl-CoA and NAD^+ declines, which can significantly impair histone acetylation and gene expression (Peleg et al., 2016; Pouikli et al., 2021). Furthermore, the activity of chromatin remodelers is highly coupled to mitochondrial metabolism and ATP availability, which decreases due to mitochondrial dysfunction (Morrison, 2020), contributing to widespread chromatin conformation and transcriptional changes.

Cellular repair, autophagy, and senescence

In addition to DNA and mitochondrial repair, several other mechanisms contribute to cellular repair, maintaining cell structure and function. These include protein quality control to ensure proteostasis, membrane repair through exocytosis and lipid remodeling, and autophagy to remove damaged cellular components. During aging, the accumulation of misfolded proteins is detected and repaired by protein quality control mechanisms. Although the cell membrane is critical for cellular structure homeostasis, its role in aging is not well understood. A recent study confirmed that plasma membrane damage can induce premature senescence (Suda et al., 2024). Autophagy is a self-scavenging mechanism that breaks down and recycles cellular components, and impaired autophagy leads to the accumulation of cellular debris. Ultimately, the failure of cellular repair results in cell death or senescence.

Protein quality control

Protein quality control is critical to maintaining proteostasis. Molecular chaperone proteins or sensor proteins in the ER play a central role in detecting misfolded proteins. If the misfolded proteins cannot be corrected by molecular chaperones, they undergo several pathways for degradation, including ER-associated degradation, ubiquitin-proteasomal or other protease degradation, and autophagy (Dubnikov et al., 2017; Chen et al., 2023). As cells age, the decline in protein quality control results in the accumulation of protein aggregates in a tissue-specific manner (Chen et al., 2024).

- *ER stress and the unfolded protein response (UPR):* The endoplasmic reticulum (ER) is the cellular organelle responsible for protein folding and modification. Oxidative stress causes protein misfolding through oxidation and modification of protein structure, which overwhelms the ER and triggers the UPR. The UPR has three primary mechanisms: (1) PERK activation to reduce overall protein synthesis and further activate ATF4 promoting gene expression involved in redox balance and amino acid metabolism; (2) IRE1 activation to splice XBP1 mRNA, producing a transcription factor that upregulates chaperones and ER-associated degradation components; and (3) cleavage of ATF6 to release ATF6f which controls the transcription of XBP1 (Chen et al., 2023). MiRNAs have been reported to play various regulatory roles in ER stress and UPR activation during aging (Demirel-Yalciner et al., 2021). The ATP-dependent chromatin remodelers SWI/SNF and RSC are critical for the activation of the UPR and the expression of other protein quality control proteins (Sahu et al., 2021). Under starvation conditions, the de-ubiquitinating protein BAP1 can downregulate ER stress and UPR-related protein expression through H2A de-ubiquitination, thereby avoiding overwhelming ER stress and cell death (Dai et al., 2017).

- *Molecular chaperone.* Molecular chaperones are a group of proteins that interact with other proteins, stabilizing them and assisting in achieving their proper three-dimensional structure, but they are not part of the final functional complex (Hartl et al., 2011). Chaperones facilitate the de novo folding of newly synthesized proteins, refold misfolded proteins, prevent protein aggregation, assist in protein transport across membranes, support multi-protein complex assembly, and target irreparable proteins for degradation via the proteasome or autophagy pathways. Many chaperones belong to the heat shock protein family, which is induced under stress conditions. The disruption of proteostasis during aging suppresses chaperone activity, leading to G1/S cell cycle arrest and senescence (Moreno et al., 2019). Notably, histone chaperones play a critical role in regulating chromatin conformation by escorting histones during nucleosome assembly, modification, recycling, and degradation (Hammond et al., 2017).
- *Ubiquitin-Proteasome System (UPS):* UPS is a primary pathway for degrading and recycling damaged, misfolded, or unneeded proteins in cells. Target proteins are modified by the attachment of one or more ubiquitin molecules through a cascade of reactions catalyzed by three enzymes: E1, the ubiquitin-activating enzyme, which activates ubiquitin using ATP; E2, the ubiquitin-conjugating enzyme, which carries activated ubiquitin; and E3, the ubiquitin ligase, which transfers ubiquitin from E2 to the target protein. E3 ligases determine which proteins are tagged, making them key regulators of protein degradation. The ubiquitinated proteins are directed to the 26S proteasome for degradation into small peptides (Sun-Wang et al., 2020). Meanwhile, cells have deubiquitinases to remove ubiquitin from proteins, reversing the process to increase protein stability. Ubiquitination is indeed an important mechanism for histone modification (Vaughan et al., 2021; Yadav et al., 2022; Mandal et al., 2024). Though not all ubiquitinated histones are degraded, ubiquitination is essential for epigenetic regulation and chromatin conformation maintenance. During aging, ubiquitin proteome remodeling occurs, and increased deubiquitinase activity leads to a global decrease in ubiquitination, which disrupts the proteostasis balance and shortens the lifespan in *C. elegans* (Koyuncu et al., 2021).

Autophagy

Autophagy is a cellular process through which cells degrade and recycle damaged organelles, proteins, nucleic acids, and other cellular debris in lysosomes to maintain cellular homeostasis. Depending on how cellular debris is delivered to the lysosome, autophagy is classified into three types. In chaperone-mediated autophagy, molecular chaperones bind to target proteins and transport them to the lysosome for degradation. In microautophagy, the lysosome directly engulfs small portions of the cytoplasm by membrane invagination to capture cytoplasmic components for degradation. Macroautophagy is the major type of autophagy, which can degrade and recycle large cellular components. It is characterized by the formation of double-membrane vesicles around the targets, called autophagosomes. Autophagosomes fuse with the lysosome to form an autolysosome, where the engulfed material is degraded and recycled. A basal level of autophagy is essential for maintaining cell health, and the overall autophagy level declines with age (Tabibzadeh, 2023). Under stress conditions, autophagy is upregulated to eliminate damaged cellular structures, facilitating repair and recovery. However, prolonged or excessive autophagy can drive cellular senescence and even lead to cell death (Aman et al., 2021; Xiang et al., 2023).

Notably, autophagy plays a pivotal role in maintaining nucleic acid homeostasis for both RNA and DNA. Cytosolic RNAs, including mRNAs, rRNAs, and other ncRNAs, have been identified in plant vacuoles and delivered to lysosomes for degradation (Hickl et al., 2021). Various RNA-protein complexes, such as stress granules and RISC, are regulated by autophagy. In Drosophila, the unloaded RISC component Ago1 is selectively degraded via autophagy, which may influence the degradation of associated mRNAs, miRNAs, or siRNAs. A specialized RNA degradation pathway, known as RNautophagy, utilizes SIDT2 to bind CAG-repeat RNA motifs and transport mRNA to lysosomes for degradation—a process independent of proteolysis (Abildgaard et al., 2020). Furthermore, autophagy also plays a crucial role in mtDNA damage and repair. When mtDNA is released into the cytosol of stressed cells, TFAM (a mitochondrial transcription factor and mtDNA-binding protein) interacts with LC3, triggering autophagy and suppressing inflammatory signaling induced by cytosolic mtDNA (Liu et al., 2024b). In addition, autophagy activation prevents the opening of the mitochondrial permeability transition pore and inhibits the release of endonuclease G from the mitochondria, thereby preventing subsequent nuclear DNA damage (Chao et al., 2021). A recent study revealed another connection between genomic DNA damage and autophagy (Lascaux et al., 2024). Topoisomerase I (TOP1), a DNA repair enzyme that resolves torsional stress in DNA, forms a DNA-protein complex known as the TOP1 cleavage complex (TOP1cc). The autophagy receptor TEX264 can bind and transport TOP1cc to lysosomes, facilitating its degradation and thereby maintaining genomic stability. Autophagy is even more important in cytosolic DNA clearance in senescent cells. The damaged chromatin in senescent cells is released into the cytosol, forming cytoplasmic chromatin fragments, which can be degraded in autolysosomes (Han et al., 2020).

Senescence

Senescence is a state of a cell that has undergone permanent cell cycle arrest but still remains alive. It occurs naturally during development or in response to various stresses, such as DNA damage and oxidative stress. In addition, senescent cells secrete various proinflammatory factors, known as the senescence-associated secretory phenotype (SASP). The p53/p21/p16 pathway is the key molecular pathway for senescence development, which can be activated by DNA damage, oxidative stress, or oncogenic stresses (Di Micco et al., 2021). The NF-κB pathway is another major pathway activated during senescence to control SASP (Chien et al., 2011). Senescence is critical to prevent the proliferation of damaged or dysfunctional cells, playing a vital role in tumor suppression, tissue remodeling, and wound healing. However, the accumulation of senescent cells over time contributes to aging and age-related diseases (Huang et al., 2022a).

Senescent cells undergo extensive epigenetic remodeling at multiple levels, resulting in altered gene expression to secure the senescent phenotype (Dasgupta et al., 2024). First, chromatin compartments (euchromatin vs. heterochromatin) are rearranged, with SASP-related genes remaining activated in euchromatin. A highly compacted chromatin structure, known as senescence-associated heterochromatin foci (SAHF), forms within heterochromatin and contributes to permanent gene silencing, particularly of genes involved in cell cycle progression (Narita, 2007). SAHF is characterized by histone modification markers linked to transcriptional repression, such as H3K9me3, H3K27me3, H4K20me3, and H4K16Ac. The histone variant macroH2A, deposited with the assistance of the HIRA histone chaperone complex, accumulates at SAHF, reinforcing chromatin compaction and gene repression. Next, the large-scale 3D chromatin structure—including topologically associated domains and chromatin loops—is reorganized. This restructuring alters enhancer-promoter interactions within chromosomes, which is critical for the expression of SASP genes. Furthermore, newly activated enhancer elements are characterized by significant changes in histone modifications, often accompanied by the transcription of eRNAs. In addition, nucleosome architecture is altered, with a decrease in canonical histones and an increase in histone variants. While overall DNA methylation levels may not significantly change, the methylation pattern is modified, promoting the expression of SASP-related genes by hypomethylating their promoters. Finally, beyond the significant impact from chromatin conformation changes, the expression of SASP genes is finely tuned by numerous ncRNAs (Panda et al., 2017; Miyata et al., 2021; Montes et al., 2021).

Epigenetic dysregulation and cellular repair in the aged kidney

Healthy kidney aging and epigenetic dysregulation

As time progresses, the kidney undergoes inevitable aging, leading to a gradual decline in renal function. The concept of healthy kidney aging is characterized by decreased renal blood flow resulting from vascular structural changes, reduced glomerular filtration rate (GFR) due to nephron loss, alterations in interstitial and glomerular structures, and diminished tubular function affecting electrolyte and acid-base balance, alongside the development of renal fibrosis. These dysregulations are closely linked to dynamic changes in various epigenetic regulators across different types of renal cells. Current research has examined changes in DNA methylation, histone modifications, ncRNAs, and RNA modifications during kidney aging. However, the roles of ATP-dependent chromatin remodeling remain to be elucidated.

DNA methylation

Similar to other organs, the DNA methylation pattern in the kidney undergoes significant changes during aging, which has been examined by multiple epigenetic clocks (Day et al., 2013; Horvath, 2013; Sagy et al., 2024). Indeed, the kidney is among the organs where biological age can be accurately "measured" by epigenetic clocks, and the correlation between kidney and blood DNA methylation changes enables the potential to predict kidney aging through peripheral blood tests (Day et al., 2013; Horvath, 2013; Pavanello et al., 2022; Yang et al., 2024b). One important application of epigenetic clock tests is in assessing the aging status of kidney transplant allografts (Cristoferi et al., 2022; Pavanello et al., 2022), which can dramatically impact the one-year posttransplant outcome (Heylen et al., 2019). In addition, age-related changes in kidney gene expression and kidney lesions are influenced by DNA methylation (Rowland et al., 2019). For instance, the promoter region of N-cadherin becomes hypermethylated in aged kidneys, leading to its reduced transcription, which may potentially affect the structural integrity of the kidney (Akintola et al., 2008). Notably, the WNT/β-catenin pathway is the top hypermethylated pathway in aged kidneys, indicating its involvement in age-related renal pathologies such as interstitial fibrosis and glomerulosclerosis (Heylen et al., 2019). Furthermore, the declined expression of key antiaging proteins Nrf2 and Klotho is dependent on the activity of DNMTs in aged kidneys, which is associated with their promoter hypermethylation (Gao et al., 2022).

Histone modifications

Several histone modification changes have been reported in kidney aging, including H4K20Me3, H3K9Me3, and H3K27Me3 (Sarg et al., 2002; Abrass et al., 2011; Han and Sun, 2020; Adams-Sherrod et al., 2024). Kidney aging is associated with an overall increase in H4K20Me3 (Sarg et al., 2002). H3K27Me3 levels rise at the promoters of both Klotho and Col3a1, coinciding with decreased levels of the demethyltransferase JMJD3 and the methyltransferase Ezh2, respectively (Abrass et al., 2011; Han and Sun, 2020). The induction of H3K27Me3 leads to reduced expression of Klotho, a critical antiaging factor. In contrast, the Col3a1 promoter shows reduced H3K9Me3 in aged kidneys. The combined effects of decreased H3K9Me3 and increased H3K27Me3 result in enhanced transcription of Collagen III, contributing to renal fibrosis. However, H3K27Me3 is decreased in the Lamc2 gene promoter, causing its induction in aged kidneys (Denisenko et al., 2018). In addition, Sirt1, a histone deacetylase important for lifespan regulation, is induced in aged kidneys, although its downstream effectors remain uncharacterized (Abrass et al., 2011). Notably, recent studies highlight sex-specific differences in histone modification patterns in the kidney, particularly in histone methylation (H3K9 and H3K27) and histone methyltransferases (Adams-Sherrod et al., 2024). Although histone acetyltransferases and HDACs display age- and sex-dependent differences, changes in H3K9 acetylation appear minimal. This suggests that histone modifications at specific promoter regions may play a significant role in regulating aging-related gene expression.

NcRNAs

The differential expression of miRNAs during aging has been profiled in rodent kidneys using microarray analysis (Bai et al., 2011; Ichii et al., 2012; Kwekel et al., 2015; Yanai et al.,

2022). Aging kidneys exhibit distinct miRNA expression patterns compared to younger kidneys. Certain miRNAs, such as miR-29, miR-335, and miR-34a, are upregulated with age and are associated with fibrosis, mitochondrial dysfunction, and cellular senescence (Bai et al., 2011; Kwekel et al., 2015). MiR-503-5p is elevated in both mouse kidneys and human serum, suggesting its potential as a biomarker for age-related renal impairment (Yanai et al., 2022). In addition, the high expression of miR-146a in the kidney interstitium promotes inflammatory cell infiltration and is related to chronic inflammation in aging kidneys (Ichii et al., 2012). Moreover, a small RNA-seq analysis of young and aged kidneys identifies the significant downregulation of miR-181 family miRNAs. The miR-181a reduction then activates the NF-κB pathway to regulate cellular senescence and SASP (Zhang et al., 2023).

The dynamic changes in lncRNAs during kidney aging have been examined through RNA deep sequencing, with more precise cell-specific sequencing conducted recently (Li et al., 2022; Kim et al., 2024). Overall, lncRNAs exhibit cell-specific expression patterns, and age-related lncRNA changes reflect this specificity. For example, the age-related increase in Meg3 occurs exclusively in glomerular endothelial cells. In contrast, multiple cell types in aged kidneys show a decrease in GM26802 and an increase in GM14964. The functions of several lncRNAs in kidney aging have been explored. GM43360, which is downregulated in aged kidneys, may reduce G1/S cell cycle arrest and suppress cellular senescence (Li et al., 2022). Similarly, TUG-1, which also declines with age, promotes mitochondrial biogenesis by inducing PGC-1α expression (Zhu et al., 2024). In renal progenitor cells, HOTAIR inhibits p15 expression by inducing H3K27me3 modification, influencing cell cycle arrest and senescence (Picerno et al., 2022). It is important to note that these findings are based on rodent studies. Given the limited conservation of lncRNAs across species, it is essential to verify their roles in human cells or tissues to ensure their relevance to human kidney aging.

RNA modification

Despite the numerous types of RNA modifications, m^6A is the only modification characterized in kidney aging to date. The overall m^6A level is reduced in total RNA from aged kidneys, accompanied by a decline in the expression of the m^6A methyltransferase METTL3 (Zhang et al., 2023, 2024b; Zhu et al., 2024). Several downstream effectors of m^6A modification have been identified, including lncRNA TUG1, LONP1 mRNA (a key mitochondrial matrix protease), and miR-181a, which contribute to mitochondrial dysfunction, kidney fibrosis, and cellular senescence. In addition, although the role of Ψ in the kidney remains unclear, a mutation in dyskerin—a key component for pseudouridylation—can lead to nephrotic syndromes such as focal segmental glomerulosclerosis and mesangial proliferative glomerulonephritis (Balogh et al., 2020).

Epigenetic dysregulation in age-related kidney diseases

Aging significantly impacts kidney health, increasing susceptibility to hypertensive nephropathy and diabetic nephropathy. Older adults are at a higher risk of developing acute kidney injury (AKI), with impaired recovery processes that promote progression to chronic kidney disease (CKD). In addition, elderly individuals face higher rates of kidney transplant failure and an elevated risk of developing renal cell carcinoma (RCC). Conversely, kidney lesions from various renal diseases can accelerate renal cell senescence and premature aging. Epigenetic dysregulation plays a critical role in driving premature kidney aging and aging-related renal diseases. Moreover, epigenetic changes in aged kidneys can interfere with the efficacy of medicines, complicating disease management in the elderly.

CKD

CKD is highly prevalent in the elderly, with age being one of the strongest risk factors. CKD is characterized by a progressively declining glomerular filtration rate (GFR) and is associated with renal pathologies such as tubular atrophy, interstitial fibrosis, and glomerulosclerosis. Diabetes and hypertension are two leading causes of CKD. Chromatin conformation regulation, particularly DNA methylation, plays a critical role in promoting CKD progression. The genome-wide DNA methylation changes in CKD have been examined by a few labs, both globally or in a cell-specific manner, correlating differential methylation patterns with kidney function and histopathological changes (Wing et al., 2014; Gluck et al., 2019; Schlosser et al., 2021; Yan et al., 2024; Sagy et al., 2024). Through combined analysis with histone modification markers, Dr. Susztak and her colleagues identified significant alterations in DNA methylation at gene regulatory elements within open chromatin regions, particularly enhancers (Yan et al., 2024). These changes may further affect transcription factor binding and gene expression related to renal fibrosis, solute carriers, and metabolism. Inhibition of DNMT1 protected against diabetic nephropathy by suppressing inflammation, suggesting an overall pathogenic role of DNA methylation in this model (Chen et al., 2019).

Histone modifications, particularly acetylation and methylation, undergo significant changes in CKD. Under diabetic conditions, acetylation of several histone lysine residues, including H3K9, H3K18, and H3K23, is induced. Notably, H3K9 acetylation has been reported to regulate renal inflammation, apoptosis, and fibrosis (Kourtidou and Tziomalos, 2023). Recent studies have also emphasized the critical role of histone deacetylases (HDACs) in CKD, with HDAC inhibitors representing a promising avenue for therapeutic development (Liu, 2021). Changes in histone methylation patterns in CKD are more complex. CKD promotes chromatin accessibility, which is associated with the reorganization of histone methylation marks linked to active gene transcription (e.g., H3K4me3, H3K36me3) and gene repression (e.g., H3K9me3, H3K27me3) (Yan et al., 2024). Alterations in histone methylation have been reported to widely influence CKD progression by affecting processes such as renal fibrosis, inflammation, oxidative stress, and glomerular pathology (Kourtidou and Tziomalos, 2023). Although the function of histone methylation changes could be gene-specific, one recent study found that the suppression of Set7 methyltransferase can mitigate diabetic glomerular pathology, suggesting the therapeutic potential of targeting specific methyltransferases or demethylases (Maxwell et al., 2024). In addition, a recent study reports the inhibition of Glis1 by histone lactylation to promote fibrosis in diabetic kidneys (Chen et al., 2025), which may link histone modification to metabolic reprogramming in CKD.

Furthermore, CKD is characterized by significant changes in ncRNA expression in the kidney, blood, and urine, which have been systematically profiled using microarrays, RNA-seq, or single-cell sequencing. One promising therapeutic direction is to utilize differentially expressed circulating or urinary ncRNAs—particularly small ncRNA signatures—as biomarkers for CKD diagnosis and prognosis (Muralidharan et al., 2017; Gu et al., 2021; Wang et al., 2021b). Over the past two decades, numerous miRNAs, lncRNAs, and circRNAs have been identified as important regulators of CKD pathogenesis, such as miR-21, miR-192, NEAT1, TUG1, and circHIPK3 (Kato et al., 2009; Meng et al., 2013; Li and Susztak, 2016; Yang et al., 2020; Liu et al., 2022). Despite these progressions, therapeutic development remains limited because of the challenges in nucleic acid delivery technologies.

It is important to note that CKD patients experience pre-mature aging or accelerated biological aging, as indicated by distinct DNA methylation patterns in their blood cells (Li et al., 2023b; Neytchev et al., 2024). This accelerated aging can be mitigated by kidney transplantation but not by dialysis (Neytchev et al., 2024). Various factors, including enhanced oxidative stress, elevated advanced glycation end-products, increased cellular senescence, and suppressed autophagy, contribute to CKD progression and premature aging. To this end, epigenetic mechanisms are highly involved in the regulation of key molecular pathways such as mTOR, P53/p21, NF-κB, and Klotho. For example, the activation of the P53/P21 pathway, which governs senescence and autophagy regulation, is intensively modulated by different epigenetic processes. The promoter of P21 undergoes demethylation associated with DNMT1 reduction, accompanied by increased histone acetylation and significant changes in histone methylation patterns, leading to enhanced P21 expression and the activation of senescence (Li et al., 2016; Al-Dabet et al., 2022). In addition, P53 activation induces miR-214, which suppresses autophagy and exacerbates cellular injury through targeting ULK1 in DKD (Ma et al., 2020).

Currently, the role of ATP-dependent chromatin remodelers and RNA modifications in CKD remains largely unclear. Although the chromatin remodeler INO80 has been reported to regulate renal tubular cell apoptosis under hypoxic conditions and decrease in the kidney after ureter obstruction, no significant change in INO80 was observed in the kidneys of 5/6 nephrectomy (a model for hypertension and kidney fibrosis) (Miura et al., 2023). Emerging studies suggest that METTL3-mediated m^6A modification plays a pro-injurious role in podocytes under diabetic conditions, and while the m^6A modification pattern change has been characterized in CKD, the downstream mechanism has not been fully explored (Jiang et al., 2022; Tsai et al., 2024). Overall, CKD is characterized by the dysregulation of multiple layers of epigenetic mechanisms, which form an epigenetic memory of pathological changes. These mechanisms represent promising targets for future therapeutic interventions aimed at slowing CKD progression and mitigating premature aging (Mimura et al., 2024).

AKI-to-CKD transition

Aging not only increases the incidence of AKI but also impairs recovery, promoting the transition to CKD and end-stage kidney disease (Kim et al., 2019). Despite the diverse injurious factors that induce AKI, such as ischemia, sepsis, and nephrotoxins, its progression to CKD is characterized by renal tubular epithelial cell injury and degeneration, inflammation, and renal fibrosis (He et al., 2017). Epigenetic modifications—including ncRNA expression, DNA methylation, and histone modifications—undergo dynamic changes during AKI and the subsequent transition to CKD (Guo et al., 2017; Sharifian et al., 2018; Connor et al., 2020; Mahtal et al., 2022; Tanemoto et al., 2022; van Zonneveld et al., 2023; Puri et al., 2024; Xiao et al., 2024; Wei et al., 2024a). These epigenetic "memories," particularly those associated with hypoxic injury and metabolic dysregulation, are critical contributors to maladaptive kidney repair and CKD development (Tanemoto et al., 2022). Generally, DNA methylation profiling identifies differentially methylated regions (DMRs) in AKI to CKD, but the function of the

DMRs is sequence-dependent. For example, hypermethylation of the gene promoters of HOXA5 and RASAL1 promotes fibrosis, while hypermethylation of the miR-219a-2 gene promoter exerts antifibrotic effects (Bechtel et al., 2010; Xiao et al., 2024; Wei et al., 2024a). The induction of HDAC3 plays a significant role in driving inflammation and fibroblast activation. Although the involvement of histone acetylation changes in this process remains unclear, NF-κB acetylation and activation have been identified as key downstream mechanisms (Wang et al., 2024). Notably, HDAC inhibitors have demonstrated antifibrotic effects in animal models (Choi et al., 2018a; Wang et al., 2024). In terms of histone methylation, H3K9 methylation has been shown to promote renal fibrosis by repressing Klotho transcription, a process that can be inhibited by targeting the methyltransferase G9a (Irifuku et al., 2016). The chromatin remodeling factor INO80 regulates renal tubular cell apoptosis by inhibiting P53, E2F1, and PMAIP1. INO80 also mediates the exchange of histone variant H2A.Z for H2A at the PMAIP1 promoter, contributing to apoptosis suppression (Miura et al., 2023). Interestingly, while these genes are known regulators of senescence, their pro-senescence roles were not further explored in the study. Numerous miRNAs have been implicated in the AKI-to-CKD transition, with a recent study highlighting their cell-type-specific functions (Connor et al., 2020; Mahtal et al., 2022). Moreover, a few lncRNAs, such as NEAT1 and H19, contribute to CKD development by interacting with miRNAs (Dong et al., 2022; Ma et al., 2022). Currently, only m^6A RNA modification has been characterized in the transition to CKD (Jung et al., 2024). The key m^6A methyltransferase, METTL3, is induced by TGF-β and plays a pro-fibrotic role.

Remarkably, recent studies have highlighted the critical role of cellular senescence in the AKI-to-CKD transition (Mylonas et al., 2021; Li et al., 2023c). Acute injury can trigger cellular senescence in the kidney (Yang et al., 2022), while the accumulation of senescent cells also increases with age (Mylonas et al., 2021). In the early stages of injury, senescent cells may contribute to preserving kidney structure. However, persistent senescence and the continued accumulation of these cells drive inflammation, maladaptive tubular repair, interstitial fibrosis, and vascular dysfunction through SASP, ultimately promoting CKD development (Harris et al., 2023; Li et al., 2023c; Chao et al., 2024). The induction of senescence during the AKI-to-CKD transition is regulated by various epigenetic mechanisms. For instance, hypomethylation of BCL9, CYP1B1, and CDK6 gene promoters, mediated by complement component C5a, promotes senescence following kidney ischemia (Castellano et al., 2019). In addition, a recent study identified histone H3K9 crotonylation, a short-chain lysine acylation catalyzed by ACSS2, as a pro-injurious factor driving inflammation, senescence, and fibrosis, independent of H3K9 acetylation (Li et al., 2024b).

Renal cell carcinoma (RCC)

Aging is a significant risk factor for RCC, the most common form of kidney cancer. Progressive epigenetic changes associated with aging can alter tumor suppressor gene expression, leading to malignant transformation. The loss of von Hippel-Lindau (VHL) is a primary driver of RCC, with promoter hypermethylation of *VHL* accounting for 7%–10% of cases (Lasseigne and Brooks, 2018). Other key RCC driver genes include several histone modifiers and ATP-dependent chromatin remodelers, such as subunits of the SWI/SNF chromatin remodeling complex (PBRM1, ARID1a), histone demethylases (KDM5a, KDM5c, UTX), a histone methyltransferase (SETD2), and a deubiquitinase (BAP1), highlighting the critical role of chromatin dynamics in RCC pathogenesis (Grammatikaki et al., 2023). In addition to genetic drivers, lncRNAs such as *MALAT1*, *HOTAIR*, and *NEAT1* are highly expressed in RCC and may act as oncogenes (Hirata et al., 2015; Pan et al., 2018; Pei et al., 2019). Another layer of epigenetic regulation involves m^6A modification, which is regulated by VHL and plays a role in tumor growth (Zhang et al., 2024a). For RCC diagnosis, several miRNAs (miR-210, miR-378, miR-451, and miR-1233) show promise as potential biomarkers (Grammatikaki, et al., 2023). Currently, epigenetic-based therapies, including DNMT inhibitors and HDAC inhibitors, are under investigation in phase I or II clinical trials for RCC treatment (Angulo et al., 2021).

Medical efficacy in elderly

Kidney aging can affect medical efficacy in two significant ways. First, as a vital organ for detoxification, age-related decline in kidney function can slow the excretion of medications, potentially increasing their toxicity and side effects (AlQashqri, 2023). This has led to the proposal of deprescription strategies to better align with the health conditions of elderly patients (Mohottige et al., 2021). Second, age-associated dysregulation of gene expression can alter target protein levels and cellular states (e.g., accumulation of senescent cells), diminishing treatment effectiveness. For instance, methylation of the *EPO* gene promoter can reduce EPO expression, potentially impacting the response to prolyl hydroxylase domain (PHD) inhibitors used in anemia treatment (Sato et al., 2019). To address these challenges, the concept of personalized medicine has been introduced, with the epigenetic clock proposed as a tool to assess the biological age of individual patients (Gigliotti et al., 2024). However, for many currently available drugs, the impact of aging on their efficacy remains unclear, highlighting the need for further research in this area.

AI disclosure

During the preparation of this work, the author(s) used ChatGPT 4.0 to edit the English language. After using this tool/service, the author(s) reviewed and edited the content as needed and take(s) full responsibility for the content of the publication.

References

Abildgaard, M.H., Brynjólfsdóttir, S.H., Frankel, L.B., 2020. The autophagy–RNA interplay: degradation and beyond. Trends Biochem. Sci. 45 (10), 845–857. doi:10.1016/j.tibs.2020.07.007.

Abrass, C.K., Hansen, K., Popov, V., Denisenko, O., 2011. Alterations in chromatin are associated with increases in collagen III expression in aging nephropathy. Am. J. Physiol. Renal Physiol. 300 (2). doi:10.1152/ajprenal.00237.2010.

Adams-Sherrod, G.A., Brooks, H.L., Kumar, P., 2024. Sex-specific modulation of renal epigenetic and injury markers in aging kidney. Am. J. Physiol. Renal Physiol. 327 (3). doi:10.1152/ajprenal.00140.2024.

Ahmed, I., Yang, S.-H., Ogden, S., Zhang, W., Li, Y., Sharrocks, A.D., 2023. eRNA profiling uncovers the enhancer landscape of oesophageal adenocarcinoma and reveals new deregulated pathways. eLife 12. doi:10.7554/elife.80840

Akintola, A.D., Crislip, Z.L., Catania, J.M., Chen, G., Zimmer, W.E., Burghardt, R.C., Parrish, A.R., 2008. Promoter methylation is associated with the age-dependent loss of N-cadherin in the rat kidney. Am. J. Physiol. Renal Physiol. 294 (1). doi:10.1152/ajprenal.00285.2007.

Al-Dabet, M.M., Shahzad, K., Elwakiel, A., Sulaj, A., Kopf, S., Bock, F., Gadi, I., Zimmermann, S., Rana, R., Krishnan, S., Gupta, D., Manoharan, J., Fatima, S., Nazir, S., Schwab, C., Baber, R., Scholz, M., Geffers, R., Mertens, P.R.,

Nawroth, P.P., Griffin, J.H., Keller, M., Dockendorff, C., Kohli, S., Isermann, B., 2022. Reversal of the renal hyperglycemic memory in diabetic kidney disease by targeting sustained tubular p21 expression. Nat. Commun. 13 (1). doi:10.1038/s41467-022-32477-9.

AlQashqri, H., 2023. Renally inappropriate medications in the old population: prevalence, risk factors, adverse outcomes, and potential interventions. Cureus 15 (11). doi:10.7759/cureus.49111.

Alvarez-Guardia, D., Palomer, X., Coll, T., Davidson, M.M., Chan, T.O., Feldman, A.M., Laguna, J.C., Vázquez-Carrera, M., 2010. The p65 subunit of NF-kappaB binds to PGC-1alpha, linking inflammation and metabolic disturbances in cardiac cells. Cardiovasc. Res. 87 (3), 449–458. doi:10.1093/cvr/cvq080.

Aman, Y., Schmauck-Medina, T., Hansen, M., Morimoto, R.I., Simon, A.K., Bjedov, I., Palikaras, K., Simonsen, A., Johansen, T., Tavernarakis, N., Rubinsztein, D.C., Partridge, L., Kroemer, G., Labbadia, J., Fang, E.F., 2021. Autophagy in healthy aging and disease. Nat. Aging 1 (8), 634–650. doi:10.1038/s43587-021-00098-4.

Angulo, J.C., Manini, C., López, J.I., Pueyo, A., Colás, B., Ropero, S., 2021. The role of epigenetics in the progression of clear cell renal cell carcinoma and the basis for future epigenetic treatments. Cancers 13 (9). doi:10.3390/cancers13092071.

Bai, X.-Y., Ma, Y., Ding, R., Fu, B., Shi, S., Chen, X.-M., 2011. miR-335 and miR-34a promote renal senescence by suppressing mitochondrial antioxidative enzymes. J. Am. Soc. Nephrol. 22 (7), 1252–1261. doi:10.1681/ASN.2010040367.

Balaban, R.S., Nemoto, S., Finkel, T., 2005. Mitochondria, oxidants, and aging. Cell 120 (4), 483–495. doi:10.1016/j.cell.2005.02.001.

Balogh, E., Chandler, J.C., Varga, M., Tahoun, M., Menyhárd, D.K., Schay, G., Goncalves, T., Hamar, R., Légrádi, R., Szekeres, Á., Gribouval, O., Kleta, R., Stanescu, H., Bockenhauer, D., Kerti, A., Williams, H., Kinsler, V., Di, W.-L., Curtis, D., Kolatsi-Joannou, M., Hammid, H., Szőcs, A., Perczel, K., Maka, E., Toldi, G., Sava, F., Arrondel, C., Kardos, M., Fintha, A., Hossain, A., D'Arco, F., Kaliakatsos, M., Koeglmeier, J., Mifsud, W., Moosajee, M., Faro, A., Jávorszky, E., Rudas, G., Saied, M.H., Marzouk, S., Kelen, K., Götze, J., Reusz, G., Tulassay, T., Dragon, F., Mollet, G., Motameny, S., Thiele, H., Dorval, G., Nürnberg, P., Perczel, A., Szabó, A.J., Long, D.A., Tomita, K., Antignac, C., Waters, A.M., Tory, K., 2020. Pseudouridylation defect due to DKC1 and NOP10 mutations causes nephrotic syndrome with cataracts, hearing impairment, and enterocolitis. Proc. Natl. Acad. Sci. U. S. A. 117 (26), 15137–15147. doi:10.1073/pnas.2002328117.

Barrès, R., Osler, M.E., Yan, J., Rune, A., Fritz, T., Caidahl, K., Krook, A., Zierath, J.R., 2009. Non-CpG methylation of the PGC-1α promoter through DNMT3B controls mitochondrial density. Cell Metab. 10 (3), 189–198. doi:10.1016/j.cmet.2009.07.011.

Bechtel, W., McGoohan, S., Zeisberg, E.M., Müller, G.A., Kalbacher, H., Salant, D.J., Müller, C.A., Kalluri, R., Zeisberg, M., 2010. Methylation determines fibroblast activation and fibrogenesis in the kidney. Nat. Med. 16 (5), 544–550. doi:10.1038/nm.2135.

Bergeron, D., Faucher-Giguère, L., Emmerichs, A.-K., Choquet, K., Song, K.S., Deschamps-Francoeur, G., Fafard-Couture, É., Rivera, A., Couture, S., Churchman, L.S., Heyd, F., Elela, S.A., Scott, M.S., 2023. Intronic small nucleolar RNAs regulate host gene splicing through base pairing with their adjacent intronic sequences. Genome Biol. 24 (1). doi:10.1186/s13059-023-03002-y.

Bernabeu, E., McCartney, D.L., Gadd, D.A., Hillary, R.F., Lu, A.T., Murphy, L., Wrobel, N., Campbell, A., Harris, S.E., Liewald, D., Hayward, C., Sudlow, C., Cox, S.R., Evans, K.L., Horvath, S., McIntosh, A.M., Robinson, M.R., Vallejos, C.A., Marioni, R.E., 2023. Refining epigenetic prediction of chronological and biological age. Genome Med. 15 (1). doi:10.1186/s13073-023-01161-y.

Booth, B.J., Nourreddine, S., Katrekar, D., Savva, Y., Bose, D., Long, T.J., Huss, D.J., Mali, P., 2023. RNA editing: expanding the potential of RNA therapeutics. Mol. Ther. 31 (6), 1533–1549.

Borchardt, E.K., Martinez, N.M., Gilbert, W.V., 2020. Regulation and function of RNA pseudouridylation in human cells. Annu. Rev. Genet. 54, 309–336. doi:10.1146/annurev-genet-112618-043830.

Bradshaw, P.C., 2021. Acetyl-coa metabolism and histone acetylation in the regulation of aging and lifespan. Antioxidants 10 (4). doi:10.3390/antiox10040572.

Bratic, A., Larsson, N.-G., 2013. The role of mitochondria in aging. J. Clin. Invest. 123 (3), 951–957. doi:10.1172/jci64125.

Bratkovič, T., Bozič, J., Rogelj, B., 2020. Functional diversity of small nucleolar RNAs. Nucleic Acids Res. 48 (4), 1627–1651. doi:10.1093/nar/gkz1140.

Burman, J.L., Pickles, S., Wang, C., Sekine, S., Vargas, J.N.S., Zhang, Z., Youle, A.M., Nezich, C.L., Wu, X., Hammer, J.A., Youle, R.J., 2017. Mitochondrial fission facilitates the selective mitophagy of protein aggregates. J. Cell Biol. 216 (10), 3231–3247. doi:10.1083/jcb.201612106.

Cai, D., Han, J.-D.J., 2021. Aging-associated lncRNAs are evolutionarily conserved and participate in NFκB signaling. Nat. Aging. 1 (5), 438–453. doi:10.1038/s43587-021-00056-0.

Cai, L.-J., Tu, L., Huang, X.-M., Huang, J., Qiu, N., Xie, G.-H., Liao, J.-X., Du, W., Zhang, Y.-Y., Tian, J.-Y., 2020. LncRNA MALAT1 facilitates inflammasome activation via epigenetic suppression of Nrf2 in Parkinson's disease. Mol. Brain. 13 (1). doi:10.1186/s13041-020-00656-8.

Castellano, G., Franzin, R., Sallustio, F., Stasi, A., Banelli, B., Romani, M., De Palma, G., Lucarelli, G., Divella, C., Battaglia, M., Crovace, A., Staffieri, F., Grandaliano, G., Stallone, G., Ditonno, P., Cravedi, P., Cantaluppi, V., Gesualdo, L., 2019. Complement component C5a induces aberrant epigenetic modifications in renal tubular epithelial cells accelerating senescence by Wnt4/βcatenin signaling after ischemia/reperfusion injury. Aging. 11 (13), 4382–4406. doi:10.18632/aging.102059.

Cedar, H., Bergman, Y., 2009. Linking DNA methylation and histone modification: patterns and paradigms. Nat. Rev. Genet. 10 (5), 295–304. doi:10.1038/nrg2540.

Celen, A.B., Sahin, U., 2020. Sumoylation on its 25th anniversary: mechanisms, pathology, and emerging concepts. FEBS J. 287 (15), 3110–3140. doi:10.1111/febs.15319.

Chao, C.-T., Kuo, F.-C., Lin, S.-H., 2024. Epigenetically regulated inflammation in vascular senescence and renal progression of chronic kidney disease. Semin. Cell Dev. Biol. 154, 305–315. doi:10.1016/j.semcdb.2022.09.012.

Chao, T., Shih, H.-T., Hsu, S.-C., Chen, P.-J., Fan, Y.-S., Jeng, Y.-M., Shen, Z.-Q., Tsai, T.-F., Chang, Z.-F., 2021. Autophagy restricts mitochondrial DNA damage-induced release of ENDOG (endonuclease G) to regulate genome stability. Autophagy 17 (11), 3444–3460. doi:10.1080/15548627.2021.1874209.

Chen, G., Chen, H., Ren, S., Xia, M., Zhu, J., Liu, Y., Zhang, L., Tang, L., Sun, L., Liu, H., Dong, Z., 2019. Aberrant DNA methylation of mTOR pathway genes promotes inflammatory activation of immune cells in diabetic kidney disease. Kidney Int. 96 (2), 409–420. doi:10.1016/j.kint.2019.02.020.

Chen, J., He, J., Wang, X., Bai, L., Yang, X., Chen, J., He, Y., Chen, K., 2025. Glis1 inhibits RTEC cellular senescence and renal fibrosis by downregulating histone lactylation in DKD. Life Sci. 361. doi:10.1016/j.lfs.2024.123293

Chen, L., Dahlstrom, J.E., Lee, S.-H., Rangasamy, D., 2012. Naturally occurring endo-siRNA silences LINE-1 retrotransposons in human cells through DNA methylation. Epigenetics 7 (7), 758–771. doi:10.4161/epi.20706.

Chen, X., Shi, C., He, M., Xiong, S., Xia, X., 2023. Endoplasmic reticulum stress: molecular mechanism and therapeutic targets. Signal Transduct. Target. Ther. 8 (1). doi:10.1038/s41392-023-01570-w.

Chen, Y.R., Harel, I., Singh, P.P., Ziv, I., Moses, E., Goshtchevsky, U., Machado, B.E., Brunet, A., Jarosz, D.F., 2024. Tissue-specific landscape of protein aggregation and quality control in an aging vertebrate. Dev. Cell 59 (14). doi:10.1016/j.devcel.2024.04.014.

Cheng, Y., Wang, S., Zhang, H., Lee, J.-S., Ni, C., Guo, J., Chen, E., Wang, S., Acharya, A., Chang, T.-C., Buszczak, M., Zhu, H., Mendell, J.T., 2024. A non-canonical role for a small nucleolar RNA in ribosome biogenesis and senescence. Cell 187 (17). doi:10.1016/j.cell.2024.06.019.

Chevalier, F.P., Rorteau, J., Ferraro, S., Martin, L.S., Gonzalez-Torres, A., Berthier, A., Kholti, N.E., Lamartine, J., 2022. MiR-30a-5p alters epidermal terminal differentiation during aging by regulating BNIP3L/NIX-dependent mitophagy. Cells 11 (5). doi:10.3390/cells11050836.

Chien, Y., Scuoppo, C., Wang, X., Fang, X., Balgley, B., Bolden, J.E., Premsrirut, P., Luo, W., Chicas, A., Lee, C.S., Kogan, S.C., Lowe, S.W., 2011. Control of the senescence-associated secretory phenotype by NF-κB promotes senescence and enhances chemosensitivity. Genes Dev. 25 (20), 2125–2136. doi:10.1101/gad.17276711.

Chini, C.C.S., Cordeiro, H.S., Tran, N.L.K., Chini, E.N., 2024. NAD metabolism: role in senescence regulation and aging. Aging Cell 23 (1). doi:10.1111/acel.13920.

Chocron, E.S., Munkácsy, E., Pickering, A.M., 2019. Cause or casualty: the role of mitochondrial DNA in aging and age-associated disease. Biochim. Biophys. Acta Mol. Basis Dis. 1865 (2), 285–297.

Choi, H.S., Song, J.H., Kim, I.J., Joo, S.Y., Eom, G.H., Kim, I., Cha, H., Cho, J.M., Ma, S.K., Kim, S.W., Bae, E.H., 2018a. Histone deacetylase inhibitor, CG200745 attenuates renal fibrosis in obstructive kidney disease. Sci. Rep. 8 (1). doi:10.1038/s41598-018-30008-5.

Choi, J., Indrisiunaite, G., Demirci, H., Ieong, K.-W., Wang, J., Petrov, A., Prabhakar, A., Rechavi, G., Dominissini, D., He, C., Ehrenberg, M., Puglisi, J.D., 2018b. 2′-O-methylation in mRNA disrupts tRNA decoding during translation elongation. Nat. Struct. Mol. Biol. 25 (3), 208–216. doi:10.1038/s41594-018-0030-z.

Clapier, C.R., Iwasa, J., Cairns, B.R., Peterson, C.L., 2017. Mechanisms of action and regulation of ATP-dependent chromatin-remodelling complexes. Nat. Rev. Mol. Cell Biol. 18 (7), 407–422. doi:10.1038/nrm.2017.26.

Cohen-Berkman, M., Dudkevich, R., Ben-Hamo, S., Fishman, A., Salzberg, Y., Ben-Asher, H.W., Lamm, A.T., Henis-Korenblit, S., 2020. Endogenous siRNAs promote proteostasis and longevity in germlineless c. Elegans. eLife 9. doi:10.7554/elife.50896

Collins, P.L., Purman, C., Porter, S.I., Nganga, V., Saini, A., Hayer, K.E., Gurewitz, G.L., Sleckman, B.P., Bednarski, J.J., Bassing, C.H., Oltz, E.M., 2020. DNA double-strand breaks induce H2Ax phosphorylation domains in a contact-dependent manner. Nat. Commun. 11 (1). doi:10.1038/s41467-020-16926-x.

Connor, K.L., Teenan, O., Cairns, C., Banwell, V., Thomas, R.A.B., Rodor, J., Finnie, S., Pius, R., Tannahill, G.M., Sahni, V., Savage, C.O.S., Hughes, J., Harrison, E.M., Henderson, R.B., Marson, L.P., Conway, B.R., Wigmore, S.J., Denby, L., 2020. Identifying cell-enriched miRNAs in kidney injury and repair. JCI Insight 5 (24). doi:10.1172/jci.insight.140399.

Cristoferi, H., Giacon, T.A., Boer, K., van Baardwijk, M., Neri, F., Campisi, M., Kimenai, H.J.A.N., Clahsen van - Groningen, M.C., Pavanello, S., Furian, L., Minnee, R.C., 2022. The applications of DNA methylation as a biomarker in kidney transplantation: a systematic review. Clin. Epigenetics 14 (1). doi:10.1186/s13148-022-01241-7.

Cui, L., Ma, R., Cai, J., Guo, C., Chen, Z., Yao, L., Wang, Y., Fan, R., Wang, X., Shi, Y., 2022. RNA modifications: importance in immune cell biology and related diseases. Signal Transduct. Target. Ther. 7 (1). doi:10.1038/s41392-022-01175-9.

Dabin, J., Fortuny, A., Polo, S.E., 2016. Epigenome maintenance in response to DNA damage. Mol. Cell 62 (5), 712–727. doi:10.1016/j.molcel.2016.04.006.

Dai, F., Lee, H., Zhang, Y., Zhuang, L., Yao, H., Xi, Y., Xiao, Z.-D., You, M.J., Li, W., Su, X., Gan, B., 2017. BAP1 inhibits the ER stress gene regulatory network and modulates metabolic stress response. Proc. Natl. Acad. Sci. U. S. A. 114 (12), 3192–3197. doi:10.1073/pnas.1619588114.

Dasgupta, N., Arnold, R., Equey, A., Gandhi, A., Adams, P.D., 2024. The role of the dynamic epigenetic landscape in senescence: orchestrating SASP expression. Npj Aging 10 (1). doi:10.1038/s41514-024-00172-2.

Day, K., Waite, L.L., Thalacker-Mercer, A., West, A., Bamman, M.M., Brooks, J.D., Myers, R.M., Absher, D., 2013. Differential DNA methylation with age displays both common and dynamic features across human tissues that are influenced by CpG landscape. Genome Biol. 14 (9). doi:10.1186/gb-2013-14-9-r102.

Demirel-Yalciner, T., Sozen, E., Ozer, N.K., 2021. Endoplasmic reticulum stress and miRNA impairment in aging and age-related diseases. Front. Aging 2. doi:10.3389/fragi.2021.790702

Denisenko, O., Mar, D., Trawczynski, M., Bomsztyk, K., 2018. Chromatin changes trigger laminin genes dysregulation in aging kidneys. Aging 10 (5), 1133–1145. doi:10.18632/aging.101453.

Di Micco, R., Krizhanovsky, V., Baker, D., d'adda di Fagagna, F., 2021. Cellular senescence in ageing: from mechanisms to therapeutic opportunities. Nat. Rev. Mol. Cell Biol. 22 (2), 75–95. doi:10.1038/s41580-020-00314-w.

Dong, X., Cao, R., Li, Q., Yin, L., 2022. The long noncoding RNA-H19 mediates the progression of fibrosis from acute kidney injury to chronic kidney disease by regulating the miR-196a/Wnt/β-catenin signaling. Nephron. 146 (2), 209–219. doi:10.1159/000518756.

Drazkowska, K., Tomecki, R., Warminski, M., Baran, N., Cysewski, D., Depaix, A., Kasprzyk, R., Kowalska, J., Jemielity, J., Sikorski, P.J., 2022. 2′-O-Methylation of the second transcribed nucleotide within the mRNA 5′ cap impacts the protein production level in a cell-specific manner and contributes to RNA immune evasion. Nucleic Acids Res. 50 (16), 9051–9071. doi:10.1093/nar/gkac722.

Druzhyna, N.M., Wilson, G.L., LeDoux, S.P., 2008. Mitochondrial DNA repair in aging and disease. Mech. Ageing Dev. 129 (7–8), 383–390. doi:10.1016/j.mad.2008.03.002.

Dubnikov, T., Ben-Gedalya, T., Cohen, E., 2017. Protein quality control in health and disease. Cold Spring Harb. Perspect. Biol. 9 (3). doi:10.1101/cshperspect.a023523.

Eberharter, A., Becker, P.B., 2002. Histone acetylation: a switch between repressive and permissive chromatin. Second in review on chromatin dynamics. EMBO Rep. 3 (3), 224–229. doi:10.1093/embo-reports/kvf053.

English, J., Son, J.M., Cardamone, M.D., Lee, C., Perissi, V., 2020. Decoding the rosetta stone of mitonuclear communication. Pharmacol. Res. 161, 105161. doi:10.1016/j.phrs.2020.105161.

Erales, J., Marchand, V., Panthu, B., Gillot, S., Belin, S., Ghayad, S.E., Garcia, M., Laforêts, F., Marcel, V., Baudin-Baillieu, A., Bertin, P., Couté, Y., Adrait, A., Meyer, M., Therizols, G., Yusupov, M., Namy, O., Ohlmann, T., Motorin, Y., Catez, F., Diaz, J.-J., 2017. Evidence for rRNA 2′-O-methylation plasticity: control of intrinsic translational capabilities of human ribosomes. Proc. Natl. Acad. Sci. U. S. A. 114 (49), 12934–12939. doi:10.1073/pnas.1707674114.

Eustermann, S., Patel, A.B., Hopfner, K.-P., He, Y., Korber, P., 2024. Energy-driven genome regulation by ATP-dependent chromatin remodellers. Nat. Rev. Mol. Cell Biol. 25 (4), 309–332. doi:10.1038/s41580-023-00683-y.

Field, A.E., Robertson, N.A., Wang, T., Havas, A., Ideker, T., Adams, P.D., 2018. DNA methylation clocks in aging: categories, causes, and consequences. Mol. Cell 71 (6), 882–895. doi:10.1016/j.molcel.2018.08.008.

Gallo Cantafio, M.E., Torcasio, R., Viglietto, G., Amodio, N., 2023. Non-coding RNA-dependent regulation of mitochondrial dynamics in cancer pathophysiology. Non-coding RNA 9 (1). doi:10.3390/ncrna9010016.

Gao, Q., Chen, F., Zhang, L., Wei, A., Wang, Y., Wu, Z., Cao, W., 2022. Inhibition of DNA methyltransferase aberrations reinstates antioxidant aging suppressors and ameliorates renal aging. Aging Cell 21 (1). doi:10.1111/acel.13526.

Gao, Y., Fang, J., 2021. RNA 5-methylcytosine modification and its emerging role as an epitranscriptomic mark. RNA Biol. 18 (S1), 117–127. doi:10.1080/15476286.2021.1950993.

Gast, M., Rauch, B.H., Haghikia, A., Nakagawa, S., Haas, J., Stroux, A., Schmidt, D., Schumann, P., Weiss, S., Jensen, L., Kratzer, A., Kraenkel, N., Müller, C., Börnigen, D., Hirose, T., Blankenberg, S., Escher, F., Kühl, A.A., Kuss, A.W., Meder, B., Landmesser, U., Zeller, T., Poller, W., 2019. Long noncoding RNA NEAT1 modulates immune cell functions and is suppressed in early onset myocardial infarction patients. Cardiovasc. Res. 115 (13), 1886–1906. doi:10.1093/cvr/cvz085.

Ghafouri-Fard, S., Shoorei, H., Taheri, M., 2020. Non-coding RNAs are involved in the response to oxidative stress. Biomed. Pharmacother. 127. doi:10.1016/j.biopha.2020.110228

Gigliotti, G., Joshi, R., Khalid, A., Widmer, D., Boccellino, M., Viggiano, D., 2024. Epigenetics, microbiome and personalized medicine: focus on kidney disease. Int. J. Mol. Sci. 25 (16). doi:10.3390/ijms25168592.

Giles, K.A., Gould, C.M., Du, Q., Skvortsova, K., Song, J.Z., Maddugoda, M.P., Achinger-Kawecka, J., Stirzaker, C., Clark, S.J., Taberlay, P.C., 2019. Integrated epigenomic analysis stratifies chromatin remodellers into distinct functional groups. Epigenetics Chromatin. 12 (1). doi:10.1186/s13072-019-0258-9.

Giordani, C., Silvestrini, A., Giuliani, A., Olivieri, F., Rippo, M.R., 2021. MicroRNAs as factors in bidirectional cross-talk between mitochondria and the nucleus during cellular senescence. Front. Physiol. 12. doi:10.3389/fphys.2021.734976

Giorgi, C., Marchi, S., Simoes, I.C.M., Ren, Z., Morciano, G., Perrone, M., Patalas-Krawczyk, P., Borchard, S., Jędrak, P., Pierzynowska, K., Szymański, J., Wang, D.Q., Portincasa, P., Węgrzyn, G., Zischka, H., Dobrzyn, P., Bonora, M., Duszynski, J., Rimessi, A., Karkucinska-Wieckowska, A., Dobrzyn, A., Szabadkai, G., Zavan, B., Oliveira, P.J., Sardao, V.A., Pinton, P., Wieckowski, M.R., 2018. Mitochondria and reactive oxygen species in aging and age-related diseases. Int. Rev. Cell Mol. Biol. 340, 209–344.

Gluck, C., Qiu, C., Han, S.Y., Palmer, M., Park, J., Ko, Y.-A., Guan, Y., Sheng, X., Hanson, R.L., Huang, J., Chen, Y., Park, A.S.D., Izquierdo, M.C., Mantzaris, I., Verma, A., Pullman, J., Li, H., Susztak, K., 2019. Kidney cytosine methylation changes improve renal function decline estimation in patients with diabetic kidney disease. Nat. Commun. 10 (1). doi:10.1038/s41467-019-10378-8.

Goncharov, A.O., Shender, V.O., Kuznetsova, K.G., Kliuchnikova, A.A., Moshkovskii, S.A., 2022. Interplay between A-to-I editing and splicing of RNA: a potential point of application for cancer therapy. Int. J. Mol. Sci. 23 (9). doi:10.3390/ijms23095240.

Gong, F., Miller, K.M., 2019. Histone methylation and the DNA damage response. Mutat. Res. Rev. Mutat. Res. 780, 37–47.

Gong, S., Qiao, H., Wang, J.-Y., Huang, S.-Y., He, S.-W., Zhao, Y., Tan, X.-R., Ye, M.-L., Li, J.-Y., Liang, Y.-L., Huang, S.-W., Chen, J., Zhu, X.-H., Liu, N., Li, Y.-Q., 2024. Ac4C modification of lncRNA SIMALR promotes nasopharyngeal carcinoma progression through activating eEF1A2 to facilitate ITGB4/ITGA6 translation. Oncogene 43 (38), 2868–2884. doi:10.1038/s41388-024-03133-x.

Goto, N., Suke, K., Yonezawa, N., Nishihara, H., Handa, T., Sato, Y., Kujirai, T., Kurumizaka, H., Yamagata, K., Kimura, H., 2024. ISWI chromatin remodeling complexes recruit NSD2 and H3K36me2 in pericentromeric heterochromatin. J. Cell Biol. 223 (8). doi:10.1083/jcb.202310084.

Grammatikaki, S., Katifelis, H., Farooqi, A.A., Stravodimos, K., Karamouzis, M.V., Souliotis, K., Varvaras, D., Gazouli, M., 2023. An overview of epigenetics in clear cell renal cell carcinoma. In Vivo 37 (1), 1–10. doi:10.21873/invivo.13049.

Greenberg, M.V.C., Bourc'his, D., 2019. The diverse roles of DNA methylation in mammalian development and disease. Nat. Rev. Mol. Cell Biol. 20 (10), 590–607. doi:10.1038/s41580-019-0159-6.

Greer, E.L., Shi, Y., 2012. Histone methylation: a dynamic mark in health, disease and inheritance. Nat. Rev. Genet. 13 (5), 343–357. doi:10.1038/nrg3173.

Grunstein, M., 1997. Histone acetylation in chromatin structure and transcription. Nature 389 (6649), 349–352. doi:10.1038/38664.

Gu, Y.-Y., Lu, F.-H., Huang, X.-R., Zhang, L., Mao, W., Yu, X.-Q., Liu, X.-S., Lan, H.-Y., 2021. Non-coding RNAs as biomarkers and therapeutic targets for diabetic kidney disease. Front. Pharmacol. 11. doi:10.3389/fphar.2020.583528

Guo, C., Dong, G., Liang, X., Dong, Z., 2019. Epigenetic regulation in AKI and kidney repair: mechanisms and therapeutic implications. Nat. Rev. Nephrol. 15 (4), 220–239. doi:10.1038/s41581-018-0103-6.

Guo, C., Pei, L., Xiao, X., Wei, Q., Chen, J.-K., Ding, H.-F., Huang, S., Fan, G., Shi, H., Dong, Z., 2017. DNA methylation protects against cisplatin-induced kidney injury by regulating specific genes, including interferon regulatory factor 8. Kidney Int. 92 (5), 1194–1205.

Guo, Y., Guan, T., Shafiq, K., Yu, Q., Jiao, X., Na, D., Li, M., Zhang, G., Kong, J., 2023. Mitochondrial dysfunction in aging. Ageing Res. Rev. 88. doi:10.1016/j.arr.2023.101955

Hakem, R., 2008. DNA-damage repair; the good, the bad, and the ugly. EMBO J. 27 (4), 589–605. doi:10.1038/emboj.2008.15.

Hammond, C.M., Strømme, C.B., Huang, H., Patel, D.J., Groth, A., 2017. Histone chaperone networks shaping chromatin function. Nat. Rev. Mol. Cell Biol. 18 (3), 141–158. doi:10.1038/nrm.2016.159.

Han, J.-J., Wang, X.-Q., Zhang, X.-A., 2022. Functional interactions between lncRNAs/circRNAs and miRNAs: insights into rheumatoid arthritis. Front. Immunol. 13. doi:10.3389/fimmu.2022.810317.

Han, X., Chen, H., Gong, H., Tang, X., Huang, N., Xu, W., Tai, H., Zhang, G., Zhao, T., Gong, C., Wang, S., Yang, Y., Xiao, H., 2020. Autolysosomal degradation of cytosolic chromatin fragments antagonizes oxidative stress-induced senescence. J. Biol. Chem. 295 (14), 4451–4463. doi:10.1074/jbc.RA119.010734.

Han, X., Sun, Z., 2020. Epigenetic regulation of KL (klotho) via H3K27me3 (histone 3 lysine [K] 27 trimethylation) in renal tubule cells. Hypertension 75 (5), 1233–1241. doi:10.1161/HYPERTENSIONAHA.120.14642.

Hannum, G., Guinney, J., Zhao, L., Zhang, L., Hughes, G., Sadda, S., Klotzle, B., Bibikova, M., Fan, J.-B., Gao, Y., Deconde, R., Chen, M., Rajapakse, I., Friend, S., Ideker, T., Zhang, K., 2013. Genome-wide methylation profiles reveal quantitative views of human aging rates. Mol. Cell 49 (2), 359–367. doi:10.1016/j.molcel.2012.10.016.

Harman, D., 1956. Aging: a theory based on free radical and radiation chemistry. J. Gerontol. 11 (3), 298–300. doi:10.1093/geronj/11.3.298.

Harris, A.S., Aratani, S., Johmura, Y., Suzuki, N., Dan, L., Nakanishi, M., 2023. In vivo dynamics of senescence in rhabdomyolysis-induced acute kidney injury. Biochem. Biophys. Res. Commun. 673, 121–130. doi:10.1016/j.bbrc.2023.06.046.

Harrison, L.J., Bose, D., 2022. Enhancer RNAs step forward: new insights into enhancer function. Development 149 (16). doi:10.1242/dev.200398.

Hartl, F.U., Bracher, A., Hayer-Hartl, M., 2011. Molecular chaperones in protein folding and proteostasis. Nature 475 (7356), 324–332. doi:10.1038/nature10317.

He, L., Wei, Q., Liu, J., Yi, M., Liu, Y., Liu, H., Sun, L., Peng, Y., Liu, F., Venkatachalam, M.A., Dong, Z., 2017. AKI on CKD: heightened injury, suppressed repair, and the underlying mechanisms. Kidney Int. 92 (5), 1071–1083.

Herridge, R.P., Dolata, J., Migliori, V., de Santis Alves, C., Borges, F., Schorn, A.J., van Ex, F., Lin, A., Bajczyk, M., Parent, J.-S., Leonardi, T., Hendrick, A., Kouzarides, T., Martienssen, R.A., 2024. Pseudouridine guides germline small RNA transport and epigenetic inheritance. Nat. Struct. Mol. Biol. doi:10.1038/s41594-024-01392-6.

Hewitt, G., Jurk, D., Marques, F.D.M., Correia-Melo, C., Hardy, T., Gackowska, A., Anderson, R., Taschuk, M., Mann, J., Passos, J.F., 2012. Telomeres are favoured targets of a persistent DNA damage response in ageing and stress-induced senescence. Nat. Commun. 3. doi:10.1038/ncomms1708

Heylen, L., Thienpont, B., Busschaert, P., Sprangers, B., Kuypers, D., Moisse, M., Lerut, E., Lambrechts, D., Naesens, M., 2019. Age-related changes in DNA methylation affect renal histology and post-transplant fibrosis. Kidney Int. 96 (5), 1195–1204. doi:10.1016/j.kint.2019.06.018.

Hickl, D., Drews, F., Girke, C., Zimmer, D., Mühlhaus, T., Hauth, J., Nordström, K., Trentmann, O., Neuhaus, E.H., Scheuring, D., Fehlmann, T., Keller, A., Simon, M., Möhlmann, T., 2021. Differential degradation of RNA species by autophagy-related pathways in Arabidopsis. J. Exp. Bot. 72 (20), 6867–6881. doi:10.1093/jxb/erab321.

Hirata, H., Hinoda, Y., Shahryari, V., Deng, G., Nakajima, K., Tabatabai, Z.L., Ishii, N., Dahiya, R., 2015. Long noncoding RNA MALAT1 promotes aggressive renal cell carcinoma through Ezh2 and interacts with miR-205. Cancer Res. 75 (7), 1322–1331. doi:10.1158/0008-5472.CAN-14-2931.

Hong, Y.A., Kim, J.E., Jo, M., Ko, G.-J., 2020. The role of sirtuins in kidney diseases. Int. J. Mol. Sci. 21 (18), 1–21. doi:10.3390/ijms21186686.

Horvath, S., 2013. DNA methylation age of human tissues and cell types. Genome Biol. 14 (10). doi:10.1186/gb-2013-14-10-r115.

Horvath, S., Oshima, J., Martin, G.M., Lu, A.T., Quach, A., Cohen, H., Felton, S., Matsuyama, M., Lowe, D., Kabacik, S., Wilson, J.G., Reiner, A.P., Maierhofer, A., Flunkert, J., Aviv, A., Hou, L., Baccarelli, A.A., Li, Y., Stewart, J.D., Whitsel, E.A., Ferrucci, L., Matsuyama, S., Raj, K., 2018. Epigenetic clock for skin and blood cells applied to hutchinson gilford progeria syndrome and ex vivo studies. Aging 10 (7), 1758–1775. doi:10.18632/aging.101508.

Hu, B., Zhong, L., Weng, Y., Peng, L., Huang, Y., Zhao, Y., Liang, X.-J., 2020. Therapeutic siRNA: state of the art. Signal Transduct. Target. Ther. 5 (1). doi:10.1038/s41392-020-0207-x.

Hu, W., Chan, C.S., Wu, R., Zhang, C., Sun, Y., Song, J.S., Tang, L.H., Levine, A.J., Feng, Z., 2010. Negative regulation of tumor suppressor p53 by microRNA miR-504. Mol. Cell 38 (5), 689–699. doi:10.1016/j.molcel.2010.05.027.

Hu, W.L., Jin, L., Xu, A., Wang, Y.F., Thorne, R.F., Zhang, X.D., Wu, M., 2018. GUARDIN is a p53-responsive long non-coding RNA that is essential for genomic stability. Nat. Cell Biol. 20 (4), 492–502. doi:10.1038/s41556-018-0066-7.

Huang, W., Hickson, L.J., Eirin, A., Kirkland, J.L., Lerman, L.O., 2022a. Cellular senescence: the good, the bad and the unknown. Nat. Rev. Nephrol. 18 (10), 611–627. doi:10.1038/s41581-022-00601-z.

Huang, X., Guo, H., Wang, L., Yang, L., Shao, Z., Zhang, W., 2022b. Recent advances in crosstalk between N6-methyladenosine (m6A) modification and circular RNAs in cancer. Mol. Ther. Nucleic Acids 27, 947–955. doi:10.1016/j.omtn.2022.01.013.

Huang, Z.-H., Du, Y.-P., Wen, J.-T., Lu, B.-F., Zhao, Y., 2022c. snoRNAs: functions and mechanisms in biological processes, and roles in tumor pathophysiology. Cell Death Discov. 8 (1). doi:10.1038/s41420-022-01056-8.

Hung, T., Wang, Y., Lin, M.F., Koegel, A.K., Kotake, Y., Grant, G.D., Horlings, H.M., Shah, N., Umbricht, C., Wang, P., Wang, Y., Kong, B., Langerød, A., Børresen-Dale, A.-L., Kim, S.K., van de Vijver, M., Sukumar, S., Whitfield, M.L., Kellis, M., Xiong, Y., Wong, D.J., Chang, H.Y., 2011. Extensive and coordinated transcription of noncoding RNAs within cell-cycle promoters. Nat. Genet. 43 (7), 621–629. doi:10.1038/ng.848.

Hyndman, K.A., 2020. Histone deacetylases in kidney physiology and acute kidney injury. Semin. Nephrol. 40 (2), 138–147.

Ichii, O., Otsuka, S., Sasaki, N., Namiki, Y., Hashimoto, Y., Kon, Y., 2012. Altered expression of microRNA miR-146a correlates with the development of chronic renal inflammation. Kidney Int. 81 (3), 280–292. doi:10.1038/ki.2011.345.

Ikura, T., Tashiro, S., Kakino, A., Shima, H., Jacob, N., Amunugama, R., Yoder, K., Izumi, S., Kuraoka, I., Tanaka, K., Kimura, H., Ikura, M., Nishikubo, S., Ito, T., Muto, A., Miyagawa, K., Takeda, S., Fishel, R., Igarashi, K., Kamiya, K., 2007. DNA damage-dependent acetylation and ubiquitination of H2AX enhances chromatin dynamics. Mol. Cell. Biol. 27 (20), 7028–7040. doi:10.1128/mcb.00579-07.

Imai, S.-I., Guarente, L., 2016. It takes two to tango: nad+ and sirtuins in aging/longevity control. Npj Aging Mech. Dis. 2 (1). doi:10.1038/npjamd.2016.17.

Irifuku, T., Doi, S., Sasaki, K., Doi, T., Nakashima, A., Ueno, T., Yamada, K., Arihiro, K., Kohno, N., Masaki, T., 2016. Inhibition of H3K9 histone methyltransferase G9a attenuates renal fibrosis and retains klotho expression. Kidney Int. 89 (1), 147–157. doi:10.1038/ki.2015.291.

Jastroch, M., Divakaruni, A.S., Mookerjee, S., Treberg, J.R., Brand, M.D., 2010. Mitochondrial proton and electron leaks. Essays Biochem. 47, 53–67. doi:10.1042/bse0470053.

Jiang, L., Liu, X., Hu, X., Gao, L., Zeng, H., Wang, X., Huang, Y., Zhu, W., Wang, J., Wen, J., Meng, X., Wu, Y., 2022. A modification of TIMP2 mRNA promotes podocyte injury in diabetic nephropathy. Mol. Ther. 30 (4), 1721–1740.

Jin, G., Xu, M., Zou, M., Duan, S., 2020. The processing, gene regulation, biological functions, and clinical relevance of N4-acetylcytidine on RNA: a systematic review. Mol. Ther. Nucleic Acids 20, 13–24. doi:10.1016/j.omtn.2020.01.037.

Jung, H.R., Lee, J., Hong, S.-P., Shin, N., Cho, A., Shin, D.-J., Choi, J.W., Kim, J.-I., Lee, J.P., Cho, S.-Y., 2024. Targeting the m6A RNA methyltransferase METTL3 attenuates the development of kidney fibrosis. Exp. Mol. Med. 56 (2), 355–369. doi:10.1038/s12276-024-01159-5.

Kato, M., Arce, L., Natarajan, R., 2009. MicroRNAs and their role in progressive kidney diseases. Clin. J. Am. Soc. Nephrol. 4 (7), 1255–1266. doi:10.2215/CJN.00520109.

Kazak, L., Reyes, A., Holt, I.J., 2012. Minimizing the damage: repair pathways keep mitochondrial DNA intact. Nat. Rev. Mol. Cell Biol. 13 (10), 659–671. doi:10.1038/nrm3439.

Kelly, G., Kataura, T., Panek, J., Ma, G., Salmonowicz, H., Davis, A., Kendall, H., Brookes, C., Ayine-Tora, D.M., Banks, P., Nelson, G., Dobby, L., Pitrez, P.R., Booth, L., Costello, L., Richardson, G.D., Lovat, P., Przyborski, S., Ferreira, L., Greaves, L., Szczepanowska, K., von Zglinicki, T., Miwa, S., Brown, M., Flagler, M., Oblong, J.E.,

Bascom, C.C., Carroll, B., Reynisson, J., Korolchuk, V.I., 2024. Suppressed basal mitophagy drives cellular aging phenotypes that can be reversed by a p62-targeting small molecule. Dev. Cell 59 (15), 1924–1939. doi:10.1016/j.devcel.2024.04.020.

Khoshnevis, S., Dreggors-Walker, R.E., Marchand, V., Motorin, Y., Ghalei, H., 2022. Ribosomal RNA 20-O-methylations regulate translation by impacting ribosome dynamics. Proc. Natl. Acad. Sci. U. S. A. 119 (12). doi:10.1073/pnas.2117334119.

Kim, E., Kim, Y.K., Lee, S.-J.V., 2021. Emerging functions of circular RNA in aging. Trends Genet. 37 (9), 819–829. doi:10.1016/j.tig.2021.04.014.

Kim, G.D., Shin, S.-I., Jung, S.W., An, H., Choi, S.Y., Eun, M., Jun, C.-D., Lee, S., Park, J., 2024. Cell type- and age-specific expression of lncRNAs across kidney cell types. J. Am. Soc. Nephrol. 35 (7), 870–885. doi:10.1681/ASN.0000000000000354.

Kim, K.H., Lee, C.B., 2024. Socialized mitochondria: mitonuclear crosstalk in stress. Exp. Mol. Med. 56 (5), 1033–1042. doi:10.1038/s12276-024-01211-4.

Kim, M.-G., Yang, J., Ko, Y.S., Lee, H.Y., Oh, S.W., Cho, W.Y., Jo, S.-K., 2019. Impact of aging on transition of acute kidney injury to chronic kidney disease. Sci. Rep. 9 (1). doi:10.1038/s41598-019-54585-1.

Kim, T.-K., Hemberg, M., Gray, J.M., 2015. Enhancer RNAs: a class of long noncoding RNAs synthesized at enhancers. Cold Spring Harb. Perspect. Biol. 7 (1). doi:10.1101/cshperspect.a018622.

Kinner, A., Wu, W., Staudt, C., Iliakis, G., 2008. Gamma-H2AX in recognition and signaling of DNA double-strand breaks in the context of chromatin. Nucleic Acids Res. 36 (17), 5678–5694. doi:10.1093/nar/gkn550.

Kinser, H.E., Pincus, Z., 2020. MicroRNAs as modulators of longevity and the aging process. Hum. Genet. 139 (3), 291–308. doi:10.1007/s00439-019-02046-0.

Komar, D., Juszczynski, P., 2020. Rebelled epigenome: histone H3S10 phosphorylation and H3S10 kinases in cancer biology and therapy. Clin. Epigenetics 12 (1). doi:10.1186/s13148-020-00941-2.

Konno, M., Koseki, J., Asai, A., Yamagata, A., Shimamura, T., Motooka, D., Okuzaki, D., Kawamoto, K., Mizushima, T., Eguchi, H., Takiguchi, S., Satoh, T., Mimori, K., Ochiya, T., Doki, Y., Ofusa, K., Mori, M., Ishii, H., 2019. Distinct methylation levels of mature microRNAs in gastrointestinal cancers. Nat. Commun. 10 (1). doi:10.1038/s41467-019-11826-1.

Kooistra, S.M., Helin, K., 2012. Post-translational modifications: molecular mechanisms and potential functions of histone demethylases. Nat. Rev. Mol. Cell Biol. 13 (5), 297–311. doi:10.1038/nrm3327.

Kourtidou, C., Tziomalos, K., 2023. The role of histone modifications in the pathogenesis of diabetic kidney disease. Int. J. Mol. Sci. 24 (6). doi:10.3390/ijms24066007.

Koyuncu, S., Loureiro, R., Lee, H.J., Wagle, P., Krueger, M., Vilchez, D., 2021. Rewiring of the ubiquitinated proteome determines ageing in C. elegans. Nature 596 (7871), 285–290. doi:10.1038/s41586-021-03781-z.

Krishnan, V., Chow, M.Z.Y., Wang, Z., Zhang, L., Liu, B., Liu, X., Zhou, Z., 2011. Histone H4 lysine 16 hypoacetylation is associated with defective DNA repair and premature senescence in Zmpste24-deficient mice. Proc. Natl. Acad. Sci. U. S. A. 108 (30), 12325–12330. doi:10.1073/pnas.1102789108.

Kristensen, L.S., Andersen, M.S., Stagsted, L.V.W., Ebbesen, K.K., Hansen, T.B., Kjems, J., 2019. The biogenesis, biology and characterization of circular RNAs. Nat. Rev. Genet. 20 (11), 675–691. doi:10.1038/s41576-019-0158-7.

Kudrin, P., Singh, A., Meierhofer, D., Kuśnierczyk, A., Ørom, U.A.V., 2024. N4-acetylcytidine (ac4C) promotes mRNA localization to stress granules. EMBO Rep. 25 (4), 1814–1834. doi:10.1038/s44319-024-00098-6.

Kumar, M., Lu, Z., Takwi, A.A.L., Chen, W., Callander, N.S., Ramos, K.S., Young, K.H., Li, Y., 2011. Negative regulation of the tumor suppressor p53 gene by microRNAs. Oncogene 30 (7), 843–853. doi:10.1038/onc.2010.457.

Kwekel, J.C., Vijay, V., Desai, V.G., Moland, C.L., Fuscoe, J.C., 2015. Age and sex differences in kidney microRNA expression during the life span of F344 rats. Biol. Sex Differ. 6 (1). doi:10.1186/s13293-014-0019-1.

Lascaux, P., Hoslett, G., Tribble, S., Trugenberger, C., Antičević, I., Otten, C., Torrecilla, I., Koukouravas, S., Zhao, Y., Yang, H., Aljarbou, F., Ruggiano, A., Song, W., Peron, C., Deangeli, G., Domingo, E., Bancroft, J., Carrique, L., Johnson, E., Vendrell, I., Fischer, R., Ng, A.W.T., Ngeow, J., D'Angiolella, V., Raimundo, N., Maughan, T., Popović, M., Milošević, I., Ramadan, K., 2024. TEX264 drives selective autophagy of DNA lesions to promote DNA repair and cell survival. Cell 187 (20). doi:10.1016/j.cell.2024.08.020.

Lasseigne, B.N., Brooks, J.D., 2018. The role of DNA methylation in renal cell carcinoma. Mol. Diagn. Ther. 22 (4), 431–442. doi:10.1007/s40291-018-0337-9.

Le, M.T.N., Teh, C., Shyh-Chang, N., Xie, H., Zhou, B., Korzh, V., Lodish, H.F., Lim, B., 2009. MicroRNA-125b is a novel negative regulator of p53. Genes Dev. 23 (7), 862–876. doi:10.1101/gad.1767609.

Lee, H.-S., Park, J.-H., Kim, S.-J., Kwon, S.-J., Kwon, J., 2010. A cooperative activation loop among SWI/SNF, gamma-H2AX and H3 acetylation for DNA double-strand break repair. EMBO J. 29 (8), 1434–1445. doi:10.1038/emboj.2010.27.

Lee, J.-H., Kim, E.W., Croteau, D.L., Bohr, V.A., 2020. Heterochromatin: an epigenetic point of view in aging. Exp. Mol. Med. 52 (9), 1466–1474. doi:10.1038/s12276-020-00497-4.

Lee, S., Kopp, F., Chang, T.-C., Sataluri, A., Chen, B., Sivakumar, S., Yu, H., Xie, Y., Mendell, J.T., 2016. Noncoding RNA NORAD regulates genomic stability by sequestering PUMILIO proteins. Cell 164 (1–2), 69–80. doi:10.1016/j.cell.2015.12.017.

Lee, W.L., Sinha, A., Lam, L.N., Loo, H.L., Liang, J., Ho, P., Cui, L., Chan, C.S.C., Begley, T., Kline, K.A., Dedon, P., 2023. An RNA modification enzyme directly senses reactive oxygen species for translational regulation in Enterococcus faecalis. Nat. Commun. 14 (1). doi:10.1038/s41467-023-39790-x.

Lenart, P., Novak, J., Bienertova-Vasku, J., 2018. PIWI-piRNA pathway: setting the pace of aging by reducing DNA damage. Mech. Ageing Dev. 173, 29–38. doi:10.1016/j.mad.2018.03.009.

Li, J., Gao, F., Wei, L., Chen, L., Qu, N., Zeng, L., Luo, Y., Huang, X., Jiang, H., 2022. Predict the role of lncRNA in kidney aging based on RNA sequencing. BMC Genom. 23 (1). doi:10.1186/s12864-022-08479-8.

Li, J., Huang, S., Shi, L., Chen, G., Liu, X., Liu, M., Guo, G., 2024a. Interaction between long noncoding RNA and microRNA in lung inflammatory diseases. Immun. Inflamm. Dis. 12 (1). doi:10.1002/iid3.1129.

Li, J., Wang, L., Hahn, Q., Nowak, R.P., Viennet, T., Orellana, E.A., Roy Burman, S.S., Yue, H., Hunkeler, M., Fontana, P., Wu, H., Arthanari, H., Fischer, E.S., Gregory, R.I., 2023a. Structural basis of regulated m7G tRNA modification by METTL1–WDR4. Nature. 613 (7943), 391–397. doi:10.1038/s41586-022-05566-4.

Li, K.Y., Tam, C.H.T., Liu, H., Day, S., Lim, C.K.P., Wing Yee, S., Huang, C., Jiang, G., Shi, M., Lee, H.M., Lan, H.-Y., Szeto, C.-C., Hanson, R.L., Nelson, R.G., Susztak, K., Chan, J.C.N., Yip, K.Y., Ma, R.C.W., 2023b. DNA methylation markers for kidney function and progression of diabetic kidney disease. Nat. Commun. 14 (1). doi:10.1038/s41467-023-37837-7.

Li, L., Xiang, T., Guo, J., Guo, F., Wu, Y., Feng, H., Liu, J., Tao, S., Fu, P., Ma, L., 2024b. Inhibition of ACSS2-mediated histone crotonylation alleviates kidney fibrosis via IL-1β-dependent macrophage activation and tubular cell senescence. Nat. Commun. 15 (1). doi:10.1038/s41467-024-47315-3.

Li, S., Livingston, M.J., Ma, Z., Hu, X., Wen, L., Ding, H.-F., Zhou, D., Dong, Z., 2023c. Tubular cell senescence promotes maladaptive kidney repair and chronic kidney disease after cisplatin nephrotoxicity. JCI Insight 8 (8). doi:10.1172/jci.insight.166643.

Li, S.Y., Susztak, K., 2016. The long noncoding RNA Tug1 connects metabolic changes with kidney disease in podocytes. J. Clin. Invest. 126 (11), 4072–4075.

Li, X., Ding, D., Yao, J., Zhou, B., Shen, T., Qi, Y., Ni, T., Wei, G., 2019. Chromatin remodeling factor BAZ1A regulates cellular senescence in both cancer and normal cells. Life Sci. 229, 225–232.

Li, X., Li, C., Li, X., Cui, P., Li, Q., Guo, Q., Han, H., Liu, S., Sun, G., 2016. Involvement of histone lysine methylation in p21 gene expression in rat kidney in vivo and rat mesangial cells in vitro under diabetic conditions. J. Diabetes Res. 2016. doi:10.1155/2016/3853242

Li, Y., Yi, Y., Gao, X., Wang, X., Zhao, D., Wang, R., Zhang, L.-S., Gao, B., Zhang, Y., Zhang, L., Cao, Q., Chen, K., 2024c. 2′-O-methylation at internal sites on mRNA promotes mRNA stability. Mol. Cell 84 (12). doi:10.1016/j.molcel.2024.04.011.

Lima, T., Li, T.Y., Mottis, A., Auwerx, J., 2022. Pleiotropic effects of mitochondria in aging. Nat. Aging 2 (3), 199–213. doi:10.1038/s43587-022-00191-2.

Liu, C., Dou, X., Zhao, Y., Zhang, L., Zhang, L., Dai, Q., Liu, J., Wu, T., Xiao, Y., He, C., 2024a. IGF2BP3 promotes mRNA degradation through internal m7G modification. Nat. Commun. 15 (1). doi:10.1038/s41467-024-51634-w.

Liu, F., Huang, J., Zhang, C., Xie, Y., Cao, Y., Tao, L., Tang, H., Lin, J., Hammes, H.-P., Huang, K., Yi, F., Su, H., Zhang, C., 2022. Regulation of podocyte injury by CircHIPK3/FUS complex in diabetic kidney disease. Int. J. Biol. Sci. 18 (15), 5624–5640. doi:10.7150/ijbs.75994.

Liu, H., 2021. The roles of histone deacetylases in kidney development and disease. Clin. Exp. Nephrol. 25 (3), 215–223. doi:10.1007/s10157-020-01995-5.

Liu, H., Zhen, C., Xie, J., Luo, Z., Zeng, L., Zhao, G., Lu, S., Zhuang, H., Fan, H., Li, X., Liu, Z., Lin, S., Jiang, H., Chen, Y., Cheng, J., Cao, Z., Dai, K., Shi, J., Wang, Z., Hu, Y., Meng, T., Zhou, C., Han, Z., Huang, H., Zhou, Q., He, P., Feng, D., 2024b. TFAM is an autophagy receptor that limits inflammation by binding to cytoplasmic mitochondrial DNA. Nat. Cell Biol. 26 (6), 878–891. doi:10.1038/s41556-024-01419-6.

Liu, J., Yao, L., Zhang, M., Jiang, J., Yang, M., Wang, Y., 2019. Downregulation of LncRNA-XIST inhibited development of non-small cell lung cancer by activating miR-335/SOD2/ROS signal pathway mediated pyroptotic cell death. Aging 11 (18), 7830–7846. doi:10.18632/aging.102291.

Ljungman, M., Parks, L., Hulbatte, R., Bedi, K., 2019. The role of H3K79 methylation in transcription and the DNA damage response. Mutat. Res. Rev. Mutat. Res. 780, 48–54.

Lou, M.-M., Tang, X.-Q., Wang, G.-M., He, J., Luo, F., Guan, M.-F., Wang, F., Zou, H., Wang, J.-Y., Zhang, Q., Xu, M.-J., Shi, Q.-L., Shen, L.-B., Ma, G.-M., Wu, Y., Zhang, Y.-Y., Liang, A.-B., Wang, T.-H., Xiong, L.-L., Wang, J., Xu, J., Wang, W.-Y., 2021. Long noncoding RNA BS-DRL1 modulates the DNA damage response and genome stability by interacting with HMGB1 in neurons. Nat. Commun. 12 (1). doi:10.1038/s41467-021-24236-z.

Lu, A.T., Fei, Z., Haghani, A., Robeck, T.R., Zoller, J.A., Li, C.Z., Lowe, R., Yan, Q., Zhang, J., Vu, H., Ablaeva, J., Acosta-Rodriguez, V.A., Adams, D.M., Almunia, J., Aloysius, A., Ardehali, R., Arneson, A., Baker, C.S., Banks, G., Belov, K., Bennett, N.C., Black, P., Blumstein, D.T., Bors, E.K., Breeze, C.E., Brooke, R.T., Brown, J.L., Carter, G.G., Caulton, A., Cavin, J.M., Chakrabarti, L., Chatzistamou, I., Chen, H., Cheng, K., Chiavellini, P., Choi, O.W., Clarke, S.M., Cooper, L.N., Cossette, M.L., Day, J., DeYoung, J., DiRocco, S., Dold, C., Ehmke, E.E., Emmons, C.K., Emmrich, S., Erbay, E., Erlacher-Reid, C., Faulkes, C.G., Ferguson, S.H., Finno, C.J., Flower, J.E., Gaillard, J.M., Garde, E., Gerber, L., Gladyshev, V.N., Gorbunova, V., Goya, R.G., Grant, M.J., Green, C.B., Hales, E.N., Hanson, M.B., Hart, D.W., Haulena, M., Herrick, K., Hogan, A.N., Hogg, C.J., Hore, T.A., Huang, T., Izpisua Belmonte, J.C., Jasinska, A.J., Jones, G., Jourdain, E., Kashpur, O., Katcher, H., Katsumata, E., Kaza, V., Kiaris, H., Kobor, M.S., Kordowitzki, P., Koski, W.R., Krützen, M., Kwon, S.B., Larison, B., Lee, S.G., Lehmann, M., Lemaitre, J.F., Levine, A.J., Li, C., Li, X., Lim, A.R., Lin, D.T.S., Lindemann, D.M., Little, T.J., Macoretta, N., Maddox, D., Matkin, C.O., Mattison, J.A., McClure, M., Mergl, J., Meudt, J.J., Montano, G.A., Mozhui, K., Munshi-South, J., Naderi, A., Nagy, M., Narayan, P., Nathanielsz, P.W., Nguyen, N.B., Niehrs, C., O'Brien, J.K., O'Tierney Ginn, P., Odom, D.T., Ophir, A.G., Osborn, S., Ostrander, E.A., Parsons, K.M., Paul, K.C., Pellegrini, M., Peters, K.J., Pedersen, A.B., Petersen, J.L., Pietersen, D.W., Pinho, G.M., Plassais, J., Poganik, J.R., Prado, N.A., Reddy, P., Rey, B., Ritz, B.R., Robbins, J., Rodriguez, M., Russell, J., Rydkina, E., Sailer, L.L., Salmon, A.B., Sanghavi, A., Schachtschneider, K.M., Schmitt, D., Schmitt, T., Schomacher, L., Schook, L.B., Sears, K.E., Seifert, A.W., Seluanov, A., Shafer, A.B.A., Shanmuganayagam, D., Shindyapina, A.V., Simmons, M., Singh, K., Sinha, I., Slone, J., Snell, R.G., Soltanmaohammadi, E., Spangler, M.L., Spriggs, M.C., Staggs, L., Stedman, N., Steinman, K.J., Stewart, D.T., Sugrue, V.J., Szladovits, B., Takahashi, J.S., Takasugi, M., Teeling, E.C., Thompson, M.J., Van Bonn, B., Vernes, S.C., Villar, D., Vinters, H.V., Wallingford, M.C., Wang, N., Wayne, R.K., Wilkinson, G.S., Williams, C.K., Williams, R.W., Yang, X.W., Yao, M., Young, B.G., Zhang, B., Zhang, Z., Zhao, P., Zhao, Y., Zhou, W., Zimmermann, J., Ernst, J., Raj, K., Horvath, S., 2023. Universal DNA methylation age across mammalian tissues. Nat. Aging 3 (9), 1144–1166. doi:10.1038/s43587-023-00462-6.

Lu, C., Zhou, D., Wang, Q., Liu, W., Yu, F., Wu, F., Chen, C., 2020. Crosstalk of MicroRNAs and oxidative stress in the pathogenesis of cancer. Oxid. Med. Cell. Longev. 2020. doi:10.1155/2020/2415324

Luo, L., Martin, S.C., Parkington, J., Cadena, S.M., Zhu, J., Ibebunjo, C., Summermatter, S., Londraville, N., Patora-Komisarska, K., Widler, L., Zhai, H., Trendelenburg, A.-U., Glass, D.J., Shi, J., 2019. HDAC4 controls muscle homeostasis through deacetylation of myosin heavy chain, PGC-1α, and Hsc70. Cell Rep. 29 (3). doi:10.1016/j.celrep.2019.09.023.

Ma, T., Li, H., Liu, H., Peng, Y., Lin, T., Deng, Z., Jia, N., Chen, Z., Wang, P., 2022. Neat1 promotes acute kidney injury to chronic kidney disease by facilitating tubular epithelial cells apoptosis via sequestering miR-129-5p. Mol. Ther. 30 (10), 3313–3332.

Ma, Z., Li, L., Livingston, M.J., Zhang, D., Mi, Q., Zhang, M., Ding, H.-F., Huo, Y., Mei, C., Dong, Z., 2020. p53/microRNA-214/ULK1 axis impairs renal tubular autophagy in diabetic kidney disease. J. Clin. Invest. 130 (9), 5011–5026.

Mah, L.-J., El-Osta, A., Karagiannis, T.C., 2010. GammaH2AX as a molecular marker of aging and disease. Epigenetics 5 (2), 129–136.

Mahtal, N., Lenoir, O., Tinel, C., Anglicheau, D., Tharaux, P.-L., 2022. MicroRNAs in kidney injury and disease. Nat. Rev. Nephrol. 18 (10), 643–662. doi:10.1038/s41581-022-00608-6.

Majidinia, M., Mir, S.M., Mirza-Aghazadeh-Attari, M., Asghari, R., Kafil, H.S., Safa, A., Mahmoodpoor, A., Yousefi, B., 2020. MicroRNAs, DNA damage response and ageing. Biogerontology 21 (3), 275–291. doi:10.1007/s10522-020-09862-2.

Mandal, K., Tomar, S.K., Santra, M.K., 2024. Decoding the ubiquitin language: orchestrating transcription initiation and gene expression through chromatin remodelers and histones. Gene 904. doi:10.1016/j.gene.2024.148218

Mattick, J.S., Amaral, P.P., Carninci, P., Carpenter, S., Chang, H.Y., Chen, -L.-L., Chen, R., Dean, C., Dinger, M.E., Fitzgerald, K.A., Gingeras, T.R., Guttman, M., Hirose, T., Huarte, M., Johnson, R., Kanduri, C., Kapranov, P., Lawrence, J.B., Lee, J.T., Mendell, J.T., Mercer, T.R., Moore, K.J., Nakagawa, S., Rinn, J.L., Spector, D.L., Ulitsky, I., Wan, Y., Wilusz, J.E., Wu, M., 2023. Long non-coding RNAs: definitions, functions, challenges and recommendations. Nat. Rev. Mol. Cell Biol. 24 (6), 430–447. doi:10.1038/s41580-022-00566-8.

Maxwell, S., Okabe, J., Kaipananickal, H., Rodriguez, H., Khurana, I., Al-Hasani, K., Chow, B.S.M., Pitsillou, E., Karagiannis, T.C., Jandeleit-Dahm, K., Ma, R.C.W., Huang, Y., Chan, J.C.N., Cooper, M.E., El-Osta, A., 2024. Set7 methyltransferase and phenotypic switch in diabetic glomerular endothelial cells. J. Am. Soc. Nephrol. 35 (6), 733–748. doi:10.1681/ASN.0000000000000345.

Melo, C.A., Drost, J., Wijchers, P.J., van de Werken, H., de Wit, E., Vrielink, J.A.F.O., Elkon, R., Melo, S.A., Léveillé, N., Kalluri, R., de Laat, W., Agami, R., 2013. ERNAs are required for p53-dependent enhancer activity and gene transcription. Mol. Cell 49 (3), 524–535. doi:10.1016/j.molcel.2012.11.021.

Meng, X.-M., Chung, A.C.K., Lan, H.Y., 2013. Role of the TGF-β/BMP-7/Smad pathways in renal diseases. Clin. Sci. 124 (4), 243–254. doi:10.1042/CS20120252.

Michalak, E.M., Burr, M.L., Bannister, A.J., Dawson, M.A., 2019. The roles of DNA, RNA and histone methylation in ageing and cancer. Nat. Rev. Mol. Cell Biol. 20 (10), 573–589. doi:10.1038/s41580-019-0143-1.

Michelini, F., Pitchiaya, S., Vitelli, V., Sharma, S., Gioia, U., Pessina, F., Cabrini, M., Wang, Y., Capozzo, I., Iannelli, F., Matti, V., Francia, S., Shivashankar, G.V., Walter, N.G., d'adda di Fagagna, F., 2017. Damage-induced lncRNAs control the DNA damage response through interaction with DDRNAs at individual double-strand breaks. Nat. Cell Biol. 19 (12), 1400–1411. doi:10.1038/ncb3643.

Mimura, I., Chen, Z., Natarajan, R., 2024. Epigenetic alterations and memory: key players in the development/progression of chronic kidney disease promoted by acute kidney injury and diabetes. Kidney Int. Available from: https://www.sciencedirect.com/science/article/pii/S0085253824009189#sec8. doi:10.1016/j.kint.2024.10.031.

Mitra, R., Lin, C.-C., Eischen, C.M., Bandyopadhyay, S., Zhao, Z., 2015. Concordant dysregulation of miR-5p and miR-3p arms of the same precursor microRNA may be a mechanism in inducing cell proliferation and tumorigenesis: a lung cancer study. RNA. 21 (6), 1055–1065. doi:10.1261/rna.048132.114.

Miura, R., Mimura, I., Saigusa, H., Yamazaki, T., Tanemoto, F., Kurata, Y., Sato, D., Tanaka, T., Nangaku, M., 2023. Chromatin remodeling factor, INO80, inhibits PMAIP1 in renal tubular cells via exchange of histone variant H2A.Z. for H2A. Sci. Rep. 13 (1). doi:10.1038/s41598-023-40540-8.

Miyata, K., Imai, Y., Hori, S., Nishio, M., Loo, T.M., Okada, R., Yang, L., Nakadai, T., Maruyama, R., Fujii, R., Ueda, K., Jiang, L., Zheng, H., Toyokuni, S., Sakata, T., Shirahige, K., Kojima, R., Nakayama, M., Oshima, M., Nagayama, S., Seimiya, H., Hirota, T., Saya, H., Hara, E., Takahashi, A., 2021. Pericentromeric noncoding RNA changes DNA binding of CTCF and inflammatory gene expression in senescence and cancer. Proc. Natl. Acad. Sci. U. S. A. 118 (35). doi:10.1073/pnas.2025647118.

Mohamed, J.S., Hajira, A., Pardo, P.S., Boriek, A.M., 2014. MicroRNA-149 inhibits PARP-2 and promotes mitochondrial biogenesis via SIRT-1/PGC-1α network in skeletal muscle. Diabetes 63 (5), 1546–1559. doi:10.2337/db13-1364.

Mohottige, D., Manley, H.J., Hall, R.K., 2021. Less is more: deprescribing medications in older adults with kidney disease: a review. Kidney360 2 (9), 1510–1522. doi:10.34067/KID.0001942021.

Mongelli, A., Mengozzi, A., Geiger, M., Gorica, E., Mohammed, S.A., Paneni, F., Ruschitzka, F., Costantino, S., 2023. Mitochondrial epigenetics in aging and cardiovascular diseases. Front. Cardiovasc. Med. 10. doi:10.3389/fcvm.2023.1204483.

Montes, M., Lubas, M., Arendrup, F.S., Mentz, B., Rohatgi, N., Tumas, S., Harder, L.M., Skanderup, A.J., Andersen, J.S., Lund, A.H., 2021. The long non-coding RNA MIR31HG regulates the senescence associated secretory phenotype. Nat. Commun. 12 (1). doi:10.1038/s41467-021-22746-4.

Morales, V., Richard-Foy, H., 2000. Role of histone N-terminal tails and their acetylation in nucleosome dynamics. Mol. Cell. Biol. 20 (19), 7230–7237.

Moreno, D.F., Jenkins, K., Morlot, S., Charvin, G., Csikasz-Nagy, A., Aldea, M., 2019. Proteostasis collapse, a hallmark of aging, hinders the chaperone-start network and arrests cells in G1. eLife 8. doi:10.7554/elife.48240

Morrison, A.J., 2020. Chromatin-remodeling links metabolic signaling to gene expression. Mol. Metab. 38. doi:10.1016/j.molmet.2020.100973

Muralidharan, J., Ramezani, A., Hubal, M., Knoblach, S., Shrivastav, S., Karandish, S., Scott, R., Maxwell, N., Ozturk, S., Beddhu, S., Kopp, J.B., Raj, D.S., 2017. Extracellular microRNA signature in chronic kidney disease. Am. J. Physiol. Renal Physiol. 312 (6). doi:10.1152/ajprenal.00569.2016.

Mylonas, K.J., O'Sullivan, E.D., Humphries, D., Baird, D.P., Docherty, M.-H., Neely, S.A., Krimpenfort, P.J., Melk, A., Schmitt, R., Ferreira-Gonzalez, S., Forbes, S.J., Hughes, J., Ferenbach, D.A., 2021. Cellular senescence inhibits renal regeneration after injury in mice, with senolytic treatment promoting repair. Sci. Transl. Med. 13 (594). doi:10.1126/scitranslmed.abb0203.

Narita, M., 2007. Cellular senescence and chromatin organisation. Br. J. Cancer 96 (5), 686–691. doi:10.1038/sj.bjc.6603636.

Nemoto, S., Fergusson, M.M., Finkel, T., 2005. SIRT1 functionally interacts with the metabolic regulator and transcriptional coactivator PGC-1α. J. Biol. Chem. 280 (16), 16456–16460. doi:10.1074/jbc.M501485200.

Neytchev, O., Erlandsson, H., Witasp, A., Nordfors, L., Qureshi, A.R., Iseri, K., Morohoshi, H., Selman, C., Ebert, T., Kublickiene, K., Stenvinkel, P., Shiels, P.G., 2024. Epigenetic clocks indicate that kidney transplantation and not dialysis mitigate the effects of renal ageing. J. Intern. Med. 295 (1), 79–90. doi:10.1111/joim.13724.

Nishikura, K., 2016. A-to-I editing of coding and non-coding RNAs by ADARs. Nat. Rev. Mol. Cell Biol. 17 (2), 83–96. doi:10.1038/nrm.2015.4.

Ozata, D.M., Gainetdinov, I., Zoch, A., O'Carroll, D., Zamore, P.D., 2019. PIWI-interacting RNAs: small RNAs with big functions. Nat. Rev. Genet. 20 (2), 89–108. doi:10.1038/s41576-018-0073-3.

Pal, S., Tyler, J.K., 2016. Epigenetics and aging. Sci. Adv. 2 (7). doi:10.1126/sciadv.1600584.

Palikaras, K., Lionaki, E., Tavernarakis, N., 2015. Balancing mitochondrial biogenesis and mitophagy to maintain energy metabolism homeostasis. Cell Death Differ. 22 (9), 1399–1401. doi:10.1038/cdd.2015.86.

Pan, Y., Wu, Y., Hu, J., Shan, Y., Ma, J., Ma, H., Qi, X., Jia, L., 2018. Long noncoding RNA HOTAIR promotes renal cell carcinoma malignancy through alpha-2, 8-sialyltransferase 4 by sponging microRNA-124. Cell Prolif. 51 (6). doi:10.1111/cpr.12507.

Panda, A.C., Abdelmohsen, K., Gorospe, M., 2017. SASP regulation by noncoding RNA. Mech. Ageing Dev. 168, 37–43.

Pandolfini, L., Barbieri, I., Bannister, A.J., Hendrick, A., Andrews, B., Webster, N., Murat, P., Mach, P., Brandi, R., Robson, S.C., Migliori, V., Alendar, A., d'Onofrio, M., Balasubramanian, S., Kouzarides, T., 2019. METTL1 promotes let-7 MicroRNA processing via m7G methylation. Mol. Cell 74 (6). doi:10.1016/j.molcel.2019.03.040.

Park, J.-A., Kim, A.-J., Kang, Y., Jung, Y.-J., Kim, H.K., Kim, K.-C., 2011. Deacetylation and methylation at histone H3 lysine 9 (H3K9) coordinate chromosome condensation during cell cycle progression. Mol. Cells 31 (4), 343–349. doi:10.1007/s10059-011-0044-4.

Paul, D., Sinha, A.N., Ray, A., Lal, M., Nayak, S., Sharma, A., Mehani, B., Mukherjee, D., Laddha, S.V., Suri, A., Sarkar, C., Mukhopadhyay, A., 2017. A-to-I editing in human miRNAs is enriched in seed sequence, influenced by sequence contexts and significantly hypoedited in glioblastoma multiforme. Sci. Rep. 7 (1). doi:10.1038/s41598-017-02397-6.

Pavanello, S., Campisi, M., Rigotti, P., Di Bello, M., Nuzzolese, E., Neri, F., Furian, L., 2022. DNA methylation—and telomere—based biological age estimation as markers of biological aging in donors kidneys. Front. Med. 9. doi:10.3389/fmed.2022.832411

Pei, H., Zhang, L., Luo, K., Qin, Y., Chesi, M., Fei, F., Bergsagel, P.L., Wang, L., You, Z., Lou, Z., 2011. MMSET regulates histone H4K20 methylation and 53BP1 accumulation at DNA damage sites. Nature 470 (7332), 124–128. doi:10.1038/nature09658.

Pei, J., Cooper, H., Flieder, D.B., Talarchek, J.N., Al-Saleem, T., Uzzo, R.G., Dulaimi, E., Patchefsky, A.S., Testa, J.R., Wei, S., 2019. NEAT1-TFE3 and KAT6A-TFE3 renal cell carcinomas, new members of MiT family translocation renal cell carcinoma. Mod. Pathol. 32 (5), 710–716. doi:10.1038/s41379-018-0191-7.

Peleg, S., Feller, C., Ladurner, A.G., Imhof, A., 2016. The metabolic impact on histone acetylation and transcription in ageing. Trends Biochem. Sci. 41 (8), 700–711. doi:10.1016/j.tibs.2016.05.008.

Petri, B.J., Klinge, C.M., 2023. m6A readers, writers, erasers, and the m6A epitranscriptome in breast cancer. J. Mol. Endocrinol. 70 (2). doi:10.1530/JME-22-0110.

Petty, E., Pillus, L., 2013. Balancing chromatin remodeling and histone modifications in transcription. Trends Genet. 29 (11), 621–629.

Piatek, M.J., Werner, A., 2014. Endogenous siRNAs: regulators of internal affairs. Biochem. Soc. Trans. 42 (4), 1174–1179. doi:10.1042/BST20140068.

Picca, A., Faitg, J., Auwerx, J., Ferrucci, L., D'Amico, D., 2023. Mitophagy in human health, ageing and disease. Nat. Metab. 5 (12), 2047–2061. doi:10.1038/s42255-023-00930-8.

Picerno, A., Giannuzzi, F., Curci, C., De Palma, G., Di Chiano, M., Simone, S., Franzin, R., Gallone, A., Di Lorenzo, V.F., Stasi, A., Pertosa, G.B., Sabbà, C., Gesualdo, L., Sallustio, F., 2022. The long non-coding RNA HOTAIR controls the self-renewal, cell senescence, and secretion of anti-aging protein α-klotho in human adult renal progenitor cells. Stem Cells 40 (10), 963–975. doi:10.1093/stmcls/sxac054.

Potter, M.L., Hill, W.D., Isales, C.M., Hamrick, M.W., Fulzele, S., 2021. MicroRNAs are critical regulators of senescence and aging in mesenchymal stem cells. Bone 142. doi:10.1016/j.bone.2020.115679

Pouikli, A., Parekh, S., Maleszewska, M., Nikopoulou, C., Baghdadi, M., Tripodi, I., Folz-Donahue, K., Hinze, Y., Mesaros, A., Hoey, D., Giavalisco, P., Dowell, R., Partridge, L., Tessarz, P., 2021. Chromatin remodeling due to degradation of citrate carrier impairs osteogenesis of aged mesenchymal stem cells. Nat. Aging 1 (9), 810–825. doi:10.1038/s43587-021-00105-8.

Pradeepa, M.M., Grimes, G.R., Kumar, Y., Olley, G., Taylor, G.C.A., Schneider, R., Bickmore, W.A., 2016. Histone H3 globular domain acetylation identifies a new class of enhancers. Nat. Genet. 48 (6), 681–686. doi:10.1038/ng.3550.

Puri, B., Majumder, S., Gaikwad, A.B., 2024. Novel dysregulated long non-coding RNAs in the acute kidney injury-to-chronic kidney diseases transition unraveled by transcriptomic analysis. Pharmacol. Res. Perspect. 12 (6). doi:10.1002/prp2.70036.

Qian, J., Zhou, X., Tanaka, K., Takahashi, A., 2023. Alteration in the chromatin landscape during the DNA damage response: continuous rotation of the gear driving cellular senescence and aging. DNA Repair 131. doi:10.1016/j.dnarep.2023.103572

Queiroz, A.L., Lessard, S.J., Ouchida, A.T., Araujo, H.N., Gonçalves, D.A., Simões Fróes Guimarães, D.S.P., Teodoro, B.G., So, K., Espreafico, E.M., Hirshman, M.F., Alberici, L.C., Kettelhut, I.D.C., Goodyear, L.J., Silveira, L.R., 2021. The MicroRNA miR-696 is regulated by SNARK and reduces mitochondrial activity in mouse skeletal muscle through Pgc1α inhibition. Mol. Metab. 51. doi:10.1016/j.molmet.2021.101226

Rackham, O., Shearwood, A.-M.J., Mercer, T.R., Davies, S.M.K., Mattick, J.S., Filipovska, A., 2011. Long noncoding RNAs are generated from the mitochondrial genome and regulated by nuclear-encoded proteins. RNA 17 (12), 2085–2093. doi:10.1261/rna.029405.111.

Rappe, A., Vihinen, H.A., Suomi, F., Hassinen, A.J., Ehsan, H., Jokitalo, E.S., McWilliams, T.G., 2024. Longitudinal autophagy profiling of the mammalian brain reveals sustained mitophagy throughout healthy aging. EMBO J. 43 (23), 6199–6231. doi:10.1038/s44318-024-00241-y.

Ray Chaudhuri, A.R., Nussenzweig, A., 2017. The multifaceted roles of PARP1 in DNA repair and chromatin remodelling. Nat. Rev. Mol. Cell Biol. 18 (10), 610–621. doi:10.1038/nrm.2017.53.

Ren, B., Guan, M.-X., Zhou, T., Cai, X., Shan, G., 2023. Emerging functions of mitochondria-encoded noncoding RNAs. Trends Genet. 39 (2), 125–139. doi:10.1016/j.tig.2022.08.004.

Rizza, S., Cardaci, S., Montagna, C., Di Giacomo, G., De Zio, D., Bordi, M., Maiani, E., Campello, S., Borreca, A., Puca, A.A., Stamler, J.S., Cecconi, F., Filomeni, G., 2018. S-nitrosylation drives cell senescence and aging in mammals by controlling mitochondrial dynamics and mitophagy. Proc. Natl. Acad. Sci. U. S. A. 115 (15). doi:10.1073/pnas.1722452115.

Rodell, R., Robalin, N., Martinez, N.M., 2024. Why U matters: detection and functions of pseudouridine modifications in mRNAs. Trends Biochem. Sci. 49 (1), 12–27. doi:10.1016/j.tibs.2023.10.008.

Rossetto, D., Avvakumov, N., Côté, J., 2012. Histone phosphorylation: a chromatin modification involved in diverse nuclear events. Epigenetics 7 (10), 1098–1108. doi:10.4161/epi.21975.

Rossiello, F., Jurk, D., Passos, J.F., d'Adda di Fagagna, F., 2022. Telomere dysfunction in ageing and age-related diseases. Nat. Cell Biol. 24 (2), 135–147. doi:10.1038/s41556-022-00842-x.

Rowe, L.A., Degtyareva, N., Doetsch, P.W., 2008. DNA damage-induced reactive oxygen species (ROS) stress response in Saccharomyces cerevisiae. Free Radic. Biol. Med. 45 (8), 1167–1177. doi:10.1016/j.freeradbiomed.2008.07.018.

Rowland, J., Akbarov, A., Eales, J., Xu, X., Dormer, J.P., Guo, H., Denniff, M., Jiang, X., Ranjzad, P., Nazgiewicz, A., Prestes, P.R., Antczak, A., Szulinska, M., Wise, I.A., Zukowska-Szczechowska, E., Bogdanski, P., Woolf, A.S., Samani, N.J., Charchar, F.J., Tomaszewski, M., 2019. Uncovering genetic mechanisms of kidney aging through transcriptomics, genomics, and epigenomics. Kidney Int. 95 (3), 624–635. doi:10.1016/j.kint.2018.10.029.

Ryu, H.-Y., Hochstrasser, M., 2021. Histone sumoylation and chromatin dynamics. Nucleic Acids Res. 49 (11), 6043–6052. doi:10.1093/nar/gkab280.

Sagy, N., Meyrom, N., Beckerman, P., Pleniceanu, O., Bar, D.Z., 2024. Kidney-specific methylation patterns correlate with kidney function and are lost upon kidney disease progression. Clin. Epigenetics 16 (1). doi:10.1186/s13148-024-01642-w.

Sahu, R.K., Singh, S., Tomar, R.S., 2021. The ATP-dependent SWI/SNF and RSC chromatin remodelers cooperatively induce unfolded protein response genes during endoplasmic reticulum stress. Biochim. Biophys. Acta Gene Regul. Mech. 1864, 11–12.

Sarg, B., Koutzamani, E., Helliger, W., Rundquist, I., Lindner, H.H., 2002. Postsynthetic trimethylation of histone H4 at lysine 20 in mammalian tissues is associated with aging. J. Biol. Chem. 277 (42), 39195–39201.

Sartorelli, V., Lauberth, S.M., 2020. Enhancer RNAs are an important regulatory layer of the epigenome. Nat. Struct. Mol. Biol. 27 (6), 521–528. doi:10.1038/S41594-020-0446-0.

Sato, K., Kumagai, N., Suzuki, N., 2019. Alteration of the DNA methylation signature of renal erythropoietin-producing cells governs the sensitivity to drugs targeting the hypoxia-response pathway in kidney disease progression. Front. Genet. 10. doi:10.3389/fgene.2019.01134

Schlosser, P., Tin, A., Matias-Garcia, P.R., Thio, C.H.L., Joehanes, R., Liu, H., Weihs, A., Yu, Z., Hoppmann, A., Grundner-Culemann, F., Min, J.L., Adeyemo, A.A., Agyemang, C., Ärnlöv, J., Aziz, N.A., Baccarelli, A., Bochud, M., Brenner, H., Breteler, M.M.B., Carmeli, C., Chaker, L., Chambers, J.C., Cole, S.A., Coresh, J., Corre, T., Correa, A., Cox, S.R., de Klein, N., Delgado, G.E., Domingo-Relloso, A., Eckardt, K.-U., Ekici, A.B., Endlich, K., Evans, K.L., Floyd, J.S., Fornage, M., Franke, L., Fraszczyk, E., Gao, X., Gào, X., Ghanbari, M., Ghasemi, S., Gieger, C., Greenland, P., Grove, M.L., Harris, S.E., Hemani, G., Henneman, P., Herder, C., Horvath, S., Hou, L., Hurme, M.A., Hwang, S.-J., Jarvelin, M.-R., Kardia, S.L.R., Kasela, S., Kleber, M.E., Koenig, W., Kooner, J.S., Kramer, H., Kronenberg, F., Kühnel, B., Lehtimäki, T., Lind, L., Liu, D., Liu, Y., Lloyd-Jones, D.M., Lohman, K., Lorkowski, S., Lu, A.T., Marioni, R.E., März, W., McCartney, D.L., Meeks, K.A.C., Milani, L., Mishra, P.P., Nauck, M., Navas-Acien, A., Nowak, C., Peters, A., Prokisch, H., Psaty, B.M., Raitakari, O.T., Ratliff, S.M., Reiner, A.P., Rosas, S.E., Schöttker, B., Schwartz, J., Sedaghat, S., Smith, J.A., Sotoodehnia, N., Stocker, H.R., Stringhini, S., Sundström, J., Swenson, B.R., Tellez-Plaza, M., van Meurs, J.B.J., van Vliet-ostaptchouk, J.V., Venema, A., Verweij, N., Walker, R.M., Wielscher, M., Winkelmann, J., Wolffenbuttel, B.H.R., Zhao, W., Zheng, Y., Loh, M., Snieder, H., Levy, D., Waldenberger, M., Susztak, K., Köttgen, A., Teumer, A., 2021. Meta-analyses identify DNA methylation associated with kidney function and damage. Nat. Commun. 12 (1). doi:10.1038/s41467-021-27234-3.

Schmitt, A.M., Garcia, J.T., Hung, T., Flynn, R.A., Shen, Y., Kun, Q., Payumo, A.Y., Peres-da-Silva, A., Broz, D.K., Baum, R., Guo, S., Chen, J.K., Attardi, L.D., Chang, H.Y., 2016. An inducible long noncoding RNA amplifies DNA damage signaling. Nat. Genet. 48 (11), 1370–1376. doi:10.1038/ng.3673.

Schoberleitner, I., Bauer, I., Huang, A., Andreyeva, E.N., Sebald, J., Pascher, K., Rieder, D., Brunner, M., Podhraski, V., Oemer, G., Cázarez-García, D., Rieder, L., Keller, M.A., Winkler, R., Fyodorov, D.V., Lusser, A., 2021. CHD1 controls H3.3 incorporation in adult brain chromatin to maintain metabolic homeostasis and normal lifespan. Cell Rep. 37 (1), 109769. doi:10.1016/j.celrep.2021.109769.

Sendinc, E., Shi, Y., 2023. RNA m6A methylation across the transcriptome. Mol. Cell 83 (3), 428–441.

Shang, R., Lee, S., Senavirathne, G., Lai, E.C., 2023. microRNAs in action: biogenesis, function and regulation. Nat. Rev. Genet. 24 (12), 816–833. doi:10.1038/s41576-023-00611-y.

Sharifian, R., Okamura, D.M., Denisenko, O., Zager, R.A., Johnson, A., Gharib, S.A., Bomsztyk, K., 2018. Distinct patterns of transcriptional and epigenetic alterations characterize acute and chronic kidney injury. Sci. Rep. 8 (1). doi:10.1038/s41598-018-35943-x.

Shen, H., An, O., Ren, X., Song, Y., Tang, S.J., Ke, X.-Y., Han, J., Tay, D.J.T., Ng, V.H.E., Molias, F.B., Pitcheshwar, P., Leong, K.W., Tan, K.-K., Yang, H., Chen, L., 2022. ADARs act as potent regulators of circular transcriptome in cancer. Nat. Commun. 13 (1). doi:10.1038/s41467-022-29138-2.

Shihabudeen Haider Ali, M.S., Cheng, X., Moran, M., Haemmig, S., Naldrett, M.J., Alvarez, S., Feinberg, M.W., Sun, X., 2019. LncRNA Meg3 protects endothelial function by regulating the DNA damage response. Nucleic Acids Res. 47 (3), 1505–1522. doi:10.1093/nar/gky1190.

Shpilka, T., Haynes, C.M., 2018. The mitochondrial UPR: mechanisms, physiological functions and implications in ageing. Nat. Rev. Mol. Cell Biol. 19 (2), 109–120. doi:10.1038/nrm.2017.110.

Silva, B., Arora, R., Bione, S., Azzalin, C.M., 2021. TERRA transcription destabilizes telomere integrity to initiate break-induced replication in human ALT cells. Nat. Commun. 12 (1). doi:10.1038/s41467-021-24097-6.

Snyder, N.A., Silva, G.M., 2021. Deubiquitinating enzymes (DUBs): regulation, homeostasis, and oxidative stress response. J. Biol. Chem. 297 (3). doi:10.1016/j.jbc.2021.101077.

Soto-Palma, C., Niedernhofer, L.J., Faulk, C.D., Dong, X., 2022. Epigenetics, DNA damage, and aging. J. Clin. Invest. 132 (16). doi:10.1172/JCI158446.

Srinivas, U.S., Tan, B.W.Q., Vellayappan, B.A., Jeyasekharan, A.D., 2019. ROS and the DNA damage response in cancer. Redox Biol. 25, 101084. doi:10.1016/j.redox.2018.101084.

Sriraman, A., Debnath, T.K., Xhemalce, B., Miller, K.M., 2020. Making it or breaking it: DNA methylation and genome integrity. Essays Biochem. 64 (5), 687–703. doi:10.1042/EBC20200009.

Statello, L., Guo, C.-J., Chen, -L.-L., Huarte, M., 2021. Gene regulation by long non-coding RNAs and its biological functions. Nat. Rev. Mol. Cell Biol. 22 (2), 96–118. doi:10.1038/s41580-020-00315-9.

Stoccoro, A., Coppedè, F., 2021. Mitochondrial dna methylation and human diseases. Int. J. Mol. Sci. 22 (9). doi:10.3390/ijms22094594.

Su, N., Yu, X., Duan, M., Shi, N., 2025. Recent advances in methylation modifications of microRNA. Genes Dis. 12 (1). doi:10.1016/j.gendis.2023.101201.

Su, Q., Liu, Y., Lv, X.-W., Dai, R.-X., Yang, X.-H., Kong, B.-H., 2020. LncRNA TUG1 mediates ischemic myocardial injury by targeting miR-132-3p/HDAC3 axis. Am. J. Physiol. Heart Circ. Physiol. 318 (2). doi:10.1152/ajpheart.00444.2019.

Suda, K., Moriyama, Y., Razali, N., Chiu, Y., Masukagami, Y., Nishimura, K., Barbee, H., Takase, H., Sugiyama, S., Yamazaki, Y., Sato, Y., Higashiyama, T., Johmura, Y., Nakanishi, M., Kono, K., 2024. Plasma membrane damage limits replicative lifespan in yeast and induces premature senescence in human fibroblasts. Nat. Aging 4 (3), 319–335. doi:10.1038/s43587-024-00575-6.

Summer, R., Shaghaghi, H., Schriner, D., Roque, W., Sales, D., Cuevas-Mora, K., Desai, V., Bhushan, A., Ramirez, M.I., Romero, F., 2019. Activation of the mTORC1/PGC-1 axis promotes mitochondrial biogenesis and induces cellular senescence in the lung epithelium. Am. J. Physiol. Lung Cell. Mol. Physiol. 316 (6). doi:10.1152/ajplung.00244.2018.

Sun-Wang, J.L., Ivanova, S., Zorzano, A., 2020. The dialogue between the ubiquitin-proteasome system and autophagy: implications in ageing. Ageing Res. Rev. 64. doi:10.1016/j.arr.2020.101203

Swahari, V., Nakamura, A., Hollville, E., Hung, Y.-H., Kanke, M., Kurtz, C.L., Caravia, X.M., Roiz-Valle, D., He, S., Krishnamurthy, J., Kapoor, S., Prasad, V., Flowers, C., Beck, M., Baran-Gale, J., Sharpless, N., López-Otín, C., Sethupathy, P., Deshmukh, M., 2024. miR-29 is an important driver of aging-related phenotypes. Commun. Biol. 7 (1). doi:10.1038/s42003-024-06735-z.

Swarbrick, A., Woods, S.L., Shaw, A., Balakrishnan, A., Phua, Y., Nguyen, A., Chanthery, Y., Lim, L., Ashton, L.J., Judson, R.L., Huskey, N., Blelloch, R., Haber, M., Norris, M.D., Lengyel, P., Hackett, C.S., Preiss, T., Chetcuti, A., Sullivan, C.S., Marcusson, E.G., Weiss, W., L'Etoile, N., Goga, A., 2010. miR-380-5p represses p53 to control cellular survival and is associated with poor outcome in MYCN-amplified neuroblastoma. Nat. Med. 16 (10), 1134–1140. doi:10.1038/nm.2227.

Tabibzadeh, S., 2023. Role of autophagy in aging: the good, the bad, and the ugly. Aging Cell 22 (1). doi:10.1111/acel.13753.

Tanemoto, F., Nangaku, M., Mimura, I., 2022. Epigenetic memory contributing to the pathogenesis of AKI-to-CKD transition. Front. Mol. Biosci. 9. doi:10.3389/fmolb.2022.1003227

Tian, S., Huang, S., Wu, S., Guo, W., Li, J., He, X., 2010. MicroRNA-1285 inhibits the expression of p53 by directly targeting its 3′ untranslated region. Biochem. Biophys. Res. Commun. 396 (2), 435–439. doi:10.1016/j.bbrc.2010.04.112.

Tilstra, J.S., Clauson, C.L., Niedernhofer, L.J., Robbins, P.D., 2011. NF-κB in aging and disease. Aging Dis. 2 (6), 449–465.

Tsai, Y.-C., Hsieh, T.-H., Liao, Y.-R., Tsai, M.-T., Lin, T.-P., Lee, D.-Y., Park, J., Kim, D., Susztak, K., Yang, S.-F., Lin, C.-C., Li, S.-Y., 2024. METTL3-mediated N6-methyladenosine mRNA modification and cGAS-STING pathway activity in kidney fibrosis. J. Am. Soc. Nephrol. 35 (10), 1312–1329. doi:10.1681/ASN.0000000000000428.

Uckelmann, M., Sixma, T.K., 2017. Histone ubiquitination in the DNA damage response. DNA Repair 56, 92–101.

Ugalde, A.P., Ramsay, A.J., de la Rosa, J., Varela, I., Mariño, G., Cadiñanos, J., Lu, J., Freije, J.M., López-Otín, C., 2011. Aging and chronic DNA damage response activate a regulatory pathway involving miR-29 and p53. EMBO J. 30 (11), 2219–2232. doi:10.1038/emboj.2011.124.

Unnikrishnan, A., Freeman, W.M., Jackson, J., Wren, J.D., Porter, H., Richardson, A., 2019. The role of DNA methylation in epigenetics of aging. Pharmacol. Ther. 195, 172–185.

Valesyan, S., Jora, M., Addepalli, B., Limbach, P.A., 2024. tRNA generates 5-methylcytidine in the variable loop. Proc. Natl. Acad. Sci. U. S. A. 121 (46). doi:10.1073/pnas.2317857121.

van Zonneveld, A.J., Zhao, Q., Rotmans, J.I., Bijkerk, R., 2023. Circulating non-coding RNAs in chronic kidney disease and its complications. Nat. Rev. Nephrol. 19 (9), 573–586. doi:10.1038/s41581-023-00725-w.

Vaughan, R.M., Kupai, A., Rothbart, S.B., 2021. Chromatin regulation through ubiquitin and ubiquitin-like histone modifications. Trends Biochem. Sci. 46 (4), 258–269. doi:10.1016/j.tibs.2020.11.005.

Victorelli, S., Salmonowicz, H., Chapman, J., Martini, H., Vizioli, M.G., Riley, J.S., Cloix, C., Hall-Younger, E., Espindola-Netto, J.M., Jurk, D., Lagnado, A.B., Gomez, L.S., Farr, J.N., Saul, D., Reed, R., Kelly, G., Eppard, M., Greaves, L.C., Dou, Z., Pirius, N., Szczepanowska, K., Porritt, R.A., Huang, H., Huang, T.Y., Mann, D.A., Masuda, C.A., Khosla, S., Dai, H., Kaufmann, S.H., Zacharioudakis, E., Gavathiotis, E., LeBrasseur, N.K., Lei, X., Sainz, A.G., Korolchuk, V.I., Adams, P.D., Shadel, G.S., Tait, S.W.G., Passos, J.F., 2023. Apoptotic stress causes mtDNA release during senescence and drives the SASP. Nature 622 (7983), 627–636. doi:10.1038/s41586-023-06621-4.

Wagner, V., Kern, F., Hahn, O., Schaum, N., Ludwig, N., Fehlmann, T., Engel, A., Henn, D., Rishik, S., Isakova, A., Tan, M., Sit, R., Neff, N., Hart, M., Meese, E., Quake, S., Wyss-Coray, T., Keller, A., 2024. Characterizing expression changes in noncoding RNAs during aging and heterochronic parabiosis across mouse tissues. Nat. Biotechnol. 42 (1), 109–118. doi:10.1038/s41587-023-01751-6.

Wang, K., Liu, H., Hu, Q., Wang, L., Liu, J., Zheng, Z., Zhang, W., Ren, J., Zhu, F., Liu, G.-H., 2022. Epigenetic regulation of aging: implications for interventions of aging and diseases. Signal Transduct. Target. Ther. 7 (1). doi:10.1038/s41392-022-01211-8.

Wang, S.-H., Zhu, X.-L., Wang, F., Chen, S.-X., Chen, Z.-T., Qiu, Q., Liu, W.-H., Wu, M.-X., Deng, B.-Q., Xie, Y., Mai, J.-T., Yang, Y., Wang, J.-F., Zhang, H.-F., Chen, Y.-X., 2021a. LncRNA H19 governs mitophagy and restores mitochondrial respiration in the heart through Pink1/Parkin signaling during obesity. Cell Death Dis. 12 (6). doi:10.1038/s41419-021-03821-6.

Wang, S., Wu, W., Claret, F.X., 2017. Mutual regulation of microRNAs and DNA methylation in human cancers. Epigenetics 12 (3), 187–197. doi:10.1080/15592294.2016.1273308.

Wang, X., Ramat, A., Simonelig, M., Liu, M.-F., 2023. Emerging roles and functional mechanisms of PIWI-interacting RNAs. Nat. Rev. Mol. Cell Biol. 24 (2), 123–141. doi:10.1038/s41580-022-00528-0.

Wang, Y.-N., Yang, C.-E., Zhang, D.-D., Chen, Y.-Y., Yu, X.-Y., Zhao, Y.-Y., Miao, H., 2021b. Long non-coding RNAs: a double-edged sword in aging kidney and renal disease. Chem. Biol. Interact. 337. doi:10.1016/j.cbi.2021.109396

Wang, Y., Jiao, B., Hu, Z., Wang, Y., 2024. Critical role of histone deacetylase 3 in the regulation of kidney inflammation and fibrosis. Kidney Int. 105 (4), 775–790. doi:10.1016/j.kint.2024.01.010.

Watanabe, R., Kanno, S.-I., Roushandeh, A.M., Ui, A., Yasui, A., 2017. Nucleosome remodelling, DNA repair and transcriptional regulation build negative feedback loops in cancer and cellular ageing. Philos. Trans. R. Soc. Lond. B Biol. Sci. 372, 1731. doi:10.1098/rstb.2016.0473.

Watanabe, T., Lin, H., 2014. Posttranscriptional regulation of gene expression by Piwi proteins and piRNAs. Mol. Cell 56 (1), 18–27.

Wei, Q., Huang, J., Livingston, M.J., Wang, S., Dong, G., Xu, H., Zhou, J., Dong, Z., 2024b. Pseudogene GSTM3P1 derived long non-coding RNA promotes ischemic acute kidney injury by target directed microRNA degradation of kidney-protective mir-668. Kidney Int. 106 (4), 640–657.

Wei, Q., Xiao, X., Huo, E., Guo, C., Zhou, X., Hu, X., Dong, C., Shi, H., Dong, Z., 2024a. Hypermethylation and suppression of microRNA219a-2 activates the ALDH1L2/GSH/PAI-1 pathway for fibronectin degradation in renal fibrosis. Mol. Ther. doi:10.1016/j.ymthe.2024.09.020.

Wijesinghe, S.N., Nicholson, T., Tsintzas, K., Jones, S.W., 2021. Involvements of long noncoding RNAs in obesity-associated inflammatory diseases. Obes. Rev. 22 (4). doi:10.1111/obr.13156.

Wilkinson, K.A., Henley, J.M., 2010. Mechanisms, regulation and consequences of protein SUMOylation. Biochem. J. 428 (2), 133–145. doi:10.1042/BJ20100158.

Wilkinson, K.D., 2000. Ubiquitination and deubiquitination: targeting of proteins for degradation by the proteasome. Semin. Cell Dev. Biol. 11 (3), 141–148. doi:10.1006/scdb.2000.0164.

Wing, M.R., Devaney, J.M., Joffe, M.M., Xie, D., Feldman, H.I., Dominic, E.A., Guzman, N.J., Ramezani, A., Susztak, K., Herman, J.G., Cope, L., Harmon, B., Kwabi-Addo, B., Gordish-Dressman, H., Go, A.S., He, J., Lash, J.P., Kusek, J.W., Raj, D.S., 2014. DNA methylation profile associated with rapid decline in kidney function: findings from the CRIC study. Nephrol. Dial. Transplant. 29 (4), 864–872. doi:10.1093/ndt/gft537.

Wu, N.N., Zhang, Y., Ren, J., 2019. Mitophagy, mitochondrial dynamics, and homeostasis in cardiovascular aging. Oxid. Med. Cell. Longev. 2019. doi:10.1155/2019/9825061

Xia, X., Wang, Y., Zheng, J.C., 2023. Internal m7G methylation: a novel epitranscriptomic contributor in brain development and diseases. Mol. Ther. Nucleic Acids 31, 295–308. doi:10.1016/j.omtn.2023.01.003.

Xiang, Y., Fu, Y., Wu, W., Tang, C., Dong, Z., 2023. Autophagy in acute kidney injury and maladaptive kidney repair. Burns Trauma. 11. doi:10.1093/burnst/tkac059

Xiao, J., Liu, Y., Yi, J., Liu, X., 2021. LINC02257, an enhancer RNA of prognostic value in colon adenocarcinoma, correlates with multi-omics immunotherapy-related analysis in 33 cancers. Front. Mol. Biosci. 8. doi:10.3389/fmolb.2021.646786

Xiao, X., Wang, W., Guo, C., Wu, J., Zhang, S., Shi, H., Kwon, S., Chen, J., Dong, Z., 2024. Hypermethylation leads to the loss of HOXA5, resulting in JAG1 expression and NOTCH signaling contributing to kidney fibrosis. Kidney Int. 106 (1), 98–114. doi:10.1016/j.kint.2024.02.023.

Xie, L., Zhong, X., Cao, W., Liu, J., Zu, X., Chen, L., 2023. Mechanisms of NAT10 as ac4C writer in diseases. Mol. Ther. Nucleic Acids 32, 359–368. doi:10.1016/j.omtn.2023.03.023.

Xiong, Q., Zhang, Y., 2023. Small RNA modifications: regulatory molecules and potential applications. J. Hematol. Oncol. 16 (1). doi:10.1186/s13045-023-01466-w.

Xiong, W., Zhao, Y., Wei, Z., Li, C., Zhao, R., Ge, J., Shi, B., 2023. N1-methyladenosine formation, gene regulation, biological functions, and clinical relevance. Mol. Ther. 31 (2), 308–330. doi:10.1016/j.ymthe.2022.10.015.

Yadav, P., Subbarayalu, P., Medina, D., Nirzhor, S., Timilsina, S., Rajamanickam, S., Eedunuri, V.K., Gupta, Y., Zheng, S., Abdelfattah, N., Huang, Y., Vadlamudi, R., Hromas, R., Meltzer, P., Houghton, P., Chen, Y., Rao, M.K., 2022. M6A RNA methylation regulates histone ubiquitination to support cancer growth and progression. Cancer Res. 82 (10), 1872–1889. doi:10.1158/0008-5472.CAN-21-2106.

Yamada, T., Mizuno, K.-I., Hirota, K., Kon, N., Wahls, W.P., Hartsuiker, E., Murofushi, H., Shibata, T., Ohta, K., 2004. Roles of histone acetylation and chromatin remodeling factor in a meiotic recombination hotspot. EMBO J. 23 (8), 1792–1803. doi:10.1038/sj.emboj.7600138.

Yan, Y., Liu, H., Abedini, A., Sheng, X., Palmer, M., Li, H., Susztak, K., 2024. Unraveling the epigenetic code: human kidney DNA methylation and chromatin dynamics in renal disease development. Nat. Commun. 15 (1). doi:10.1038/s41467-024-45295-y.

Yanai, K., Kaneko, S., Ishii, H., Aomatsu, A., Hirai, K., Ookawara, S., Morishita, Y., 2022. MicroRNA expression profiling in age-dependent renal impairment. Front. Med. 9. doi:10.3389/fmed.2022.849075

Yang, L., Tang, L., Min, Q., Tian, H., Li, L., Zhao, Y., Wu, X., Li, M., Du, F., Chen, Y., Li, W., Li, X., Chen, M., Gu, L., Sun, Y., Xiao, Z., Shen, J., 2024a. Emerging role of RNA modification and long noncoding RNA interaction in cancer. Cancer Gene Ther. 31 (6), 816–830. doi:10.1038/s41417-024-00734-2.

Yang, L., Wang, B., Guo, F., Huang, R., Liang, Y., Li, L., Tao, S., Yin, T., Fu, P., Ma, L., 2022. FFAR4 improves the senescence of tubular epithelial cells by AMPK/SirT3 signaling in acute kidney injury. Signal Transduct. Target. Ther. 7 (1). doi:10.1038/s41392-022-01254-x.

Yang, P.-L., Lai, T.-S., Chou, Y.-H., Lai, L.-C., Lin, S.-L., Chen, Y.-M., 2024b. DNA methylation in peripheral blood is associated with renal aging and renal function decline: a national community study. Clin. Epigenetics 16 (1). doi:10.1186/s13148-024-01694-y.

Yang, X.-J., Seto, E., 2007. HATs and HDACs: from structure, function and regulation to novel strategies for therapy and prevention. Oncogene 26 (37), 5310–5318. doi:10.1038/sj.onc.1210599.

Yang, Y.-L., Xue, M., Jia, Y.-J., Hu, F., Zheng, Z.-J., Wang, L., Si, Z.-K., Xue, Y.-M., 2020. Long noncoding RNA NEAT1 is involved in the protective effect of Klotho on renal tubular epithelial cells in diabetic kidney disease through the ERK1/2 signaling pathway. Exp. Mol. Med. 52 (2), 266–280. doi:10.1038/s12276-020-0381-5.

Yelland, J.N., Bravo, J.P.K., Black, J.J., Taylor, D.W., Johnson, A.W., 2023. A single 2′-O-methylation of ribosomal RNA gates assembly of a functional ribosome. Nat. Struct. Mol. Biol. 30 (1), 91–98. doi:10.1038/s41594-022-00891-8.

You, H., Li, H., Gou, W., 2023. lncRNA HOTAIR promotes ROS generation and NLRP3 inflammasome activation by inhibiting Nrf2 in diabetic retinopathy. Medicine 102 (37). doi:10.1097/MD.0000000000035155.

Yue, Y., Ren, L., Zhang, C., Miao, K., Tan, K., Yang, Q., Hu, Y., Xi, G., Luo, G., Yang, M., Zhang, J., Hou, Z., An, L., Tian, J., 2022. Mitochondrial genome undergoes de novo DNA methylation that protects mtDNA against oxidative damage during the peri-implantation window. Proc. Natl. Acad. Sci. U. S. A. 119 (30). doi:10.1073/pnas.2201168119.

Yurikova, O.Y., Aisina, D.E., Niyazova, R.E., Atambayeva, S.A., Labeit, S., Ivashchenko, A.T., 2019. The interaction of miRNA-5p and miRNA-3p with the mRNAs of orthologous genes. Mol. Biol. 53 (4), 612–623. doi:10.1134/s0026893319040174.

Zhang, C., Shen, S., Xu, L., Li, M., Tian, B., Yao, L., Zhu, X., 2024b. LONP1 alleviates ageing-related renal fibrosis by maintaining mitochondrial homeostasis. J. Cell. Mol. Med. 28 (17). doi:10.1111/jcmm.70090.

Zhang, C., Yi, X., Hou, M., Li, Q., Li, X., Lu, L., Qi, E., Wu, M., Qi, L., Jian, H., Qi, Z., Lv, Y., Kong, X., Bi, M., Feng, S., Zhou, H., 2023. The landscape of m1A modification and its posttranscriptional regulatory functions in primary neurons. eLife 12. doi:10.7554/elife.85324

Zhang, C., Yu, M., Hepperla, A.J., Zhang, Z., Raj, R., Zhong, H., Zhou, J., Hu, L., Fang, J., Liu, H., Liang, Q., Jia, L., Liao, C., Xi, S., Simon, J.M., Xu, K., Liu, Z., Nam, Y., Kapur, P., Zhang, Q., 2024a. Von Hippel Lindau tumor suppressor controls m6A-dependent gene expression in renal tumorigenesis. J. Clin. Invest. 134 (8). doi:10.1172/JCI175703.

Zhang, H., Lu, R., Huang, J., Li, L., Cao, Y., Huang, C., Chen, R., Wang, Y., Huang, J., Zhao, X., Yu, J., 2024c. N4-acetylcytidine modifies primary microRNAs for processing in cancer cells. Cell. Mol. Life Sci. 81 (1). doi:10.1007/s00018-023-05107-w.

Zhang, L.-S., Liu, C., Ma, H., Dai, Q., Sun, H.-L., Luo, G., Zhang, Z., Zhang, L., Hu, L., Dong, X., He, C., 2019. Transcriptome-wide mapping of internal N7-methylguanosine methylome in mammalian mRNA. Mol. Cell 74 (6). doi:10.1016/j.molcel.2019.03.036.

Zhang, W., Qu, J., Liu, G.-H., Belmonte, J.C.I., 2020. The ageing epigenome and its rejuvenation. Nat. Rev. Mol. Cell Biol. 21 (3), 137–150. doi:10.1038/s41580-019-0204-5.

Zhang, Y., Ni, X., Wei, L., Yu, Y., Zhu, B., Bai, Y., Pei, X., Gao, F., Guo, L., Yong, Z., Zhao, W., 2023. METTL3 alleviates D-gal-induced renal tubular epithelial cellular senescence via promoting miR-181a maturation. Mech. Ageing Dev. 210, 111774. doi:10.1016/j.mad.2022.111774.

Zhao, Y., Rai, J., Li, H., 2023. Regulation of translation by ribosomal RNA pseudouridylation. Sci. Adv. 9 (33). doi:10.1126/sciadv.adg8190.

Zhou, K.I., Pecot, C.V., Holley, C.L., 2024. -methylation (Nm) in RNA: progress, challenges, and future directions. RNA. 30 (5), 570–582. doi:10.1261/rna.079970.124.

Zhou, W.-Y., Cai, Z.-R., Liu, J., Wang, D.-S., Ju, H.-Q., Xu, R.-H., 2020. Circular RNA: metabolism, functions and interactions with proteins. Mol. Cancer 19 (1). doi:10.1186/s12943-020-01286-3.

Zhu, Y., Yang, B., Chen, S., Chen, G., Zeng, X., Min, H., Xu, L., 2024. M6A RNA methylation-mediated TUG1 stability maintains mitochondrial homeostasis during kidney aging by epigenetically regulating PGC1-α expression. Antioxid. Redox Signal 41 (16-18), 993–1013. doi:10.1089/ars.2024.0631.

CHAPTER

6

The influence of acute kidney injury on aging

Gonzalo Ramírez-Guerrero[a,b,c] *and Mitchell Rosner*[d]

[a]International Renal Research Institute of Vicenza (IRRIV), Vicenza, Italy
[b]Carlos Van Buren Hospital, Nephrology and Dialysis Unit, Valparaíso, Chile
[c]Department of Medicine, Universidad de Valparaíso, Valparaíso, Chile
[d]Division of Nephrology, Department of Medicine, University of Virginia Health System, Charlottesville, VA, United States

Learning objectives

- Understand and list the common etiologies of acute kidney injury in elderly patients (age > 65 years).
- Recognize the structural and functional changes in the kidney that occur with age, which increase the susceptibility to AKI in the elderly.
- Understand how repair processes in the kidney are altered by aging.
- Describe the diagnostic processes for AKI in the elderly and how changes in the elderly lead to unique challenges in the diagnosis of AKI.
- Describe the management of AKI in the elderly using both nondialytic and dialytic modalities.

Introduction

Aging is a continuous and multifactorial process influenced by genetic and environmental parameters. Many studies have used arbitrary cut-off points to define the term "elderly," such as over 60, 65, or 70 years. Nevertheless, most prospective epidemiological studies define the "elderly population" as the age group >65 years (Ferrucci et al., 2008). Caring for the elderly population presents unique challenges for clinicians due to issues such as frailty, comorbidities, polypharmacy, and ethical concerns. These issues have become more

Aging and the Kidney
https://doi.org/10.1016/B978-0-443-34069-7.00007-0

prevalent and complex in an ever-growing population of patients. With a global increase in life expectancy, there is an estimated tripling in the number of people aged 80 years and above between 2019 and 2050. For example, Australia's elderly population increased by 35% between 2009 and 2019 ("Population Division: World Population Prospects," 2019; *Australian Bureau of Statistics: Disability, Ageing and Carers Australia: Summary of Findings*, 2018). Patients aged 80 years and above constitute a significant proportion of ICU admissions in Europe (5%–12%) and North America (20%) (Rai et al., 2023). Not surprisingly, higher ICU and hospital mortality rates have been reported in the elderly patient population, secondary to the more complex medical and surgical nature of admissions when compared to younger patients (Reinikainen et al., 2007; Ryan et al., 2008; Fuchs et al., 2012). As a result of this combination of factors (rising age with less organ reserve, increasing comorbid conditions, increased frailty, increased polypharmacy), the incidence of acute kidney injury (AKI) is increasing in older patients and is associated with poorer outcomes (Hsu et al., 2007; Waikar et al., 2006a; Xue et al., 2006). As has been extensively discussed in the literature, the development of AKI in ICU and hospitalized patients is associated with increased mortality, increased days in the ICU, increased ventilator days, higher costs, and long-term morbidity and mortality (Li et al., 2020b; Chronopoulos et al., 2010a; Li et al., 2017, 2020a; Rewa and Bagshaw, 2014).

This chapter will focus on AKI in elderly patients. Specifically, it will discuss its epidemiology, mechanisms, and relationship to the aging kidney. In addition, the benefits and risks of extracorporeal therapies to treat AKI in this group of patients will be reviewed.

Epidemiology of AKI in elderly patients

AKI is a systemic disease that is a frequent and severe complication in critically ill patients due to its high morbidity, mortality, and economic impact (Chertow et al., 2005; Uchino et al., 2005). In addition, the incidence of AKI in elderly patients has been increasing, particularly in those with chronic kidney disease (CKD). Patients with both CKD and AKI tend to be older, have ischemic heart disease, and are less likely to recover kidney function than patients with AKI alone (Anderson et al., 2011). Elderly patients represent the largest segment of individuals admitted to the ICU. Fifty-five percent of all ICU bed days in the United States are occupied by patients aged > 65 years (Angus et al., 2004). The epidemiology of AKI in this group is complex due to the high number and heterogeneity of comorbidities accompanying these patients (Fonarow and Heywood, 2006). For example, in patients hospitalized for heart failure and CKD, up to 45% experience AKI (Fonarow and Heywood, 2006). An analysis of Medicare beneficiaries in the United States reported an increase in AKI episodes from 13.6 (66–69 years) to 18.1 (70–74 years), 24.9 (75–79 years), 34.2 (80–84 years), and 46.9 (85 years and older) per 1000 patient-years, respectively (Xue et al., 2006; "Acute kidney injury," 2013). A report from Taiwan indicated an incidence of AKI in 52.8% of all elderly patients receiving major surgery associated with ICU admissions (Chao et al., 2012), while a study in China reported a 14.8% incidence of AKI among patients >80 years, with most cases secondary to sepsis (Wen et al., 2013). Similarly, in a more recent study among elderly men in China, there was a high risk of AKI in patients admitted to the ICU (39.0%), with the main etiologies being infections (39.6%), hypovolemia (23.8%), and cardiovascular events (15.9%)

TABLE 6.1 Studies showing the incidence and mortality of AKI in elderly patients.

Author	Year	Total number of patients	Patients with AKI	AKI incidence (%)	Diagnostic criteria	Average age (years)	Mortality (%)
(Xu et al., 2021)	2021	30,194	2505	8.3%	KDIGO	65	–
(Pongsittisak et al., 2020)	2020	624	158	22.7%	KDIGO	76	34.8%
(Formica et al., 2018)	2018	18,804	149	0.8% in >65 years	KDIGO	>65	67.8%
(Li et al., 2020a)	2019	1711	668	39%	KDIGO	87	25.7%
(Funk et al., 2016)	2016	424	424	N/D	KDIGO	>80	18.0%
(Sun et al., 2023)	2023	7775	511	6.57%	KDIGO	73	N/D
(Ebert et al., 2023)	2023	1901	383	20%	KDIGO	80.4	N/D
(Turgutalp et al., 2017)	2017	3229	236	7.3%	KDIGO	69.6/81.2	23.5%/31%
(Hu et al., 2021)	2021	36,445	7621	20.91%	KDIGO	75	9.71%
(Bani Hani et al., 2023)	2023	168	55	32.7%	KDIGO	84	19%
(Hatakeyama et al., 2024)	2024	12,361/17,008	1431/2096	11.6%/12.3%	KDIGO	69/80	N/D

N/D, No Data.

(Li et al., 2020b). The above findings confirm that there exists a three- to eightfold, age-dependent increase in the frequency of community-acquired AKI in patients older than 60 years (Table 6.1) (Feest et al., 1993).

For elderly patients who survive an AKI episode, it is estimated that 31.3% did not recover kidney function compared to 26% of younger patients. These patients eventually develop CKD (Rosner, 2013; Schmitt et al., 2008a). Ishani et al. reported that patients 67 years and older with an episode of AKI had a 54% risk of developing CKD, and this increased to 216% for patients with underlying CKD (Ishani et al., 2009). Other groups reported recovery in kidney function in 40% of AKI patients by day 28. Approximately half died by day 60, and relatively few survived to 1 year (Palevsky et al., 2008, 2009).

Common etiologies of AKI in elderly patients

Comorbid conditions, such as renovascular disease, congestive heart failure, hypertension, and diabetes, accumulate with age and increase susceptibility to AKI. These conditions often necessitate procedures or medications (e.g., nephrotoxic contrast, ACE inhibitors, antibiotics, nonsteroidal antiinflammatory drugs (NSAIDs)) that can stress or directly damage the kidneys. Furthermore, age-related structural and functional changes in the kidneys, including decreased glomerular filtration rate and diminished kidney reserve, reduce the ability to cope with acute stress and increase the likelihood of clinically significant AKI when an exposure occurs.

Several studies have shown that the etiologies of AKI in older patients are similar to those in the general population. Nevertheless, there are some unique issues in the elderly population, such as sepsis, which is more common among persons older than 60 years and is frequently associated with AKI. Furthermore, AKI related to urinary tract obstruction (due to prostatic disease or cancers) and hypovolemic etiologies is also more prevalent in older age (Anderson et al., 2011; Cardinale et al., 2022). Importantly, AKI in the elderly is often multifactorial, with a predominance of iatrogenic insults (procedures and medication use) in patients with less kidney reserve compared to younger counterparts (Waikar et al., 2006b). In addition, once AKI is established, these patients report poorer renal recovery when dialysis is required, an increased risk of rehospitalization, and progression toward CKD or ESRD (Schmitt et al., 2008a; Ishani et al., 2009; Turgutalp et al., 2017).

Two studies (IRACIBLE cohort study and Liaño group) have reported etiologies of AKI that appear to increase with age: obstructive causes (12% for <65 years, 15% for 65%–75% years, 23% for >75 years), hypovolemia without nephrotoxic drugs (14% for <65 years. 15% for 65–75 years, 19% for >75 years) and cardio-renal syndrome (6% for <65 years, 9% for 65–75 years, 15% for >75 years) (Cardinale et al., 2022; Pascual and Liaño, 1998).

Specific etiologies

1. Hemodynamic instability and ischemic causes
    - Hypotension and Hypovolemia: Hypoperfusion of the kidneys is common due to dehydration, heart failure, or other etiologies of hypotension (autonomic instability, medications) and is a primary cause, which is often exacerbated by age-related changes in renal blood flow regulation and vascular resistance that increase the susceptibility to tubular ischemia (Anderson et al., 2011; Chao et al., 2013).
    - Cardiovascular Surgery: AKI is commonly observed following major surgeries, especially cardiac and vascular procedures, where the kidney may experience ischemia-reperfusion injury (Chao et al., 2013; Panesso, 2021).
2. Sepsis-associated AKI
    - Sepsis: Elderly patients are more susceptible to infections, which frequently result in AKI due to sepsis. Sepsis contributes to both systemic inflammatory responses and direct kidney damage, potentially through immune dysregulation and heightened inflammatory markers (Anderson et al., 2011; Coca, 2010).
3. Medication-related nephrotoxicity
    - Polypharmacy and Nephrotoxic Drugs: The elderly are often prescribed multiple drugs, including NSAIDs, angiotensin-converting enzyme (ACE) inhibitors, diuretics, and contrast agents, which pose significant nephrotoxic risks. Drug toxicity accounts

for a large proportion of AKI cases among elderly patients due to impaired renal autoregulation and reduced kidney function (Panesso, 2021; Coca, 2010).

- Contrast-induced nephropathy (CIN): Frequently following diagnostic procedures, CIN is particularly concerning in the elderly due to preexisting kidney impairment and dehydration. Preventive measures, such as adequate hydration, are recommended before and after contrast administration.

4. Structural and functional changes in aging kidneys

- Reduced renal reserve: Age-associated renal changes, such as glomerulosclerosis, reduced nephron number, and vascular sclerosis, reduce the kidney's ability to respond to stress, making elderly kidneys more susceptible to injury from relatively minor insults (Anderson et al., 2011; Chao et al., 2013).
- Chronic conditions: Comorbidities like diabetes, hypertension, and CKD further compromise renal function. These conditions amplify the risk of AKI and also predispose the kidney to more severe and long-lasting damage postinjury (Panesso, 2021; Coca, 2010).

5. Postrenal causes

- Obstructive uropathy: Benign prostatic hyperplasia and cancers of the bladder or prostate, as well as cervical cancer and intraabdominal lymphoma (compressive lymphadenopathy), increase the likelihood of urinary obstruction and AKI (Chao et al., 2013; Panesso, 2021).

These etiologies highlight the complex interplay of hemodynamic factors, increased vulnerability due to structural kidney changes, and polypharmacy in the elderly, all of which contribute to a higher incidence and severity of AKI in this population.

Underlying factors associated with AKI in elderly patients

As the kidneys age, they experience a size reduction, with approximately a 10% decrease in kidney mass per decade after age 50, mainly due to cortical tissue loss associated with glomerulosclerosis, although the medulla remains primarily unaffected. Histological changes with aging include tubular atrophy, interstitial fibrosis, and mononuclear cell infiltration (Panesso, 2021; Long et al., 2005; Aalami et al., 2003). Glomerulosclerosis, a critical factor in CKD progression, often results from podocyte injury and has been linked to systemic atherosclerosis, which exacerbates intrarenal vascular disease (Floege et al., 1997; Kasiske, 1987). Structural alterations in arterial tone can lead to glomerular damage, albuminuria, and reduced GFR (Hashimoto and Ito, 2011; Chirinos et al., 2019). Tubular atrophy, aggravated by decreased blood flow and peritubular capillary rarefaction, reduces kidney function. Aging renal tubules have lower capacities for sodium reabsorption and urine concentration, making elderly patients more prone to dehydration and prerenal AKI (Schelling, 2016; Luckey and Parsa, 2003; Perazella and Mahnensmith, 1997). Reduced GFR in the elderly, even without preexisting kidney disease, results from decreased renal plasma flow and vascular changes that restrict filtration, with cortical atrophy and vascular lesions in small arteries

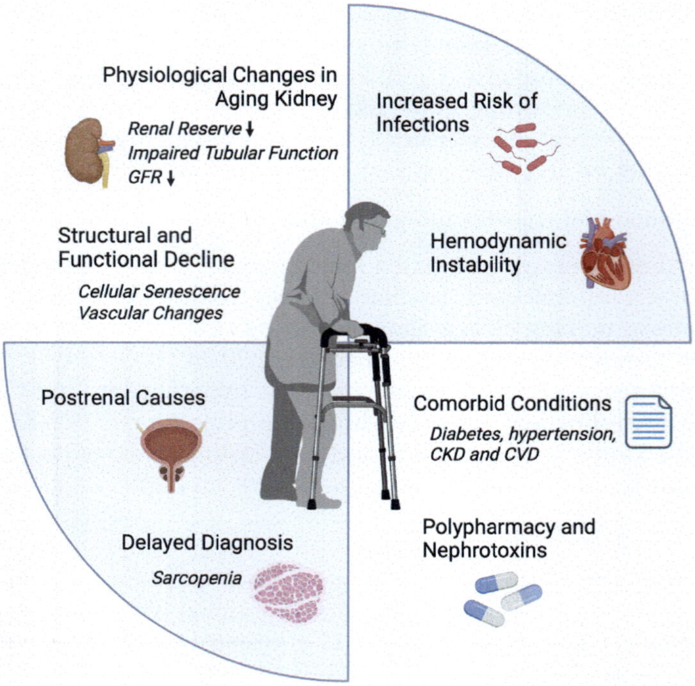

FIG. 6.1 Causes of increased susceptibility to AKI in elderly patients. This figure summarizes the multifactorial causes of heightened susceptibility to acute kidney injury in elderly patients. Key factors include physiological changes in the aging kidney (e.g., reduced renal reserve, impaired tubular function, and decreased glomerular filtration rate), structural and functional decline (vascular changes and cellular senescence), comorbid conditions (e.g., diabetes, hypertension, CKD, and cardiovascular disease), polypharmacy and nephrotoxic agents, hemodynamic instability, increased risk of infections, postrenal causes (e.g., urinary obstruction), and challenges in early diagnosis due to sarcopenia. Together, these factors illustrate the unique vulnerability of this population to AKI and its complications.

further compounding this decline (Hollenberg et al., 1974). A progressive loss in renal functional reserve limits the kidney's adaptive response to physiological stress, heightening AKI risk (Panesso, 2021). In addition, elderly kidneys show a blunted vasodilatory response and an intact vasoconstrictive response, which may increase susceptibility to AKI during low perfusion states and with renin-angiotensin system inhibition (Hollenberg et al., 1974). Finally, due to muscle mass loss, serum creatinine levels may underestimate the actual GFR in older adults, making it challenging to assess renal function accurately and increasing the risk of nephrotoxicity if dosing is not adjusted (Fig. 6.1) (Panesso, 2021).

Altered repair after AKI in elderly patients

Various factors contribute to the reduced repair capacity of the aging kidney following injury, including impaired angiogenesis, reduced proliferative capacity, cellular senescence, and a compromised immune response. Regarding angiogenesis, aging kidneys show a decrease in glomerular and peritubular capillary proliferation, attributed to lower levels of vascular endothelial growth factor, which is essential for blood vessel formation. In addition, there are higher levels of thrombospondin-1, an inhibitor of angiogenesis, thus diminishing the kidney's repair ability (Kang et al., 2001). Furthermore, the proliferative capacity of the renal tubular epithelium, essential for repairing damaged tissue, is limited in aging kidneys, likely due to cellular senescence. In this state, cells remain metabolically active but cannot divide, with the accumulation of the cell cycle inhibitor protein $p16^{INK4a}$ playing a role in reducing proliferation as well as the capacity for repair (Panesso, 2021; Schmitt et al., 2008b; Braun et al., 2012). Cellular senescence further complicates recovery, as senescent cells accumulate in aging tissues, releasing proinflammatory and pro-fibrotic factors that harm surrounding healthy cells, creating an environment that promotes inflammation and fibrosis instead of repair (Childs et al., 2015). Finally, the aging process is associated with low-grade chronic inflammation, along with a decline in immune function or "immunosenescence," which reduces the effectiveness of immune cells involved in tissue repair. Collectively, these factors impair the kidney's regenerative capacity, increasing the risk of progression to CKD following AKI in older adults (Franceschi et al., 2018; Rodwell et al., 2004).

Diagnosis of AKI in elderly patients

Diagnosing AKI in elderly patients poses significant challenges due to the limitations of traditional biomarkers such as serum creatinine. The current diagnosis of AKI is based on an acute deterioration in GFR, reflected by an increase in serum creatinine levels and/or a decline in urine output. Small increases in creatinine are associated with increased mortality (Chertow et al., 2005). Operationally, international consensus criteria defined AKI according to the Kidney Disease: Improving Global Outcomes (KDIGO) guidelines. Nevertheless, muscle mass heavily influences serum creatinine, which declines with age, leading to lower baseline levels of serum creatinine in older adults. Thus physiological decline in glomerular filtration rate may result in minimal increases in serum creatinine. The KDIGO diagnostic criteria for AKI, which rely on absolute or relative changes in serum creatinine, may fail to identify cases in older individuals with reduced muscle reserves (Chao et al., 2012; Waikar and Bonventre, 2009).

In addition, the slower rise and peak of serum creatinine in this population further delay diagnosis, potentially missing critical windows for intervention (Chao et al., 2012, 2013; Waikar and Bonventre, 2009; Siew et al., 2011). This diagnostic gap is concerning given the high prevalence of AKI in elderly patients. Therefore it is reasonable that older patients might be disadvantaged under the KDIGO guidelines for AKI diagnosis due to lower muscle mass on average (Odden et al., 2009). Oliguria has been defined in the KDIGO guidelines as diuresis of <0.5 ml/kg/hour for 6 h. In one group, including urine output in the diagnosis of AKI increased the incidence of AKI from 8% to 60% ("Clinical practice guideline for acute kidney injury. Notice," 2012; Ronco et al., 2010; Quan et al., 2016). The utility of using changes in urine output more consistently in the diagnosis of AKI in the elderly is not known. Hemodynamic parameters, intravascular hypovolemia/hypervolemia, and levels of hormones such as aldosterone and antidiuretic hormone influence urine output. Therefore it may be an unspecific marker of renal function. However, reduced urine output is associated with worse outcomes in critical patients, including greater mortality, ICU admission, and hospitalization in patients with AKI based solely on oliguria. The risk of mortality increases 2.84 (1.41–5.70) to 7.85 (2.76–22.33) times with the combined diagnosis of AKI that includes creatinine and urine output (Quan et al., 2016; Kellum et al., 2015; Mizota et al., 2016).

Alternative biomarkers, such as cystatin C, have emerged as promising tools to address some limitations. Unlike serum creatinine, cystatin C is unaffected by muscle mass, making it a more reliable indicator of kidney function in populations with reduced muscle mass, including the elderly. It is produced constantly by all nucleated cells and is exclusively eliminated through GFR, offering a stable and accurate reflection of renal function. Studies have shown that cystatin C can detect AKI earlier than serum creatinine, particularly in elderly patients, and provides predictive value for adverse outcomes such as progression to severe AKI, CKD, or mortality. Furthermore, using cystatin C in conjunction with serum creatinine has enhanced diagnostic accuracy, allowing for the early identification of AKI in older adults. This combined approach may improve clinical outcomes by enabling timely interventions (Coca, 2010; Kister et al., 2023; Yokota et al., 2018).

Ultrasonography, especially point-of-care ultrasound (PoCUS), has emerged as a valuable diagnostic tool in detecting postrenal (obstructive) AKI. PoCUS is a bedside imaging modality that enables the immediate assessment of hydronephrosis, the cardinal sign of obstructive AKI. According to Gaudreau-Simard et al., in a population with a mean age of 72 years, PoCUS demonstrated a sensitivity of 85% and a specificity of 78% in detecting hydronephrosis in AKI patients, making it a reliable diagnostic option. The prevalence of hydronephrosis in their study cohort was 33%, highlighting the importance of imaging in evaluating AKI causes. PoCUS's portability and real-time imaging capabilities are particularly beneficial for elderly patients (Gaudreau-Simard et al., 2024).

Despite its utility, PoCUS remains underutilized in clinical practice, with only 2% of AKI cases in the study cohort undergoing PoCUS. This gap represents a significant opportunity for improvement in diagnosing and managing AKI in elderly patients. In settings where PoCUS was utilized, it effectively supported clinical decision-making by identifying or ruling out urinary obstruction, thus expediting appropriate interventions. Moreover, the study highlighted that PoCUS, when integrated into emergency and internal medicine practices, reduces diagnostic delays and allows for more tailored management, particularly in elderly populations prone to rapid clinical deterioration (Gaudreau-Simard et al., 2024).

Managing AKI in elderly patients

Nondialytic management of AKI

Many risk factors contributing to AKI in elderly patients are nonmodifiable. Beyond advanced age, these factors include inherent characteristics such as gender, genetic predispositions (polymorphisms that elevate AKI risk), and multiple comorbidities such as heart failure, diabetes, hypertension, obesity, and CKD. Consequently, the cornerstone of AKI prevention begins with assessing an individual's risk of developing this condition. Several validated risk assessment models have been designed for clinical scenarios where the primary insult's timing are predictable, such as postoperative states after cardiac and vascular surgeries, percutaneous coronary interventions, or contrast medium administration. These models incorporate key clinical variables into logistic regression frameworks to estimate the overall risk of AKI (Englberger et al., 2010; Jorge-Monjas et al., 2016; Inohara et al., 2015). It is important to note that these scoring systems have good negative predictive power but are more limited in their positive predictive power.

Assessing AKI risk before potential renal insult offers notable benefits. First, it facilitates the application of preventive strategies, such as the early implementation of the KDIGO bundle for AKI prevention. Second, it enhances the informed consent process by providing patients with more precise information about associated risks. Finally, it aids quality improvement initiatives by comparing expected versus observed AKI rates following a known procedure (Englberger et al., 2010; Jorge-Monjas et al., 2016; Inohara et al., 2015).

Nondialytic management of AKI focuses on strategies to prevent progression to worsening stages of AKI, minimize complications, and promote recovery. Management typically emphasizes fluid, electrolyte, and medication management. Avoiding volume overload is critical as it is linked to poor outcomes in AKI patients. The REVERSE-AKI trial demonstrated the feasibility of restrictive fluid management to achieve a negative fluid balance, reducing the need for renal replacement therapy (RRT) in nonhypovolemic patients with AKI, while also lowering adverse event rates (Vaara et al., 2021:Meyhoff et al., 2022; National Heart, Lung, and Blood Institute PETAL Clinical Trials Network et al., 2023; Vaara et al., 2022).

Nevertheless, daily and cumulative fluid balance monitoring is crucial, as fluid overload is strongly associated with increased mortality in critically ill patients (Payen et al., 2008; Garzotto et al., 2016). In addition, the integrity of the endothelial glycocalyx is also a key consideration during fluid therapy, as injury to this structure may exacerbate vascular permeability, leading to fluid leakage into extravascular spaces (Milford and Reade, 2019; Woodcock and Woodcock, 2012). Thus the rate and volume of fluid administration must be tailored to individual patient needs to avoid complications like interstitial edema and delayed renal recovery. Combining vasopressors with fluid therapy, especially norepinephrine as the first-line vasopressor, can reduce fluid requirements while maintaining hemodynamic stability, further improving outcomes.

Fluid composition also requires careful consideration. Balanced crystalloids are generally preferred over 0.9% saline to minimize the risks of hyperchloremia and subsequent kidney injury, as supported by evidence from trials like SMART and SALT-ED (Semler et al., 2018; Self et al., 2018). Albumin may be considered in patients requiring substantial fluid replacement; however, its routine use in resuscitation remains debated. No data support its routine use for volume resuscitation in sepsis, and data to inform a suggested cut-off value for crystalloid infusion above which albumin should be considered as part of resuscitation fluid are limited (Zarbock et al., 2023). Finally, another solution for managing severe acidosis is 4.2% sodium bicarbonate. The BICAR-ICU study (median age: 66 years) found that treatment with intravenous 4.2% sodium bicarbonate for severe metabolic acidemia ($pH < 7.20$) and moderate-to-severe AKI in the ICU reduced the primary composite outcome (death from any cause by day 28 and the presence of at least one organ failure at day 7) and 28-day mortality (Jaber et al., 2018).

Renal replacement therapy in elderly patients

The initiation of dialysis in elderly patients with AKI is a complex decision, balancing potential survival benefits against the risks and the broader implications for quality of life.

While dialysis is often essential to correct severe metabolic derangements, manage fluid overload, and address life-threatening electrolyte imbalances, its utility in critically ill older adults is less clear. Evidence suggests that in elderly patients, particularly those over 70 years, dialysis may not significantly improve survival outcomes and, in some cases, may even accelerate mortality or increase the burden of end-of-life distress. A Brazilian study highlighted that no survival benefit was observed in patients over 70 years undergoing dialysis for AKI compared to those managed without it, especially in those with multiple comorbidities or requiring intensive care (Teles et al., 2019). Similarly, data from a US-based cohort found that in frail older adults, dialysis initiation at lower creatinine thresholds was associated with higher mortality rates, raising questions about its benefit in this subgroup (Akbar and Moss, 2014; Wilson et al., 2014).

The risks associated with dialysis in elderly patients are substantial. Complications such as hemodynamic instability, infections related to catheter placement, bleeding due to anticoagulation, and altered drug clearance are more prevalent in this group (Teles et al., 2019). Moreover, dialysis does not address the underlying pathophysiology of AKI or comorbid conditions, which are often the primary drivers of poor outcomes. The increased prevalence of frailty and reduced physiological reserves in elderly patients further diminishes the likelihood of recovering renal function or achieving meaningful survival benefits (Akbar and Moss, 2014).

From an ethical perspective, initiating dialysis in older patients demands a patient-centered approach. The concept of shared decision-making is paramount, focusing on aligning treatment options with the patient's values, goals, and quality-of-life expectations. Time-limited trials (TLTs) of dialysis have emerged as a practical strategy to navigate this decision-making process. TLTs involve initiating dialysis for a predetermined period with clearly defined clinical milestones and reevaluation points. This approach allows both clinicians and families to assess the effectiveness of dialysis while retaining the option to withdraw treatment if it fails to achieve agreed-upon goals (Akbar and Moss, 2014; Scherer and Holley, 2016). TLTs also serve to reduce conflict among care teams and families, providing a framework for integrating palliative care services and ensuring that the patient's dignity is preserved.

While dialysis is often perceived as a technological imperative, there is growing recognition of the need to move beyond a default approach to treatment in elderly AKI patients. Instead, a comprehensive evaluation of the patient´s overall prognosis, comorbidities, and functional status should guide the decision. Studies consistently show that elderly patients initiating dialysis often experience reduced quality of life, and a significant proportion of survivors report outcomes comparable to death, with prolonged hospital stays and high dependency (Teles et al., 2019; Akbar and Moss, 2014). As such, the nephrology community is increasingly calling for a reevaluation of dialysis ethics in this population, advocating for more nuanced and individualized care.

Prognosis after AKI in elderly patients

Recovery of renal function and prognosis of AKI in the elderly: AKI is no longer viewed as entirely reversible. While prerenal AKI may leave minimal impact, recovery after AKI is often incomplete, ranging from subclinical conditions with reduced renal functional reserve to dialysis-dependent ESRD, which accounts for over 40% of cases in some studies (Bhandari and Turney, 1996; Schiffl, 2006; Liaño et al., 2007). Elderly patients, particularly those over 65 years, are about 28% less likely to recover renal function and face up to a 20-fold higher risk of developing CKD compared to younger patients (Schmitt et al., 2008a; Parikh et al., 2008). These outcomes are influenced by intrinsic changes in aging kidneys, as described previously, and the high prevalence of comorbidities in older populations. The role of managing these comorbidities in improving recovery remains insufficiently studied (Kashani et al., 2017).

Mortality after AKI in elderly patients: AKI significantly increases short- and long-term mortality in elderly patients. Short-term mortality, defined as death within 90 days of AKI onset, varies between 20% and 45%, with higher rates for hospital-acquired AKI compared to community-acquired cases (Pascual and Liaño, 1998; Yılmaz and Erdem, 2010). Worse outcomes are observed in intrinsic (renal) AKI compared to prerenal AKI and in cases of oliguria or anuria (Coca, 2010; Yılmaz and Erdem, 2010; Oweis and Alshelleh, 2018). Mortality data for non-RRT-requiring AKI in elderly patients is mixed, with some studies reporting no increase, while others link higher mortality to age and comorbidities (Lameire et al., 1987; Ali et al., 2007). In ICU settings, mortality rates for elderly AKI patients range from 31% to 80%, driven by variations in treatment intensity, disease severity, and follow-up duration (Table 6.1) (Chronopoulos et al., 2010b). While advanced age can be an independent risk factor for death, frailty and multiorgan dysfunction are more strongly associated (Bagshaw et al., 2009). Long-term mortality, occurring beyond 3 months, is particularly severe for elderly patients requiring dialysis, with up to 66% dying within a year (Acuna et al., 2007; Rhee et al., 2016). These findings are complicated by confounding factors that reduce their clinical predictive value.

Quality of life after AKI in elderly patients: Health-related quality of life (HRQoL) after AKI in elderly patients is rarely studied. The POST-RENAL study found that AKI survivors had significantly lower physical and mental HRQoL compared to the general population, with age and poor renal function at follow-up identified as key predictors (Wang et al., 2015). However, other studies suggest that comorbidities play a more critical role in determining HRQoL than age (Landoni et al., 2006; Stephen et al., 2006). These findings underscore the need for systematic HRQoL assessments, particularly in long-term follow-ups, to address the impact of age and severe comorbidities after AKI.

Conclusions

The aging population has made AKI a critical challenge in elderly care, marked by higher incidence, limited recovery, and progression to CKD. Age-related renal changes, polypharmacy, and comorbidities amplify their vulnerability, while traditional diagnostic tools, like serum creatinine, often delay intervention. Therapeutic strategies, including nuanced use of RRT and personalized fluid management, emphasize the importance of aligning care with patient values and long-term outcomes. Focusing on individualized, evidence-based approaches is essential to improve survival and quality of life in this growing population.

References

Aalami, O.O., Fang, T.D., Song, H.M., Nacamuli, R.P., 2003. Physiological features of aging persons. Arch. Surg. 138 (10), 1068–1076.

Acuna, K., Costa, E., Grover, A., Camelo, A., Santos Junior, R., 2007. Clinical-epidemiological characteristics of adults and elderly admitted to an intensive care unit of the Amazon (Rio Branco, Acre). Rev. Bras. Ter. Intensiva 19 (3), 304–309.

Akbar, S., Moss, A.H., 2014. The ethics of offering dialysis for AKI to the older patient: time to re-evaluate? Clin. J. Am. Soc. Nephrol. 9 (9), 1652–1656.

Ali, T.Z., Khan, I., Simpson, W., Prescott, G., Townend, J., Smith, W., MacLeod, A., 2007. Incidence and outcomes in acute kidney injury: a comprehensive population-based study. J. Am. Soc. Nephrol. 18 (4), 1292–1298.

Anderson, S., Eldadah, B., Halter, J.B., Hazzard, W.R., Himmelfarb, J., Horne, F.M.F., et al., 2011. Acute kidney injury in older adults. J. Am. Soc. Nephrol. 22 (1), 28–38.

Angus, D.C., Barnato, A.E., Linde-Zwirble, W.T., Weissfeld, L.A., Watson, R.S., Rickert, T., Rubenfeld, G.D., 2004. Use of intensive care at the end of life in the United States: an epidemiologic study. Crit. Care Med. 32 (3), 638–643.

Australian Bureau of Statistics, 2018. Disability, Ageing and Carers, Australia: Summary of Findings. Australian Bureau of Statistics, Canberra.

Bagshaw, S.M., Webb, S.A.R., Delaney, A., George, C., Pilcher, D., Hart, G.K., Bellomo, R., 2009. Very old patients admitted to intensive care in Australia and New Zealand: a multi-centre cohort analysis. Crit. Care 13 (2), R45.

Bani Hani, A., et al., 2023. Incidence, risk factors and outcomes of acute kidney injury in surgical intensive care unit octogenarians at the Jordan University Hospital. BMC Geriatr. 23 (1), 266.

Bhandari, S., Turney, J.H., 1996. Survivors of acute renal failure who do not recover renal function. QJM 89 (6), 415–421.

Braun, H., Schmidt, B.M.W., Raiss, M., Baisantry, A., Mircea-Constantin, D., Wang, S., et al., 2012. Cellular senescence limits regenerative capacity and allograft survival. J. Am. Soc. Nephrol. 23 (9), 1467–1473.

Cardinale, A., Messikh, Z., Antoine, V., Aglae, C., Reboul, P., Cariou, S., et al., 2022. Specificity of severe AKI aetiology and care in the elderly: the IRACIBLE prospective cohort study. J. Nephrol. 35 (8), 2097–2108.

Chang-Panesso, M., 2021. Acute kidney injury and aging. Pediatr. Nephrol. 36 (10), 2997–3006.

Chao, C.T., Lin, Y.F., Tsai, H.B., Wu, V.C., Ko, W.J., 2013. Acute kidney injury network staging in geriatric postoperative acute kidney injury patients: shortcomings and improvements. J. Am. Coll. Surg. 217 (2), 240–250.

Chao, C.T., Wu, V.C., Lai, C.F., Shiao, C.C., Huang, T.M., Wu, P.C., et al., 2012. Advanced age affects the outcome-predictive power of RIFLE classification in geriatric patients with acute kidney injury. Kidney Int. 82 (8), 920–927.

Chertow, G.M., Burdick, E., Honour, M., Bonventre, J.V., Bates, D.W., 2005. Acute kidney injury, mortality, length of stay, and costs in hospitalized patients. J. Am. Soc. Nephrol. 16 (11), 3365–3370.

Childs, B.G., Durik, M., Baker, D.J., van Deursen, J.M., 2015. Cellular senescence in aging and age-related disease: from mechanisms to therapy. Nat. Med. 21 (12), 1424–1435.

Chirinos, J.A., Segers, P., Hughes, T., Townsend, R., 2019. Large-artery stiffness in health and disease: JACC state-of-the-art review. J. Am. Coll. Cardiol. 74 (9), 1237–1263.

Chronopoulos, A., Cruz, D.N., Ronco, C., 2010a. Hospital-acquired acute kidney injury in the elderly. Nat. Rev. Nephrol. 6 (3), 141–149.

Chronopoulos, A., Rosner, M.H., Cruz, D.N., Ronco, C., 2010b. Acute kidney injury in elderly intensive care patients: a review. Intensive Care Med. 36 (9), 1454–1464.

Clinical practice guideline for acute kidney injury. Notice, 2012. Kidney Int. Suppl., 2, pp. 1–141.

Coca, S.G., 2010. Acute kidney injury in elderly persons. Am. J. Kidney Dis. 56 (1), 122–131.

Ebert, N., et al., 2023. Incidence of hospital-acquired acute kidney injury and trajectories of glomerular filtration rate in older adults. BMC Nephrol. 24 (1), 226.

Englberger, L., Suri, R.M., Li, Z., Dearani, J.A., Park, S.J., Sundt, T.M., Schaff, H.V., 2010. Validation of clinical scores predicting severe acute kidney injury after cardiac surgery. Am. J. Kidney Dis. 56 (4), 623–631.

Feest, T.G., Round, A., Hamad, S., 1993. Incidence of severe acute renal failure in adults: results of a community-based study. BMJ 306 (6876), 481–483.

Ferrucci, L., Giallauria, F., Guralnik, J.M., 2008. Epidemiology of aging. Radiol. Clin. North Am. 46 (4), 643–652.

Floege, J., Hackmann, B., Kliem, V., Kriz, W., Alpers, C.E., Johnson, R.J., et al., 1997. Age-related glomerulosclerosis and interstitial fibrosis in Milan normotensive rats: a podocyte disease. Kidney Int. 51 (1), 230–243.

Fonarow, G.C., Heywood, J.T., 2006. The confounding issue of comorbid renal insufficiency. Am. J. Med. 119 (12), S17–S25.

Formica, M., et al., 2018. Acute kidney injury and chronic kidney disease in the elderly and polypharmacy. Blood Purif. 46 (4), 332–336.

Franceschi, C., Garagnani, P., Parini, P., Giuliani, C., Santoro, A., 2018. Inflammaging: a new immune-metabolic viewpoint for age-related diseases. Nat. Rev. Endocrinol. 14 (10), 576–590.

Fuchs, L., Chronaki, C.E., Park, S., Novack, V., Baumfeld, Y., Scott, D., et al., 2012. ICU admission characteristics and mortality rates among elderly and very elderly patients. Intensive Care Med. 38 (10), 1654–1661.

Funk, I., et al., 2016. Clinical course of acute kidney injury in elderly individuals above 80 years. Kidney Blood Press. Res. 41 (6), 947–955.

Garzotto, F., Ostermann, M., Martín-Langerwerf, D., Sánchez-Sánchez, M., Teng, J., Robert, R., et al., 2016. The dose response multicentre investigation on fluid assessment (DoReMIFA) in critically ill patients. Crit. Care 20 (1), 196.

Gaudreau-Simard, M., Saiyin, T., McInnes, M.D.F., Ruller, S., Clark, E.G., Wooller, K., et al., 2024. Test characteristics of point-of-care ultrasonography in patients with acute kidney injury. Ultrasound J. 16 (1), 3.

Hashimoto, J., Ito, S., 2011. Central pulse pressure and aortic stiffness determine renal hemodynamics: pathophysiological implication for microalbuminuria in hypertension. Hypertension 58 (5), 839–846.

Hatakeyama, Y., et al., 2024. Differences in characteristics and risk factors for acute kidney injury between elderly and very elderly patients: a retrospective review. Clin. Exp. Nephrol. 28 (11), 1097–1110.

Hollenberg, N.K., Adams, D.F., Solomon, H.S., Rashid, A., Abrams, H.L., Merrill, J.P., 1974. Senescence and the renal vasculature in normal man. Circ. Res. 34 (3), 309–316.

Hsu, C.-Y., McCulloch, C.E., Fan, D., Ordoñez, J.D., Chertow, G.M., Go, A.S., 2007. Community-based incidence of acute renal failure. Kidney Int. 72 (2), 208–212.

Hu, W., et al., 2021. The incidence, characteristics, and use of suspected nephrotoxic drugs in elderly patients with community-acquired acute kidney injury. Clin. Interv. Aging 16, 35–42.

Inohara, T., Kohsaka, S., Abe, T., Miyata, H., Numasawa, Y., Ueda, I., et al., 2015. Development and validation of a pre-percutaneous coronary intervention risk model of contrast-induced acute kidney injury with an integer scoring system. Am. J. Cardiol. 115 (12), 1636–1642.

Ishani, A., Xue, J.L., Himmelfarb, J., Eggers, P.W., Kimmel, P.L., Molitoris, B.A., Collins, A.J., 2009. Acute kidney injury increases risk of ESRD among elderly. J. Am. Soc. Nephrol. 20 (1), 223–228.

Jaber, S., Paugam, C., Futier, E., Lefrant, J.-Y., Lasocki, S., Lescot, T., et al., 2018. Sodium bicarbonate therapy for patients with severe metabolic acidaemia in the intensive care unit (BICAR-ICU): a multicenter, open-label, randomized controlled, phase 3 trial. Lancet 392 (10141), 31–40.

Jorge-Monjas, P., Bustamante-Munguira, J., Lorenzo, M., Heredia-Rodríguez, M., Fierro, I., Gómez-Sánchez, E., et al., 2016. Predicting cardiac surgery–associated acute kidney injury: the CRATE score. J. Crit. Care 31 (1), 130–138.

Kang, D.H., Anderson, S., Kim, Y.G., Mazzalli, M., Suga, S., Jefferson, J.A., et al., 2001. Impaired angiogenesis in the aging kidney: vascular endothelial growth factor and thrombospondin-1 in renal disease. Am. J. Kidney Dis. 37 (3), 601–611.

Kashani, K., Shao, M., Li, G., Williams, A.W., Rule, A.D., Kremers, W.K., et al., 2017. No increase in the incidence of acute kidney injury in a population-based annual temporal trends epidemiology study. Kidney Int. 92 (3), 721–728.

Kasiske, B.L., 1987. Relationship between vascular disease and age-associated changes in the human kidney. Kidney Int. 31 (5), 1153–1159.

Kellum, J.A., Sileanu, F.E., Murugan, R., Lucko, N., Shaw, A.D., Clermont, G., 2015. Classifying AKI by urine output versus serum creatinine level. J. Am. Soc. Nephrol. 26 (9), 2231–2238.

Kidney Disease: Improving Global Outcomes (KDIGO) Acute Kidney Injury Work Group, 2012. KDIGO clinical practice guideline for acute kidney injury. Kidney Int. Suppl. 2 (1), 1–138.

Landoni, G., Zangrillo, A., Franco, A., Aletti, G., Roberti, A., Calabrò, M.G., et al., 2006. Long-term outcome of patients who require renal replacement therapy after cardiac surgery. Eur. J. Anaesthesiol. 23 (1), 17–22.

Kister, T.S., Schmidt, M., Heuft, L., Federbusch, M., Haase, M., Kaiser, T., 2023. Laboratory diagnostic of acute kidney injury and its progression: risk of underdiagnosis in female and elderly patients. J. Clin. Med. 12 (3), 1092.

Lameire, N., Matthys, E., Vanholder, R., De Keyser, K., Pauwels, W., Nachtergaele, H., et al., 1987. Causes and prognosis of acute renal failure in elderly patients. Nephrol. Dial. Transpl. 2 (5), 316–322.

Li, Q., Mao, Z., Hu, P., Kang, H., Zhou, F., 2020a. Analysis of the short-term prognosis and risk factors of elderly acute kidney injury patients in different KDIGO diagnostic windows. Aging Clin. Exp. Res. 32 (5), 851–860.

Li, Q., Zhao, M., Wang, X., 2017. The impact of transient and persistent acute kidney injury on short-term outcomes in very elderly patients. Clin. Interv. Aging 12, 1013–1020.

Li, Q., Zhao, M., Zhou, F., 2020b. Hospital-acquired acute kidney injury in very elderly men: clinical characteristics and short-term outcomes. Aging Clin. Exp. Res. 32 (6), 1121–1128.

Liaño, F., Felipe, C., Tenorio, M.-T., Rivera, M., Abraira, V., Sáez-de-Urturi, J.-M., et al., 2007. Long-term outcome of acute tubular necrosis: a contribution to its natural history. Kidney Int. 71 (7), 679–686.

Long, D.A., Mu, W., Price, K.L., Johnson, R.J., 2005. Blood vessels and the aging kidney. Nephron Exp. Nephrol. 101 (3), e95–e99.

Luckey, A.E., Parsa, C.J., 2003. Fluid and electrolytes in the aged. Arch. Surg. 138 (10), 1055–1060.

Meyhoff, T.S., Hjortrup, P.B., Wetterslev, J., Sivapalan, P., Laake, J.H., Cronhjort, M., et al., 2022. Restriction of intravenous fluid in ICU patients with septic shock. N. Engl. J. Med. 386, 2459–2470.

Milford, E.M., Reade, M.C., 2019. Resuscitation fluid choices to preserve the endothelial glycocalyx. Crit. Care 23 (1), 259.

Mizota, T., Minamisawa, S., Imanaka, Y., Fukuda, K., 2016. Oliguria without serum creatinine increase after living donor liver transplantation is associated with adverse post-operative outcomes. Acta Anaesthesiol. Scand. 60 (7), 874–881.

Odden, M.C., Shlipak, M.G., Tager, I.B., 2009. Serum creatinine and functional limitation in elderly persons. J. Gerontol. A Biol. Sci. Med. Sci. 64 (3), 370–376.

Oweis, A.O., Alshelleh, S.A., 2018. Incidence and outcomes of acute kidney injury in octogenarians in Jordan. BMC Res. Notes 11 (1), 844.

Palevsky, P.M., O'Connor, T.Z., Chertow, G.M., Crowley, S.T., Zhang, J.H., Kellum, J.A., 2009. Intensity of renal replacement therapy in acute kidney injury: perspective from within the Acute Renal Failure Trial Network Study. Crit. Care 13 (4), 310.

Palevsky, P.M., Zhang, J.H., O'Connor, T.Z., Chertow, G.M., Crowley, S.T., Choudhury, D., et al., 2008. Intensity of renal support in critically ill patients with acute kidney injury. N. Engl. J. Med. 359 (1), 7–20.

Panesso, M., 2021. Acute kidney injury and aging. Pediatr. Nephrol. 36 (10), 2997–3006.

Parikh, C.R., Coca, S.G., Wang, Y., Masoudi, F.A., Krumholz, H.M., 2008. Long-term prognosis of acute kidney injury after acute myocardial infarction. Arch. Intern. Med. 168 (9), 987–995.

Pascual, J., Liaño, F., 1998. Causes and prognosis of acute renal failure in the very old. J. Am. Geriatr. Soc. 46 (6), 721–725.

Payen, D., de Pont, A.C., Sakr, Y., Spies, C., Reinhart, K., Vincent, J.L., 2008. A positive fluid balance is associated with a worse outcome in patients with acute renal failure. Crit. Care 12 (3), R74.

Perazella, M.A., Mahnensmith, R.L., 1997. Hyperkalemia in the elderly: drugs exacerbate impaired potassium homeostasis. J. Gen. Intern. Med 12 (10), 646–656.

Pongsittisak, W., et al., 2020. Acute kidney injury outcomes of elderly and nonelderly patients in the medical intensive care unit of a university hospital in a developing country. Crit. Care Res. Pract. 2020, 2391683.

Population Division, 2019. World Population Prospects 2019: Ten Key Findings. United Nations, Department of Economic and Social Affairs, New York.

Quan, S., Pannu, N., Wilson, T., Ball, C., Tan, Z., Tonelli, M., et al., 2016. Prognostic implications of adding urine output to serum creatinine measurements for staging of acute kidney injury after major surgery: a cohort study. Nephrol. Dial. Transpl. 31 (12), 2049–2056.

Rai, S., Brace, C., Ross, P., Darvall, J., Haines, K., Mitchell, I., et al., 2023. Characteristics and outcomes of very elderly patients admitted to intensive care: a retrospective multicenter cohort analysis. Crit. Care Med. 51 (10), 1328–1338.

Reinikainen, M., Uusaro, A., Niskanen, M., Ruokonen, E., Kari, A., 2007. Intensive care of the elderly in Finland. Acta Anaesthesiol. Scand. 51 (5), 522–529.

Rewa, O., Bagshaw, S.M., 2014. Acute kidney injury—epidemiology, outcomes and economics. Nat. Rev. Nephrol. 10 (4), 193–207.

Rhee, H., Jang, K.S., Park, J.M., Kim, I.Y., Kim, J.H., Song, S.H., et al., 2016. Short- and long-term mortality rates of elderly acute kidney injury patients who underwent continuous renal replacement therapy. PLoS One 11 (11), e0167067.

Rodwell, G.E.J., Sonu, R., Zahn, J.M., Lund, J., Wilhelmy, J., Wang, L., et al., 2004. A transcriptional profile of aging in the human kidney. PLoS Biol. 2 (12), e427.

Ronco, C., Grammaticopoulos, S., Rosner, M., De Cal, M., Soni, S., Lentini, P., Piccinni, P., 2010. Oliguria, creatinine and other biomarkers of acute kidney injury. In: Ronco, C., Bellomo, R., Kellum, J.A. (Eds.), Critical Care Nephrology. second ed. Karger, Basel, pp. 118–127.

Rosner, M.H., 2013. Acute kidney injury in the elderly. Clin. Geriatr. Med. 29 (3), 565–578.

Ryan, D., Connelly, S., Chiu, M., Garcia, C., Iwashyna, T.J., 2008. The very elderly in intensive care: admission characteristics and mortality. Crit. Care Resusc. 10 (2), 106–110.

Schelling, J.R., 2016. Tubular atrophy in the pathogenesis of chronic kidney disease progression. Pediatr. Nephrol. 31 (5), 693–706.

Scherer, J.S., Holley, J.L., 2016. The role of time-limited trials in dialysis decision making in critically ill patients. Clin. J. Am. Soc. Nephrol. 11 (2), 344–353.

Schiffl, H., 2006. Renal recovery from acute tubular necrosis requiring renal replacement therapy: a prospective study in critically ill patients. Nephrol. Dial. Transpl. 21 (5), 1248–1252.

Schmitt, R., Coca, S., Kanbay, M., Tinetti, M.E., Cantley, L.G., 2008a. Recovery of kidney function after acute kidney injury in the elderly: a systematic review and meta-analysis. Am. J. Kidney Dis. 52 (2), 262–271.

Schmitt, R., Marlier, A., Cantley, L.G., 2008b. Zag expression during aging suppresses proliferation after kidney injury. J. Am. Soc. Nephrol. 19 (12), 2375–2383.

Self, W.H., Semler, M.W., Wanderer, J.P., Wang, L., Byrne, D.W., Collins, S.P., et al., 2018. Balanced crystalloids versus saline in noncritically ill adults. N. Engl. J. Med. 378 (9), 819–828.

Semler, M.W., Self, W.H., Wanderer, J.P., Ehrenfeld, J.M., Wang, L., Byrne, D.W., et al., 2018. Balanced crystalloids versus saline in critically ill adults. N. Engl. J. Med. 378 (9), 829–839.

National Heart, Lung, and Blood Institute PETAL Clinical Trials Network, Shapiro, N.I., Douglas, I.S., Brower, R.G., Brown, S.M., Exline, M.C., et al., 2023. Early restrictive or liberal fluid management for sepsis-induced hypotension. N. Engl. J. Med. 388, 499–510.

Siew, E.D., Ware, L.B., Ikizler, T.A., 2011. Biological markers of acute kidney injury. J. Am. Soc. Nephrol. 22 (5), 810–820.

Stephen, J., Simpson, K., Allison, M., 2006. Long-term quality of life and hospital mortality in patients treated with intermittent or continuous hemodialysis for acute renal and respiratory failure. Ren. Fail. 28 (4), 323–330.

Sun, Q., et al., 2023. Risk factors of perioperative acute kidney injury in elderly patients: a single-center retrospective study. Int. Urol. Nephrol. 55 (2), 459–467.

Teles, F., de Mendonça, A., Marinho, A., Garcia, T., Balbi, A., Ponce, D., Abrão, J., 2019. The impact of dialysis on critically ill elderly patients with acute kidney injury: an analysis by propensity score matching. Braz. J. Nephrol. 41 (1), 14–22.

Turgutalp, K., et al., 2017. Clinical outcomes of acute kidney injury developing outside the hospital in elderly. Int. Urol. Nephrol. 49 (1), 113–121.

Uchino, S., Kellum, J.A., Bellomo, R., Doig, G.S., Morimatsu, H., Morgera, S., et al., 2005. Acute renal failure in critically ill patients: a multinational, multicenter study. JAMA 294 (7), 813–818.

United Nations, Department of Economic and Social Affairs, Population Division, 2019. World Population Prospects 2019: Ten Key Findings. United Nations, New York.

Vaara, S.T., Forni, L.G., Joannidis, M., 2022. Subphenotypes of acute kidney injury in adults. Curr. Opin. Crit. Care 28 (6), 599–604.

Vaara, S.T., Ostermann, M., Bitker, L., Schneider, A., Poli, E., Hoste, E., et al., 2021. Restrictive fluid management versus usual care in acute kidney injury (REVERSE-AKI): a pilot randomized controlled feasibility trial. Intensive Care Med. 47, 665–673.

Waikar, S.S., Bonventre, J.V., 2009. Creatinine kinetics and the definition of acute kidney injury. J. Am. Soc. Nephrol. 20 (3), 672–679.

Waikar, S.S., Curhan, G.C., Wald, R., McCarthy, E.P., Chertow, G.M., 2006a. Declining mortality in patients with acute renal failure, 1988 to 2002. J. Am. Soc. Nephrol. 17 (4), 1143–1150.

Waikar, S.S., Wald, R., Chertow, G.M., Curhan, G.C., Winkelmayer, W.C., Liangos, O., et al., 2006b. Validity of international classification of diseases, ninth revision, clinical modification codes for acute renal failure. J. Am. Soc. Nephrol. 17 (6), 1688–1694.

Wang, A.Y., Bellomo, R., Cass, A., Finfer, S., Gattas, D., Myburgh, J., et al., 2015. Health-related quality of life in survivors of acute kidney injury: the prolonged outcomes study of the randomized evaluation of normal versus augmented level replacement therapy study outcomes. Nephrology 20 (7), 492–498.

Wen, J., Cheng, Q., Zhao, J., Ma, Q., Song, T., Liu, S., et al., 2013. Hospital-acquired acute kidney injury in Chinese very elderly persons. J. Nephrol. 26 (3), 572–579.

Wilson, F.P., Yang, W., Machado, C.A., Mariani, L.H., Borovskiy, Y., Berns, J.S., Feldman, H.I., 2014. Dialysis versus nondialysis in patients with AKI: a propensity-matched cohort study. Clin. J. Am. Soc. Nephrol. 9 (4), 673–681.

Woodcock, T.E., Woodcock, T.M., 2012. Revised Starling equation and the glycocalyx model of transvascular fluid exchange: an improved paradigm for prescribing intravenous fluid therapy. Br. J. Anaesth 108 (3), 384–394.

Xu, L., et al., 2021. Is acute kidney injury age-dependent in older adults: an observational study in two centers from North China. BMC Geriatr. 21 (1), 7.

Xue, J.L., Daniels, F., Star, R.A., Kimmel, P.L., Eggers, P.W., Molitoris, B.A., Himmelfarb, J., Collins, A.J., 2006. Incidence and mortality of acute renal failure in Medicare beneficiaries, 1992 to 2001. J. Am. Soc. Nephrol. 17 (4), 1135–1142.

Yılmaz, R., Erdem, Y., 2010. Acute kidney injury in the elderly population. Int. Urol. Nephrol. 42 (1), 259–271.

Yokota, L.G., Sampaio, B.M., Rocha, E.P., Balbi, A.L., Prado, I.R.S., Ponce, D., 2018. Acute kidney injury in elderly patients: narrative review on incidence, risk factors, and mortality. Int. J. Nephrol. Renovasc. Dis. 11, 217–224.

Zarbock, A., Nadim, M.K., Pickkers, P., Gomez, H., Bell, S., Joannidis, M., et al., 2023. Sepsis-associated acute kidney injury: consensus report of the 28th Acute Disease Quality Initiative workgroup. Nat. Rev. Nephrol. 19 (6), 401–417.

CHAPTER

7

Nutritional considerations and aging

Yoko Narasaki[a,b], *Connie M. Rhee*[a,b,c], *and Kamyar Kalantar-Zadeh*[c,d]

[a]Department of Medicine, David Geffen School of Medicine at UCLA, Los Angeles, CA, United States

[b]Nephrology Section, Veterans Affairs Greater Los Angeles Healthcare System, Los Angeles, CA, United States

[c]Division of Nephrology, Hypertension, and Kidney Transplantation, University of California Irvine, Orange, CA, United States

[d]Division of Nephrology and Hypertension, The Lundquist Institute at Harbor-UCLA Medical Center, Torrance, CA, United States

Introduction

With healthy aging, natural alterations in physical functions and vital cofactors necessary for optimal enzyme function may occur with varying degrees in each individual. Despite the significant alterations in the aging gastrointestinal tract (GIT), the majority of digestive and absorptive capacity appears to be preserved at a moderate intake of macronutrients in healthy aging. When it comes to the postabsorption stage, optimal nutrient metabolism is typically altered, which is characterized by impaired glucose disposal, decreased muscle protein synthesis (MPS), and altered lipid dynamics.

Among the lifestyle factors, dietary modification is a powerful strategy for healthy aging by regulating nutrient signaling, gut microbiota, and energy metabolism. Many studies have found the significant antiaging potential of dietary patterns, such as the Mediterranean diet and Dietary Approaches to Stop Hypertension (DASH). Indeed, the dietary guidelines for the general population recommend following a dietary pattern that shares similar characteristics with these dietary patterns, such as encouraging the intake of fresh fruits and vegetables, whole grains, healthy fats, and lean proteins.

Diet plays an important role in overall health and particularly in preventing kidney-related issues. Yet, findings from studies do not show a consistent relationship between dietary intake and kidney health. However, emerging evidence suggests that adherence to healthy dietary patterns such as the DASH diet, Mediterranean diet, and plant-based diet, along with

Aging and the Kidney
https://doi.org/10.1016/B978-0-443-34069-7.00011-2

dietary intakes of specific nutrients significant in these diets (i.e., lower in saturated fatty acids [SFAs], sodium, glycemic load, and phosphorus load; while higher in plant-based protein, polyunsaturated fatty acids [PUFAs], fiber, potassium, and antioxidants), is related to better kidney function in people, including those in the latter stages of life.

In this chapter, we review the current evidence regarding (1) the impact of protein-energy wasting (PEW) malnutrition on kidney health outcomes and (2) the effects of dietary protein and amino acids, other macronutrients (e.g., carbohydrates, fats), and dietary patterns on kidney function among those in the later stages of life.

Changes in nutrition metabolism with aging

Along with major physiological changes in health conditions with aging (i.e., immune system, musculoskeletal system, cardiovascular system, central nervous system), the natural aging process impacts the digestive system/GIT.

Effect of the aging GIT on nutrition, digestion and absorption, metabolism, and gut microbiome

Alterations in the aging GIT include chewing impairment, decreased stomach acid secretion (i.e., gastric acid, pancreatic lipase, bile salts), delayed gastric emptying, and morphological changes to the small intestine (Fig. 7.1) (Milan and Cameron-Smith, 2015). Moreover,

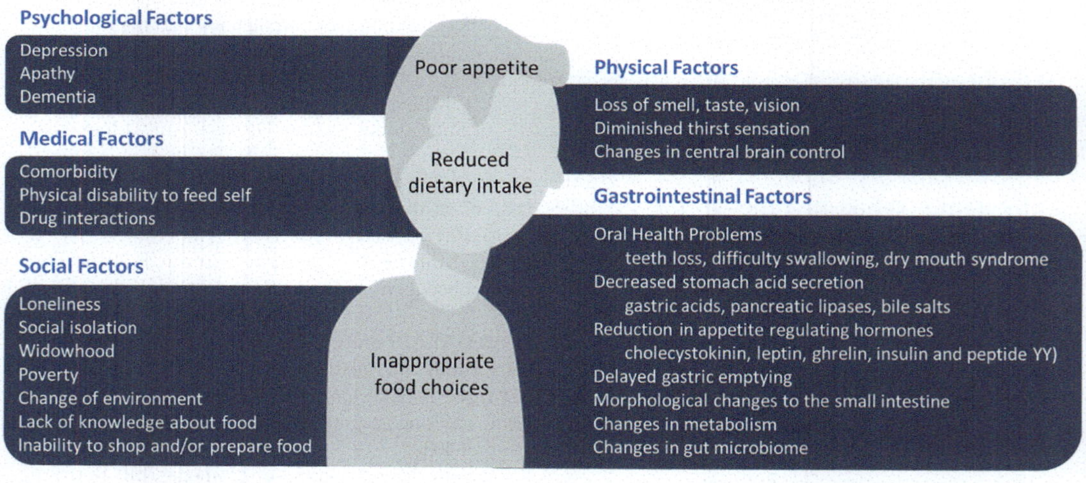

FIG. 7.1 Factors impacting dietary intake among the elderly. Multiple factors potentially impact dietary intake in the elderly population. Changes in the aging gastrointestinal tract include oral health problems, decreased stomach acid secretion, reduction in appetite-regulating hormones, delayed gastric emptying, morphological changes to the small intestine, and changes in metabolism and the gut microbiome. These gastrointestinal factors, as well as physiological, psychological, medical, and social factors, all potentially contribute to poor appetite, inappropriate food choices, and reduced dietary intake in the elderly population.

there are reductions in appetite-regulating hormones such as cholecystokinin, leptin, ghrelin, insulin and peptide YY, contributing to less appetite, hungry, or cravings for food, and lower dietary intakes compared to their younger counterparts (de Boer et al., 2013; Rémond et al., 2015). Physiological and psychological changes and social factors are also associated with an alteration of food intake during aging (de Boer et al., 2013).

In contrast to the hypothesis that these factors lead to a reduction in digestion and absorption in the older population, GIT function seems to be well preserved with aging with respect to the digestion and absorption of macronutrients such as protein, fat, and carbohydrates, while this may not, per se, pertain to micronutrients (Milan and Cameron-Smith, 2015). In the elderly, glucose absorption is typically preserved (Russell, 2000), although it should be noted that some individuals have slightly impaired glucose absorption, especially those with decreased kidney function (Arora et al., 1989) and in the setting of larger carbohydrate loads (Feibusch and Holt, 1982). Similarly, there is little evidence of impaired protein digestion and absorption with aging at moderate intake (Russell, 2000) and even with higher protein intake (Cheng et al., 1978) while some conflicting results were found with higher protein intake (Werner and Hambraeus, 1971). Studies examining whether fat digestion and absorption differ between younger and older adults have also reported inconsistent findings. Some reported that the age-related differences were due to a decline in kidney function (Schaefer et al., 1995) in the setting of hospitalization and malnourished conditions (Saltzman and Mason, 1992) or with higher fat intake (Werner and Hambraeus, 1971). Meanwhile, studies have shown that the absorption of some important micronutrients, such as calcium, vitamin D, and vitamin B12, declines with age (Milan and Cameron-Smith, 2015). Taken together, the changes in nutrient digestion and absorption may depend largely on health status and the prevalence of comorbidities and may not be a function of aging itself (Milan and Cameron-Smith, 2015).

In the latter stage of metabolism, following the process of digestion and absorption, changes in macronutrient metabolism in older adults are readily apparent. Impairment of glucose homeostasis is reported, likely due to tissue insulin resistance (Fink et al., 1983). Although there are confounding factors such as BMI, physical activity levels, and habitual diet, aging per se seems to be associated with decreased peripheral insulin sensitivity (Elahi and Muller, 2000). Possibly the most important contributing factor to altered protein metabolism in aging is the anabolic resistance or inadequate stimulation of MPS in response to protein intake (Cuthbertson et al., 2005). The patterns of protein intake often seen in older adults, such as insufficient amounts of intake and uneven or inconsistent consumption throughout the day, as well as factors including concurrent alterations in digestive function and insulin responsiveness, are all known to impact protein metabolism and ultimately MPS (Milan and Cameron-Smith, 2015). Studies have shown clear evidence of altered postprandial lipid metabolism, determined by the increase in most lipid levels in blood (i.e., cholesterol, TG, LDL) and prolonged and exaggerated TG levels as a result of high-fat intake (Milan and Cameron-Smith, 2015). Hormonal and metabolic mechanisms involved in the clearance and storage of ingested lipids are likely key determinants of age-related differences in lipid metabolism (Milan and Cameron-Smith, 2015).

The gut microbiome changes in response to alterations in diet, health conditions and chronic disease, body composition, and natural aging. Studies have reported that the microbiota in the elderly have higher proportions of the phylum Bacteroidetes, while younger adults have higher proportions of Firmicutes (Mariat et al., 2009).

Consequences of the aging GIT on nutritional status

PEW is a condition of metabolism and nutritional derangements, which is frequently observed in those suffering from other conditions such as sarcopenia (i.e., loss of muscle mass and function) and frailty (i.e., multisystem impairment associated with increased vulnerability to stressors) (Narasaki et al., 2021). Changes in eating patterns and GIT function in the elderly are associated with a higher risk of malnutrition and PEW, especially among older chronic kidney disease (CKD) patients who have additional risk factors for PEW due to impaired kidney function (i.e., uremia-induced catabolism, acidosis, and persistent inflammation) (Koppe and Fouque, 2019; Wu et al., 2019; Chao et al., 2019). PEW is, in turn, associated with a higher risk of infection, frailty, depression, low quality of life, hospitalization, cardiovascular disease, and death (Ikizler et al., 2013).

Impact of dietary intake on kidney health in the elderly with or without CKD

Macronutrients

Recommended dietary protein intake (DPI)

In general, while a protein intake of 0.8 g/kg/d has been traditionally recommended for adults of all ages based on the amount of need (0.6 g/kg/d) and an additional "buffer" amount to ensure safe intake (0.2 g/kg/d) (Kovesdy et al., 2013), there have been recommendations for higher dietary protein intake (DPI) of at least 1.0 g/kg/d for older adults to optimally preserve lean body mass, various body functions, and overall health status (Volkert et al., 2019). This paradigm shift toward recommending higher intake among the elderly population is based on epidemiological studies and clinical trials that support the benefits of higher protein intake for older adults in terms of bone mass density (Promislow et al., 2002; Rapuri et al., 2003), slower rates of bone loss (Hannan et al., 2000), fewer health problems (Vellas et al., 1997), and greater lean body mass. Alteration in body composition (i.e., increased body fat and decreased lean body mass) is one of the changes that occurs with healthy aging. Short to longer-term follow-up of protein intake in clinical trials demonstrated that diets containing the RDA levels of protein (0.8 g/kg/d) resulted in reduced urinary nitrogen excretion over time among older adults during a period of 18 days (Morse et al., 2001) to up to 14 weeks (Campbell et al., 2001). In the latter trial, although whole body composition and weight did not change over the course of the 14 weeks of intervention, mid-thigh muscle area was significantly decreased, which suggests the RDA for protein may not be adequate for the metabolic and physiological needs of older adults (Campbell et al., 2001). Association of higher DPI with the maintenance of lean body mass has been found in many observational studies and in a systematic review (Yaegashi et al., 2021). For example, over a 3-year follow-up among 2066 healthy older adults who participated in the Health, Aging, and Body Composition Study, the loss of lean body mass among those in the highest quintile of protein intake was approximately 40% lower compared to that in those in the lowest quintile of protein intake (Houston et al., 2008). The latter studies also observed that greater protein intake, irrespective of its source (plant vs. animal protein) (Li et al., 2019; Chen et al., 2023) and higher protein intake with more even distribution across meals (Farsijani et al., 2016) were associated with higher lean body mass in older adults.

DPI and its short-term effect on kidney function

While there are concerns about the kidney health or safety of prescribing a high protein intake, particularly in older adults, there are sparse and inconsistent data regarding the safety of high protein diets on kidney status in healthy individuals, including those who are older (Table 7.1). One of the major functions of the kidney in protein metabolism is to eliminate waste products from protein intake. Therefore it is not surprising that the ability to compensate for increased amino acids or DPI declines in most cases of the healthy older population (Walrand et al., 2008) in response to changes in kidney function with aging, such as lower average glomerular filtration rate (GFR) and renal plasma flow (Narasaki et al., 2021). Indeed, a randomized crossover feeding trial of a high versus usual protein diet for 10 days among 10 healthy younger and 9 older participants showed a lack of a physiological increase in GFR that would be expected with high protein intake among the older participants with normal age-related decline in their GFR (Walrand et al., 2008). On the other hand, it is also possible that a decline in the ability to handle high protein intake is not per se applicable to all elderly adults or that the decline is within the normal range, and that the kidney function reserve in healthy elderly adults may be preserved until the eighth decade of life because of individual differences in aging. This was confirmed by a study comparing GFRs after an overnight amino acid infusion in 15 participants of younger age and 10 participants of older age, in which there was no statistically significant difference in the increase in GFR following amino acid infusion among the older group versus the younger group (Fliser et al., 1993).

DPI and its moderate- to long-term effects on kidney function

With respect to the intermediate- to long-term effect of high protein intake on kidney function in healthy older adults, inconsistent results such as no effect (Halbesma et al., 2009; Beasley et al., 2014), protective effect (Higashiyama et al., 2010; Kubo et al., 2023), and adverse effect have been reported (Table 7.1) (Cirillo et al., 2014). With respect to the studies showing no association, among the 8461 adults aged 28–75 years who participated in the Prevention of Renal and Vascular End-stage Disease (PREVEND) prospective community-based cohort study, DPI estimated using 24-h urinary urea nitrogen was not associated with eGFR decline over the 6.4 years of follow-up (Halbesma et al., 2009). Notably, this cohort, consisting of only a small portion (~9%) of those with impaired kidney function (defined as eGFR < 60 ml/min/1.73 m^2), observed that either higher or lower protein intake was associated with a higher risk of cardiovascular events, and lower intake was associated with a higher risk of all-cause and cardiovascular mortality. Another prospective cohort study with 6.4 years of follow-up, in which total, animal, and vegetable protein intake was ascertained by FFQ, found no association with change in eGFR in 3623 adults aged ≥ 65 years after adjusting for demographic and lifestyle characteristics and comorbidities (Beasley et al., 2014). Although this study included one-quarter (23%) of those with impaired kidney function (defined as eGFR < 60 ml/min/1.73 m^2), there was no evidence for effect modification by baseline eGFR.

There are several explanations for the discrepancy found in the studies examining the kidneys' ability to adapt to the increases in protein intake or the relationship of dietary protein with kidney function (Cirillo et al., 2014). One of the possible explanations is the

TABLE 7.1 Selected studies on the quantity and quality of dietary protein intake and kidney function in the short term (upper panel) and moderate-to-long term (lower panel).

Author	Population (*N*)	Study design	Intervention/ Exposure	Duration/ Follow-up	Kidney function outcome	Results
Kidney function (short term)						
Fliser et al., J. Am. Soc. Nephrol., 1993	Adults of young age with a median of 26 years ($N = 15$) and those of old age with a median age of 70 years ($N = 10$)	nRCT	Amino acid infusion	Overnight	GFR (insulin clearance) and ERPF (para-amino-hippurate clearance)	No statistically significant difference in amino acid-infused GFR between the older and younger groups.
Walrand et al., Am. J. Physiol. Endocrinol. Metab., 2008	Younger adults aged 24 ± 1 years ($N = 10$) and older adults aged 70 ± 2 years ($N = 9$)	RCT	High vs. usual protein diet (3.0 vs. 1.5 g/kg fat-free mass/day)	10 days	GFR	Lower GFR was observed in the older group compared to the younger group. A significant increase in GFR following a high-protein diet occurred only in the younger group.
Wagner et al., J. Am. Diet. Assoc., 2007	Younger adults aged 25–40 ($N = 12$) and older adults aged 55–75 years ($N = 10$)	CT	High vs. Low protein diet (2.0 vs. 0.5 g/kg/day)	1 week/ diet	GFR	The older group, mainly women, showed an increase in glomerular filtration rate after the high-protein diet compared to the low-protein diet; the younger group did not.
Kidney function (moderate-to-long term)						
Knight et al., Ann. Intern. Med., 2003	Women aged 42–68 years with normal renal function (eGFR ≥ 80 mL/min/1.73 m^2, $N = 1135$) and with mild renal insufficiency ($55 \leq$ eGFR < 80 mL/min/1.73 m^2, $N = 489$) from the Nurses' Health Study	PC	Protein intake ascertained by a semi-quantitative FFQ	11 years	eGFR decline	Total protein intake was not associated with eGFR decline among women with normal renal function, but higher intake of total and nondairy animal protein was associated with a greater decline in eGFR among women with mild renal insufficiency.

Halbesma et al., J. Am. Soc. Nephrol., 2009	Adults aged 28–75 years from the Prevention of Renal and Vascular End-stage Disease (PREVEND) study (N = 8461)	PC	Protein intake estimated from 24-h urinary urea nitrogen excretion (Maroni formula)	6.4 years	eGFR decline, where eGFR is calculated using the MDRD study equation	No association between total protein intake and eGFR decline.
Higashiyama et al., J. Epidemiol., 2010	Adults aged ≥ 30 years, including those aged ≥ 80 years (N = 7404), from the National Survey on Circulatory Disorders and the National Nutrition Survey	CS	Total animal and vegetable protein intake ascertained by a household food weighing method	NA	Presence of CKD; eGFR calculated using the abbreviated MDRD study equation	Higher protein intake (total, animal, vegetable) was associated with higher GFR in both sexes and a low prevalence of CKD in women.
Cirillo et al., Nephrol. Dial. Transplant., 2014	Adults aged 45–64 years (N = 1522) from Gubbio Study	CS/PC	Protein intake estimated using 24-hour urinary urea nitrogen excretion	12 years	eGFR decline, where eGFR was calculated using the CKD-EPI equation	Higher protein intake was associated cross-sectionally with higher GFR, but longitudinally with greater GFR decline over time.
Beasley et al., Nutrition 2014	Adults aged ≥ 65 years (N = 3623) from the Cardiovascular Health Study	PC	Dietary protein intake ascertained by FFQ	6.4 years	Rapid decline in kidney function, as defined by (ΔeGFR-cysC > 3 mL•min•1.73 m^2), where eGFR was estimated using equations based on cystatin C or creatinine along with cystatin C	Protein intake (total, animal, vegetable) was not associated with a change in eGFR.
Gopinath et al., ACI Rep., 2016	Adults aged ≥ 50 years (N = 1185)	CS	Dietary low/reduced-fat dairy food and dietary calcium intake ascertained by FFQ	NA	Prevalence and 10-year incidence of CKD	Highest quintile of dietary low/reduced fat dairy food consumption versus the lowest quintile was associated with a reduced risk of CKD. Increasing the total intake of dietary calcium was also associated with a reduced risk of CKD.

Continued

TABLE 7.1 Selected studies on the quantity and quality of dietary protein intake and kidney function in the short term (upper panel) and moderate-to-long term (lower panel)—cont'd

Author	Population (N)	Study design	Intervention/ Exposure	Duration/ Follow-up	Kidney function outcome	Results
Haring et al., J. Ren. Nutr., 2017	Adults aged 44–66 years (N = 11,952) from the Atherosclerosis Risk in Communities (ARIC) Study	PC	Total animal, vegetable protein intake, and specific dietary protein sources ascertained by FFQ	23 years (median)	Incident of CKD stage 3 (a decrease in eGFR of ≥25% from baseline, resulting in an eGFR < 60 ml/ min/1.73 m^2), where eGFR was calculated using the 2009 CKD-EPI equation	There were varied associations between the type of protein and specific dietary protein sources with the risk of incident CKD, with red and processed meat being adversely associated with CKD risk, and total (tendency), vegetable—particularly nuts, low-fat dairy products, and legumes—being protective against the development of CKD.
Bernier-Jean, Nephrol. Dial. Transplant., 2021	Adult women aged > 70 years (N = 1374) from the Longitudinal Study of Aging Women	PC	Plant-sourced protein and animal protein obtained by FFQ	10 years	Decline in eGFR	Older women consuming a diet that is richer in plant-sourced protein experience a slower decline in kidney function. The intake of animal protein was not associated with eGFR decline.
Kubo et al., Environ. Health Prev. Med., 2023	Adults aged 40–74 years (N = 3277) from the Circulatory Risk in Communities Study	PC	Total, animal, and vegetable protein intake was ascertained by the brief-type self-administered diet history questionnaire	8.1 years (median)	Development/Incident of CKD (eGFR < 60 ml/ min/1.73 m^2): GFR was calculated using the CKD-EPI equation with the Japanese coefficient	Higher protein intake, more specifically animal protein intake, was associated with a lower risk of CKD.

Lu et al., BMJ Open, 2023	Adults aged 50 + years with (N = 1452) and without diabetes (N = 8,316) from the Guangzhou Biobank Cohort Study	CS	Portion of consumption of red meat, poultry, fish, seafood, and processed meat per week	NA	eGFR, prevalent CKD (eGFR < 60 mL/min/1.73 m^2)	Higher processed meat intake was associated with lower eGFR overall, in both those with and without diabetes. Higher fish and seafood intake was associated with higher eGFR among those with diabetes and lower eGFR among those without diabetes.
Mirzababaei et al., Sci. Rep., 2024	Women aged 30–65 years with diabetic nephropathy (N = 105) or without diabetic nephropathy (N = 105)	CC	High vs. low consumption of red, processed, and white meat ascertained by FFQ	NA	Developing kidney damage (i.e., microalbuminuria, severe albuminuria, higher BUN levels) and diabetic nephropathy	Higher consumption of red and processed meat sources was associated with microalbuminuria, severe albuminuria, higher BUN levels, and higher odds of diabetic nephropathy.

Abbrev.: CC, Case-control study; CS, Cross-sectional cohort study; CKD, chronic kidney disease; CKD-EPI, Chronic Kidney Disease Epidemiology; CT, Crossover trial; eGFR, estimated glomerular filtration rate; FFQ, food frequency questionnaire; MDRD, Modification of Diet in Renal Disease; NA, not applicable or not available; nRCT, nonrandomized controlled trial; PC, prospective cohort study; RCT, randomized controlled trial.

different equations used for calculation of estimated GFR (eGFR). It is known that eGFR calculated using the abbreviated Modification of Diet in Renal Disease (MDRD) equation has low accuracy for values ≥ 60 ml/min/1.73 m² (Stevens et al., 2006). Moreover, given the nature of serum creatinine as an imprecise biomarker of kidney function that is influenced by nonrenal factors (i.e., muscle mass), nephron loss can be present with or without changes in serum creatinine levels (Hommos et al., 2017). Thus it should be emphasized that there is the possibility that older adults may lack kidney function reserve or the ability to augment GFR in the setting of high protein diets even if they have normal GFR levels (Narasaki et al., 2021). Other areas which may contribute to this discrepancy across studies include the differential follow-up periods, including too abbreviated follow-up to adequately detect a sizeable eGFR decline or to evaluate the effects of DPI on eGFR, as well as the lack of normalization of protein intake (i.e., DPI scaled to ideal body weight rather than actual intake) (Cirillo et al., 2014). In summary, although short-term intervention studies indicate that high protein intake induces the upregulation of eGFR regardless of the age and some studies over relatively longer periods suggest the advantage of higher protein intake in healthy elderly individuals, there should be caution with respect to the potential risk of consuming this diet over long-term periods until further studies can rigorously evaluate the long-term safety and efficacy of higher protein intake in healthy aging adults.

Source of DPI and its effect on kidney function

Growing evidence on the source of dietary protein has shown the advantages of diets consisting of plant-based proteins rather than animal-based proteins in older adults. With respect to studies suggesting the benefits of plant-based protein, a cross-sectional cohort study consisting of 1185 adults aged ≥ 50 years found an association between the highest quintile of dietary low/reduced-fat dairy food versus the lowest quintile and a lower risk of prevalence of CKD (Gopinath et al., 2016). Prospective studies have also confirmed this favorable relationship of plant-based protein on kidney function. A study using the Atherosclerosis Risk in Communities (ARIC) cohort found an association of higher total plant-based protein intake, but not total animal-based protein intake, with a lower risk of incident CKD after a median follow-up of 23 years (Haring et al., 2017). This study also found varied associations of specific dietary protein sources with the risk of incident CKD, such that consumption of red meat and processed meat was adversely associated with CKD risk, whereas nuts, low-fat dairy products, and legumes were associated with a lower risk of developing CKD. In the Longitudinal Study of Aging Women cohort, which included 1374 women aged > 70 years, it was observed that the consumption of a diet richer in plant-based protein was associated with a slower decline in eGFR after 10 years of follow-up, while intake of animal protein was not associated with a decline in eGFR (Bernier-Jean et al., 2021). Regarding evidence supporting the harmful effects of consuming higher animal-based proteins in older adults, a cross-sectional relationship between higher processed meat, fish, and seafood intake and lower eGFR was seen among 9768 adults aged ≥ 50 years (Lu et al., 2023). A case-control study including women aged 30–65 years with or without diabetic nephropathy (N = 105 and 105, respectively) showed that higher consumption of red meat and processed meat was associated with microalbuminuria, severe albuminuria, higher BUN levels, and higher odds of diabetic nephropathy (Mirzababaei et al., 2024).

Protein restriction and supplemented protein restriction

While higher protein intake could potentially be associated with favorable kidney function and/or a lack of kidney dysfunction in healthy older adults without CKD or underlying kidney disease risk factors, this does not per se apply to those at risk for nephron loss or with kidney disease. Reduced DPI has favorable effects on kidney health, which include not only the ability to prevent and correct contributors to and/or early markers of kidney damage (i.e., reduction in glomerular hyperfiltration, proteinuria, eGFR decline) but may also confer improvements in metabolic disturbances and the symptom burden that occurs with kidney failure (i.e., better control of phosphorus and potassium homeostasis, decreased metabolic acidosis, lipid balance, reduced inflammation, and lower uremic toxin burden) (Yan et al., 2018; Morris et al., 2020; Koppe and Fouque, 2019). A prospective cohort study among 1674 older women showed differential relationships between DPI and kidney function based on the presence or absence of preexisting decreased kidney function, such that total protein intake was not associated with eGFR decline among women with normal renal function (eGFR ≥ 80 mL/min/1.73 m^2), but higher intake of total and nondairy animal protein was associated with greater decline of eGFR among women with mild renal insufficiency (55 ≤ eGFR < 80 mL/min/1.73 m^2) (Knight et al., 2003).

There is ongoing uncertainty regarding at what level of kidney function higher protein intake has more favorable versus adverse effects on kidney health due to a limited evidence base, particularly with respect to differences across individuals of various ages. However, there is growing evidence supporting low-protein diets as a cornerstone in reducing the risk of ESKD in people with CKD, including those who are elderly. In patients with CKD up to the age of 70 years, a retrospective cohort study suggested that low-protein diets can reduce patients' morbidity, preserve renal function, relieve uremic symptoms, improve nutritional status, postpone the initiation of dialysis for 6 months, and entail substantial cost-savings (Eyre et al., 2008). Another study compared $N = 61$ patients treated with a low-protein diet for ≥ six months prior to their transition to dialysis treatment versus $N = 61$ patients not treated with low-protein diets, matched for sex, age, dialysis modality, diabetes, and initiation of dialysis.

The safety of low-protein diets is often debated in patients with CKD. For example, the MDRD study, a large randomized controlled trial of dietary protein and phosphorus restriction on CKD outcomes, which examined 1585 patients aged 18–70 years old, showed a small but significant decline in nutrition indicators, essentially muscle mass, due to the adverse effect of inadequate protein and energy intake (Kopple et al., 1997). Loss of lean body mass is unavoidable in cases where the energy intake is insufficient, even when protein intake is adequate (Kopple et al., 1986). Thus the importance of nutritional counseling to ensure an energy intake of 30–35 kcal/kg/d, as well as maintenance of a neutral nitrogen balance, should be emphasized through regular nutritional follow-ups by a renal dietitian in order to detect early signs of malnutrition when a low-protein diet is prescribed (Bauer et al., 2013). Under those conditions, the development of malnutrition during a low-protein diet is extremely rare. As a safety precaution, malnourished patients, patients under stress conditions such as those with recent hospitalization or surgery, and elderly CKD patients with stable kidney function (i.e., not with CKD progression or advanced CKD stage) with the presence of poor nutrition status or PEW should avoid or defer a low-protein diet

(Bauer et al., 2013; Piccoli et al., 2023). Individual risk assessment and appropriate nutritional monitoring should be used to guide the patient's decision-making process and whether to support prioritization of low-protein diets or not (Piccoli et al., 2023).

A very low protein diet (VLPD, 0.3–0.4 g/kg/d of protein) supplemented with essential amino acids or ketoacid analogs (KAs, up to 0.6 g/kg/d) under close supervision is another dietary regimen beyond regular LPDs. Given that KAs can be utilized without releasing nitrogenous waste into the body, using KAs paired with VLPD can be used to reduce CKD progression while also reducing nitrogen waste and maintaining adequate amino acid levels (Koppe and Fouque, 2019). Patients with advanced NDD-CKD aged > 70 years who participated in a randomized control trial showed that a VLPD (0.3 g/kg/d of protein) with KAs, EAAs, and vitamins delayed dialysis initiation by approximately 11 months versus a control group in whom DPI was not restricted, although both groups showed comparable mortality rates (Brunori et al., 2007).

Carbohydrate intake

While it is well recognized that DPI increases renal blood flow and GFR and may lead to lower kidney function, particularly in the setting of decreased nephron mass and in those with a risk of kidney disease, there is much less evidence regarding the effects of carbohydrate and fat intake on kidney function. A randomized controlled trial of 163 overweight/obese adults aged ≥ 30 years (mean age 52 ± 11 years) without underlying diabetes or kidney disease revealed the short-term implications of the amount and type of carbohydrate on kidney function (Juraschek et al., 2016). After each five-week period of cross-feeding of four types of diets, namely combinations of high versus low glycemic index diets and high versus low carbohydrate diets (defined by the proportion of total energy intake), lower carbohydrate consumption resulted in a rise in GFR, and concurrent receipt of low glycemic index with low carbohydrate diets had additive effects on increasing GFR while maintaining constant body weights.

Reports on the long-term effects of carbohydrate intake and kidney function are also limited. With respect to the quantity and quality of carbohydrates, there are studies suggesting a link between higher carbohydrate intake, especially those related to greater GI, and the risk of CKD in healthy or overweight/obese individuals. In an observational study including 2600 adults aged ≥ 50 years, the highest quartile of dietary GI intake, ascertained by FFQ, was associated with a higher risk of having eGFR < 60 ml/min/1.73 m^2, while the highest quartile of dietary cereal fiber intake was associated with a lower risk of having eGFR < 60 ml/min/1.73 m^2 compared to the lowest quartile of each intake (Gopinath et al., 2016). In addition to these cross-sectional associations, longitudinal analyses found that higher baseline intake of energy-dense, nutrient-poor sources of carbohydrates (e.g., cookies) was associated with a higher risk of 5-year incidence of CKD. A metaanalysis including 1687 participants from nine randomized controlled trials among the overweight/obese population without CKD showed an association between a low-carbohydrate diet versus a control diet and an increase in eGFR (Oyabu et al., 2016). In a prospective cohort including 6746 participants without diabetes mellitus and 1058 with diabetes mellitus aged 40–69 years, diets rich in carbohydrates, ascertained by 24-h dietary recall FFQ, were associated with a higher risk of CKD development (defined as a composite of eGFR ≤ 60 ml/min/1.73 m^2 and development of proteinuria) only among those without diabetes after approximately 10 years of follow-up

(Nam et al., 2019). In the same cohort study among adults aged 40–69 years, participants on a diet with a low fat-to-carbohydrate ratio were associated with a higher risk of CKD after a median follow-up of 11.4 years, suggesting that limiting excessive high-carbohydrate and low-fat intake is important to prevent CKD development (Kim et al., 2021).

An increasing body of evidence suggests the risk of consuming sugar or its alternatives on cardiometabolic diseases. Limited studies examining the associations between the consumption of sugar-sweetened beverages and CKD risk among older adults are inconsistent. A prospective study among 63,257 adults aged 45–74 years showed no association between soda intake, ascertained by 24-h dietary recall, and the risk of ESKD over a mean follow-up of 16.8 years (Lew et al., 2018). In contrast, another prospective population-based cohort study analyzed data from 127,830 adults aged 40–69 years, which showed an association between lower consumption of sugar-sweetened beverages or artificially sweetened beverages and a reduced risk of developing CKD after a median follow-up of 10.5 years (Heo et al., 2024). A metaanalysis including six studies with a total of 25,455 adults examining sugar-sweetened beverages and three studies with a total of 19,995 adults examining artificially sweetened beverages concluded that either sugar or artificially sweetened beverage consumption above seven servings per week was associated with an increased risk of CKD (Lo et al., 2021). Fructose is a type of sugar that naturally exists in fruits and honey but is preferentially added to sugar-sweetened soft drinks and sodas as a component of high-fructose corn syrup in the modern food industry (Nakagawa and Kang, 2021). In animal models, high-fructose consumption has been shown to cause glomerular hypertrophy, subtle renal damage (Boot-Handford and Heath, 1981) and accelerated progression of CKD (Gersch et al., 2007). Evidence from human studies also indicates that higher fructose intake plays a role in adverse CKD outcomes. In an examination of over ten healthy younger adults, high-fructose corn syrup increased vascular resistance in the kidney (Chapman et al., 2020).

Several mechanisms could be speculated with respect to the association between dietary carbohydrate intake and kidney function. For example, it has been suggested that the short-term rise in GFR and long-term risk of incident CKD observed with lower carbohydrate consumption may simply be due to the substitution of dietary protein for dietary carbohydrate. Because metabolic derangements, such as insulin resistance, are known risk factors for CKD, metabolic abnormalities accompanied by higher dietary carbohydrate intake may play a role. Moreover, other factors related to higher carbohydrate intake, especially those that are greatly refined and higher GI carbohydrates (i.e., systemic inflammation, oxidative stress, and alteration in gut microbiota), may contribute to the association between higher carbohydrate intake and higher incident CKD in the long-term (Nam et al., 2019).

Fat intake

Similar to DPI, the quantity and the type of dietary fat intake seem to be important in kidney health. Among experimental animal models examining higher dietary fat intake, those with study periods of less than eight weeks (i.e., four to eight weeks) have not identified adverse CKD outcomes, but those with longer study periods (i.e., eight to twelve weeks) have shown alterations in kidney structure and function. Kidney mass did not change in rats fed high-fat and/or high-sugar diets (e.g., excess lard, sucrose, or a combination of lard + sucrose) over a four-week and eight-week period, although there was a significant increase in weight and abdominal fat over these time periods (Pranprawit et al., 2013). In another study of rats, feeding a high-fat diet versus standard chow over a six-week period was found to increase adiposity and renal mass, while there was no evidence of early kidney injury ascertained by urinary and plasma biomarkers (urine-to-protein creatinine ratio, plasma cystatin C) nor changes in renal histology (Crinigan et al., 2015). In contrast, relatively longer intake of high-fat diets containing dietary fat ranging from 15% (Dwyer et al., 1995) to 30% (Altunkaynak et al., 2008) to 60% (Deji et al., 2009) of total energy intake derived from saturated fatty acid sources (including lard, beef tallow, and coconut oil) led to renal fat accumulation with concomitant changes in kidney structure and function.

It has been noted that different types of dietary fat have resulted in varying effects on kidney health. A study of rats fed a low-dose regimen (5%) of lipid-enriched diets with three different sources of fat (e.g., canola oil, fish oil, and butter) versus a control diet suggests that even low levels of supplementation of different types of fat can modify age-related changes in kidney function over a chronic nutritional regimen (Valente Gamba et al., 2001). In this study, while a faster onset of increased proteinuria, age-related decline in GFR, and renal blood flow was shown in all lipid-enriched diet groups compared to the control group, deterioration in GFR and renal blood flow was most marked in those receiving butter and fish oil, and the lowest GFR and renal blood flow were observed in those receiving butter by the 18th month. Epidemiological studies have also shown the effects of the type of dietary fat on kidney outcomes in the older population. In a cross-sectional study among 5042 adults aged 45–84 years from the Multi-Ethnic Study of Atherosclerosis, greater low-fat daily intake was associated with a lower urinary albumin-to-creatinine ratio (Nettleton et al., 2008). Similarly, higher intake of animal fat and two or more servings per week of red meat were found to be associated with an increased risk of microalbuminuria among 3348 women with a median age of 67 years, followed over 11 years in the Nurses' Health Study (Lin et al., 2010a). More specifically, in terms of the subtypes of dietary fatty acids, the most favorable effects were observed with total PUFAs, n-6 PUFAs, and n-3 PUFAs found in fish oil as eicosapentaenoic and docosahexaenoic acids, while adverse effects were found with SFAs. For example, greater intake of SFAs was associated with a higher risk of albuminuria in a study of 19,256 adults aged ≥ 45 years from the Reasons for Geographic and Racial Differences in Stroke (REGARDS) cohort (Lin et al., 2010b). In this study, however, greater intake of SFAs was not associated with eGFR. < 60 ml/min/1.73 m^2 and neither total nor other subtypes of dietary fat were associated with high albuminuria or eGFR < 60 ml/min/1.73 m^2. A population-based study among 2600 adults aged ≥ 50 years with or without moderate CKD, increased intake of dietary n-3 PUFAs and fish ascertained by FFQ was associated with the lower prevalence of CKD (Gopinath et al., 2011b). In 1074 adults aged 40–79 years with incident ESKD and 3230 matched controls, there was an inverse trend between dietary total and n-6 PUFAs intake and incident ESKD assessed from FFQs (Malhotra et al., 2016). The benefits of PUFAs have also been demonstrated in the older CKD population: among 4480 NHANES participants with decreased kidney function, those with low intakes of dietary patterns in which cholesterols and total PUFAs comprised >50% of dietary nutrient intake were more likely to have late-stage CKD (Lin et al., 2022).

In summary, limited studies suggest that although dietary fat intake has not been shown to lead to acute changes in renal hemodynamics nor adverse kidney effects in the short-term, the chronic metabolic perturbations (i.e., persistent hyperglycemia, obesity, inflammation) induced by a high-fat diet may contribute to kidney damage over time.

Micronutrients

Potassium intake

Given that potassium is an essential nutrient needed for the maintenance of normal cellular function (i.e., cardiac electrophysiology, skeletal muscle contraction, nerve conduction, maintaining osmotic equilibrium, and activation of enzymes in various metabolic processes), it is encouraged to consume higher dietary potassium in the general population regardless of age (Services, December 2020). On the contrary, among CKD patients, although potassium restriction has been the standard of care due to the hypothesis that higher dietary potassium intake contributes to hyperkalemia, there has been a shift in recommendations from a previous paradigm of universal potassium restriction to now potassium liberalization and individualization (Ikizler et al., 2020). With respect to the effects of dietary potassium intake on kidney function, it is known that increased dietary potassium intake inhibits vascular smooth muscle cell proliferation, oxidative stress, platelet aggregation, glomerulosclerosis, and tubular damage, and increases kallikrein secretion and GFR, while decreased potassium intake activates the renin-angiotensin-aldosterone system (Takase et al., 2024).

In the older population without CKD, epidemiological studies describe blunted or significant associations between dietary potassium intake and the progression of CKD. Dietary potassium intake, ascertained using FFQ, was not associated with albuminuria or eGFR decline among more than 3000 women with a median age of 67 years who participated in the Nurses' Health Study (Lin et al., 2010a), as well as 21,636 adults aged ≥ 45 years who participated in the Reasons for Geographic and Racial Differences in Stroke (REGARDS) Study (Aaron et al., 2011). Many studies have shown the disadvantage of low potassium intake on CKD progression among elderly people, using urinary potassium excretion as an estimation method for dietary potassium intake. A cross-sectional analysis of data from the Health Examinee (HEXA) cohort of the Korean Genome and Epidemiologic Study (KoGES), including both adults with eGFR < 60 ($N = 3053$) and eGFR ≥ 60 ($N = 156{,}658$) aged 40–69 years, observed that the lowest quartiles of potassium intake, ascertained using FFQ, were associated with higher odds for advanced CKD (eGFR < 45 mL/min/1.73 m^2) (Kim et al., 2018). Prospective studies have also found an association between low potassium intake and the risk of CKD progression. For example, the PREVEND study, a prospective population-based cohort consisting of 5315 adults aged 28–75 years, showed that low urinary potassium excretion was associated with an increased risk of developing CKD after a median follow-up of 10.3 years (Kieneker et al., 2016). In 9778 Hispanic/Latino adults aged 18–74 years, lower potassium intake was associated with an increased risk of developing CKD after a mean follow-up of 6.2 years (Swift et al., 2022). The benefits of higher potassium intake on CKD outcomes were also found in the elderly population. In the overall and subgroup analysis of participants aged 18–44, 45–64, and ≥ 65 years from the Gubbio Study, higher urinary potassium was associated with less eGFR decline (Lo et al., 2021). Similar findings have been observed in 317,162 adults aged 40–69 years from South Korea, as well as across subgroup analyses based on age < 60 versus ≥ 60 years after a median follow-up of 11.9 years (Kim et al., 2024).

Data showing the absence of or a weak relationship between dietary potassium intake and serum potassium levels also supports the liberalization of dietary potassium intake. Indeed, in 95 NDD-CKD patients with a median age of 67 years, dietary potassium ascertained by

3-day food records was not associated with serum potassium or hyperkalemia (Ramos et al., 2021). With respect to data looking at the association between dietary potassium intake and CKD progression, the multicenter, prospective Korean Cohort Study for Outcome in Patients with CKD (KNOW-CKD) cohort study found that low urinary potassium excretion, measured using three metrics (i.e., spot urinary potassium-to-creatinine ratio, spot urinary potassium concentration, and 24-h urinary potassium excretion), was associated with CKD progression among 1821 NDD-CKD patients aged 20–75 years with 5376 person-years of follow-up (Kim et al., 2019). Another prospective cohort study among over five thousand people with CKD stage 2 aged ≥ 40 years showed that dietary potassium intake, ascertained by FFQ in patients with hypertension, was associated with a lower risk of CKD development and eGFR decline after a mean follow-up of 47.8 months (Mun et al., 2019).

Sodium intake

Although it remains uncertain whether dietary sodium intake is associated with CKD progression, dietary sodium restriction is routinely recommended for CKD patients. In addition to mechanisms involving increased blood pressure, increased sympathetic tone, oxidative stress, inflammation, endothelial dysfunction, vascular stiffness, and fibrosis are all known pathways through which high sodium intake might impair kidney function (Takase et al., 2024).

In terms of the association of dietary sodium intake with incident CKD among the older population, lower dietary sodium intake was found to be associated with a reduced risk of eGFR decline over 11 years of follow-up among 3296 women with a median age of 67 years (Lin et al., 2010a). On the other hand, another population-based prospective cohort study consisting of 465,288 adults aged 37–73 years observed that a higher self-reported frequency of adding salt to foods was associated with a higher risk of CKD after a median follow-up of 11.8 years (Tang et al., 2023). Interestingly, another prospective community-based cohort study in adults aged 40–69 years found that not only high but also low sodium intake was associated with an increased risk of CKD in participants with hypertension (Yoon et al., 2018). Given the inherent features of the sodium-based mechanism underlying the maintenance of cellular homeostasis in the human body, excessive limitation of sodium intake may not be beneficial in the long term (Yoon et al., 2018).

There are mixed reports on the relationship between dietary sodium intake and kidney function in older CKD patients. In scenarios of relatively short-term exposure (i.e., mean follow-up of 1.5 years) (Mazarova et al., 2016) and/or patients with only slight kidney impairment rather than moderate or severe stages of CKD (Nomura et al., 2017), dietary sodium intake may not always be associated with CKD progression. The results from an RCT among older NDD-CKD patients showed that restriction of sodium intake reduces proteinuria among 20 hypertensive CKD stage 3–4 patients with a mean age of 68.5 years (McMahon et al., 2013; Campbell et al., 2014). A metaanalysis of RCTs, including some studies with a mean age of ≥ 65 years, also confirmed that moderate salt restriction significantly reduces proteinuria/albuminuria in patients with CKD stages 1–4 (Garofalo et al., 2018). Other studies among older NDD-CKD patients showed that high-sodium intake is associated with an increased risk of kidney failure (Nerbass et al., 2015; Cury et al., 2022). The conflicting findings regarding the association between sodium or potassium and kidney health are possibly due to the differential sodium sensitivity in varying patient characteristics (i.e., hypertension, older age) (Yoon et al., 2018) and the close interaction between sodium and potassium. From this point of view, results from studies including older adults showing that a high urinary sodium-to-potassium ratio was associated with faster kidney function decline (Deriaz et al., 2019; Hattori et al., 2020) and incident CKD (Swift et al., 2022) suggest that lowering sodium and increasing potassium in the diet may contribute to CKD prevention.

Phosphorus intake

Studies have reported a close relationship between dietary phosphorus intake and kidney dysfunction.

Given the important roles of phosphorus in a number of biological processes, phosphorus homeostasis is tightly regulated by the balance of phosphorus absorption, renal excretion, and exchanges from bone and soft tissues. Previous studies have demonstrated a close relationship between high dietary phosphorus intake and high serum phosphorus levels (de Boer et al., 2009) as well as the significant linkage of high serum phosphorus levels with the risk of cardiovascular disease (Dhingra et al., 2007; Muntner et al., 2002; Achinger and Ayus, 2006; Hruska et al., 2007) and death (Chang et al., 2014; Kestenbaum et al., 2005) among populations with and without CKD. Limited data have evaluated the association between dietary phosphorus intake and kidney function, suggesting the risk of incident CKD induced by excessively high (Yoon et al., 2017) and low (Lee et al., 2021) dietary phosphorus intake among older adults aged 40–69 years. Higher phosphorus is naturally present in foods rich in protein, such as dairy products, meat, poultry, fish, and legumes, while processed foods containing phosphorus additives also contribute to the higher intake of phosphorus from the diet. It is well known that the different phosphorus bioavailability found in each food results in different effects on kidney outcomes (Narasaki et al., 2020; Kalantar-Zadeh et al., 2010). Indeed, a cross-sectional analysis examining the bioavailability of phosphorus and kidney function among a total of 3962 adults aged 21–84 years showed that higher phosphorus intake from food additives, but not from those naturally found in foods, was associated with worse kidney function (Duong et al., 2022). The potential mechanisms underlying the deleterious effects of high dietary phosphorus intake on kidney function include inhibition of nitric oxide synthesis in endothelial cells, increases in inflammation, inflammatory mediators, and endothelial dysfunction. Moreover, fibroblast growth factor-23 (FGF-23) induced by higher serum phosphorus levels, as well as the confounding effects of concomitant nutrients such as sodium and potassium, may also affect kidney function.

Fiber intake

Higher dietary fiber intake may have reno-protective effects in aged populations, directly through increasing insulin sensitivity, reducing oxidative stress, ameliorating systemic inflammation, and indirectly by contributing to other recognized risk factors for the decline in kidney function (i.e., diabetes, hypertension, dyslipidemia, and atherosclerosis) (Díaz-López et al., 2013). Cross-sectional (Díaz-López et al., 2013) and longitudinal (Heo et al., 2023) relationships between higher fiber intake and decreased risk of CKD were found in older adults aged 55–80 years who participated in the PREvención con DIeta MEDiterránea (PREDIMED) study (Díaz-López et al., 2013) and in subgroup analyses based on age (<60 vs. ≥ 60 years) in the UK Biobank prospective cohort after a median follow-up of 9.9 years (Heo et al., 2023), respectively.

Types of diet

Dietary approaches to stop hypertension diet

The Dietary Approaches to Stop Hypertension (DASH) diet is a healthy, balanced eating plan initially designed to help prevent or treat hypertension, which focuses on increased fruits, vegetables, whole grains, and low-fat dairy products; it also includes fish, poultry, beans, and nuts, whereas sugar-sweetened foods, red meat, and fats are limited (Appel et al., 1997). Following this plan, the DASH approach provides a diet rich in potassium, calcium, magnesium, fiber, and protein and is low in saturated fat and sodium (Appel et al., 1997). The benefit of this diet has been demonstrated in a number of studies, which are not limited to the primary objective of showing benefits on blood pressure management but have also been expanded to other health benefits, including reduction in type 2 diabetes, cardiovascular disease, stroke, and death (Narasaki and Rhee, 2022).

Cross-sectional (Crews et al., 2015, Lee et al., 2017) and prospective (Lin et al., 2011; Smyth et al., 2016, Rebholz et al., 2016b; Liu et al., 2017) studies among middle-aged to elderly adults, as well as a metaanalysis (Mozaffari et al., 2020), consistently showed the beneficial effects of the DASH diet on kidney function and in preventing incident CKD. For example, consuming a DASH diet and its individual components (i.e., lower intake of red and processed meat as well as higher intakes of nuts, legumes, and low-fat dairy products) was associated with a lower risk for the incidence of CKD among 14,882 participants aged 45–64 years in the Atherosclerosis Risk in Communities (ARIC) Study after a median follow-up of 23 years (Rebholz et al., 2016a).

Mediterranean diet

The Mediterranean diet is one of the most recognized types of diets for overall health and the prevention of chronic disease, modeled after the historic diet of the island of Crete. The Mediterranean diet shares many characteristics with the DASH diet by encouraging plant-based foods such as fruits, vegetables, whole grains, nuts, and beans/legumes, but it is distinguished by focusing on healthy fat consumption, specifically from olives/olive oil (Gallieni and Cupisti, 2016). With respect to the relationship between the Mediterranean diet and kidney function in the older population, a cross-sectional study among 1100 adults with or without CKD aged 70 years showed that adherence to a Mediterranean diet was associated with a lower likelihood of CKD (Huang et al., 2013). Moreover, a prospective study among 900 adults aged > 40 years demonstrated that a Mediterranean diet was associated with a reduced incidence of CKD and eGFR decline after a mean follow-up of 6.9 years (Khatri et al., 2014). In an RCT among community-dwelling adults aged 55–80 years with multiple cardiovascular risk factors, it was found that a Mediterranean diet had similar beneficial effects on kidney function compared to a low-fat diet (Díaz-López et al., 2012).

Plant-dominant low-protein diet (PLADO) and plant-focused nutrition in patients with diabetes and CKD diet (PLAFOND)

Plant-based diets have also garnered particular interest with respect to the potential health benefits. In the area of kidney health among the older population, a dietary pattern characterized by high consumption of whole grains, fruits, vegetables, and low-fat dairy foods was associated with lower urinary albumin-to-creatinine ratios in a cross-sectional analysis of the

MESA cohort among 5042 adults aged 45–84 years (Nettleton et al., 2008). A community-based prospective cohort study among 9229 adults aged 40–69 years also found that a diet rich in vegetables and fruit was associated with decreased risk of incident CKD after a mean follow-up of 8.2 years (Jhee et al., 2019). Typically, greater intake of fruits and vegetables is associated with lower dietary acid load (Scialla and Anderson, 2013). From this point of view, a prospective cohort study including 15,055 adults aged 45–64 years demonstrated that dietary acid load was associated with a higher risk of incident CKD, while its individual components such as a higher dietary intake of magnesium and vegetable sources of protein were associated with a lower risk of incident CKD after a median follow-up of 21 years (Rebholz et al., 2015).

Other characteristics (specific food or component)

Processed food

A global rise in ultra-processed food (UPF) consumption has been linked to various health concerns (Baker et al., 2020). Given the complex industrial processing of foods to include chemicals that improve their flavor, color, preservatives, and antioxidants, with few substances derived from natural food, UPFs are typically affordable and accessible (i.e., lower price, ready to consume, and hyper-palatable) and have poor nutritional value due to having lower favorable nutrients (dietary fiber and micronutrients) and greater unfavorable nutrients or components (refined carbohydrates, added sugars, SFAs, trans fatty acids, sodium, additives, and advanced glycation end products) than non-UPF foods (Rey-García et al., 2021). Several studies have shown a significant association between UPFs and kidney disease. Among 1312 community-dwelling elderly individuals, high UPF consumption was associated with a greater decline in kidney function after six years of follow-up (Rey-García et al., 2021). The prevalence of CKD was higher among adults aged 40–69 years with higher UPF intake (Kityo and Lee, 2022). Various studies (Cai et al., 2022; Du et al., 2022; Gu et al., 2023) and a metaanalysis (Xiao et al., 2024) found that higher UPF intake was also associated with incident CKD. In a prospective cohort of 2616 adults aged 21–74 years with CKD, greater consumption of UPFs was associated with CKD progression over a median follow-up of 7 years in the overall cohort and in those with CKD stages 1–2, but not in those with CKD stages 3a–5, potentially due to the diminished CKD progression by a low-protein diet (Sullivan et al., 2023).

Alcohol

As other dietary components usually do, alcohol consumption seems to have differential effects depending on how it is consumed. It is well known that excessive drinking of alcohol has adverse health consequences. Kidney disease is not the exception, and heavy alcohol consumption may cause kidney damage through oxidative damage, inflammatory injury, renin-angiotensin system activation, abnormal immunoreactivity, and renal tubular dysfunction (Fan et al., 2019). On the other hand, alcohol in moderation (i.e., up to 1 drink or 2 drinks/day for women and men, respectively) has had an inverse association with the development of CKD, which may be explained by the favorable effects of alcohol consumption on risk factors of cardiovascular disease, including endothelial dysfunction and insulin resistance. Alcohol consumption has been shown to be associated with increasing paraoxonase activity (Van Der Gaag et al., 1999) and inhibition of lipoprotein oxidation (Watson et al., 1995) as well as higher serum high-density lipoprotein cholesterol (HDL-C) levels (Schaeffner et al., 2003). Moreover, ethanol and nonalcoholic wine components, especially polyphenols, have been shown to influence oxidative balance and endothelial function (Presti et al., 2007).

Most studies in the elderly population found either no association (Menon et al., 2010; Foster et al., 2015) or a protective association (Buja et al., 2011; Funakoshi et al., 2012; Koning et al., 2015; Kimura et al., 2018; Okada et al., 2019; Hu et al., 2020; Kimura et al., 2023) between moderate alcohol consumption and incident CKD, while some studies showed a relationship between excessive alcohol consumption and a higher risk of prevalent and incident CKD (Shankar et al., 2006; Kimura et al., 2023; Buja et al., 2011). Heavy drinking (≥4 servings) was associated with a higher prevalence of CKD and 5-year incident CKD in a population-based study of adults aged 43–86 years (Shankar et al., 2006).

Although studies suggest the protective effects of moderate alcohol consumption on incident CKD and may have underestimated the deleterious effects of heavy alcohol consumption due to limited sample sizes in the largest alcohol consumption group (Kimura et al., 2023), potential differential consequences across sexes (Kimura et al., 2018; Kimura et al., 2023; Buja et al., 2011), and different types of alcohol, as well as the harmful aspects of alcohol consumption on global disease burden (especially all-cause mortality and cancers), should be further evaluated.

Polyphenols

With respect to a nonalcoholic component of wine, polyphenols are known as a favorable dietary component against chronic diseases, mainly due to their antioxidant and antiinflammatory properties (Guerreiro et al., 2022). With regard to kidney disease, animal studies have shown the beneficial effects of wine polyphenol, resveratrol, and quercetin. Exposure to resveratrol seemed to attenuate oxidative stress (Orellana et al., 2002) and suppress proteinuria and hyperlipidemia in rats (Nihei et al., 2001). Another study in rats observed that quercetin administration reduced oxidative stress and improved kidney function (Satyanarayana et al., 2001). Fruits and vegetables are also rich in a number of other polyphenols, and experimental models including animal studies have shown the potential benefits of consuming polyphenols on kidney health (Ashkar et al., 2022).

Conclusion

Healthy aging generally preserves the ability to digest and absorb macronutrients, but postabsorptive changes, such as reduced insulin sensitivity, anabolic resistance of muscle protein synthesis, altered lipid handling, and shifts in the gut microbiome, create vulnerability to PEW, sarcopenia, frailty, and adverse kidney outcomes. These risks are especially pronounced in individuals with CKD.

Evidence consistently supports plant-dominant, minimally processed dietary patterns such as the DASH and Mediterranean diets. These emphasize vegetables, fruits, whole grains, legumes, nuts, unsaturated fats, fiber, potassium, and antioxidants while limiting sodium, saturated fat, refined high-glycemic carbohydrates, phosphorus additives, sugar-sweetened beverages, and UPFs.

Protein intake is central to maintaining lean mass. For community-dwelling older adults without CKD, at least 1.0 g/kg/day—distributed evenly across meals and emphasizing plant sources or low-fat dairy—is recommended. Short-term hyperfiltration responses are usually well-tolerated. In contrast, older adults with CKD or those with reduced nephron reserve benefit from dietitian-guided protein restriction (0.6–0.8 g/kg/day, or very-low-protein regimens with supplementation when appropriate). Adequate energy intake, around 30–35 kcal/kg/day, is essential to prevent muscle loss.

Carbohydrate quality matters. A lower glycemic load with higher cereal or total fiber intake is linked to better outcomes, while excess refined sugars, particularly fructose-rich sweeteners, are harmful. For fats, limiting saturated fatty acids and prioritizing polyunsaturated fats is favorable, while moderate fish intake is generally beneficial.

Micronutrient management requires individualization. Potassium from whole foods may be protective but must be monitored in CKD. Sodium restriction reduces proteinuria, although extreme restriction may not suit all. Phosphorus additives potentiate worsening kidney disease and vascular calcification. Excessive alcohol use may be harmful. Polyphenol-rich foods may provide additional antiinflammatory benefits.

Clinically, routine screening for PEW and sarcopenia, coupled with personalized, pattern-based counseling, helps preserve muscle, protect kidney function, and improve the quality of life in older adults.

References

Aaron, K.J., Campbell, R.C., Judd, S.E., Sanders, P.W., Muntner, P., 2011. Association of dietary sodium and potassium intakes with albuminuria in normal-weight, overweight, and obese participants in the Reasons for Geographic and Racial Differences in Stroke (REGARDS) study. Am. J. Clin. Nutr. 19383207. 94 (4), 1071–1078. Available from: http://www.ajcn.org/content/94/4/1071.full.pdf+html. doi:10.3945/ajcn.111.013094.

Achinger, S.G., Ayus, J.C., 2006. Left ventricular hypertrophy: is hyperphosphatemia among dialysis patients a risk factor? J. Am. Soc. Nephrol. 10466673. 17 (3), S255–S261. https://journals.lww.com/jasn/pages/default.aspx. doi:10.1681/ASN.2006080923.

Altunkaynak, M.E., Özbek, E., Altunkaynak, B.Z., Can, I., Unal, D., Unal, B., 2008. The effects of high-fat diet on the renal structure and morphometric parametric of kidneys in rats. J. Anat. 14697580. 212 (6), 845–852. doi:10.1111/j.1469-7580.2008.00902.x.

Appel, L.J., Moore, T.J., Obarzanek, E., Vollmer, W.M., Svetkey, L.P., Sacks, F.M., Bray, G.A., Vogt, T.M., Cutler, J.A., Windhauser, M.M., Lin, P.H., Karanja, N., Simons-Morton, D., McCullough, M., Swain, J., Steele, P., Evans, M.A., Miller, E.R., Harsha, D.W., 1997. A clinical trial of the effects of dietary patterns on blood pressure. N. Engl. J. Med. 00284793. 336 (16), 1117–1124. doi:10.1056/NEJM199704173361601.

Arora, S., Kassarjian, Z., Krasinski, S.D., Croffey, B., Kaplan, M.M., Russell, R.M., 1989. Effect of age on tests of intestinal and hepatic function in healthy humans. Gastroenterology. 00165085. 96 (6), 1560–1565. doi:10.1016/0016-5085(89)90527-1.

Ashkar, F., Bhullar, K.S., Wu, J., 2022. The effect of polyphenols on kidney disease: targeting Mitochondria. Nutrients. 20726643. 14 (15). Available from: http://www.mdpi.com/journal/nutrients/. doi:10.3390/nu14153115.

Baker, P., Machado, P., Santos, T., Sievert, K., Backholer, K., Hadjikakou, M., Russell, C., Huse, O., Bell, C., Scrinis, G., Worsley, A., Friel, S., Lawrence, M., 2020. Ultra-processed foods and the nutrition transition: global, regional and national trends, food systems transformations and political economy drivers. Obes. Rev. 1467789X. 21 (12). Available from: http://onlinelibrary.wiley.com/journal/10.1111/(ISSN)1467-789X. doi:10.1111/obr.13126.

Bauer, J., Biolo, G., Cederholm, T., Cesari, M., Cruz-Jentoft, A.J., Morley, J.E., Phillips, S., Sieber, C., Stehle, P., Teta, D., Visvanathan, R., Volpi, E., Boirie, Y., 2013. Evidence-based recommendations for optimal dietary protein intake in older people: a position paper from the prot-age study group. J. Am. Med. Dir. Assoc. 15389375. 14 (8), 542–559. doi:10.1016/j.jamda.2013.05.021.

Beasley, J.M., Katz, R., Shlipak, M., Rifkin, D.E., Siscovick, D., Kaplan, R., 2014. Dietary protein intake and change in estimated GFR in the Cardiovascular Health Study. Nutrition. 18731244. 30 (7–8), 794–799. Available from: www.elsevier.com/locate/nut. doi:10.1016/j.nut.2013.12.006.

Bernier-Jean, A., Prince, R.L., Lewis, J.R., Craig, J.C., Hodgson, J.M., Lim, W.H., Teixeira-Pinto, A., Wong, G., 2021. Dietary plant and animal protein intake and decline in estimated glomerular filtration rate among elderly women: a 10-year longitudinal cohort study. Nephrol. Dial. Transplant. 14602385. 36 (9), 1640–1647. Available from: http://ndt.oxfordjournals.org/. doi:10.1093/ndt/gfaa081.

Boot-Handford, R.P., Heath, H., 1981. The effect of dietary fructose and diabetes on the rat kidney. Br. J. Exp. Pathol. 62 (4), 398–406.

Brunori, G., Viola, B.F., Parrinello, G., De Biase, V., Como, G., Franco, V., Garibotto, G., Zubani, R., Cancarini, G.C., 2007. Efficacy and safety of a very-low-protein diet when postponing dialysis in the elderly: a prospective randomized multicenter controlled study. Am. J. Kidney Dis. 02726386. 49 (5), 569–580. doi:10.1053/j.ajkd.2007.02.278.

Buja, A., Scafato, E., Baggio, B., Sergi, G., Maggi, S., Rausa, G., Basile, A., Manzato, E., Ghirini, S., Perissinotto, E., 2011. Renal impairment and moderate alcohol consumption in the elderly. Results from the Italian Longitudinal Study on Aging (ILSA). Public Health Nutr. 1368-9800. 14 (11), 1907–1918. doi:10.1017/s1368980011000863.

Cai, Q., Duan, M.J., Dekker, L.H., Carrero, J.J., Avesani, C.M., Bakker, S.J.L., De Borst, M.H., Navis, G.J., 2022. Ultraprocessed food consumption and kidney function decline in a population-based cohort in the Netherlands. Am. J. Clin. Nutr. 19383207. 116 (1), 263–273. Available from: http://www.ajcn.org/contents-by-date.2005.shtml. doi:10.1093/ajcn/nqac073.

Campbell, K.L., Johnson, D.W., Bauer, J.D., Hawley, C.M., Isbel, N.M., Stowasser, M., Whitehead, J.P., Dimeski, G., McMahon, E., 2014. A randomized trial of sodium-restriction on kidney function, fluid volume and adipokines in CKD patients. BMC Nephrol. 14712369. 15 (1). Available from: http://www.biomedcentral.com/bmcnephrol/. doi:10.1186/1471-2369-15-57.

Campbell, W.W., Trappe, T.A., Wolfe, R.R., Evans, W.J., 2001. The recommended dietary allowance for protein may not be adequate for older people to maintain skeletal muscle. J. Gerontol. A Biol. Sci. Med. Sci. 1079-5006. 56 (6), M373. doi:10.1093/gerona/56.6.m373.

Chang, A.R., Lazo, M., Appel, L.J., Gutiérrez, O.M., Grams, M.E., 2014. High dietary phosphorus intake is associated with all-cause mortality: results from NHANES III1-3. Am. J. Clin. Nutr. 19383207. 99 (2), 320–327. Available from: http://ajcn.nutrition.org/content/99/2/320.full.pdf+html. doi:10.3945/ajcn.113.073148.

Chao, C.T., Wang, J., Huang, J.W., Chan, D.C., Chien, K.L., 2019. Frailty predicts an increased risk of end-stage renal disease with risk competition by mortality among 165,461 diabetic kidney disease patients. Aging Dis. 21525250. 10 (6), 1270–1281. Available from: http://www.aginganddisease.org/. doi:10.14336/AD.2019.0216.

Chapman, C.L., Grigoryan, T., Vargas, N.T., Reed, E.L., Kueck, P.J., Pietrafesa, L.D., Bloomfield, A.C., Johnson, B.D., Schlader, Z.J., 2020. High-fructose corn syrup-sweetened soft drink consumption increases vascular resistance in the kidneys at rest and during sympathetic activation. Am. J. Physiol. Renal Physiol. 15221466. 318 (4), F1053. Available from: https://journals.physiology.org/doi/10.1152/ajprenal.00374.2019. doi:10.1152/AJPRENAL.00374.2019.

Chen, S., Lin, X., Ma, J., Li, M., Chen, Y., Fang, A.P., Zhu, H.L., 2023. Dietary protein intake and changes in muscle mass measurements in community-dwelling middle-aged and older adults: a prospective cohort study. Clin. Nutr. 15321983. 42 (12), 2503–2511. Available from: http://www.elsevier-international.com/journals/clnu/. doi:10.1016/j.clnu.2023.10.017.

Cheng, A.H.R., Gomez, A., Bergan, J.G., Lee, T.C., Monckeberg, F., Chichester, C.O., 1978. Comparative nitrogen balance study between young and aged adults using three levels of protein intake from a combination wheat-soy-milk mixture. Am. J. Clin. Nutr. 00029165. 31 (1), 12–22. doi:10.1093/ajcn/31.1.12.

Cirillo, M., Lombardi, C., Chiricone, D., De Santo, N.G., Zanchetti, A., Bilancio, G., 2014. Protein intake and kidney function in the middle-age population: contrast between cross-sectional and longitudinal data. Nephrol. Dial. Transplant. 0931-0509. 29 (9), 1733–1740. doi:10.1093/ndt/gfu056.

Crews, D.C., Kuczmarski, M.F., Miller, E.R., Zonderman, A.B., Evans, M.K., Powe, N.R., 2015. Dietary habits, poverty, and chronic kidney disease in an urban population. J. Ren. Nutr. 10512276. 25 (2), 103–110. Available from: http://www.sciencedirect.com/science/journal/10512276. doi:10.1053/j.jrn.2014.07.008.

Crinigan, C., Calhoun, M., Sweazea, K.L., 2015. Short-term high fat intake does not significantly alter markers of renal function or inflammation in young male Sprague-Dawley rats. J. Nutr. Metab. 20900732. 2015. Available from: www.hindawi.com/journals/jnume/. doi:10.1155/2015/157520.

Cury, C.M., Banin, V.B., Dos Reis, P.F., Caramori, J.C.T., Barretti, P., de Andrade, L.G.M., Martin, L.C., 2022. Association between urinary sodium excretion and hard outcomes in non-dialysis chronic kidney disease patients. BMC Nephrol. 14712369. 23 (1). Available from: https://bmcnephrol.biomedcentral.com/. doi:10.1186/s12882-022-02911-7.

Cuthbertson, D., Smith, K., Babraj, J., Leese, G., Waddell, T., Atherton, P., Wackerhage, H., Taylor, P.M., Rennie, M.J., 2005. Anabolic signaling deficits underlie amino acid resistance of wasting, aging muscle. FASEB J. 19 (3), 422–424. doi:10.1096/fj.04-2640fje.

de Boer, A., Horst, G.J.T., Lorist, M.M., 2013. Physiological and psychosocial age-related changes associated with reduced food intake in older persons. Ageing Res. Rev. 18729649. 12 (1), 316–328. doi:10.1016/j.arr.2012.08.002.

de Boer, I.H., Rue, T.C., Kestenbaum, B., 2009. Serum phosphorus concentrations in the third national health and nutrition examination survey (NHANES III). Am. J. Kidney Dis. 02726386. 53 (3), 399–407. doi:10.1053/j.ajkd.2008.07.036.

Deji, N., Kume, S., Araki, S.I., Soumura, M., Sugimoto, T., Isshiki, K., Chin-Kanasaki, M., Sakaguchi, M., Koya, D., Haneda, M., Kashiwagi, A., Uzu, T., 2009. Structural and functional changes in the kidneys of high-fat diet-induced obese mice. Am. J. Physiol. Renal Physiol. 15221466. 296 (1), F118. Available from: http://ajprenal.physiology.org/cgi/reprint/296/1/F118. doi:10.1152/ajprenal.00110.2008.

Deriaz, D., Guessous, I., Vollenweider, P., Devuyst, O., Burnier, M., Bochud, M., Ponte, B., 2019. Estimated 24-h urinary sodium and sodium-to-potassium ratio are predictors of kidney function decline in a population-based study. J. Hypertens. 0263-6352. 37 (9), 1853–1860. doi:10.1097/hjh.0000000000002098.

Dhingra, R., Sullivan, L.M., Fox, C.S., Wang, T.J., D'Agostino, R.B., Gaziano, J.M., Vasan, R.S., 2007. Relations of serum phosphorus and calcium levels to the incidence of cardiovascular disease in the community. Arch. Intern. Med. 15383679. 167 (9), 879–885. Available from: http://archinte.ama-assn.org/cgi/reprint/167/9/879. doi:10.1001/archinte.167.9.879.

Díaz-López, A., Bulló, M., Basora, J., Martínez-González, M.A., Guasch-Ferré, M., Estruch, R., Wärnberg, J., Serra-Majem, L., Arós, F., Lapetra, J., Ros, E., Pintó, X., Covas, M.I., Salas-Salvadó, J., 2013. Cross-sectional associations between macronutrient intake and chronic kidney disease in a population at high cardiovascular risk. Clin. Nutr. 15321983. 32 (4), 606–612. doi:10.1016/j.clnu.2012.10.013.

Díaz-López, A., Bulló, M., Martínez-González, M.A., Guasch-Ferré, M., Ros, E., Basora, J., Covas, M.I., López-Sabater, M.D.C., Salas-Salvadó, J., 2012. Effects of Mediterranean diets on kidney function: a report from the PREDIMED trial. Am. J. Kidney Dis. 15236838. 60 (3), 380–389. doi:10.1053/j.ajkd.2012.02.334.

Du, S., Kim, H., Crews, D.C., White, K., Rebholz, C.M., 2022. Association between ultraprocessed food consumption and risk of incident CKD: a prospective cohort study. Am. J. Kidney Dis. 15236838. 80 (5), 589. Available from: http://www.elsevier.com/inca/publications/store/6/2/3/2/7/6/index.htt. doi:10.1053/j.ajkd.2022.03.016.

Duong, C.N., Akinlawon, O.J., Gung, J., Noel, S.E., Bigornia, S., Flanagan, K., Pourafshar, S., Lin, P.H., Davenport, C.A., Pendergast, J., Scialla, J.J., Tucker, K.L., 2022. Bioavailability of phosphorus and kidney function in the Jackson Heart Study. Am. J. Clin. Nutr. 19383207. 116 (2), 541–550. Available from: http://www.ajcn.org/contents-by-date.2005.shtml. doi:10.1093/ajcn/nqac116.

Dwyer, T.M., Mizelle, H.L., Cockrell, K., Buhner, P., 1995. Renal sinus lipomatosis and body composition in hypertensive, obese rabbits. Int. J. Obes. 03070565. 19 (12), 869–874.

Elahi, D., Muller, D.C., 2000. Carbohydrate metabolism in the elderly. Eur. J. Clin. Nutr. 0954-3007. 54 (S3), S112. doi:10.1038/sj.ejcn.1601032.

Eyre, S., Attman, P.O., Haraldsson, B., 2008. Positive effects of protein restriction in patients with chronic kidney disease. J. Ren. Nutr. 10512276. 18 (3), 269–280. doi:10.1053/j.jrn.2007.11.013.

Fan, Z., Yun, J., Yu, S., Yang, Q., Song, L., 2019. Alcohol consumption can be a "double-edged sword" for chronic kidney disease patients. Med. Sci. Monit. 1643-3750. 25, 7059–7072. doi:10.12659/msm.916121.

Farsijani, S., Morais, J.A., Payette, H., Gaudreau, P., Shatenstein, B., Gray-Donald, K., Chevalier, S., 2016. Relation between mealtime distribution of protein intake and lean mass loss in free-living older adults of the NuAge study. Am. J. Clin. Nutr. 19383207. 104 (3), 694–703. Available from: http://ajcn.nutrition.org/content/104/3/694.full.pdf. doi:10.3945/ajcn.116.130716.

Feibusch, J.M., Holt, P.R., 1982. Impaired absorptive capacity for carbohydrate in the aging human. Dig. Dis. Sci. 15732568. 27 (12), 1095–1100. doi:10.1007/BF01391447.

Fink, R.I., Kolterman, O.G., Griffin, J., Olefsky, J.M., 1983. Mechanisms of insulin resistance in aging. J. Clin. Invest. 00219738. 71 (6), 1523–1535. doi:10.1172/JCI110908.

Fliser, D., Zeier, M., Nowack, R., Ritz, E., 1993. Renal functional reserve in healthy elderly subjects. J. Am. Soc. Nephrol. 1046-6673. 3 (7), 1371–1377. doi:10.1681/asn.v371371.

Foster, M.C., Hwang, S.J., Massaro, J.M., Jacques, P.F., Fox, C.S., Chu, A.Y., 2015. Lifestyle factors and indices of kidney function in the framingham heart study. Am. J. Nephrol. 14219670. 41 (4–5), 267–274. Available from: www.karger.ch/journals/ajn/ajn_jh.htm. doi:10.1159/000430868.

Funakoshi, Y., Omori, H., Onoue, A., Mihara, S., Ogata, Y., Katoh, T., 2012. Association between frequency of drinking alcohol and chronic kidney disease in men. Environ. Health Prev. Med. 1342-078X. 17 (3), 199–204. doi:10.1007/s12199-011-0238-6.

Gallieni, M., Cupisti, A., 2016. DASH and Mediterranean diets as nutritional interventions for CKD patients. Am. J. Kidney Dis. 02726386. 68 (6), 828–830. doi:10.1053/j.ajkd.2016.09.001.

Garofalo, C., Borrelli, S., Provenzano, M., De Stefano, T., Vita, C., Chiodini, P., Minutolo, R., De Nicola, L., Conte, G., 2018. Dietary salt restriction in chronic kidney disease: a meta-analysis of randomized clinical trials. Nutrients. 20726643. 10 (6). Available from: http://www.mdpi.com/2072-6643/10/6/732/pdf. doi:10.3390/nu10060732.

Gersch, M.S., Mu, W., Cirillo, P., Reungjui, S., Zhang, L., Roncal, C., Sautin, Y.Y., Johnson, R.J., Nakagawa, T., 2007. Fructose, but not dextrose, accelerates the progression of chronic kidney disease. Am. J. Physiol. Renal Physiol. 15221466. 293 (4), F1256. Available from: http://ajprenal.physiology.org/cgi/reprint/293/4/F1256. doi:10.1152/ajprenal.00181.2007.

Gopinath, B., Harris, D.C., Flood, V.M., Burlutsky, G., Mitchell, P., 2011b. Consumption of long-chain n-3 PUFA, α-linolenic acid and fish is associated with the prevalence of chronic kidney disease. Br. J. Nutr. 105 (9), 1361–1368.

Gopinath, B., Harris, D.C., Flood, V.M., Burlutsky, G., Mitchell, P., 2016. Associations between dairy food consumption and chronic kidney disease in older adults. Sci. Rep. 20452322. 6. Available from: www.nature.com/srep/index.html. doi:10.1038/srep39532.

Gu, Y., Li, H., Ma, H., Zhang, S., Meng, G., Zhang, Q., Liu, L., Hongmei, W., Zhang, T., Wang, X., Zhang, J., Sun, S., Wang, X., Zhou, M., Jia, Q., Song, K., Liu, Q., Huang, T., Borné, Y., Wang, Y., Qi, L., Niu, K., 2023. Consumption of ultraprocessed food and development of chronic kidney disease: the Tianjin chronic low-grade systemic inflammation and health and UK biobank cohort studies. Am. J. Clin. Nutr. 00029165. 117 (2), 373–382. doi:10.1016/j.ajcnut.2022.11.005.

Guerreiro, Í., Ferreira-Pêgo, C., Carregosa, D., Santos, C.N., Menezes, R., Fernandes, A.S., Costa, J.G., 2022. Polyphenols and their metabolites in renal diseases: an overview. Foods. 23048158. 11 (7). Available from: https://www.mdpi.com/2304-8158/11/7/1060/pdf. doi:10.3390/foods11071060.

Halbesma, N., Bakker, S.J.L., Jansen, D.F., Stolk, R.P., De Zeeuw, D., De Jong, P.E., Gansevoort, R.T., 2009. High protein intake associates with cardiovascular events but not with loss of renal function. J. Am. Soc. Nephrol. 15333450. 20 (8), 1797–1804. Available from: http://jasn.asnjournals.org/cgi/reprint/20/8/1797. doi:10.1681/ASN.2008060649.

Hannan, M.T., Tucker, K.L., Dawson-Hughes, B., Cupples, L.A., Felson, D.T., Kiel, D.P., 2000. Effect of dietary protein on bone loss in elderly men and women: the Framingham Osteoporosis Study. J. Bone Miner. Res. 08840431. 15 (12), 2504–2512. doi:10.1359/jbmr.2000.15.12.2504.

Haring, B., Selvin, E., Liang, M., Coresh, J., Grams, M.E., Petruski-Ivleva, N., Steffen, L.M., Rebholz, C.M., 2017. Dietary protein sources and risk for incident chronic kidney disease: results from the atherosclerosis risk in communities (ARIC) study. J. Ren. Nutr. 10512276. 27 (4), 233–242. Available from: http://www.sciencedirect.com/science/journal/10512276. doi:10.1053/j.jrn.2016.11.004.

Hattori, H., Hirata, A., Kubo, S., Nishida, Y., Nozawa, M., Kawamura, K., Hirata, T., Kubota, Y., Sata, M., Kuwabara, K., Higashiyama, A., Kadota, A., Sugiyama, D., Miyamatsu, N., Miyamoto, Y., Okamura, T., 2020. Estimated 24 h urinary sodium-to-potassium ratio is related to renal function decline: a 6-year cohort study of Japanese urban residents. Int. J. Environ. Res. Public Health. 1660-4601. 17 (16), 5811. doi:10.3390/ijerph17165811.

Heo, G.Y., Kim, H.J., Kalantar, D., Jung, C.Y., Kim, H.W., Park, J.T., Chang, T.I., Yoo, T.H., Kang, S.W., Rhee, C.M., Kalantar-Zadeh, K., Han, S.H., 2023. Association between fiber intake and risk of incident chronic kidney disease: the UK biobank study. J. Nutr. Health Aging. 17604788. 27 (11), 1018–1027. Available from: https://www.springer.com/journal/12603. doi:10.1007/s12603-023-1998-6.

Heo, G.Y., Koh, H.B., Park, J.T., Han, S.H., Yoo, T.H., Kang, S.W., Kim, H.W., 2024. Sweetened beverage intake and incident chronic kidney disease in the UK biobank study. JAMA Netw. Open. 25743805. 7 (2), E2356885. Available from: https://jamanetwork.com/journals/jamanetworkopen. doi:10.1001/jamanetworkopen.2023.56885.

Higashiyama, A., Watanabe, M., Kokubo, Y., Ono, Y., Okayama, A., Okamura, T., 2010. Relationships between protein intake and renal function in a Japanese general population: NIPPON DATA90. J. Epidemiol. 1349-9092. 20 (Supplement_III), S537. doi:10.2188/jea.je20090222.

Hommos, M.S., Glassock, R.J., Rule, A.D., 2017. Structural and functional changes in human kidneys with healthy aging. J. Am. Soc. Nephrol. 15333450. 28 (10), 2838–2844. Available from: http://jasn.asnjournals.org/content/28/10/2838.full.pdf+html. doi:10.1681/ASN.2017040421.

Houston, D.K., Nicklas, B.J., Ding, J., Harris, T.B., Tylavsky, F.A., Newman, A.B., Jung, S.L., Sahyoun, N.R., Visser, M., Kritchevsky, S.B., 2008. Dietary protein intake is associated with lean mass change in older, community-dwelling adults: the health, aging, and body composition (Health ABC) study. Am. J. Clin. Nutr. 00029165. 87 (1), 150–155. Available from: http://www.ajcn.org/cgi/reprint/87/1/150. doi:10.1093/ajcn/87.1.150.

Hruska, K.A., Saab, G., Mathew, S., Lund, R., 2007. Renal osteodystrophy, phosphate homeostasis, and vascular calcification. Semin. Dial. 1525139X. 20 (4), 309–315. doi:10.1111/j.1525-139X.2007.00300.x.

Hu, E.A., Lazo, M., Rosenberg, S.D., Grams, M.E., Steffen, L.M., Coresh, J., Rebholz, C.M., 2020. Alcohol consumption and incident kidney disease: results from the atherosclerosis risk in communities study. J. Ren. Nutr. 10512276. 30 (1), 22–30. Available from: http://www.sciencedirect.com/science/journal/10512276. doi:10.1053/j.jrn.2019.01.011.

Huang, X., Juan Jiménez-Moleón, J., Lindholm, B., Cederholm, T., Ärnlöv, J., Risérus, U., Sjögren, P., Jesús Carrero, J., Diet, M., 2013. Kidney function, and mortality in men with CKD. Clin. J. Am. Soc. Nephrol. 1555-9041. 8 (9), 1548–1555. doi:10.2215/cjn.01780213.

Ikizler, T.A., Burrowes, J.D., Byham-Gray, L.D., Campbell, K.L., Carrero, J.J., Chan, W., Fouque, D., Friedman, A.N., Ghaddar, S., Goldstein-Fuchs, D.J., Kaysen, G.A., Kopple, J.D., Teta, D., Wang, A.Y.-M., Cuppari, L., 2020. KDOQI clinical practice guideline for nutrition in CKD: 2020 update. Am. J. Kidney Dis. 15236838. 76 (3), S1. Available from: http://www.elsevier.com/inca/publications/store/6/2/3/2/7/6/index.htt. doi:10.1053/j.ajkd.2020.05.006.

Ikizler, T.A., Cano, N.J., Franch, H., Fouque, D., Himmelfarb, J., Kalantar-Zadeh, K., Kuhlmann, M.K., Stenvinkel, P., Terwee, P., Teta, D., Wang, A.Y.M., Wanner, C., 2013. Prevention and treatment of protein energy wasting in chronic kidney disease patients: a consensus statement by the International Society of Renal Nutrition and Metabolism. Kidney Int. 15231755. 84 (6), 1096–1107. Available from: https://www.journals.elsevier.com/kidney-international. doi:10.1038/ki.2013.147.

Jhee, J.H., Kee, Y.K., Park, J.T., Chang, T.I., Kang, E.W., Yoo, T.H., Kang, S.W., Han, S.H., 2019. A diet rich in vegetables and fruit and incident CKD: a community-based prospective cohort study. Am. J. Kidney Dis. 15236838. 74 (4), 491–500. Available from: http://www.elsevier.com/inca/publications/store/6/2/3/2/7/6/index.htt. doi:10.1053/j.ajkd.2019.02.023.

Juraschek, S.P., Chang, A.R., Appel, L.J., Anderson, C.A.M., Crews, D.C., Thomas, L., Charleston, J., Miller, E.R., 2016. Effect of glycemic index and carbohydrate intake on kidney function in healthy adults. BMC Nephrol. 14712369. 17 (1), 1–10. Available from: http://www.biomedcentral.com/bmcnephrol/. doi:10.1186/s12882-016-0288-5.

Kalantar-Zadeh, K., Gutekunst, L., Mehrotra, R., Kovesdy, C.P., Bross, R., Shinaberger, C.S., Noori, N., Hirschberg, R., Benner, D., Nissenson, A.R., Kopple, J.D., 2010. Understanding sources of dietary phosphorus in the treatment of patients with chronic kidney disease. Clin. J. Am. Soc. Nephrol. 1555905X. 5 (3), 519–530. Available from: http://cjasn.asnjournals.org/cgi/reprint/5/3/519. doi:10.2215/CJN.06080809.

Kestenbaum, B., Sampson, J.N., Rudser, K.D., Patterson, D.J., Seliger, S.L., Young, B., Sherrard, D.J., Andress, D.L., 2005. Serum phosphate levels and mortality risk among people with chronic kidney disease. J. Am. Soc. Nephrol. 10466673. 16 (2), 520–528. Available from: https://journals.lww.com/jasn/pages/default.aspx. doi:10.1681/ASN.2004070602.

Khatri, M., Moon, Y.P., Scarmeas, N., Gu, Y., Gardener, H., Cheung, K., Wright, C.B., Sacco, R.L., Nickolas, T.L., Elkind, M.S.V., 2014. The association between a Mediterranean-style diet and kidney function in the northern manhattan study cohort. Clin. J. Am. Soc. Nephrol. 1555905X. 9 (11), 1868–1875. Available from: http://cjasn.asnjournals.org/content/9/11/1868.full.pdf. doi:10.2215/CJN.01080114.

Kieneker, L.M., Bakker, S.J.L., de Boer, R.A., Navis, G.J., Gansevoort, R.T., Joosten, M.M., 2016. Low potassium excretion but not high sodium excretion is associated with increased risk of developing chronic kidney disease. Kidney Int. 15231755. 90 (4), 888–896. Available from: https://www.journals.elsevier.com/kidney-international. doi:10.1016/j.kint.2016.07.012.

Kim, H.J., Koh, H.B., Heo, G.Y., Kim, H.W., Park, J.T., Chang, T.I., Yoo, T.H., Kang, S.W., Kalantar-Zadeh, K., Rhee, C., Han, S.H., 2024. Higher potassium intake is associated with a lower risk of chronic kidney disease: population-based prospective study. Am. J. Clin. Nutr. 19383207. 119 (4), 1044–1051. Available from: https://www.sciencedirect.com/science/journal/00029165. doi:10.1016/j.ajcnut.2024.02.004.

Kim, H., Lee, H., Kwon, S.H., Jeon, J.S., Noh, H., Han, D.C., Kim, H., 2021. Relationship between carbohydrate-to-fat intake ratio and the development of chronic kidney disease: a community-based prospective cohort study. Clin. Nutr. 15321983. 40 (10), 5346–5354. Available from: http://www.elsevier-international.com/journals/clnu/. doi:10.1016/j.clnu.2021.09.001.

Kim, H.W., Park, J.T., Yoo, T.H., Lee, J., Chung, W., Lee, K.B., Chae, D.W., Ahn, C., Kang, S.W., Choi, K.H., Han, S.H., 2019. Urinary Potassium excretion and progression of CKD. Clin. J. Am. Soc. Nephrol. 1555905X. 14 (3), 330–340. Available from: https://cjasn.asnjournals.org/content/14/3/330.full.pdf. doi:10.2215/CJN.07820618.

Kim, J., Lee, J., Kim, K.N., Oh, K.H., Ahn, C., Lee, J., Kang, D., Park, SK., 2018. Association between dietary mineral intake and chronic kidney disease: The Health Examinees (HEXA) study. Int. J. Environ. Res. Public Health 15 (7), 1342.

Kimura, Y., Yamamoto, R., Shinzawa, M., Aoki, K., Tomi, R., Ozaki, S., Yoshimura, R., Shimomura, A., Iwatani, H., Isaka, Y., Iseki, K., Tsuruya, K., Fujimoto, S., Narita, I., Konta, T., Kondo, M., Kasahara, M., Shibagaki, Y., Asahi, K., Watanabe, T., Yamagata, K., Moriyama, T., 2023. Alcohol consumption and a decline in glomerular filtration rate: the Japan specific health checkups study. Nutrients. 2072-6643. 15 (6), 1540. doi:10.3390/nu15061540.

Kimura, Y., Yamamoto, R., Shinzawa, M., Isaka, Y., Iseki, K., Yamagata, K., Tsuruya, K., Yoshida, H., Fujimoto, S., Asahi, K., Moriyama, T., Watanabe, T., 2018. Alcohol consumption and incidence of proteinuria: a retrospective cohort study. Clin. Exp. Nephrol. 1342-1751. 22 (5), 1133–1142. doi:10.1007/s10157-018-1568-0.

Kityo, A., Lee, S.A., 2022. The intake of ultra-processed foods and prevalence of chronic kidney disease: the health examinees study. Nutrients. 20726643. 14 (17). Available from: http://www.mdpi.com/journal/nutrients/. doi:10.3390/nu14173548.

Knight, E.L., Stampfer, M.J., Hankinson, S.E., Spiegelman, D., Curhan, G.C., 2003. The impact of protein intake on renal function decline in women with normal renal function or mild renal insufficiency. Ann. Intern. Med. 00034819. 138 (6), 460. Available from: http://annals.org/issues.aspx. doi:10.7326/0003-4819-138-6-200303180-00009.

Koning, S.H., Gansevoort, R.T., Mukamal, K.J., Rimm, E.B., Bakker, S.J.L., Joosten, M.M., 2015. Alcohol consumption is inversely associated with the risk of developing chronic kidney disease. Kidney Int. 15231755. 87 (5), 1009–1016. Available from: https://www.journals.elsevier.com/kidney-international. doi:10.1038/ki.2014.414.

Koppe, L., Fouque, D., 2019. The role for protein restriction in addition to renin-angiotensin-aldosterone system inhibitors in the management of CKD. Am. J. Kidney Dis. 02726386. 73 (2), 248–257. doi:10.1053/j.ajkd.2018.06.016.

Kopple, J.D., Levey, A.S., Greene, T., Chumlea, W.C., Gassman, J.J., Hollinger, D.L., Maroni, B.J., Merrill, D., Scherch, L.K., Schulman, G., Wang, S.R., Zimmer, G.S., 1997. Effect of dietary protein restriction on nutritional status in the modification of diet in renal disease study. Kidney Int. 00852538. 52 (3), 778–791. Available from: https://www.journals.elsevier.com/kidney-international. doi:10.1038/ki.1997.395.

Kopple, J.D., Monteon, F.J., Shaib, J.K., 1986. Effect of energy intake on nitrogen metabolism in nondialyzed patients with chronic renal failure. Kidney Int. 00852538. 29 (3), 734–742. doi:10.1038/ki.1986.59.

Kovesdy, C.P., Kopple, J.D., Kalantar-Zadeh, K., 2013. Management of protein-energy wasting in non-dialysis-dependent chronic kidney disease: reconciling low protein intake with nutritional therapy. Am. J. Clin. Nutr. 19383207. 97 (6), 1163–1177. Available from: http://ajcn.nutrition.org/content/97/6/1163.full.pdf+html. doi:10.3945/ajcn.112.036418.

Kubo, S., Imano, H., Muraki, I., Kitamura, A., Noda, H., Cui, R., Maruyama, K., Yamagishi, K., Umesawa, M., Shimizu, Y., Hayama-Terada, M., Kiyama, M., Okada, T., Iso, H., 2023. Total protein intake and subsequent risk of chronic kidney disease: the circulatory risk in communities study. Environ. Health Prev. Med. 1342-078X. 28, 32. doi:10.1265/ehpm.22-00247.

Lee, H.S., Lee, K.B., Hyun, Y.Y., Chang, Y., Ryu, S., Choi, Y., 2017. DASH dietary pattern and chronic kidney disease in elderly Korean adults. Eur. J. Clin. Nutr. 71 (6), 755–761.

Lee, J., Oh, K.H., Park, S.K., 2021. Dietary micronutrients and risk of chronic kidney disease: a cohort study with 12 year follow-up. Nutrients. 20726643. 13 (5). Available from: https://www.mdpi.com/2072-6643/13/5/1517/pdf. doi:10.3390/nu13051517.

Lew, Q.L.J., Jafar, T.H., Jin, A., Yuan, J.M., Koh, W.P., 2018. Consumption of coffee but not of other caffeine-containing beverages reduces the risk of end-stage renal disease in the Singapore Chinese Health Study. J. Nutr. 15416100. 148 (8), 1315–1322. Available from: http://jn.nutrition.org. doi:10.1093/jn/nxy075.

Li, C.Y., Fang, A.P., Ma, W.J., Wu, S.L., Li, C.L., Chen, Y.M., Zhu, H.L., 2019. Amount rather than animal vs plant protein intake is associated with skeletal muscle mass in community-dwelling middle-aged and older Chinese adults: results from the Guangzhou nutrition and health study. J. Acad. Nutr. Diet. 22122672. 119 (9), 1501–1510. Available from: http://www.elsevier.com/wps/find/journaldescription.cws_home/727057/description#description. doi:10.1016/j.jand.2019.03.010.

Lin, H.I., Chen, H.M., Hsu, C.C., Lin, H.J., Wang, J.J., Weng, S.F., Kao, Y., Huang, C.C., 2022. Associations between dietary patterns and stages of chronic kidney disease. BMC Nephrol. 14712369. 23 (1). Available from: http://www.biomedcentral.com/bmcnephrol/. doi:10.1186/s12882-022-02739-1.

Lin, J., Fung, T.T., Hu, F.B., Curhan, G.C., 2011. Association of dietary patterns with albuminuria and kidney function decline in older white women: a subgroup analysis from the nurses health study. Am. J. Kidney Dis. 02726386. 57 (2), 245–254. doi:10.1053/j.ajkd.2010.09.027.

Lin, J., Hu, F.B., Curhan, G.C., 2010a. Associations of diet with albuminuria and kidney function decline. Clin J Am Soc Nephrol, 5 (5), 836–843.

Lin, J., Judd, S., Le, A., Ard, J., Newsome, B.B., Howard, G., Warnock, D.G., Mcclellan, W., 2010b. Associations of dietary fat with albuminuria and kidney dysfunction. Am. J. Clin. Nutr. 92, 897–904.

Liu, Y., Kuczmarski, M.F., Miller, E.R., Nava, M.B., Zonderman, A.B., Evans, M.K., Powe, N.R., Crews, D.C., 2017. Dietary habits and risk of kidney function decline in an urban population. J. Ren. Nutr. 10512276. 27 (1), 16–25. Available from: http://www.sciencedirect.com/science/journal/10512276. doi:10.1053/j.jrn.2016.08.007.

Lo, W.C., Ou, S.H., Chou, C.L., Chen, J.S., Wu, M.Y., Wu, M.S., 2021. Sugar- and artificially-sweetened beverages and the risks of chronic kidney disease: a systematic review and dose–response meta-analysis. J. Nephrol. 17246059. 34 (6), 1791–1804. Available from: http://www.springer.com/medicine/nephrology/journal/40620. doi:10.1007/s40620-020-00957-0.

Lu, T.Y., Zhang, W.S., Zhu, T., Jiang, C.Q., Zhu, F., Jin, Y.L., Lam, T.H., Cheng, K.K., Xu, L., 2023. Associations of meat, fish and seafood consumption with kidney function in middle-aged to older Chinese: a cross-sectional study based on the Guangzhou Biobank Cohort Study. BMJ Open. 20446055. 13 (10). Available from: http://bmjopen.bmj.com/content/early/by/section. doi:10.1136/bmjopen-2023-073738.

Malhotra, R., Cavanaugh, K.L., Blot, W.J., Ikizler, T.A., Lipworth, L., Kabagambe, E.K., 2016. Dietary polyunsaturated fatty acids and incidence of end-stage renal disease in the Southern Community Cohort Study. BMC Nephrol. 14712369. 17 (1). Available from: http://www.biomedcentral.com/bmcnephrol/. doi:10.1186/s12882-016-0371-y.

Mariat, D., Firmesse, O., Levenez, F., Guimarães, V.D., Sokol, H., Doré, J., Corthier, G., Furet, J.-P., 2009. The Firmicutes/Bacteroidetes ratio of the human microbiota changes with age. BMC Microbiol. 1471-2180. 9 (1), 123. doi:10.1186/1471-2180-9-123.

Mazarova, A., Molnar, A.O., Akbari, A., Sood, M.M., Hiremath, S., Burns, K.D., Ramsay, T.O., Mallick, R., Knoll, G.A., Ruzicka, M., 2016. The association of urinary sodium excretion and the need for renal replacement therapy in advanced chronic kidney disease: a cohort study. BMC Nephrol. 14712369. 17 (1). Available from: http://www.biomedcentral.com/bmcnephrol/. doi:10.1186/s12882-016-0338-z.

McMahon, E.J., Bauer, J.D., Hawley, C.M., Isbel, N.M., Stowasser, M., Johnson, D.W., Campbell, K.L., 2013. A randomized trial of dietary sodium restriction in CKD. J. Am. Soc. Nephrol. 15333450. 24 (12), 2096–2103. Available from: http://jasn.asnjournals.org/content/24/12/2096.full.pdf+html. doi:10.1681/ASN.2013030285.

Menon, V., Katz, R., Mukamal, K., Kestenbaum, B., de Boer, I.H., Siscovick, D.S., Sarnak, M.J., Shlipak, M.G., 2010. Alcohol consumption and kidney function decline in the elderly: alcohol and kidney disease. Nephrol. Dial. Transplant. 0931-0509. 25 (10), 3301–3307. doi:10.1093/ndt/gfq188.

Milan, A.M., Cameron-Smith, D., 2015. Digestion and postprandial metabolism in the elderly. Adv. Food Nutr. Res. 76, 79–124. Available from: http://www.elsevier.com/wps/find/bookdescription.cws_home/704624/description#description. doi:10.1016/bs.afnr.2015.09.001.

Mirzababaei, A., Abaj, F., Roumi, Z., Khosroshahi, R.A., Aali, Y., Clark, C.C.T., Radmehr, M., Mirzaei, K., 2024. Consumption of red, white, and processed meat and odds of developing kidney damage and diabetic nephropathy (DN) in women: a case control study. Sci. Rep. 20452322. 14 (1). Available from: https://www.nature.com/srep/. doi:10.1038/s41598-024-59097-1.

Morris, A., Krishnan, N., Kimani, P.K., Lycett, D., 2020. Effect of dietary potassium restriction on serum potassium, disease progression, and mortality in chronic kidney disease: a systematic review and meta-analysis. J. Ren. Nutr. 10512276. 30 (4), 276–285. Available from: http://www.sciencedirect.com/science/journal/10512276. doi:10.1053/j.jrn.2019.09.009.

Morse, M.H., Haub, M.D., Evans, W.J., Campbell, W.W., 2001. Protein requirement of elderly women: nitrogen balance responses to three levels of protein intake. J. Gerontol. A Biol. Sci. Med. Sci. 1079-5006. 56 (11), M724. doi:10.1093/gerona/56.11.m724.

Mozaffari, H., Ajabshir, S., Alizadeh, S., 2020. Dietary approaches to stop hypertension and risk of chronic kidney disease: a systematic review and meta-analysis of observational studies. Clin. Nutr. 02615614. 39 (7), 2035–2044. doi:10.1016/j.clnu.2019.10.004.

Mun, K.H., Yu, G.I., Choi, B.Y., Kim, M.K., Shin, M.H., Shin, D.H., 2019. Association of dietary potassium intake with the development of chronic kidney disease and renal function in patients with mildly decreased kidney function: the Korean multi-rural communities cohort study. Med. Sci. Monit. 16433750. 25, 1061–1070. Available from: https://www.medscimonit.com/download/index/idArt/913504. doi:10.12659/MSM.913504.

Muntner, P., He, J., Hamm, L., Loria, C., Whelton, P.K., 2002. Renal insufficiency and subsequent death resulting from cardiovascular disease in the United States. J. Am. Soc. Nephrol. 10466673. 13 (3), 745–753. Available from: https://journals.lww.com/jasn/pages/default.aspx. doi:10.1681/asn.v133745.

Nakagawa, T., Kang, D.H., 2021. Fructose in the kidney: from physiology to pathology. Kidney Res. Clin. Pract. 22119140. 40 (4), 527–541. Available from: http://krcp-ksn.org/journal/view.php?doi=10.23876/j.krcp.21.138. doi:10.23876/J.KRCP.21.138.

Nam, K.H., An, S.Y., Joo, Y.S., Lee, S., Yun, H.R., Jhee, J.H., Han, S.H., Yoo, T.H., Kang, S.W., Park, J.T., 2019. Carbohydrate-rich diet is associated with increased risk of incident chronic kidney disease in non-diabetic subjects. J. Clin. Med. 20770383. 8 (6). Available from: https://www.mdpi.com/2077-0383/8/6/793/pdf. doi:10.3390/jcm8060793.

Narasaki, Y., Rhee, C.M., 2022. Chapter 15 – Effects of nutritional status and changes in nutrient intake on renal function. In: Kopple, J.D., Massry, S.G., Kalantar-Zadeh, K., D., Fouque (Eds.), Nutritional management of renal disease (4th ed., pp. xxxxxx). Academic Press.

Narasaki, Y., Rhee, C.M., Kramer, H., Kalantar-Zadeh, K., 2021. Protein intake and renal function in older patients. Curr. Opin. Clin. Nutr. Metab. Care. 14736519. 24 (1), 10–17. Available from: http://journals.lww.com/co-clinicalnutrition/pages/default.aspx. doi:10.1097/MCO.0000000000000712.

Narasaki, Y., Yamasaki, M., Matsuura, S., Morinishi, M., Nakagawa, T., Matsuno, M., Katsumoto, M., Nii, S., Fushitani, Y., Sugihara, K., Noda, T., Yoneda, T., Masuda, M., Yamanaka-Okumura, H., Takeda, E., Sakaue, H., Yamamoto, H., Taketani, Y., 2020. Phosphatemic index is a novel evaluation tool for dietary phosphorus load: A whole-foods approach. J. Ren. Nutr. 30 (6), 493–502.

Nerbass, F.B., Pecoits-Filho, R., McIntyre, N.J., McIntyre, C.W., Taal, M.W., 2015. High sodium intake is associated with important risk factors in a large cohort of chronic kidney disease patients. Eur. J. Clin. Nutr. 14765640. 69 (7), 786–790. Available from: http://www.nature.com/ejcn/index.html. doi:10.1038/ejcn.2014.215.

Nettleton, J.A., Steffen, L.M., Palmas, W., Burke, G.L., Jacobs, D.R., 2008. Associations between microalbuminuria and animal foods, plant foods, and dietary patterns in the Multiethnic Study of Atherosclerosis. Am. J. Clin. Nutr. 00029165. 87 (6), 1825–1836. Available from: http://www.ajcn.org/cgi/reprint/87/6/1825. doi:10.1093/ajcn/87.6.1825.

Nihei, T., Miura, Y., Yagasaki, K., 2001. Inhibitory effect of resveratrol on proteinuria, hypoalbuminemia and hyperlipidemia in nephritic rats. Life Sci. 00243205. 68 (25), 2845–2852. doi:10.1016/s0024-3205(01)01061-x.

Nomura, K., Asayama, K., Jacobs, L., Thijs, L., Staessen, J.A., 2017. Renal function in relation to sodium intake: a quantitative review of the literature. Kidney Int. 15231755. 92 (1), 67–78. Available from: https://www.journals.elsevier.com/kidney-international. doi:10.1016/j.kint.2016.11.032.

Okada, Y., Uehara, S., Shibata, M., Koh, H., Oue, K., Kambe, H., Morimoto, M., Sato, K.K., Hayashi, T., 2019. Habitual alcohol intake modifies relationship of uric acid to incident chronic kidney disease. Am. J. Nephrol. 14219670. 50 (1), 55–62. Available from: www.karger.ch/journals/ajn/ajn_jh.htm. doi:10.1159/000500707.

Orellana, M., Araya, J., Guajardo, V., Rodrigo, R., 2002. Modulation of cytochrome P450 activity in the kidney of rats following long-term red wine exposure. Comp. Biochem. Physiol. C Toxicol. Pharmacol. 15320456. 132 (3), 399–405. doi:10.1016/s1532-0456(02)00076-5.

Oyabu, C., Hashimoto, Y., Fukuda, T., Tanaka, M., Asano, M., Yamazaki, M., Fukui, M., 2016. Impact of low-carbohydrate diet on renal function: a meta-analysis of over 1000 individuals from nine randomised controlled trials. Br. J. Nutr. 0007-1145. 116 (4), 632–638. doi:10.1017/s0007114516002178.

Piccoli, G.B., Cederholm, T., Avesani, C.M., Bakker, S.J.L., Bellizzi, V., Cuerda, C., Cupisti, A., Sabatino, A., Schneider, S., Torreggiani, M., Fouque, D., Carrero, J.J., Barazzoni, R., 2023. Nutritional status and the risk of malnutrition in older adults with chronic kidney disease – implications for low protein intake and nutritional care: a critical review endorsed by ERN-ERA and ESPEN. Clin. Nutr. 15321983. 42 (4), 443–457. Available from: http://www.elsevier-international.com/journals/clnu/. doi:10.1016/j.clnu.2023.01.018.

Pranprawit, A., Wolber, F.M., Heyes, J.A., Molan, A.L., Kruger, M.C., 2013. Short-term and long-term effects of excessive consumption of saturated fats and/or sucrose on metabolic variables in Sprague Dawley rats: a pilot study. J. Sci. Food Agric. 10970010. 93 (13), 3191–3197. doi:10.1002/jsfa.6240.

Presti, R.L., Carollo, C., Caimi, G. 2007. Wine consumption and renal diseases: new perspectives. Nutrition 23, 598–602.

Promislow, J.H.E., Goodman-Gruen, D., Slymen, D.J., Barrett-Connor, E., 2002. Protein consumption and bone mineral density in the elderly: the Rancho Bernardo study. Am. J. Epidemiol. 00029262. 155 (7), 636–644. doi:10.1093/aje/155.7.636.

Ramos, C.I., González-Ortiz, A., Espinosa-Cuevas, A., Avesani, C.M., Carrero, J.J., Cuppari, L., 2021. Does dietary potassium intake associate with hyperkalemia in patients with chronic kidney disease? Nephrol. Dial. Transplant. 14602385. 36 (11), 2049–2057. Available from: http://ndt.oxfordjournals.org/. doi:10.1093/ndt/gfaa232.

Rapuri, P.B., Gallagher, J.C., Haynatzka, V., 2003. Protein intake: effects on bone mineral density and the rate of bone loss in elderly women. Am. J. Clin. Nutr. 00029165. 77 (6), 1517–1525. http://www.ajcn.org/contents-by-date.2005.shtml. doi:10.1093/ajcn/77.6.1517.

Rebholz, C. M., Crews, D.C., Grams, M.E., Steffen, L.M., Levey, A.S., Miller, E.R., Appel, L.J., Coresh, J., 2016b. DASH (Dietary Approaches to Stop Hypertension) Diet and Risk of Subsequent Kidney Disease. Am Kidney Dis 68, 853–861.

Rebholz, C.M., Coresh, J., Grams, M.E., Steffen, L.M., Anderson, C.A.M., Appel, L.J., Crews, D.C., 2015. Dietary acid load and incident chronic kidney disease: results from the ARIC study. Am. J. Nephrol. 14219670. 42 (6), 427–435. Available from: www.karger.ch/journals/ajn/ajn_jh.htm. doi:10.1159/000443746.

Rebholz, C.M., Crews, D.C., Grams, M.E., Steffen, L.M., Levey, A.S., Miller, E.R., 3L.J., Appel, Coresh, J., 2016a. DASH (Dietary Approaches to Stop Hypertension) Diet and Risk of Subsequent Kidney Disease. Am. J. Kidney Dis. 68, 853–861.

Rémond, D., Shahar, D.R., Gille, D., Pinto, P., Kachal, J., Peyron, M.A., Santos, C.N.D., Walther, B., Bordoni, A., Dupont, D., Tomás-Cobos, L., Vergères, G., 2015. Understanding the gastrointestinal tract of the elderly to develop dietary solutions that prevent malnutrition. Oncotarget. 19492553. 6 (16), 13858–13898. Available from: http://www.impactjournals.com/oncotarget/index.php?journal=oncotarget&page=article&op=download&path%5B%5D=4030&path%5B%5D=9606. doi:10.18632/oncotarget.4030.

Rey-García, J., Donat-Vargas, C., Sandoval-Insausti, H., Bayan-Bravo, A., Moreno-Franco, B., Banegas, J.R., Rodríguez-Artalejo, F., Guallar-Castillón, P., 2021. Ultra-processed food consumption is associated with renal function decline in older adults: a prospective cohort study. Nutrients. 20726643. 13 (2), 1–13. Available from: https://www.mdpi.com/2072-6643/13/2/428/pdf. doi:10.3390/nu13020428.

Russell, R.M., 2000. The aging process as a modifier of metabolism. Am. J. Clin. Nutr. 00029165. 72 (2), 529S. doi:10.1093/ajcn/72.2.529s.

Saltzman, J.R., Mason, J.B., 1992. Nutrition and the elderly. Curr. Opin. Gastroenterol. 02671379. 8 (2), 307–313. doi:10.1097/00001574-199204000-00018.

Satyanarayana, P.S.V., Singh, D., Chopra, K., 2001. Quercetin, a bioflavonoid, protects against oxidative stress-related renal dysfunction by cyclosporine in rats. Methods Find. Exp. Clin. Pharmacol. 03790355. 23 (4), 175–181. Available from: http://journals.prous.com/journals/servlet/xmlxsl/pk_journals.xml_journal_home_pr?p_JournalId=6. doi:10.1358/mf.2001.23.4.634641.

Schaefer, E.J., Lichtenstein, A.H., Lamon-Fava, S., McNamara, J.R., Ordovas, J.M., 1995. Lipoproteins, nutrition, aging, and atherosclerosis. Am. J. Clin. Nutr. 0002-9165. 61 (3), 726S. doi:10.1093/ajcn/61.3.726S.

Schaeffner, E.S., Kurth, T., Curhan, G.C., Glynn, R.J., Rexrode, K.M., Baigent, C., Buring, J.E., Gaziano, J.M., 2003. Cholesterol and the risk of renal dysfunction in apparently healthy men. J. Am. Soc. Nephrol. 10466673. 14 (8), 2084–2091. Available from: https://journals.lww.com/jasn/pages/default.aspx. doi:10.1681/asn.v1482084.

Scialla, J.J., Anderson, C.A.M., 2013. Dietary acid load: a novel nutritional target in chronic kidney disease? Adv. Chronic Kidney Dis. 15485609. 20 (2), 141–149. doi:10.1053/j.ackd.2012.11.001.

Shankar, A., Klein, R., Klein, B.E.K., 2006. The association among smoking, heavy drinking, and chronic kidney disease. Am. J. Epidemiol. 1476-6256. 164 (3), 263–271. doi:10.1093/aje/kwj173.

Smyth, A., Griffin, M., Yusuf, S., Mann, J.F.E., Reddan, D., Canavan, M., Newell, J., O'Donnell, M., 2016. Diet and major renal outcomes: a prospective cohort study. The NIH-AARP diet and health study. J. Ren. Nutr. 10512276. 26 (5), 288–298. doi:10.1053/j.jrn.2016.01.016.

Stevens, L.A., Coresh, J., Greene, T., Levey, A.S., 2006. Assessing kidney function—Measured and estimated glomerular filtration rate. N. Engl. J. Med. 15334406. 354 (23), 2473–2483. Available from: http://content.nejm.org/cgi/reprint/354/23/2473.pdf. doi:10.1056/NEJMra054415.

Sullivan, V.K., Appel, L.J., Anderson, C.A.M., Kim, H., Unruh, M.L., Lash, J.P., Trego, M., Sondheimer, J., Dobre, M., Pradhan, N., Rao, P.S., Chen, J., He, J., Rebholz, C.M., Cohen, D.L., Feldman, H.I., Go, A.S., Nelson, R.G., Rahman, M., Shah, V.O., Foods, U., Progression, K.D., 2023. Mortality, and cardiovascular disease risk in the CRIC study. Am. J. Kidney Dis. 15236838. 82 (2), 202–212. Available from: http://www.elsevier.com/inca/publications/store/6/2/3/2/7/6/index.htt. doi:10.1053/j.ajkd.2023.01.452.

Swift, S.L., Drexler, Y., Sotres-Alvarez, D., Raij, L., Llabre, M.M., Schneiderman, N., Horn, L.V., Lash, J.P., Mossavar-Rahmani, Y., Elfassy, T., 2022. Associations of sodium and potassium intake with chronic kidney disease in a prospective cohort study: findings from the Hispanic Community Health Study/Study of Latinos, 2008–2017. BMC Nephrol. 14712369. 23 (1). Available from: http://www.biomedcentral.com/bmcnephrol/. doi:10.1186/s12882-022-02754-2.

Takase, H., Kawakatsu, N., Hayashi, K., Kin, F., Isogaki, T., Dohi, Y., 2024. Urinary Na/K ratio is a predictor of developing chronic kidney disease in the general population. Hypertens. Res. 0916-9636. 47 (1), 225–232. doi:10.1038/s41440-023-01399-4.

Tang, R., Kou, M., Wang, X., Ma, H., Li, X., Heianza, Y., Qi, L., 2023. Self-reported frequency of adding salt to food and risk of incident chronic kidney disease. JAMA Netw. Open. 25743805. 6 (12), E2349930. Available from: https://jamanetwork.com/journals/jamanetworkopen. doi:10.1001/jamanetworkopen.2023.49930.

Valente Gamba, C., Caraviello, A.Z., Matsushita, A., Alves, G.M., da Silva, L.N., Gomes, G.N., Gil, F.Z., 2001. Effects of dietary lipids on renal function of aged rats. Braz. J. Med. Biol. Res. 0100-879X. 34 (2), 265–269. doi:10.1590/s0100-879x2001000200016.

Van Der Gaag, M.S., Van Tol, A., Scheek, L.M., James, R.W., Urgert, R., Schaafsma, G., Hendriks, H.F.J., 1999. Daily moderate alcohol consumption increases serum paraoxonase activity; a diet-controlled, randomised intervention study in middle-aged men. Atherosclerosis. 00219150. 147 (2), 405–410. doi:10.1016/S0021-9150(99)00243-9.

Vellas, B.J., Hunt, W.C., Romero, L.S., Koehler, K.M., Baumgartner, R.N., Garry, P.J., 1997. Changes in nutritional status and patterns of morbidity among free- living elderly persons: a 10-year longitudinal study. Nutrition. 08999007. 13 (6), 515–519. Available from: www.elsevier.com/locate/nut. doi:10.1016/S0899-9007(97)00029-4.

Volkert, D., Beck, A.M., Cederholm, T., Cruz-Jentoft, A., Goisser, S., Hooper, L., Kiesswetter, E., Maggio, M., Raynaud-Simon, A., Sieber, C.C., Sobotka, L., van Asselt, D., Wirth, R., Bischoff, S.C., 2019. ESPEN guideline on clinical nutrition and hydration in geriatrics. Clin. Nutr. 15321983. 38 (1), 10–47. Available from: http://www.elsevier-international.com/journals/clnu/. doi:10.1016/j.clnu.2018.05.024.

Walrand, S., Short, K.R., Bigelow, M.L., Sweatt, A.J., Hutson, S.M., Nair, K.S., 2008. Functional impact of high protein intake on healthy elderly people. Am. J. Physiol. Endocrinol. Metab. 15221555. 295 (4), E921. Available from: http://ajpendo.physiology.org/cgi/reprint/295/4/E921. doi:10.1152/ajpendo.90536.2008.

Watson, A.D., Berliner, J.A., Hama, S.Y., Du, B.N.L., Faull, K.F., Fogelman, A.M., Navab, M., 1995. Protective effect of high density lipoprotein associated paraoxonase inhibition of the biological activity of minimally oxidized low density lipoprotein. J. Clin. Invest. 00219738. 96 (6), 2882–2891. Available from: http://www.jci.org.

Werner, I., Hambraeus, L., 1971. The digestive capacity of elderly people. The effect of a high protein diet. Acta Soc. Med. Ups. 76 (5–6), 239–242.

Wu, P.Y., Chao, C.T., Chan, D.C., Huang, J.W., Hung, K.Y., 2019. Contributors, risk associates, and complications of frailty in patients with chronic kidney disease: a scoping review. Ther. Adv. Chronic Dis. 20406231. 10. Available from: http://www.sagepub.com/journalsProdDesc.nav?prodId=Journal201940. doi:10.1177/2040622319880382.

Xiao, B., Huang, J., Chen, L., Lin, Y., Luo, J., Chen, H., Lizhe, F., Tang, F., Ouyang, W., Yifan, W., 2024. Ultra-processed food consumption and the risk of incident chronic kidney disease: a systematic review and meta-analysis of cohort studies. Ren. Fail. 0886-022X. 46 (1). doi:10.1080/0886022x.2024.2306224.

Yaegashi, A., Kimura, T., Hirata, T., Tamakoshi, A., 2021. Association of dietary protein intake with skeletal muscle mass in older adults: a systematic review. Geriatr. Gerontol. Int. 1444-1586. 21 (12), 1077–1083. doi:10.1111/ggi.14291.

Yan, B., Su, X., Xu, B., Qiao, X., Wang, L., Cheungpasitporn, W., 2018. Effect of diet protein restriction on progression of chronic kidney disease: a systematic review and meta-analysis. PLOS ONE. 1932-6203. 13 (11), e0206134. doi:10.1371/journal.pone.0206134.

Yoon, C.Y., Noh, J., Lee, J., Kee, Y.K., Seo, C., Lee, M., Cha, M.U., Kim, H., Park, S., Yun, H.R., Jung, S.Y., Jhee, J.H., Han, S.H., Yoo, T.H., Kang, S.W., Park, J.T., 2018. High and low sodium intakes are associated with incident chronic kidney disease in patients with normal renal function and hypertension. Kidney Int. 15231755. 93 (4), 921–931. Available from: https://www.journals.elsevier.com/kidney-international. doi:10.1016/j.kint.2017.09.016.

Yoon, C.Y., Park, J.T., Jhee, J.H., Noh, J., Kee, Y.K., Seo, C., Lee, M., Cha, M.U., Kim, H., Park, S., Yun, H.R., Jung, S.Y., Han, S.H., Yoo, T.H., Kang, S.W., 2017. High dietary phosphorus density is a risk factor for incident chronic kidney disease development in diabetic subjects: a community-based prospective cohort study. Am. J. Clin. Nutr. 19383207. 106 (1), 311–321. Available from: http://ajcn.nutrition.org/content/106/1/311.full.pdf. doi:10.3945/ajcn.116.151654.

CHAPTER

8

Proteomics

Stephen Z. Fadem[a] and Emaad M. Abdel-Rahman[b]

[a]Department of Medicine, Section of Nephrology, Baylor College of Medicine, Houston, TX, United States

[b]Division of Nephrology, University of Virginia, Charlottesville, VA, United States

Introduction

As aging occurs, cellular changes lead to a decline in kidney function and disruption of pathways that help sustain cellular integrity. Uncovering the molecular mechanisms is key to developing therapies that will enable adaptation to the aging process. Proteins perform most of the biological functions of the cell, and thousands of them need to be identified. Proteomics aims to determine their structure, link them to their genes, understand how they are regulated and stimulated to perform, and explore how they relate to one another. It is making significant contributions to our understanding of the aging process in kidney disease. It promises to enhance our skills as clinicians by providing us with valuable tools to track the progression of aging.

Mass spectrometry emerged from the discovery of the electron in 1897 by J.J. Thomson, who built the first mass spectrometer (MS) in 1912. By the 1940s, mass spectrometers became commercially available. As MS technology advanced, it found applications in astronomy, DNA sequencing, and the complex analysis of protein sequences. Proteomics became a new specialty following the development of two-dimensional gel electrophoresis (2D gel techniques) in 1974. The term "proteomics" was coined in 1994 (Griffiths, 2008). Liquid chromatography and mass spectrometry (LC-MS) enable the separation and identification of complex protein mixtures.

The mass of a minimum of six amino acids can identify the signature of a protein. Data analysis tools can quickly identify the protein from its peptide sequence. It is estimated that the human genome codes for 19,750 proteins. Currently, 18,407 have been discovered. Artificial intelligence tools, such as AlphaFold, despite its limitations, enable scientists to predict the three-dimensional shape of a protein, given that its shape, how it folds, and how it can change shape determine its function.

Aging and the Kidney
https://doi.org/10.1016/B978-0-443-34069-7.00010-0

Advances in proteomics and machine learning have enabled researchers to develop aging clocks that measure the drift from youth of biomarkers validated as disease indicators. These are many of the hallmarks of aging that also influence kidney damage (Palmer, 2022).

Identifying biomarkers for kidney disease gives us tools to diagnose and manage kidney disease. Delving into relationships between protein production, maintenance, and degradation, as well as proteomic integration with other cellular functions, gives us a window into understanding aging, chronic kidney disease (CKD) progression, and their relationships.

AlphaFold—Google DeepMind

AlphaFold was developed by Google DeepMind and the European Bioinformatics Institute (EMBL). It is now a searchable online database (https://alphafold.ebi.ac.uk) and provides downloads for the human proteome. Analyzing the cell proteins of the kidney using current tools is advancing the understanding of normal pathways and changes related to age.

Google DeepMind is the combined effort of Google Brain and DeepMind, using artificial intelligence systems. After defeating a StarCraft II gaming champion with AlphaStar and inventing WaveNet as the text-to-speech model behind Google Assistant, it leaped to AlphaFold to accurately predict three-dimensional protein structures. AlphaFold now has 200 million protein structure predictions freely available to the public through UniProt, the standard repository of protein sequences and annotations, https://www.uniprot.org. The 2024 Nobel Prize in Chemistry was jointly awarded to Google DeepMind's Demis Hassabis and Jumper et al. (2021), and the University of Washington's David Baker, for their respective roles in computational protein design and protein structure prediction.

Proteomics and CKD

Proteomics entails analyzing plasma proteins in individuals with CKD to identify those associated with outcomes. Advances in machine learning for extracting quantitative protein information from biological samples have greatly enhanced dataset organization and the design of biomarker risk panels.

To help identify what peptides perpetuate the further loss of kidney function, 106 patients with various stages of CKD were evaluated against 66 controls. Extracted blood peptides were fractionated and analyzed using a capillary high-pressure liquid chromatography system interfaced with an electrospray ionizer and mass spectroscopy. The peptides of interest underwent matrix-assisted laser desorption-time of flight mass spectrometry (MALDI-TQF-MS) and linear ion trap mass spectrometry. The model differentiated CKD and nonCKD patients with an odds ratio of 2.018 (95% CI 1.44–2.82, $p = 0.00004$). The study demonstrated that proteomics could be useful in identifying novel plasma peptides as specific biomarkers for CKD progression (Gajjala et al., 2019).

In a large study, the proteins of 3235 participants from the Chronic Renal Insufficiency Cohort (CRIC) were evaluated for associations and pathways. A risk model consisting of 65 proteins was developed, with fourteen of these potentially useful as drug targets. The study also identified five new proteins that had not been previously reported (Dubin et al., 2023).

Further research on CKD patients involved 703 participants in the African Study of Kidney Disease and Hypertension (AASK) and 1628 participants in the Atherosclerosis Risk in Communities (ARIC) trial. Seven proteins were identified as associated with all-cause mortality in AASK, and three (β-microglobulin, spondin-1, and N-terminal pro-brain natriuretic peptide [NT-proBNP]) were also found in the validating ARIC trial (Srialluri et al., 2023).

Another example of how proteomics is furthering our knowledge of CKD pathophysiology is the study by Ramírez Medina et al. (2023). A total of 414 nondialysis CKD patients with multiple diseases were analyzed for proteomic signals using SWATH-MS, a data-independent acquisition variant that essentially isolates digested ionized peptides of samples falling within a specified mass range by liquid chromatography coupled to a tandem mass spectrometer and systematically fragments them using precursor isolation windows. This leads to multiplexed and complex fragment ion spectra. These mass spectrometric coordinates of the proteins and peptides can be mapped as peptide query parameters (PQPs). This study revealed 626 proteins and 25 biomarkers important to disease progression. It supported the role of the complement cascade in diabetic nephropathy. It also confirmed the enrichment of proteins involved in the ubiquitin-proteasome pathway.

Aging kidneys exhibit significant proteomic changes that can affect various cellular functions. Autopsy data suggest that by the eighth decade of life, kidney mass declines by 10%–30% and that the majority of the decline in renal mass occurs after age 60. Data from kidney donors confirm a decline in the elderly but suggest that cortical mass decreases while medullary mass increases. Histologic changes are also seen in the aging kidney and are characterized by changes in blood vessels, as well as glomerulosclerosis, tubular atrophy, and interstitial fibrosis. Healthy adults from 18 to 29 years old may demonstrate a 2.7% incidence of nephrosclerosis, but 73% of persons aged 70–77 have these abnormal features on biopsy.

GFR declines from 100% at age 30 to 55% at age 89. A study involving 254 healthy subjects demonstrated that the average decline in creatinine clearance was 0.75 ml/min/year. However, in up to one-third of the cases, GFR stabilized, and in some subjects, it even increased. The decline in GFR among most patients is physiological rather than indicative of disease (Glassock and Rule, 2016). The question remains as to why GFR declines in some patients while it does not in others. To address this question, transitioning from histopathology to advanced tools like mass spectrometry and sophisticated data management, such as machine learning, may provide better insights. This contextualizes the molecular changes that have been the focus of this section (Dybiec et al., 2022). Proteomic biomarkers in CKD enhance our understanding of aging mechanisms since kidney disease often reflects accelerated aging processes, and these biomarkers are frequently shared. In the next section, we will explore insights into the causes of aging from the perspective of how we can better understand and mitigate them.

Proteomics and aging

The human genome contains approximately 3.1 billion base pairs. As we identify their functions, we quickly recognize the value of proteomics. The value of integrating the two "-omics" is that single-nucleotide polymorphisms identified through a genome-wide association study can help pinpoint suspicious areas of the genome that may be implicated in causation. Confounders, the commonality of pathways, the dynamic interactions between various proteins, and the perturbations associated with translation defects make it more challenging to use proteomics to determine the direction of influence when understanding diseases. The value of proteomics lies in identifying which proteins are involved in the disease process.

The aging mechanisms in the kidney and the organism at large share much in common, and their interrelations determine protein integrity. Proteomics is valuable in studying several aging hallmarks, as it can help track misfolded proteins, identify the protein changes involved in DNA repair, and track mitochondrial changes. It also helps map signaling proteins. Identifying gut flora can aid in the use of prebiotics and probiotics to decrease post-stem cell transplant graft-versus-host reactions (Andermann et al., 2016). The molecular signatures of aging and kidney disease can help distinguish the links between the two entities and are already leading to practical therapeutic advances.

Quantifying the biological aging process may help clinicians intervene when appropriate biomarkers identify modifiable risk factors. Several "clocks" have been constructed. Epigenetic clocks have demonstrated that the percentage of methylation of cytosine-guanine (CpG) sites on DNA predicts chronological age. The use of machine learning has advanced to the point where biological age and the risk of developing health outcomes can also be determined. Newer methods can filter out immune factors that bias the predictions (Tomusiak et al., 2024).

Studying proteins offers advantages in that the proteins and their metabolites are the final determinants of the phenotype. A proteomic age clock was developed using plasma proteomic expression data from nearly 51,000 Finnish, Chinese, and UK participants from three cohorts. The cohorts were split into 70% training and 30% test sets. External validation was performed using independent datasets from China and Finland. The proteomic age clock was compared with the UK Biobank and gave similar predictive results. Six machine learning models were compared to predict chronological age using 2897 proteins. LightGBM was selected. It is an open-source gradient-boosting framework for machine learning that was developed by Microsoft. Researchers were able to create a protein model with 204 aging proteins, using LightGBM along with the Boruta algorithm to determine features and SHAP to identify and rank relevant subsets. This protein-predicted age (ProtAge) explained the variation in chronological age, was comparable to the larger 2897 protein model, and was used to calculate the ProtAgeGap—the difference between age-related proteins and chronological age. The results were comparable across all three databases (China, Finland, and the UK). The ProtAgeGap was associated with serum creatinine and serum cystatin C, C-reactive protein, serum albumin, telomere length, IGF-1, and liver enzymes. Clinically, it was related to several factors, including a slow walking pace, self-rated facial aging, sleeping ≥ 10 h a day, fatigue and insomnia, elevated blood pressure, the frailty index, reaction time, arterial stiffness, body mass index, bone mineral density, fluid intelligence, pulmonary function tests, and hand grip strength (Argentieri et al., 2024). Fluid intelligence is the ability to reason and solve newly presented problems (Horn and Cattell, 1966).

For participants over age 65 at recruitment, the top decile of the ProtAgeGap over a follow-up period of 11–16 years was associated with higher risks of osteoarthritis (59.4%), all-cause mortality (55.2%), ischemic heart disease (50.6%), type-2 diabetes (35.3%), and CKD (33.6%). Serum cystatin C had the highest association with the ProtAgeGap. The ProtAgeGap was also greater when more than one disease was present (Argentieri et al., 2024). The mismatch risks between serum creatinine and cystatin C have been evaluated elsewhere. A cohort study using the National Health and Nutrition Examination Survey (NHANES) 1999–2004 compared the highest and lowest quartiles of the serum creatinine-to-serum cystatin C ratio. A low ratio was significantly associated with all-cause mortality, cardiovascular disease, and cancer ($P < 0.001$) (Wang et al., 2024) Table 8.1).

Researchers have assessed thousands of proteins using LC-MS, multiplexed proteomic assays with modified aptamers, and proximity extension assays. Aptamers are single strands of either DNA or RNA that can fold into a three-dimensional conformation and bind to proteins. Aptamers have therapeutic potential (Nimjee et al., 2017). The proximity extension assay employs polymerase chain reactions to detect nucleic acids linked to antibodies. The interaction between the protein pairs and these antibodies enables the nucleic acid tags to trigger a measurable signal. This technique has been used to detect proteins associated with cancer, lupus, diabetes, and CKD. The National Institute on Aging conducted a literature search with a selective review of thirty-three publications identifying proteins associated with aging (Moaddel et al., 2021). From these, the authors paired the protein list to 154 proteins and utilized enrichment analysis tools to better understand their biological functions and pathways. These tools helped determine if the proteins identified were statistically related to their study paths. Moaddel's team identified 21 well-known signaling pathways involved in the aging process. These included IGF1, MAPK, HIF-1, FOXO, AGE/RAGE, and cytokine signaling pathways. IGF1 levels are associated with muscle strength and low mortality, yet IGF1 declines with age. The IGF1-Akt pathway is involved in the modulation of mTOR, which is also implicated in the aging process. MAPK is strongly associated with aging. It plays a role in cell growth and differentiation but also in apoptosis. HIF is a transcription factor that

TABLE 8.1 Molecules that have been shown to be associated with both aging and CKD.

	Molecule(s)	Description	Shared in aging & CKD	Proteomic role
1	Cystatin C	An index of kidney function	Yes	Marker of CKD, but also a biomarker of aging, frailty, and mortality
2	CKD273	A multi-peptide marker of progressive CKD	Yes	Estimates the development of microalbuminuria and CKD
3	Beta$_2$-microglobulin	Rises in advancing CKD is a surrogate for middle molecular weight uremic toxins	Yes	Increases with age and renal senescence; identified in patients with sarcopenia and cognitive decline
4	Interleukin-6	IL-6 is a cytokine associated with inflammation	Yes	Elevated in age-related decline and worsening kidney function
5	Serum albumin	A traditional marker of inflammation	Yes	Albuminuria is an indicator of frailty, comorbidity, and mortality
6	ProtAgeGap	Biological age predictor	Yes	Correlates with cystatin C, CRP, telomere length, and CKD.
7	Uremic toxins—indole, cresole, phenole sulfate	Gut-derived; fermented by bacteria, sulfated in the liver	Yes	Elevated with age; causes damage to the brain, heart, and kidneys. Probiotics may be beneficial
8	C-reactive protein	A marker of inflammation and a risk factor in CKD	Yes	Identified by age clock analysis as a marker of aging

supports erythropoiesis and angiogenesis, but it becomes dysregulated with aging. HIF2 is associated with erythropoiesis. In a low-oxygen environment, the HIF1α subunit decreases the mitochondrial production of ATP. It contributes to oxidative stress, triggering factors that translocate NF-kB and STAT3 to the nucleus, which in turn trigger pro-inflammatory cytokines. FOXO helps mediate oxidative stress but can also trigger cell cycle arrest and apoptosis. Advanced glycation end products (AGEs) are irreversible molecules that trigger an inflammatory response when bound to their receptor, RAGE. They play a role in the pathogenesis of diabetes and CKD. AGE is the reaction between sugar, which is broken down with heat, and proteins. AGE-rich foods in the diet can also trigger RAGE receptors and, in excess, can be associated with accelerated aging. Several proteins that trigger cytokines are upregulated with age. The pro-inflammatory cytokines include IL-6, IL-12, IL-1, IL-17, and IL-18, while IL-10 and IL-13 are antiinflammatory (Moaddel et al., 2021).

The pathway between an amino acid's translation into a protein and the protein's functionality is complex and subject to degradation with aging. Based on RNA coding, amino acids are linked into peptides on the ribosome, then folded, assembled, and transported to their site of action. They must be activated to participate in enzymatic activity. Post-translational modifications may create an altered protein structure with a different biological purpose. PTMs can add phosphorus, methyl, ubiquitin, or glucose to the protein. They may also modify its structure and function by cleaving, deregulating, or linking it to another protein. PTM modification of proteins identified as biomarkers could lead to misleading findings when studying the aging process. As proteomics research advances, PTM effects are being included in biomarker investigations. Measuring proteins alone is giving way to using PTM information to develop more precise biomarkers (Moaddel et al., 2021).

Implications for clinical practice

Two examples of how proteomics can advance renal patient care, particularly as we age, are included. These implications involve the gut microbiome and can be adapted to lifestyle and dietary modifications. In addition, the development of validated markers can streamline health care and research while improving outcomes.

The gut microbiome

Using LC-MS enabled Aronov and colleagues in 2011 to compare blood from dialysis patients who had undergone colectomy with blood from those with an intact colon, and to clearly separate uremic toxins in dialysis patients with and without colons (Aronov et al., 2011). This study demonstrated around 35 metabolites that were not removed by dialysis and that were high in dialysis patients but lower in those with normal kidney function. Among these metabolites were αphenylacetyl-1-glutamine, indoxyl sulfate, and p-cresol sulfate. All are nearly absent in patients without colons. Patients with normal kidney function have the precursors to these metabolites excreted in the urine. As patients age, their metabolome also changes, as reported in a study from Sun and colleagues. They profiled the gut and serum bacteria from 151 healthy subjects aged 22–111 years, finding that their influence on serum metabolites increased with age. Their study measured several clinical laboratory values, including lipid metabolism, C-reactive protein, superoxide dismutase, beta-hydroxybutyrate, homocysteine, serum creatinine, urea, and uric acid. Telomere length was also measured from leukocyte DNA. Stool samples were analyzed using LC-MS. Fecal DNA was also extracted, and a genetic analysis was performed. They used BLASTp, a protein sequence alignment tool, to compare sequences with those in the KEGG database.

Amino acid sequences could be assigned a KEGG ortholog (KO). Metagenomic species (MGS) were clusters based on characteristics of DNA sequences. The analysis showed that gut microbiota and dominant microbial species changed in different age groups. Across several ethnicities, compositional changes in microbes converged as people age. *Escherichia coli* MGSs were enriched in the elderly subjects, as were *Anaerostipes hadrus, Clostridium symbiosum*, and *O. splanchnicus,* while *Faecalibacterium prausnitzii* MGSs were enriched in the youngest participants. KO abundance was related to the tyrosine, tryptophan, and phenylalanine pathways. Tryptophan is metabolized to indole, while phenylalanine is metabolized to tyrosine and then to p-cresyl, phenol, and phenylacetylglutamine. Markers of impaired kidney function, such as phenylalanine, phenylacetylglutamine, indoxyl sulfate, and hippuric acid, correlated with serum creatinine, the blood urea nitrogen, and uric acid. The bacterial enzymes involved in indole, Hippurate, and bile acid synthesis were more abundant in the older individuals. The study identified 74 MGSs predictive of uremic toxins and bile salts significantly correlated with *E. coli, F. prausnitzii, D. piger, O. splanchnicus*, and *B. wadsworthia. Klebsiella* species and *E. coli* also correlated with worsening kidney function. (Sun et al., 2023).

Aging is associated with a decline in kidney function. Identifying bacteria and gut toxins in the elderly cohort commonly linked to uremia establishes a connection between aging and the kidneys. Many metabolites are the bacterial breakdown products of dietary amino acids. When kidney function is normal, amino acids can be easily metabolized and eliminated through the kidneys. However, their accumulation in CKD and normal aging leads to gut bacterial conversion into toxins that contribute to the pathogenesis of heart, brain, and kidney diseases (Sun et al., 2023).

The tubular transport of organic ions into the urine is an important mechanism to rid the body of uremic toxins. It is downregulated by indoxyl sulfate and upregulated by statins. The accumulation of uremic toxins due to impaired tubular transport and the ingestion of foods high in tyrosine results in its conversion by gut bacteria to phenol. Coriobacteria and Erysipelotrichales, both gram-positive anaerobic bacteria, are increased in renal failure and contain the enzyme tyrosine phenol-lyase (TPL), which can metabolize tyrosine to phenol. Phenol is then conjugated to phenyl sulfate in the liver. Phenyl sulfate is toxic to podocytes and decreases mitochondrial function. It results in a thickened glomerular basement membrane, increased inflammation, and fibrosis. Over a two-year period, the level of phenyl sulfate is related to the progression of microalbuminuria to albuminuria in diabetics. In mice, the reduction in dietary tyrosine reduces proteinuria. In addition, therapy that blocks TPL can also reduce phenol (Kikuchi et al., 2019). Polyphenols that inhibit TPL have been investigated, and quercetin was found to be the most potent. Quercetin is a flavonoid that has potential in cardiovascular and kidney disease, but clinical trials that demonstrate a clear benefit are still lacking (Kobayashi et al., 2024; Zhang et al., 2023).

A diet low in animal protein but enriched with plant fiber and protein not only reduces the filtered load on the glomerulus but also decreases the availability of α-amino acids to be metabolized by bacteria into uremic toxins like p-cresol sulfate and indoxyl sulfate. It also shifts the microbiota toward saccharolytic bacteria that can ferment fiber and carbohydrates to produce short-chain fatty acids. These SCFAs reduce inflammation and strengthen the gut barrier.

The use of probiotics containing *Lactobacillus* and *Bifidobacterium* genera may also reduce indoxyl sulfate and p-cresyl sulfate in CKD patients and may reduce not just the progression of kidney disease but also the impact of uremic toxins on the heart, brain, and kidneys (Fagundes et al., 2018). While the use of probiotic supplements is generally considered safe, they are not recommended for patients who are immunocompromised.

Health care discovery and delivery are costly and require significant investment in time and money, not only for evidence-based clinical trials but also for the recovery of research, manufacturing, and distribution costs to pharmaceutical companies, and ultimately to the health care system and the patient. Moreover, the inconvenience to patients of taking an additional medication is a concern. Shortcomings often prevent the use of therapies that can yield long-term benefits, which may not be apparent for several years. These issues can be addressed by using validated biomarkers to indicate whether a long-term advantage to therapy exists. CKD273 represents a search for just such a biomarker.

CKD273

While urine albumin-creatinine ratios have been validated and are inexpensive, they generally provide information about a disease only after the pathological process has advanced. Proteomic techniques offer an advantage because they examine many protein markers and can be studied at various levels of disease. Comparing these markers determines a manageable number that can be contrasted across several diseases and against placebos. They can also be evaluated longitudinally, at various stages of life, allowing for the trending of kidney function with advancing age. Novel biomarkers can help us manage and study not just CKD but also diabetic nephropathy and IgA nephropathy (Andrzej et al., 2011).

Peptide biomarkers identified through proteomic studies can aid in the early identification and management of diseases, especially from urine. Using CE-MS, a study examined the urine peptides from 230 uremic toxins associated with progressive CKD and 379 controls. They included indoxyl sulfate, p-cresyl sulfate, 5-methoxytryptophan, acetyl carnitine, and taurine. A cluster analysis identified 273 peptides that differentiated CKD from the control group. Its levels were associated with the presence of disease, separating CKD patients by renal function over a follow-up period of 3.6 years. They named their aggregate marker CKD273 (Argiles et al., 2013). As anticipated, CKD273 includes fragments of inflammatory proteins and breakdown products from the extracellular matrix (Mihai et al., 2016). In a proteomics analysis of 2672 patients with various stages of CKD, CKD273 performed better than urinary albumin excretion in the early stages of kidney disease. It has since been shown to be a risk factor for cardiovascular disease and may help identify patients who could benefit the most from early interventions (Pontillo et al., 2017). A cohort of 451 patients with CKD stages G1 through G5 was followed for a median of 5.5 years. CKD273 was associated with a greater than 10-fold risk in patients with stages G1 through G3B without a history of heart disease. It also estimated the development of microalbuminuria and declining kidney function (Pontillo et al., 2017). In a systematic review, CKD273 was able to predict the decline in kidney function in normoalbuminuric patients with diabetes (Lorenzo et al., 2023). CKD273 is a promising indicator of the value proteomics will have in the early identification of disease, its stratification by disease staging, and management through delineating high-risk markers, which can assist in selecting patients most likely to respond to a therapeutic intervention.

Proteomics can assist in the identification of druggable targets. In a retrospective review, it was observed that spironolactone users had a lower rate of progression to ESRD than nonusers, HR 0.66 (95% CI, 0.51–0.84; P value < 0.001). However, the incidence of hyperkalemia was higher at 3.17 (95% CI, 2.41–4.17; P value < 0.001), and offset its value (Yang et al., 2018). In the PRIORITY trial, patients with type 2 diabetes and normal albuminuria were stratified into a high-risk category to develop albuminuria, having a urinary CKD273 > 0.154. The high-risk cohort was randomized to receive spironolactone for a treatment period of 2.5 years, with the primary endpoint being the development of albuminuria. The findings indicated that the high-risk group had an HR of 3.50 (95% CI 2.50–4.90) for a decline in renal function and increased proteinuria. Spironolactone did not demonstrate efficacy in preventing proteinuria, but did illustrate the value of CKD273 (Tofte et al., 2020). Finerenone has been shown to sustain a decrease of 43% from baseline in the GFR of CKD patients with type 2 diabetes with proteinuria in a randomized double blind trial. HR was 0.82 (95% CI 0.73–0.93). The incidence of patients who discontinued the trial because of hyperkalemia was low, only 2.3%, although hyperkalemia was a side effect. Gynecomastia was not seen with finerenone. No studies thus far have been performed to see if CKD273-stratified patients will benefit from finerenone. However, dapagliflozin has been shown in a small (n = 40) randomized, controlled, crossover trial of type 2 diabetes and proteinuria to lower CKD score (−0.221; 95% CI – 0.356, – 0.087; P = 0.002), and significantly drop patients from high risk to low risk with dapagliflozin (P = 0.21) (Curovic et al., 2022). CKD273 classifier and other urinary peptide classifiers, HF2 and CAD238, have been able to demonstrate the increase in risk to patients with prediabetes, making early intervention possible and potentially increasing disease outcomes (Bakris et al., 2020) Fig. 8.1.

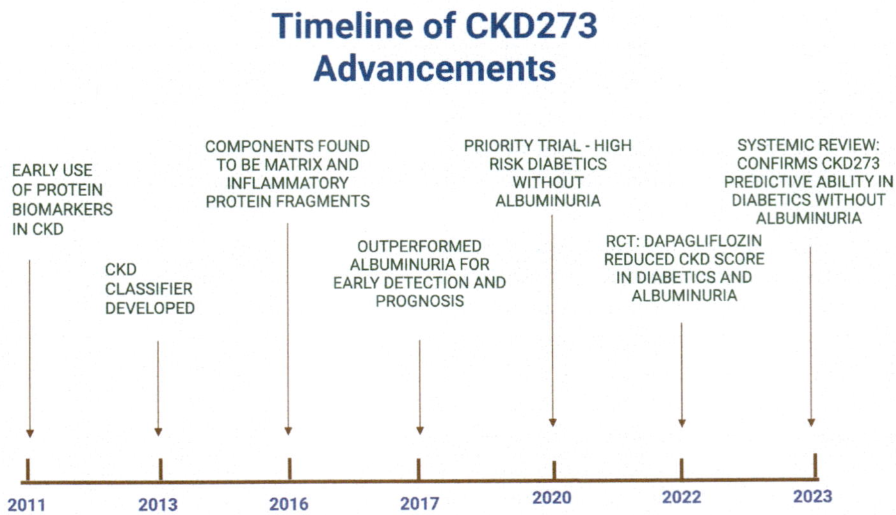

FIG. 8.1 Timeline of CKD273 Advancements. Advancements in CKD273, a multipeptide protein classifier. See text for details. Created in BioRender. Fadem, S. https://BioRender.com/p3r48aq.

Conclusion

The accumulation of protein fragments associated with aging and the decline in kidney function offers valuable insights into the molecular pathways involved in the aging process. Recent advancements in technology, particularly through the development of liquid chromatography-mass spectrometry (LC-MS) and machine learning, have facilitated the identification of these molecules and their roles in both cross-sectional and longitudinal analyses of kidney disease. It has been established that these molecules possess significant potential as biomarkers, serving as diagnostic tools in managing patients experiencing progressive CKD and aging. In particular, CKD273 and the uremic toxins demonstrate considerable promise.

AI disclosure

During the preparation of this work, the author(s) used Grammarly as a grammar and syntax checker. In no way did it influence the content of this chapter. After using this tool/service, the author(s) reviewed and edited the content as needed and take(s) full responsibility for the content of the publication.

References

Andermann, T.M., Rezvani, A., Bhatt, A.S., 2016. Microbiota Manipulation With Prebiotics and Probiotics in Patients Undergoing Stem Cell Transplantation. Curr. Hematol. Malig. Rep. 1558822X. 11 (1), 19–28. Available from: http://www.springerlink.com/content/1558-8211/. doi:10.1007/s11899-016-0302-9.

Andrzej, C., Małgorzata, O., Agnieszka, H., Anna, K., Agnieszka, K., Adam, L., Radosław, 2011. Urinary proteomic strategies in biomarkers discovery of renal diseases. J. Pre-Clin. Clin. Res. 5, 1–6.

Argentieri, M.A., Xiao, S., Bennett, D., Winchester, L., Nevado-Holgado, A.J., Ghose, U., Albukhari, A., Yao, P., Mazidi, M., Lv, J., Millwood, I., Fry, H., Rodosthenous, R.S., Partanen, J., Zheng, Z., Kurki, M., Daly, M.J., Palotie, A., Adams, C.J., Li, L., Clarke, R., Amin, N., Chen, Z., van Duijn, C.M., 2024. Proteomic aging clock predicts mortality and risk of common age-related diseases in diverse populations. Nat. Med. 1546170X. 30 (9), 2450–2460. Available from: https://www.nature.com/nm/. doi:10.1038/s41591-024-03164-7.

Argiles, À., Justyna, S., Flore, D., Nathalie, G., Mohammed, D., Ulrika, L., Lourdes, O., Christian, D., Georges, M., Klaus, M.W., Harald, M., 2013. New proteomics classifier assessing CKD and its prognosis. PLOS ONE 8, e62837.

Aronov, P.A., Luo, F.J.G., Plummer, N.S., Quan, Z., Holmes, S., Hostetter, T.H., Meyer, T.W., 2011. Colonic contribution to uremic solutes. J. Am. Soc. Nephrol. 15333450. 22 (9), 1769–1776. Available from: http://jasn.asnjournals.org/content/22/9/1769.full.pdf+html. doi:10.1681/ASN.2010121220.

Bakris, G.L., Agarwal, R., Anker, S.D., Pitt, B., Ruilope, L.M., Rossing, P., Kolkhof, P., Nowack, C., Schloemer, P., Joseph, A., Filippatos, G., 2020. Effect of finerenone on chronic kidney disease outcomes in type 2 diabetes. N. Engl. J. Med. 15334406. 383 (23), 2219–2229. Available from: http://www.nejm.org/medical-index. doi:10.1056/NEJMoa2025845.

Curovic, V.R., Mie, K.E., Teemu, J.R., Marie, F.-M., Tine, W.H., Harald, M., Peter, R., Tarunveer, S.A., Frederik, P., 2022. Dapagliflozin Improves the Urinary Proteomic Kidney-Risk Classifier CKD273 in Type 2 Diabetes with Albuminuria - a Randomized Clinical Trial. Diabetes Care 45, 2662–2668.

Dubin, R.F., Deo, R., Ren, Y., Wang, J., Zheng, Z., Shou, H., Go, A.S., Parsa, A., Lash, J.P., Rahman, M., Hsu, C.Y., Weir, M.R., Chen, J., Anderson, A., Grams, M.E., Surapaneni, A., Coresh, J., Li, H., Kimmel, P.L., Vasan, R.S., Feldman, H., Segal, M.R., Ganz, P., 2023. Proteomics of CKD progression in the chronic renal insufficiency cohort. Nat. Commun. 20411723. 14 (1). Available from: https://www.nature.com/ncomms/. doi:10.1038/s41467-023-41642-7.

Dybiec, J., Szlagor, M., Młynarska, E., Rysz, J., Franczyk, B., 2022. Structural and functional changes in aging kidneys. Int. J. Mol. Sci. 1422-0067. 23 (23), 15435. doi:10.3390/ijms232315435.

Fagundes, R.A.B., Soder, T.F., Grokoski, K.C., Benetti, F., Mendes, R.H., 2018. Probiotics in the treatment of chronic kidney disease: a systematic review. J. Bras. Nefrol. 21758239. 40 (3), 278–286. doi:10.1590/2175-8239-JBN-3931.

Gajjala, P.R., Bruck, H., Noels, H., Heinze, G., Ceccarelli, F., Kribben, A., Saez-Rodriguez, J., Marx, N., Zidek, W., Jankowski, J., Jankowski, V., 2019. Novel plasma peptide markers involved in the pathology of CKD identified using mass spectrometric approach. J. Mol. Med. 14321440. 97 (10), 1451–1463. Available from: http://link.springer.com/journal/109. doi:10.1007/s00109-019-01823-8.

Glassock, R.J., Rule, A.D., 2016. Aging and the kidneys: anatomy, physiology and consequences for defining chronic kidney disease. Nephron. 22353186. 134 (1), 25–29. Available from: http://www.karger.com/Journal/Home/223854. doi:10.1159/000445450.

Griffiths, J., 2008. A Brief History of Mass Spectrometry. Anal. Chem. 0003-2700. 80 (15), 5678–5683. doi:10.1021/ac8013065.

Horn, J.L., Cattell, R.B., 1966. Refinement and test of the theory of fluid and crystallized general intelligences. J. Educ. Psychol. 00220663. 57 (5), 253–270. doi:10.1037/h0023816.

Jumper, J., Evans, R., Pritzel, A., et al., 2021. Highly accurate protein structure prediction with AlphaFold. Nature 596 (7873), 583–589. doi:10.1038/s41586-021-03819-2.

Kikuchi, K., Saigusa, D., Kanemitsu, Y., Matsumoto, Y., Thanai, P., Suzuki, N., Mise, K., Yamaguchi, H., Nakamura, T., Asaji, K., Mukawa, C., Tsukamoto, H., Sato, T., Oikawa, Y., Iwasaki, T., Oe, Y., Tsukimi, T., Fukuda, N.N., Ho, H.J., Nanto-Hara, F., Ogura, J., Saito, R., Nagao, S., Ohsaki, Y., Shimada, S., Suzuki, T., Toyohara, T., E. Mishima, H.S., Akiyama, Y., Akiyama, Y., Ichijo, M., Matsuhashi, T., Matsuo, A., Ogata, Y., Yang, C.C., Suzuki, C., Breeggemann, M.C., Heymann, J., Shimizu, M., Ogawa, S., Takahashi, N., Suzuki, T., Owada, Y., Kure, S., Mano, N., Soga, T., Wada, T., Kopp, J.B., Fukuda, S., Hozawa, A., Yamamoto, M., Ito, S., Wada, J., Tomioka, Y., abe, T., 2019. Gut microbiome-derived phenyl sulfate contributes to albuminuria in diabetic kidney disease. Nat. Commun. 10, 1835.

Kobayashi, T., Oishi, S., Matsui, M., Hara, K., Hashimoto, H., Watanabe, K., Yoshioka, Y., Miyoshi, N., Dupont, C., 2024. Tyrosine phenol-lyase inhibitor quercetin reduces fecal phenol levels in mice. PNAS Nexus. 2752-6542. 3 (7). doi:10.1093/pnasnexus/pgae265.

Lorenzo, C., Justyna, S., Harald, M., Ralph, W., Joachim, B., Harald, R., 2023. Recent Advances in Urinary Peptide and Proteomic Biomarkers in Chronic Kidney Disease: a Systematic Review. Int. J. Mol. Sci. 24, 9156.

Mihai, S, Codrici, E, Popescu I.D., Enciu, A.M., Rusu, E., Zilisteanu, D., Albulescu, R., Anton, G., Tanase, C., 2016. Proteomic biomarkers panel: new insights in chronic kidney disease. Dis. Markers 2016, 3185232. doi:10.1155/2016/3185232. PMID: 27667892; PMCID: PMC5030443.

Moaddel, R., Ubaida-Mohien, C., Tanaka, T., Lyashkov, A., Basisty, N., Schilling, B., Semba, R.D., Franceschi, C., Gorospe, M., Ferrucci, L., 2021. Proteomics in aging research: a roadmap to clinical, translational research. Aging Cell. 14749726. 20 (4). Available from: http://onlinelibrary.wiley.com/journal/10.1111/(ISSN)1474-9726. doi:10.1111/acel.13325.

Nimjee, S.M., White, R.R., Becker, R.C., Sullenger, B.A., 2017. Aptamers as Therapeutics. Annu. Rev. Pharmacol. Toxicol. 15454304. 57, 61–79. Available from: http://arjournals.annualreviews.org/loi/pharmtox. doi:10.1146/annurev-pharmtox-010716-104558.

Palmer, R.D., 2022. Aging clocks & mortality timers, methylation, glycomic, telomeric and more. A window to measuring biological age. Aging Med. 24750360. 5 (2), 120–125. Available from: https://onlinelibrary.wiley.com/journal/24750360. doi:10.1002/agm2.12197.

Pontillo, C., Jacobs, L., Staessen, J.A., Schanstra, J.P., Rossing, P., Heerspink, H.J.L., Siwy, J., Mullen, W., Vlahou, A., Mischak, H., Vanholder, R., Zürbig, P., Jankowski, J., 2017. A urinary proteome-based classifier for the early detection of decline in glomerular filtration. Nephrol. Dial. Transplant. 14602385. 32 (9), 1510–1516. Available from: http://ndt.oxfordjournals.org/. doi:10.1093/ndt/gfw239.

Ramírez Medina, C.R., Ali, I., Baricevic-Jones, I., Odudu, A., Saleem, M.A., Whetton, A.D., Kalra, P.A., Geifman, N., 2023. Proteomic signature associated with chronic kidney disease (CKD) progression identified by data-independent acquisition mass spectrometry. Clin. Proteomics. 15590275. 20 (1). Available from: https://clinicalproteomicsjournal.biomedcentral.com/. doi:10.1186/s12014-023-09405-0.

Srialluri, N., Surapaneni, A., Schlosser, P., Chen, T.K., Schmidt, I.M., Rhee, E.P., Coresh, J., Grams, M.E., 2023. Circulating proteins and mortality in CKD: a proteomics study of the AASK and ARIC cohorts. Kidney Med. 25900595. 5 (10). Available from: https://www.journals.elsevier.com/kidney-medicine. doi:10.1016/j.xkme.2023.100714.

Sun, L., Li, Z., Hu, C., Ding, J., Zhou, Q., Pang, G., Wu, Z., Yang, R., Li, S., Li, J., Cai, J., Sun, Y., Li, R., Zhen, H., Sun, S., Zhang, J., Fang, M., Chen, Z., Lv, Y., Cao, Q., Sun, Y., Gong, R., Huang, Z., Duan, Y., Liu, H., Dong, J., Li,

J., Ruan, J., Lu, H., He, B., Li, N., Li, T., Xue, W., Li, Y., Shen, J., Yang, F., Zhao, C., Liang, Q., Zhang, M., Chen, C., Gong, H., Hou, Y., Wang, J., Zhang, Y., Yang, H., Zhu, S., Xiao, L., Jin, Z., Guo, H., Zhao, P., Brix, S., Xu, X., Jia, H., Kristiansen, K., Yang, Z., Nie, C., 2023. Age-dependent changes in the gut microbiota and serum metabolome correlate with renal function and human aging. Aging Cell. 14749726. 22 (12). Available from: http://onlinelibrary.wiley.com/journal/10.1111/(ISSN)1474-9726. doi:10.1111/acel.14028.

Tofte, N., Lindhardt, M., Adamova, K., Bakker, S.J.L., Beige, J., Beulens, J.W.J., Birkenfeld, A.L., Currie, G., Delles, C., Dimos, I., Francová, L., Frimodt-Møller, M., Girman, P., Göke, R., Havrdova, T., Heerspink, H.J.L., Kooy, A., Laverman, G.D., Mischak, H., Navis, G., Nijpels, G., Noutsou, M., Ortiz, A., Parvanova, A., Persson, F., Petrie, J.R., Ruggenenti, P.L., Rutters, F., Rychlík, I., Siwy, J., Spasovski, G., Speeckaert, M., Trillini, M., Zürbig, P., von der Leyen, H., Rossing, P., Zimmermann, S., Rädisch, B., Hävemeier, A., Busmann, A., Wittkop, U., Neuhaus, B., Ax-Smolarski, R., Zieglschmid, V., Bollweber, E., Wölk, H., Curovic, V.R., Tougaard, N.H., Eickhoff, M.K., Pilemann-Lyberg, S., Winther, S.A., Rosenlund, S.V., Hansen, T.W., von Scholten, B.J., Hansen, C.S., Zobel, E.H., Laursen, J.C., Theilade, S., Jelstrup, L., Juhl, T.R., Riis, D., Hermann, J.A., Lundgaard, A.G., Halkjær, M.L.D., Aabo, L., Lerche, T.F., Lajer, M., Stefansen, R.J., Campbell, M.A., Durban, A., Raad, J., Prigge, M., Schiemann, M., Wilson, R., Kean, S., Douglas, E., Surtees, P., Gant, C., Yeung, S.M.H., Hagedoorn, I., Flynn, J., Galloway, J., Brooksbank, K., Aparicio, C., Iliev, I.P., Nones, F., Bue, F.L., Melacini, D., Cugini, D., Prandini, S., Lecchi, V., Yakymchuk, S., Gherardi, G., Villa, A., Villa, D., Gaspari, F., Cannata, A.N., Ferrari, S., Stucchi, N., Albrechtová, Š., Eldeik, E., Amanaki, R., Fernandez-Fernandez, B., Sanchez-Rodriguez, J., Vázquez, C., Sanz, A.B., Sanchez-Niño, M.D., Ramos, A.M., Gonzalo, M., Schmidt, U., Selim, G., Gjorgovski, T., Stratrova, S.S., Stojceva-Taneva, O., Schutten-Westerneng, P., Wierbos, B., Huvers, F., De Bruin, A.K., Lapauw, B., de Man, E., Rokegem, K., Inion, S., Kreutzmann, K., Dewettinck, I., Graaf, C.B.-D., Jong, F.C.-D., Entius, J., Nannings, M., van Steenderen, S., Petry, F.W., Kilic, C., 2020. Early detection of diabetic kidney disease by urinary proteomics and subsequent intervention with spironolactone to delay progression (PRIORITY): a prospective observational study and embedded randomised placebo-controlled trial. Lancet Diabetes Endocrinol. 22138595. 8 (4), 301–312. Available from: http://www.journals.elsevier.com/the-lancet-diabetes-and-endocrinology. doi:10.1016/S2213-8587(20)30026-7.

Tomusiak, A., Floro, A., Tiwari, R., Riley, R., Matsui, H., Andrews, N., Kasler, H.G., Verdin, E., 2024. Development of an epigenetic clock resistant to changes in immune cell composition. Commun. Biol. 23993642. 7 (1). Available from: https://www.springer.com/journal/42003. doi:10.1038/s42003-024-06609-4.

Wang, S., Yang, T., Bao, Y., Zhou, L., Jing, P., Lingfeng, G., Shi, X., Wang, H., Wang, L., 2024. Association of serum creatinine-cystatin C ratio with all-cause, cardiovascular and cancer mortality in US adults: a nationwide cohort study. BMC Geriatr. 1471-2318. 24 (1). doi:10.1186/s12877-024-05546-5.

Yang, C.T., Kor, C.T., Hsieh, Y.P., 2018. Long-term effects of spironolactone on kidney function and hyperkalemia-associated hospitalization in patients with chronic kidney disease. J. Clin. Med. 20770383. 7 (11). Available from: https://www.mdpi.com/2077-0383/7/11/459/pdf. doi:10.3390/jcm7110459.

Zhang, W., Zheng, Y., Yan, F., Dong, M., Ren, Y., 2023. Research progress of quercetin in cardiovascular disease. Front. Cardiovasc. Med. 2297-055X. 10. doi:10.3389/fcvm.2023.1203713.

PART 2

Unique characteristics of kidney diseases in the elderly

CHAPTER

9

Impaired quality of life in elderly CKD patients

Zara Ijaz[a] *and Angelina Edwards*[b]

[a]Department of Internal Medicine, Houston Methodist Hospital, Houston, TX, United States

[b]Department of Medicine, Division of Nephrology, Houston Methodist Academic Institute, Houston Methodist Hospital, Weill Cornell Medical College, Houston, TX, United States

Introduction

Chronic kidney disease (CKD) is a progressive condition that affects over 800 million people worldwide (Levin et al., 2024). The care of patients living with CKD is complex and imposes a significant burden not only on their physical health but also on their mental, emotional and social well-being. Due to recent treatment advancements patients have longer life expectancies. Thus the overall quality of life has become an important focus. For CKD patients, global physical health and symptom burden, financial challenges, dependence on caregivers, and psychological stressors all impact quality of life. Specific physical challenges include cardiovascular complications, intense pruritus, treatment-related complications, cognitive decline, issues with dialysis access, and sexual dysfunction. Mentally, patients often experience depression, anxiety, and isolation.

Recognizing and managing these impairments are essential to providing high-quality and comprehensive care. Screening tools such as the Kidney Disease Quality of Life survey, the Montreal Cognitive Assessment (MoCA), and the Mini Mental Status Examination (MMSE) provide global, patient-centered assessments. Addressing these factors provides a holistic and patient-centered approach for optimal outcomes.

This chapter explores the causes, mechanisms, and screening for functional impairments experienced by patients with CKD, as well as their impact on quality of life.

Aging and the Kidney
https://doi.org/10.1016/B978-0-443-34069-7.00013-6

Causes and mechanisms of impaired quality of life among elderly patients with CKD

Cardiovascular disease

Renal impairment and cardiovascular disease (CVD) are deeply intertwined and contribute substantially to impaired quality of life. Patients with advanced CKD have a five-to-tenfold higher risk of CVD compared to those without, and it is the main cause of death in end-stage renal disease (ESRD). Classic risk factors for CVD are highly prevalent in CKD patients and include hypertension, hyperlipidemia, and diabetes. In addition, factors such as volume overload, anemia, uremia, and chronic inflammation promote vascular and myocardial changes, resulting in myocardial fibrosis, calcifications, and atherosclerosis (Jankowski et al., 2021). Overall, these conditions can negatively impact quality of life due to subsequent frequent hospitalizations, chronic fatigue, and physical and psychological stress. According to the American Heart Association, hemodialysis patient mortality is 20% per year, with over 50% attributable to CVD (Virani et al., 2023). Complications such as coronary artery disease, heart failure, sudden cardiac death, and arrhythmias contribute to increased morbidity and mortality (Zoccali et al., 2023; Tonelli et al., 2016; Banerjee et al., 2021).

Proposed management options for cardiovascular complications in ESRD patients include collaboration among cardiologists and nephrologists regarding pharmacologic interventions such as diuretics, sodium-glucose cotransporter-2 (SGLT2) inhibitors, renin-angiotensin-aldosterone system inhibitors, mineralocorticoid receptor antagonists, and beta blockers (Banerjee et al., 2021). Symptomatic management of anemia with iron supplementation, optimization of volume overload, and lifestyle modifications emphasizing low-salt diets and regular exercise have all been implicated in improving quality of life and decreasing the overall morbidity and mortality of this disease (Terpening, 2023; Banerjee et al., 2021; Banerjee and Wang, 2022; Gonzalez Suarez et al., 2025).

Pruritus

Generalized pruritus is a common symptom in patients with advanced CKD and is associated with adverse health outcomes. Patients with pruritus have a twofold increase in sleep disorders when compared to those without and a higher incidence of anxiety and depression. In addition to the psychosocial impact, persistent scratching can lead to further compromise of the skin barrier and subsequent skin infections, resulting in recurrent hospitalizations. The Stockholm Creatinine Measurements (SCREAM) Project studied the burden of pruritus in patients undergoing dialysis in Sweden between 2005 and 2021 and its associated adverse health outcomes. Of over 3000 dialysis patients enrolled, 30% experienced pruritus during the first year of dialysis and were more often elderly, female, and had lower serum albumin, elevated C-reactive protein, and higher serum calcium and phosphorus levels (Faucon et al., 2025).

In addition, an exacerbation of dermatologic conditions otherwise present in the general elderly population can also occur in patients with kidney disease. For example, xerosis (dry skin), eczema, psoriasis, and contact dermatitis can be worsened due to impaired skin barrier functionality in these patients. Specifically, CKD-related pruritus due to accumulation of uremic toxins is common. While uremia induced pruritus may be the most likely cause for these patients' itching, it is important to consider other diseases which present with pruritus, including hyperparathyroidism, liver dysfunction, and even cutaneous T-cell lymphoma (Gibbs et al., 2020; Insogna, 2018; Kwo et al., 2017).

Pruritus can significantly impact the physical health of elderly patients with CKD and certainly reduce the overall physical functioning and well-being of these patients.

Treatment-related complications

Renal replacement therapy is often initiated among the elderly with advanced kidney disease. However, dialysis-specific complications can significantly impact quality of life and cognitive reserve. The hemodynamic shifts during dialysis contribute to labile blood pressure and decreased cerebral blood flow, resulting in chronic ischemia and cerebral atrophy. One study revealed that about 25% of a group of 635 patients on hemodialysis had evidence of cerebral ischemia. The drop in cerebral blood flow was further characterized with positron-emission tomography-computed tomography (PET-CT) and showed that elderly patients on hemodialysis experience about a 10% decrease in global cerebral blood flow. In addition, higher dialyzate temperatures, ultrafiltration rates, and volumes were linked to poorer cerebral blood flow (Drew et al., 2020). The cumulative impact of hemodynamic instability and orthostatic hypotension results in cerebral atrophy, brain injury, orthostasis, and an increase in falls.

Elderly patients with CKD are vulnerable to adverse medication-related effects due to reduced GFR, polypharmacy, and potential drug interactions. Impaired kidney function interferes with the pharmacokinetics of several medications, making it challenging for clinicians to predict therapeutic responses and increasing the risk of both overdosing and underdosing. To mitigate these risks, it is important to avoid polypharmacy, simplify medication regimens, and ensure that clinicians are well-informed regarding the indications and contraindications of certain medications. Strategies to aid in decreasing these complications include starting at lower doses when prescribing new medications and adjusting dosages based on clinical response. At every visit, medication review—including over-the-counter medications, common side effects, and adherence—should be assessed (Ponticelli et al., 20155).

Cognitive decline

Up to 40% of patients with CKD have cognitive impairments. Risk factors for development include a lower estimated glomerular filtration rate (eGFR) and microalbuminuria, with the latter being a stronger risk factor. As defined, cognitive impairment is characterized as a deficit in one or more functions, such as learning, concentration, memory, and decision-making. Other manifestations of cognitive decline may include limitations in executive functions and visuospatial abilities, similar to dementia. These overall impairments may vary from mild to more severe, with subsequent compromise of activities of daily living and personal independence.

Given the multiple comorbidities associated with CKD, the pathophysiology of CKD-related cognitive decline is multifactorial. Contributing factors include clinical depression, polypharmacy, sleep disturbances, and nutritional deficiencies. Notably, cerebrovascular disease, including strokes, transient ischemic attacks, and small vessel infarcts, disproportionately affects this patient population, leading to CKD-related cognitive decline.

The accumulation of uremic toxins has also been implicated in the mechanism of cognitive decline in CKD patients. Uremic metabolites accumulate at early stages of kidney disease and as the disease progresses. These are usually cleared through dialysis; however, dialysis membranes may be less efficient at clearing larger protein-bound metabolites, such as 4-hydroxyphenylacetate, which has been identified as a potential molecule contributing to the pathogenesis of CKD-related cognitive impairment (Drew et al., 2019).

Dialysis access dysfunction

In the United States, hemodialysis remains the most common form of renal replacement therapy, with most fresh-start dialysis patients being over the age of 65. While arteriovenous fistulas are the preferred access for hemodialysis due to increased patency and lower risk of infections, patients with advanced kidney disease often experience challenges with long-term vascular access. Access complications such as stenosis, thrombosis, and infections may occur, leading to missed or truncated dialysis sessions. Patient-related factors associated with vascular access malfunction include advanced age, smoking, and diabetes. The presence of comorbidities such as coronary artery disease, congestive heart failure, and stroke reduces vascular quality and hinders the maturation of an arteriovenous fistula. One retrospective cohort study demonstrated that dialysis patients with arteriovenous access who experienced early (within one year) loss of fistula patency faced an increased risk of mortality (Wu et al., 2018). These complications usually require procedural interventions, which add to the physical and psychological burden of this chronic illness (Higgins et al., 2023).

In addition to access malfunction, physical pain, numbness, and extremity edema often interfere with daily activities and overall well-being. Chronic pain associated with cannulation during dialysis sessions is often unrecognized and underreported. Moreover, the presence of an arteriovenous fistula can interfere with simple everyday tasks such as wearing a watch, lifting objects, or performing activities requiring fine motor skills. As such, these limitations often lead to frustration, inconvenience, increased dependence on others, and a further decline in quality of life (Aitken et al., 2013; Hara et al., 2018; Lok et al., 2020).

Depression and anxiety

Due to the chronic and progressive nature of CKD, mental illnesses, including depression and anxiety, are highly prevalent among this population. A full review can be found in the chapter on depression in this book. The impact of mental health on quality of life is substantial.

A small cross-sectional study conducted in Jordan evaluated depression, anxiety, and quality of life among 103 CKD patients in outpatient nephrology clinics between 2018 and 2020. It was found that more than fifty percent of patients (58.3%) experienced depression, and about half (50.5%) experienced anxiety. A negative correlation was also noted between depression and quality of life (Alshelleh et al., 2022).

Similarly, a multicenter cross-sectional study of 1079 elderly patients with CKD throughout twenty-four provinces of China analyzed the prevalence of depression and its relationship to kidney function and health-related quality of life (HRQoL). In this study, depression was evaluated using the Geriatric Depression Scale (GDS-15), and HRQoL was measured using the Kidney Disease Quality of Life-36 (KDQOL-36) scale. The study found the prevalence of depression among participants to be 23%. It also indicated that lower eGFR was associated with higher GDS-15 scores. Furthermore, factors such as marital status, level of education, history of CVD, diabetes, CKD stage, and presence of proteinuria were independent predictors of depression in these patients. As such, patients with depression were more likely to be single, have lower education levels, and higher rates of CVD, electrolyte derangements, proteinuria, and anemia (Wang et al., 2021).

Patients with depression and anxiety frequently experience significant functional impairment, disrupted sleep cycles, weakened immune function, poor nutritional status, and an increased risk of suicidal ideation. These psychiatric conditions have also been linked to reduced social functioning, poor adherence to treatment, and a decline in physical health. Early identification and management of mental disorders are essential to protecting both the psychological and physical well-being of patients with CKD and should be deemed a crucial component of comprehensive patient care (Alshelleh et al., 2022).

In addition to anxiety and depression, many patients with CKD also experience apathy. Apathy is a distinct syndrome characterized by decreased motivation, reduced goal-directed behavior, blunted emotional expression, and limited social engagement. It can overlap with depression and is known to contribute to cognitive decline. Research has shown that patients with apathy often exhibit poor delayed memory performance and significantly lower scores in HRQoL assessments.

A study conducted across five Dutch nephrology centers involving 180 patients aged 65 and older with an estimated glomerular filtration rate of 20 mL/min/1.73 m^2 or less found that 36% of participants exhibited symptoms of apahy. Notably, in about half of these cases, apathy symptoms occurred independently of depressive symptoms. The presence of apathy was significantly associated with reduced physical and cognitive function, lower HRQoL, and a twofold increase in mortality risk over a four-year period. Furthermore, apathy contributed to greater caregiver burden and negatively impacted family members. Currently, treatment options for apathy are limited, with interventions primarily focusing on reducing patient disability rather than relying on pharmacological approaches (Voorend et al., 2024).

Social isolation

Social isolation is characterized by the absence or lack of social relationships and sparse contact with family, friends, community, and social environments. In general, adults tend to become more socially withdrawn with age due to retirement, personal medical conditions, and deaths within their families. There is a plethora of evidence to support the notion that social isolation is associated with a lower quality of life and an increased risk of developing psychological disorders (Zhou et al., 2021).

Patients with CKD often suffer debilitating symptoms in addition to treatment burdens, which inadvertently decrease their social functioning. Symptoms, including fatigue, pain, frequent dialysis treatments, and medication side effects, all play a role in hindering the social relationships of these patients. These lower levels of social functioning are highly associated with reduced quality of life and substantial mental health impairment (Sluiter et al., 2024).

Social isolation is noted to be a modifiable risk factor for CKD. In patients with kidney disease, social isolation has been linked to worsening kidney function. There are multiple mechanisms that may account for this decline in kidney function. For example, patients who are routinely social may be more inclined to take care of their health. Socially withdrawn individuals may not have loved ones to encourage them to seek medical assistance. Some studies have shown that isolated individuals have elevated levels of genes that promote inflammation, which can be detrimental to the already proinflammatory state of CKD.

To support this, a prospective study conducted in China analyzed the association between CKD and social isolation. Participants with CKD stages 3b-5 were noted to have less social participation. The study found that high levels of social isolation were connected to a rapid decline in eGFR and subsequent CKD (Zhou et al., 2021).

Studies have shown that reduced social support is associated with higher mortality rates. Enhancing social support for patients with CKD can lead to better health outcomes by promoting greater adherence to medical appointments and medication regimens, improving access to healthcare, and reducing symptoms of depression and anxiety (Fuertes et al., 2021).

To summarize, social isolation represents a significant modifiable risk factor in the progression of CKD, which contributes to a decline in overall quality of life. The cycle of worsening kidney function leading to poor social functioning, and vice versa, ultimately negatively impacts both physical and mental health. Addressing social well-being in CKD patients should be prioritized as a key area of evaluation during routine follow-up and health maintenance.

Loss of independence

Elderly adults with advanced kidney disease often experience functional decline at higher rates than those without. These patients suffer from frailty and must depend on others to carry out basic activities of daily living. Cognitive impairment, which contributes to loss of independence, is common among this population as well (Hall et al., 2016). Studies have shown that even mild cognitive impairment can be associated with decreased mobility, poor muscle strength, and increased frailty (Greinert et al., 2023). Due to these impairments, many individuals with CKD require varying levels of assistance from help with tasks such as managing medications and transportation to appointments and dialysis sessions, to more involved support with personal care needs, including toileting and hygiene (Matthews et al., 2024). The lack of independence due to functional impairments and reliance on caregivers for support significantly diminishes quality of life in CKD patients (Bowling et al., 2011).

Caregiver burden

The burden of CKD is multifaceted and extends not only to those suffering from the disease but also to their caregivers. Given the advancements in the administration of hemodialysis in patients with ESRD, patients are now living much longer. The frailty associated with old age and the multiple comorbidities of these patients necessitate their dependence on others as caregivers to help manage their health as well as activities of daily living.

Caregivers are unpaid individuals, including family members, friends, or neighbors, who provide physical, mental, or financial care for a patient with an illness. Some duties that caregivers may carry out include support with personal care, mobility, management of medications, transport to appointments, dietary needs, and emotional support. These caregivers are often subject to an increased risk of developing physical and psychological distress in their challenging role. Unfortunately, the impact of this disease on caregivers often goes unnoticed and untreated (Driehuis et al., 2025).

One qualitative study in Northern Ireland explored the caregiver-associated burden of CKD in patients on hemodialysis among two different dialysis units (Matthews et al., 2024). Researchers conducted twenty-four interviews with the caregivers over a six-month period. The study participants included a broad age range of 35–86-year-old caregivers, fourteen of whom were female and ten of whom were male. All participants were of white ethnicity. The study results showed that caregivers were negatively impacted by their responsibilities associated with caring for those with CKD. Caregivers felt overwhelmed attempting to handle personal affairs, their own household, and professional endeavors, along with being a caregiver. The demanding role left them little time or energy to fulfill their own responsibilities. Isolation also affected caregivers due to the considerable time invested in this role. Participants of the study reported social withdrawal and loss of connection to their own friends and family members. Respondents endorsed feelings of distress when observing their loved ones going through the relentless adverse effects of hemodialysis when they could do little to ease their suffering. The thoughts of not knowing who would assume their role if they were to become debilitated themselves led to increased levels of anxiety.

In the above study, a poor understanding of the complex medical aspects of kidney disease also contributed to caregiver burden. The combination of a lack of medical knowledge and new roles and responsibilities was seen as overwhelming. Insufficient understanding of multiple medications, renal diets, treatment modalities, and potential complications was a common theme among participants (Matthews et al., 2024).

Managing a renal diet can add to caregiver stress, affecting both the caregiver and the patient. However, when family members are actively supportive in providing renal-friendly meals, it can positively influence the patient's adherence to dietary guidelines.

Methods to help alleviate this significant burden on caregivers, as reported by caregivers, included the incorporation of spiritual beliefs, methods to cope with stress, and support from peers. Caregivers enrolled in the study found that relying on faith and their religious communities was comforting, in addition to implementing mindfulness and meditation in their routines. Furthermore, an emphasis on the reduction of chronic stress by identifying and applying effective coping strategies can lead to greater support for well-being and resilience throughout the chronic disease journey (Cameranesi et al., 2025).

While the highlighted study focused on patients of white background, the generalizability to other ethnic groups may be limited. Nonetheless, it provides valuable insight into the emotional and physical burdens of the caregiving experience that must be acknowledged and addressed.

Sexual dysfunction

Human sexuality is a crucial component of lifestyle quality. Sexual dysfunction among patients with CKD remains highly prevalent but is often underdiagnosed despite its negative impact on quality of life. Sexual dysfunction also affects interpersonal relations, which can be distressing to patients. In women, sexual dysfunction is defined as low sexual interest/arousal disorder, orgasmic disorders, and genito-pelvic pain disorders. In men, it is defined as erectile dysfunction, hypoactive disorder, and premature or delayed ejaculation (Wang et al., 2021). Many physiologic factors associated with sexual dysfunction progress as kidney function declines. These include vascular disease, hormonal irregularities, neuropathy, and psychiatric disorders (Palmer, 2003). Appropriate vasculature is important for adequate blood flow to the genitalia to augment sexual function. Well-known comorbidities of CKD are hypertension and diabetes which can compromise vascular and thus blood flow. CKD itself is a risk factor for atherosclerosis due to systemic inflammation and abnormalities in bone metabolism. Interestingly, erectile dysfunction may be one of the first signs of CVD in these patients. Hormonal irregularities seen in CKD patients are not fully understood. It is suggested that interference of the hypothalamic–pituitary–gonadal (HPG) axis can lead to increased luteinizing hormone (LH). Prolactin levels are noted to be elevated in these patients, which elicits negative feedback on gonadotropin-releasing hormone (GRH) release in the hypothalamus. This results in a hypogonadotropic hypogonadism, which significantly impacts sexual function in both males and females.

Ultimately, sexual dysfunction in patients with CKD arises from a combination of psychological and physiological factors, significantly impacting their quality of life. To support a more patient-centered approach to care, routine screening of patients at risk for sexual dysfunction is necessary (Wang et al., 2021).

Financial burden

The financial burden associated with CKD considerably contributes to psychological distress and diminished quality of life. Studies indicate that nearly half of CKD patients in the United States experience some form of financial hardship throughout the course of their illness. This burden is exacerbated by high medical expenses, especially among individuals under the age of 65 who do not qualify for Medicare and are not yet on dialysis (Acquah et al., 2021).

As the disease progresses, so does the economic burden, with ESRD patients incurring the highest costs, ranging from $20,000 to over $100,000 per patient each year. These costs are further increased when considering the multiple comorbidities common in this population (Chung et al., 2023).

Unfortunately, these financial constraints often lead to medication nonadherence and delayed medical care, both of which contribute to worsening physical and mental health outcomes. Emotional distress, deterioration of overall health, and food insecurity are also prevalent as patients struggle to balance the costs of healthcare and basic needs. A higher symptom burden in this context has been associated with lower HRQoL scores as well (Faye et al., 2022).

Quality of life screening tools

As late stages of CKD are often characterized by significant symptom burden, quality of life screening tools play a crucial role in evaluating the well-being of patients with CKD, and several have been validated in this population. The KDQOL-36 survey is the most used. Additional tools, such as the MoCA and MMSE, are also used to assess the cognitive aspects that may influence quality of life. Here, we will explore the effectiveness of these tools and examine their limitations.

In 2008, the Centers for Medicare and Medicaid Services (CMS) enforced annual assessments of HRQoL in ESRD patients as part of its requirements for financial coverage for ESRD facilities. The KDQOL-36, published in 2000, was deemed the recommended tool for assessing quality of life in adults with ESRD but is also used in those not on dialysis. The KDQOL-36 consists of a physical component summary, mental component summary, burden of kidney disease, symptoms and problems of kidney disease, and the effects of kidney disease. The physical component summary includes physical functioning, limitations due to physical conditions, general health, and pain, while the mental component summary consists of social functioning, role limitations due to emotional problems, vitality, and mental health (Cohen et al., 2019). Recent studies have highlighted the considerable symptom and HRQoL burden associated with CKD, validating the KDQOL-36 as an appropriate representation of CKD patients 'quality of life (Fletcher et al., 2022). Among nondialysis dependent CKD patients, those who reported increased fatigue and associated symptoms via the KDQOL-36 questionnaire had a worse trajectory of CKD progression, worse quality of life and higher risk of death and renal replacement therapy (Faye et al., 2022). Another study examined the interplay of sex, HRQoL, and demographic variables in older adults with advanced CKD. Females reported a lower score on the physical and mental portions than males. Furthermore, a lower eGFR, lower hemoglobin, elevated phosphate levels, and preexisting diabetes were associated with lower HRQoL scores in men over women. Potential explanations for this disparity may be because that men are more likely than women to underreport mental and physical weakness due to societal norms. In addition, women tend to cope more emotionally compared to men, which is overall associated with a poorer quality of life. Women may experience symptoms more intensely than men and are more likely to suffer from anxiety and depression (Chesnaye et al., 2022; Fraser and Phillips, 2024).

As previously discussed, the presence of cognitive impairment can directly impact the quality of life in patients with kidney disease. Therefore an accurate assessment of this impairment must be conducted, especially in those undergoing dialysis. Tools such as the MoCA and MMSE have been utilized and validated for detecting cognitive impairment in this population (Drew et al., 2019).

The MoCA is an exam that assesses global cognitive function, including spatiotemporal orientation, attention, visuospatial function, executive function, memory, language, naming, and abstract thinking. It was initially intended to test for mild cognitive impairment and is easy to administer to patients in-office (Ciolek and Lee, 20200). The MMSE was developed in 1975 for evaluating the mental status of hospitalized patients. Over many years, it has become a globally used tool for cognitive assessment, especially in elderly patients. The MMSE focuses on testing cognition, orientation, memory, attention, and verbal and written ability (Gallegos et al., 2022).

One study demonstrated the effectiveness of the MoCA and MMSE among other cognitive screening tools, including the Trail Making Test Part B, the Mini-Cog test, and the Digit Symbol Substitution Test. One-hundred fifty patients on dialysis were selected and underwent comprehensive testing for memory, attention, and executive function. These results were used to examine the predictive ability of the aforementioned tests. It was found that the MoCA test had the highest predictability for severe cognitive impairment (Drew et al., 2020).

The MoCA has demonstrated higher sensitivity but lower specificity in identifying severe cognitive impairment in patients undergoing dialysis. In the referenced study, a score of less than or equal to 21 on the MoCA had a sensitivity of 86% but a specificity of just 55% for detecting severe impairment. In contrast, the MMSE exhibited both lower sensitivity and specificity when compared to the MoCA. As a result, the MoCA may be preferred over the MMSE for evaluating impaired cognition (Drew et al., 2020). The MoCA is also superior to the MMSE in its evaluation of executive and visuospatial functions. However, a limitation of both tools is that their accuracy is easily influenced by the educational background and cultural differences of the patients. This can affect the reliability of the study, especially among diverse populations (Siqueira et al., 2019).

Given the limitations of these current screening tools, future opportunities include developing a cognitive screening tool specifically designed for dialysis patients. This will assist in accounting for the unique barriers and difficulties that dialysis patients may experience (Drew et al., 2020; Tiffin-Richards et al., 2014). To better accommodate individuals with varying educational backgrounds, adjusting cutoff scores according to a patient's level of education could help minimize bias and improve reliability in future testing (Angermann et al., 2017).

Managing impaired quality of life

Managing symptoms that contribute to a poor quality of life in patients with CKD is complex and requires a multidisciplinary approach. This may include coordination among various healthcare professionals and the active inclusion of patients and their families in discussions regarding symptom management. Elderly patients with CKD frequently experience distressing, multisystem symptoms such as uremia, pruritus, psychological distress, physical pain, sexual dysfunction, sleep disturbances, and cardiovascular complications (Rhee et al., 2022).

Unfortunately, the nonspecific and subtle nature of the symptoms can make recognition and categorization by clinicians rather challenging. Adding to this issue, patients may underreport their symptoms, which further complicates effective and timely management of their concerns.

It is vital that patients with CKD feel fully supported throughout their journey, listened to, understood, and actively advocated for in addressing both their symptom burden and quality of life. Effective strategies for symptom management include modalities beyond dialysis, such as conservative management and shared decision-making. While dialysis remains necessary for patients with advanced kidney disease, research suggests that it may be linked to a more rapid decline in eGFR, especially in elderly patients and those with multiple comorbidities (Kalantar-Zadeh et al., 2022).

Conservative management focuses on slowing disease progression and improving quality of life through early intervention and proactive treatment of comorbidities. For example, the use of electrolyte binders, diuretics, and dietary education aids in delaying dialysis in these patients. Strict adherence to a low-protein diet can help reduce the burden of uremic toxins and electrolyte derangements. Diets rich in fiber, fruits, and vegetables have been shown to support the gut microbiome and promote better overall health in patients with CKD (Zarantonello et al., 2021).

As discussed, cognitive decline is highly prevalent among patients with CKD. The presence of cognitive decline in CKD patients has been linked to several adverse health outcomes. These include increased frailty and fall risk, poor mobility, and decreased muscle strength (Greinert et al., 2023). Addressing the impact of cognitive impairment and methods of managing it is necessary for protecting the quality of life. General strategies to manage and care for patients experiencing CKD-related cognitive impairment include, but are not limited to, frequent office visits for follow-ups, avoidance of polypharmacy, treating mental illnesses that may arise, and coordination of interdisciplinary care between dietitians, physicians, pharmacists, nurses, and social workers. Early discussions surrounding goals of care and advance directives should be made with these patients before significant cognitive decline occurs (Drew et al., 2019; Fraser and Phillips, 2024). Interventions involving physical activity, education on their chronic disease state, enhanced nutritional interventions, and optimization of CKD-related anemia are important modifiable factors that can improve HRQoL.

For patients with CKD who are not on dialysis, proposed interventions for slowing the progression of cognitive decline include targeting albuminuria with medications such as angiotensin-converting enzyme inhibitors or angiotensin receptor blockers. One trial demonstrated that patients with reduced albuminuria had a 20%–40% lower likelihood of scoring poorly on the MMSE. In addition, the SPRINT trial showed that strict blood pressure control was linked to reduced rates of cognitive impairment (Drew et al., 2019).

The European Quality Study (EQUAL) explored symptom burden in patients before and after starting dialysis. About 450 patients were assessed for symptoms. Fatigue, decreased interest in sex, and difficulty with sexual arousal were the most common and bothersome symptoms reported. These symptoms were evaluated at the time of dialysis initiation and again at one year. It was found that only fatigue showed modest improvement, while the other symptoms remained unchanged or worsened (de Rooij et al., 2022).

Among patients with CKD receiving dialysis, interventions aimed at improving the clearance of uremic toxins may lead to cognitive improvements. Furthermore, kidney transplantation has been associated with cognitive benefits, especially within the first-year post-transplant, in both children and adults (Drew et al., 2019).

Nutritional deficiencies in vitamin D, B-complex, omega-3 fatty acids, and antioxidants have been associated with impaired cognitive function. Recent evidence suggests that addressing these deficiencies with targeted supplementation can support cognitive health and promote a healthier gut microbiome. In addition, limiting the intake of processed foods can help reduce systemic inflammation and neurotoxicity. Patients should be educated on these dietary strategies, which can contribute to improvements in cognitive function and overall quality of life (Kanbay et al., 2025).

Conclusion

In summary, CKD presents complex challenges for patients regarding quality of life. The impact goes far beyond the progressive decline in overall health associated with this disease. We have explored the array of mental, physical, and social factors contributing to diminished quality of life in these patients. The physical toll of comorbidities, including CVD and cognitive impairment, is compounded by emotional stressors, loss of independence, and social isolation. These challenges intersect and can amplify one another, exacerbating the burden of this illness.

This chapter has highlighted how these physical, emotional, and social domains play critical roles in shaping the experiences of these patients. Several screening tools aid in identifying this burden, including the KDQOL-36 and cognitive impairment examinations.

Current and future endeavors to improve the quality of life in CKD patients must include more than disease management. Integrating mental health support, as well as social and financial resources, in a personalized manner makes for a more comprehensive and inclusive care model. Prioritizing these efforts enhances not only overall health but also affirms the value and dignity of patients over the course of their illness.

References

Acquah, I., Valero-Elizondo, J., Javed, Z., Ibrahim, H.N., Patel, K.V., Ali, H.J.R., Menser, T., Khera, R., Cainzos-Achirica, M., Nasir, K., 2021. Financial hardship among nonelderly adults with CKD in the United States. Am. J. Kidney Dis. 15236838. 78 (5), 658–668. Available from: http://www.elsevier.com/inca/publications/store/6/2/3/2/7/6/index.htt. doi:10.1053/j.ajkd.2021.04.011.

Aitken, E., McLellan, A., Glen, J., Serpell, M., Mactier, R., Clancy, M., 2013. Pain resulting from arteriovenous fistulae: prevalence and impact. Clin. Nephrol. 0301-0430. 80 (11), 328–333. doi:10.5414/CN107917.

Alshelleh, S., Alhouri, A., Taifour, A., Abu-Hussein, B., Alwreikat, F., Abdelghani, M., Badran, M., Al-Asa'd, Y., Alhawari, H., Oweis, A.O., 2022. Prevelance of depression and anxiety with their effect on quality of life in chronic kidney disease patients. Sci. Rep. 20452322. 12 (1). Available from: https://www.nature.com/srep/. doi:10.1038/s41598-022-21873-2.

Angermann, S., Baumann, M., Steubl, D., Lorenz, G., Hauser, C., Suttmann, Y., Reichelt, A.-L., Satanovskij, R., Sonntag, F., Heemann, U., Grimmer, T., Schmaderer, C., Garg, P.K., 2017. Cognitive impairment in hemodialysis patients: implementation of cut-off values for the Montreal Cognitive Assessment (MoCA)-test for feasible screening. PLoS One. 1932-6203. 12 (10), e0184589. doi:10.1371/journal.pone.0184589.

Banerjee, D., Rosano, G., Herzog, C.A., 2021. Management of heart failure patient with CKD. Clin. J. Am. Soc. Nephrol. 1555905X. 16 (7), 1131–1139. Available from: https://cjasn.asnjournals.org/content/16/7/1131/full-text.pdf?with-ds=yes. doi:10.2215/CJN.14180920.

Banerjee, D., Wang, A.Y., 2022. Personalizing Heart Failure Management in Chronic Kidney Disease Patients. Nephrology, Dialysis, Transplantation 37 (11), 2055–2062. doi:10.1093/ndt/gfab026.

Bowling, C.B., Sawyer, P., Campbell, R.C., Ahmed, A., Allman, R.M., 2011. Impact of chronic kidney disease on activities of daily living in community-dwelling older adults. J. Gerontol. A Biol. Sci. Med. Sci. 1079-5006. 66A (6), 689–694. doi:10.1093/gerona/glr043.

Cameranesi, M., Mollard, R., Harasemiw, O., Curtis, S., Iman, Y., Buenafe, J., Protudjer, J.L.P., Tangri, N., MacKay, D., 2025. Lived experiences of older adults with advanced CKD and their caregivers. Kidney360. 2641-7650. 6 (5), 754–762. doi:10.34067/kid.0000000723.

Chesnaye, N.C., Meuleman, Y., de Rooij, E.N.M., Hoogeveen, E.K., Dekker, F.W., Evans, M., Pagels, A.A., Caskey, F.J., Torino, C., Porto, G., Szymczak, M., Drechsler, C., Wanner, C., Jager, K.J., 2022. Health-related quality-of-life trajectories over time in older men and women with advanced chronic kidney disease. Clin. J. Am. Soc. Nephrol.

1555905X. 17 (2), 205–214. Available from: https://cjasn.asnjournals.org/content/17/2/205. doi:10.2215/CJN.08730621.

Chung, H., Crowe, C.L., Kong, S.X., Singh, R., Farej, R., Elliott, J., Williamson, T., Willey, V.J., 2023. Descriptive study of the economic burden among patients with type 2 diabetes mellitus, chronic kidney disease, and chronic kidney disease and type 2 diabetes mellitus in a large US commercially insured population. J. Manag. Care Spec. Pharm. 23761032. 29 (1), 80–89. Available from: https://www.jmcp.org/doi/epdf/10.18553/jmcp.2023.29.1.80. doi:10.18553/jmcp.2023.29.1.80.

Ciolek, C.H., Lee, S.Y., 2020. Cognitive issues in the older adult. In: Avers, D., Wong, R.A. (eds.), Cognitive issues in the older adult, 4th ed. St. Louis, MO, Mosby, pp. 425–452. doi:10.1016/B978-0-323-60912-8.00019-1.

Cohen, D.E., Lee, A., Sibbel, S., Benner, D., Brunelli, S.M., Tentori, F., 2019. Use of the KDQOL-36™ for assessment of health-related quality of life among dialysis patients in the United States. BMC Nephrol. 14712369. 20 (1). Available from: http://www.biomedcentral.com/bmcnephrol/. doi:10.1186/s12882-019-1295-0.

de Rooij, E.N.M., Meuleman, Y., de Fijter, J.W., Jager, K.J., Chesnaye, N.C., Evans, M., Caskey, F.J., Torino, C., Porto, G., Szymczak, M., Drechsler, C., Wanner, C., Dekker, F.W., Hoogeveen, E.K., 2022. Symptom burden before and after dialysis initiation in older patients. Clin. J. Am. Soc. Nephrol. 1555905X. 17 (12), 1719–1729. Available from: http://cjasn.asnjournals.org/content/by/year. doi:10.2215/CJN.09190822.

Drew, D.A., Tighiouart, H., Rollins, J., Duncan, S., Babroudi, S., Scott, T., Weiner, D.E., Sarnak, M.J., 2020. Evaluation of screening tests for cognitive impairment in patients receiving maintenance hemodialysis. J. Am. Soc. Nephrol. 15333450. 31 (4), 855–864. Available from: https://jasn.asnjournals.org/content/jnephrol/31/4/855.full.pdf?with-ds=yes. doi:10.1681/ASN.2019100988.

Drew, D.A., Weiner, D.E., Sarnak, M.J., 2019. Cognitive Impairment in CKD: Pathophysiology, Management, and Prevention. Am. J. Kidney Dis. 74 (6), 782–790. doi:10.1053/j.ajkd.2019.05.017.

Driehuis, E., Demirhan, I., Konijn, W.S., Vogels, T.J.F.M., Goto, N.A., van Groenou, M.I.B., Verhaar, M.C., van Jaarsveld, B.C., Abrahams, A.C., 2025. Determinants of caregiver burden among spouses of patients with kidney failure: a qualitative study. Am. J. Kidney Dis. 15236838. 85 (4), 477. Available from: https://www.sciencedirect.com/science/journal/02726386. doi:10.1053/j.ajkd.2024.11.005.

Faucon, A.L., Clase, C.M., Rydell, H., Uhde, M., Barany, P., Evans, M., Carrero, J.J., 2025. Burden of CKD-associated pruritus and adverse clinical outcomes in patients receiving dialysis: the stockholm creatinine measurements (SCREAM) project. Am. J. Kidney Dis. 15236838. 85 (1), 45. Available from: https://www.sciencedirect.com/science/journal/02726386. doi:10.1053/j.ajkd.2024.05.013.

Faye, M., Legrand, K., Gall, L.L., Leffondre, K., Omorou, A.Y., De Pinho, N.A., Combe, C., Fouque, D., Jacquelinet, C., Laville, M., Liabeuf, S., Massy, Z.A., Speyer, E., Filho, R.P., Stengel, B., Frimat, L., Ayav, C., 2022. Five-year symptom trajectories in nondialysis-dependent CKD patients. Clin. J. Am. Soc. Nephrol. 1555905X. 17 (11), 1588–1597. Available from: https://cjasn.asnjournals.org/content/clinjasn/17/11/1588.full.pdf. doi:10.2215/CJN.06140522.

Fletcher, B.R., Damery, S., Aiyegbusi, O.L., Anderson, N., Calvert, M., Cockwell, P., Ferguson, J., Horton, M., Paap, M.C.S., Sidey-Gibbons, C., Slade, A., Turner, N., Kyte, D., 2022. Symptom burden and health-related quality of life in chronic kidney disease: a global systematic review and meta-analysis. PLoS Med. 15491676. 19 (4). Available from: https://journals.plos.org/plosmedicine/article/file?id=10.1371/journal.pmed.1003954&type=printable. doi:10.1371/journal.pmed.1003954.

Fraser, S.D.S., Phillips, T., 2024. Quality of life in people with chronic kidney disease: focusing on modifiable risk factors. Curr. Opin. Nephrol. Hypertens. 14736543. 33 (6), 573–582. Available from: http://journals.lww.com/co-nephrolhypertens/pages/default.aspx. doi:10.1097/MNH.0000000000001013.

Fuertes, J., Rubinstein, S., Yarandi, N., Cohen, S.D., 2021. Social support, caregivers, and chronic kidney disease. Semin. Nephrol. 41 (6), 574–579. Available from: http://www.elsevier.com/inca/publications/store/6/2/3/3/3/5/index.htt. doi:10.1016/j.semnephrol.2021.10.009.

Gallegos, M., Morgan, M.L., Cervigni, M., Martino, P., Murray, J., Calandra, M., Razumovskiy, A., Caycho-Rodríguez, T., Gallegos, W.L.A., 2022. 45 years of the mini-mental state examination (MMSE): a perspective from ibero-america. Dement. Neuropsychol. 19805764. 16 (4), 384–387. Available from: https://www.demneuropsy.com.br/wp-content/uploads/articles_xml/1980-5764-dn-2021-0097/1980-5764-dn-2021-0097.pdf. doi:10.1590/1980-5764-DN-2021-0097.

Gibbs, J., Ma, S., Kim, A., Seminario-Vidal, L., Sokol, L., Zhang, H., Zhang, X., Sagatys, E., Chen, P., Messina, J., 2020. Utility of flow cytometry and gene rearrangement analysis in tissue and blood of patients with suspected cutaneous T-cell lymphoma. Oncol. Rep. 1021-335X. 45 (1), 349–358. doi:10.3892/or.2020.7865.

Gonzalez Suarez, M.L., Arriola-Montenegro, J., Rolón, L., 2025. Hypertension Management in Patients With Advanced Chronic Kidney Disease With and Without Dialysis. Curr. Opin. Cardiol. doi:10.1097/HCO.0000000000001221.

Greinert, R., Greinert, D., Eger, A.L., Ripoll, C., Girndt, M., 2023. Subclinical cognitive impairment in chronic kidney disease is associated with frailty and reduced quality of life. Nephrol. Dial. Transplant. 14602385. 38 (5), 1151–1157. Available from: http://ndt.oxfordjournals.org/. doi:10.1093/ndt/gfac303.

Hall, R.K., Haines, C., Gorbatkin, S.M., Schlanger, L., Shaban, H., Schell, J.O., Gurley, S.B., Colón-Emeric, C.S., Bowling, C.B., 2016. Incorporating geriatric assessment into a nephrology clinic: preliminary data from two models of care. J. Am. Geriatr. Soc. 15325415. 64 (10), 2154–2158. Available from: http://www.blackwellpublishing.com/journal.asp?ref=0002-8614&site=1. doi:10.1111/jgs.14262.

Hara, Y., Sonoda, K., Hashimoto, K., Fuji, K., Yamada, Y., Kamijo, Y., 2018. Influence of arteriovenous fistula on daily living behaviors involving the upper limbs in hemodialysis patients: a cross-sectional questionnaire study. BMC Nephrol. 1471-2369. 19 (1). doi:10.1186/s12882-018-1097-9.

Higgins, M.C.S.S., Diamond, M., Mauro, D.M., Kapoor, B.S., Steigner, M.L., Fidelman, N., Aghayev, A., Chamarthy, M.R.K., Dedier, J., Dillavou, E.D., Felder, M., Lew, S.Q., Lockhart, M.E., Siracuse, J.J., Dill, K.E., Hohenwalter, E.J., 2023. ACR appropriateness Criteria® dialysis fistula malfunction. J. Am. Coll. Radiol. 1558349X. 20 (11), S382. Available from: https://www.sciencedirect.com/science/journal/15461440. doi:10.1016/j.jacr.2023.08.016.

Insogna, K.L., 2018. Primary hyperparathyroidism. N. Engl. J. Med. 15334406. 379 (11), 1050–1059. Available from: http://www.nejm.org/medical-index. doi:10.1056/NEJMcp1714213.

Jankowski, J., Floege, J., Fliser, D., Böhm, M., Marx, N., 2021. Cardiovascular disease in chronic kidney disease pathophysiological insights and therapeutic options. Circulation. 15244539. 143 (11), 1157–1172. Available from: http://circ.ahajournals.org. doi:10.1161/CIRCULATIONAHA.120.050686.

Kalantar-Zadeh, K., Lockwood, M.B., Rhee, C.M., Tantisattamo, E., Andreoli, S., Balducci, A., Laffin, P., Harris, T., Knight, R., Kumaraswami, L., Liakopoulos, V., Lui, S.F., Kumar, S., Ng, M., Saadi, G., Ulasi, I., Tong, A., Li, P.K.T., 2022. Patient-centred approaches for the management of unpleasant symptoms in kidney disease. Nat. Rev. Nephrol. 1759507X. 18 (3), 185–198. Available from: https://www.nature.com/nrneph/. doi:10.1038/s41581-021-00518-z.

Kanbay, M., Ozbek, L., Guldan, M., Abdel-Rahman, S.M., Sisman, U., Mallamaci, F., Zoccali, C., 2025. Nutrition, cognition and chronic kidney disease: a comprehensive review of interactions and interventions. Eur. J. Clin. Invest. 13652362. 55 (6). Available from: http://onlinelibrary.wiley.com/journal/10.1111/(ISSN)1365-2362. doi:10.1111/eci.70045.

Kwo, P.Y., Cohen, S.M., Lim, J.K., 2017. ACG Clinical Guideline: Evaluation of Abnormal Liver Chemistries. Am. J. Gastroenterol. 112 (1), 18–35. doi:10.1038/ajg.2016.517.

Levin, A., Ahmed, S.B., Carrero, J.J., Foster, B., Francis, A., Hall, R.K., Herrington, W.G., Hill, G., Inker, L.A., Kazancıoğlu, R., Lamb, E., Lin, P., Madero, M., McIntyre, N., Morrow, K., Roberts, G., Sabanayagam, D., Schaeffner, E., Shlipak, M., Shroff, R., Tangri, N., Thanachayanont, T., Ulasi, I., Wong, G., Yang, C.W., Zhang, L., Robinson, K.A., Wilson, L., Wilson, R.F., Kasiske, B.L., Cheung, M., Earley, A., Stevens, P.E., 2024. Executive summary of the KDIGO 2024 clinical practice guideline for the evaluation and management of chronic kidney disease: known knowns and known unknowns. Kidney Int. 15231755. 105 (4), 684–701. Available from: https://www.sciencedirect.com/science/journal/00852538. doi:10.1016/j.kint.2023.10.016.

Lok, C.E., Huber, T.S., Lee, T., Shenoy, S., Yevzlin, A.S., Abreo, K., Allon, M., Asif, A., Astor, B.C., Glickman, M.H., Graham, J., Moist, L.M., Rajan, D.K., Roberts, C., Vachharajani, T.J., Valentini, R.P., 2020. KDOQI clinical practice guideline for vascular access: 2019 update. Am. J. Kidney Dis. 15236838. 75 (4), S1. Available from: http://www.elsevier.com/inca/publications/store/6/2/3/2/7/6/index.htt. doi:10.1053/j.ajkd.2019.12.001.

Matthews, M., McKeaveney, C., Noble, H., Reid, J., Aoun, M., 2024. Exploring the unmet needs and experiences of informal caregivers of patients with end-stage kidney disease (ESKD) receiving haemodialysis – a qualitative study. PLoS One. 1932-6203. 19 (5), e0302525. doi:10.1371/journal.pone.0302525.

Palmer, B.F., 2003. Sexual dysfunction in men and women with chronic kidney disease and end-stage kidney disease. Adv. Ren. Replace. Ther. 10734449. 10 (1), 48–60. Available from: http://www.elsevier.com/inca/publications/store/6/2/3/2/7/0/index.htt. doi:10.1053/jarr.2003.50003.

Ponticelli, C., Sala, G., Glassock, R.J., 2015. Drug management in the elderly adult with chronic kidney disease: A review for the primary care physician. Mayo Clinic Proceedings 90 (5), 633–645. doi:10.1016/j.mayocp.2015.01.016.

Rhee, C.M., Edwards, D., Ahdoot, R.S., Burton, J.O., Conway, P.T., Fishbane, S., Gallego, D., Gallieni, M., Gedney, N., Hayashida, G., Ingelfinger, J., Kataoka-Yahiro, M., Knight, R., Kopple, J.D., Kumarsawami, L., Lockwood,

M.B., Murea, M., Page, V., Sanchez, J.E., Szepietowski, J.C., Lui, S.F., Kalantar-Zadeh, K., 2022. Living well with kidney disease and effective symptom management: consensus conference proceedings. Kidney Int. Rep. 24680249. 7 (9), 1951–1963. http://www.journals.elsevier.com/kidney-international-reports. doi:10.1016/j.ekir.2022.06.015.

Siqueira, G.S.A., Hagemann, P.D.M.S., Coelho, D.D.S., Santos, F.H.D., Bertolucci, P.H.F., Heyn, P.C., 2019. Can MoCA and MMSE be interchangeable cognitive screening tools? A systematic review. Gerontologist. 17585341. 59 (6), E743. Available from: http://gerontologist.oxfordjournals.org/. doi:10.1093/geront/gny126.

Sluiter, A., van Zwieten, A., Shen, J.I., Manera, K., 2024. Measuring social functioning in chronic kidney disease. Semin. Nephrol. 02709295. 44 (3–4), 151547. doi:10.1016/j.semnephrol.2024.151547.

Terpening, C.M., 2023. Prevention of cardiovascular events in patients with chronic kidney disease. Ann. Pharmacother. 15426270. 57 (12), 1425–1435. Available from: https://journals.sagepub.com/home/AOP. doi:10.1177/10600280231165774.

Tiffin-Richards, F.E., Costa, A.S., Holschbach, B., Frank, R.D., Vassiliadou, A., Krüger, T., Kuckuck, K., Gross, T., Eitner, F., Floege, J., Schulz, J.B., Reetz, K., 2014. The Montreal Cognitive Assessment (MoCA)—A sensitive screening instrument for detecting cognitive impairment in chronic hemodialysis patients. PLoS One. 19326203. 9 (10). Available from: http://www.plosone.org/article/fetchObject.action?uri=info%3Adoi%2F10.1371%2Fjournal.pone.0106700&representation=PDF. doi:10.1371/journal.pone.0106700.

Tonelli, M., Karumanchi, S.A., Thadhani, R., 2016. Epidemiology and Mechanisms of Uremia-Related Cardiovascular Disease. Circulation, 133 (5), 518–536. doi:10.1161/CIRCULATIONAHA.115.018713.

Virani, S.S., Newby, L.K., Arnold, S.V., Bittner, V., Brewer, L.P.C., Demeter, S.H., Dixon, D.L., Fearon, W.F., Hess, B., Johnson, H.M., Kazi, D.S., Kolte, D., Kumbhani, D.J., Lofaso, J., Mahtta, D., Mark, D.B., Minissian, M., Navar, A.M., Patel, A.R., Piano, M.R., Rodriguez, F., Talbot, A.W., Taqueti, V.R., Thomas, R.J., Van Diepen, S., Wiggins, B., Williams, M.S., 2023. AHA/ACC/ACCP/ASPC/NLA/PCNA guideline for the management of patients with chronic coronary disease: a report of the American Heart Association/American College of Cardiology Joint Committee on Clinical Practice Guidelines. Circulation. 15244539. 148 (9), E9. Available from: http://circ.ahajournals.org. doi:10.1161/CIR.0000000000001168.

Voorend, C.G.N., van Buren, M., Berkhout-Byrne, N.C., Kerckhoffs, A.P.M., van Oevelen, M., Gussekloo, J., Richard, E., Bos, W.J.W., Mooijaart, S.P., 2024. Apathy symptoms, physical and cognitive function, health-related quality of life, and mortality in older patients with CKD: a longitudinal observational study. Am. J. Kidney Dis. 15236838. 83 (2), 162. Available from: https://www.sciencedirect.com/science/journal/02726386. doi:10.1053/j.ajkd.2023.07.021.

Wang, C.J., Cukor, D., Johansen, K.L., 2021. Sexual Dysfunction Among Patients With Chronic Kidney Disease. Semin. Nephrol. 41 (6), 534–549. doi:10.1016/j.semnephrol.2021.10.006.

Wu, C.-K., Lin, C.-H., Hsu, C.-C., Tarng, D.-C., Kor, C.-T., Chen, Y.-C., Chia-Lin, W., Chang, C.-C., 2018. Association of early loss of primary functional patency of arteriovenous access with mortality in incident hemodialysis patients. Medicine. 0025-7974. 97 (31), e11630. doi:10.1097/md.0000000000011630.

Zarantonello, D., Rhee, C.M., Kalantar-Zadeh, K., Brunori, G., 2021. Novel conservative management of chronic kidney disease via dialysis-free interventions. Curr. Opin. Nephrol. Hypertens. 14736543. 30 (1), 97–107. Available from: http://journals.lww.com/co-nephrolhypertens/pages/default.aspx. doi:10.1097/MNH.0000000000000670.

Zhou, W., Li, Y., Ning, Y., Gong, S., Song, N., Zhu, B., Wang, J., Zhao, S., Shi, Y., Ding, X., 2021. Social isolation is associated with rapid kidney function decline and the development of chronic kidney diseases in middle-aged and elderly adults: findings from the china health and retirement longitudinal study (CHARLS). Front. Med. 2296-858X. 8. doi:10.3389/fmed.2021.782624.

Zoccali, C., Mallamaci, F., Adamczak, M., De Oliveira, R.B., Massy, Z.A., Sarafidis, P., Agarwal, R., Mark, P.B., Kotanko, P., Ferro, C.J., Wanner, C., Burnier, M., Vanholder, R., Wiecek, A., 2023. Cardiovascular complications in chronic kidney disease: a review from the European Renal and Cardiovascular Medicine Working Group of the European Renal Association. Cardiovasc. Res. 17553245. 119 (11), 2017–2032. Available from: http://cardiovascres.oxfordjournals.org/. doi:10.1093/cvr/cvad083.

CHAPTER

10

Sleep

Seki A. Balogun[a] *and Emaad M. Abdel-Rahman*[b]

[a]Geriatric Medicine Fellowship Program, University of Oklahoma, Norman, OK, United States
[b]Division of Nephrology, University of Virginia, Charlottesville, VA, United States

Introduction

Older adults are projected to make up a quarter of the population in the United States and Europe over the next two decades. In addition, they continue to be the fastest-growing sector of the population worldwide (Division, 2024). Sleep disturbances are common in older adults, occurring in about one in two people (Ayalon et al., 2004). Changes in sleep quality and the sleep-wake cycle occur with normal aging and can be difficult to differentiate from pathological issues.

The stages of normal human sleep are divided into wakefulness, non-rapid eye movement (non-REM) stages 1-3, and REM sleep. The various stages are distinguished based on the measurement of brain waves with electroencephalography (EEG), muscle tone with electromyography (EMG), and eye movements (Feinsilver, 2021).

During the wakefulness stage, there is a low-amplitude mixed-frequency signal with a predominant alpha rhythm on EEG and relatively high muscle tone on EMG.

Stage 1 non-REM sleep is characterized by the disappearance of alpha activity on EEG, a reduction in muscle tone, and a decrease in EMG amplitude, along with slow eye movements. Sleep is usually light during this phase, with easy awakening and not much restorative value.

Stage 2 non-REM sleep is characterized by sleep spindles and K-complexes on EEG and makes up about half of the total sleep time, while stage 3 non-REM sleep features large, slow delta waves and is usually the deepest and most restorative stage of sleep. The REM sleep stage has active brain waves similar to wakefulness but low muscle tone, with voluntary muscles being almost paralyzed.

With normal sleep, there are cycles lasting up to 2–3 h, transitioning between the four stages of sleep each night with some individual variability. Sleep latency (time to stage 1 non-REM sleep) is an average of about 20 min with more stage 3 non-REM sleep occurring in the first half of the night and REM sleep predominating in the latter half. Sleep efficiency is defined as the ratio of total sleep time to time in bed, and this is normally about 85% in healthy adults (Feinsilver, 2021).

Aging and the Kidney
https://doi.org/10.1016/B978-0-443-34069-7.00012-4

Changes in sleep with normal aging

In younger adults, there is typically about 8 h of total sleep per night, with a high percentage being stage 3 non-REM (deep) sleep, which gradually decreases with aging. Older adults tend to have higher percentages of wakefulness and stage 1 non-REM (light) sleep, as well as a reduction in sleep efficiency. The total sleep time in older adults is similar to that of younger adults, and sleep latency increases only minimally with normal aging. In addition, older adults often experience a change in the timing of peak sleepiness, occurring earlier in the evening with earlier awakening in the morning, a phenomenon known as "phase advance." These normal changes in sleep with aging may lead to complaints of poor sleep maintenance or "not feeling well-rested," and it is important to differentiate this from pathological sleep disorders that may also occur in this age group (Feinsilver, 2021).

Sleep disorders and chronic kidney disease

Chronic kidney disease (CKD) is highly prevalent worldwide, with an estimated prevalence of 10%, and is associated with multiple poor outcomes, including an increase in morbidity and mortality rates (Saran et al., 2015).

Sleep disorders are common in patients with CKD, especially in those with more advanced CKD and end-stage kidney disease (ESKD) on dialysis, regardless of the dialysis modality. These sleep disorders, which often result in poor sleep quality, include insomnia, sleep apnea (SA), restless leg syndrome (RLS), and changes in the sleep circadian cycle.

While most studies showed high prevalence of sleep disorders in patients with CKD and ESKD, there is heterogenicity in the prevalence of sleep disorders among various studies (Lindner et al., 2015; Sakaguchi et al., 2011; Unruh, 2007; Jurado-Gamez et al., 2007; Unruh et al., 2006; Agarwal and Light, 2011; Rosas, 2011; Pierratos and Hanly, 2011). Some of the possible rationale to explain this variability in prevalence include the difference in life styles, environmental conditions, genetic factors, and other modifiable factors as blood pressure and depression among patients in the various studies.

In a 2022 cross-sectional study, 42.5% of CKD patients, ages 19–85 years, had poor sleep and this correlated positively with increasing age (Yazıcı and Güney, 2022). It is worth noting that the relationship between sleep disorders and CKD is bidirectional where CKD is associated with sleep disorders and sleep disorders are associated with incident CKD (Koh et al., 2024).

The exact mechanisms contributing to the increased prevalence of sleep disorders in patients with CKD and ESKD are not well defined, and the data available are occasionally contradictory. Several possible contributory factors include:

1. General and comorbid conditions associated with kidney diseases include obesity, an increase in neck circumference, metabolic syndrome, lung and heart diseases, diabetes mellitus, and hypertension (Full et al., 2020).
2. Uremic toxins in predialysis CKD with associated systemic inflammation and increased inflammatory biomarkers such as interleukin-1β, interleukin-6, interleukin-18, tumor necrosis factor α, and C-reactive protein (Chiu et al., 2009; Erten et al., 2005), activation

of the sympathetic nervous system and the renin–angiotensin–aldosterone system, induction of endothelial dysfunction, and metabolic abnormalities associated with worsening kidney function, such as hypercalcemia (Virga et al., 2000), hyperphosphatemia, pruritus, and anemia (Čengić et al., 2012).

3. Hemodialysis (HD)-related electrolyte shifts, increased fluid with pharyngeal edema, postdialysis tiredness, and naps during dialysis (Pai et al., 2007). Low levels of melatonin in HD patients, along with numbness, tingling, and anxiety, further contribute to sleep disturbances in these patients (Mehra et al., 2023).

Older adults also have an increased risk of poor sleep quality. Norman and Loredo reviewed the potential changes in older adults that may explain the specific increased risk of obstructive sleep apnea (OSA). Increased risk factors for OSA, such as obesity, diabetes mellitus, and cerebrovascular strokes, were found to be more common in this population. In addition, anatomic and physiologic changes in bony structures and fat deposits in the pharyngeal walls are thought to contribute to the increased prevalence of OSA in the older adult population (Norman and Loredo, 2008).

Sleep disorders in older adults with CKD

Insomnia

Chronic insomnia is defined as frequent difficulty in falling or staying asleep with unsatisfying sleep that continues for at least 3 nights per week for at least 3 months, resulting in impaired daytime sleeping despite opportunities to sleep (Krystal et al., 2021).

Studies on the prevalence of insomnia in patients with CKD and ESKD demonstrate a high degree of variability, with prevalence ranging between 38% and 70% (Lindner et al., 2015; Lyons, 2024).

In a systematic review and metaanalysis (n = 45,796) of poor sleep and insomnia stratified by age, CKD stages, and renal replacement modality, comparing CKD (n = 34,949) and non-CKD patients (n = 12,847), the prevalence of insomnia was 48%, 46%, 61%, and 26% in patients with predialysis CKD, ESKD on HD, ESKD on peritoneal dialysis (PD), and post-kidney transplant (KTX), respectively, versus 19% in non-CKD patients (Tan et al., 2022). In addition, insomnia tended to be more prevalent with increased age, though it was not clinically significant in those above 50 years compared to those younger than 50 years.

Insomnia is also significantly associated with an increased incidence of ESKD and CKD with eGFR < 45 ml/min/1.73 m^2 (Lu et al., 2018). **Up to 86% of adults with CKD experience poor sleep quality, with a gradual increase in mean insomnia scores corresponding to increased severity of kidney disease** (Aggarwal et al., 2017).

Obstructive sleep apnea (OSA)

OSA is a chronic condition that usually presents with loud snoring during sleep and an increase in daytime sleepiness. While the presentation of OSA may be similar in older adults compared to younger adults, older adults may attribute snoring to normal aging and may not seek medical assistance. The mechanisms of OSA involve recurrent periods of airway collapse, either complete or partial, resulting in inadequate airflow, followed by a transient arousal from sleep with a return of adequate air flow.

The prevalence of OSA among adults aged 30–60 years is approximately 9% in women and 24% in men. OSA is even more common in older adults, with a prevalence rate of 37.5%–62% and a stepwise increase with aging (Norman and Loredo, 2008).

In patients with CKD, the prevalence of both obstructive and central sleep apnea is higher compared to the general population. The overall prevalence of moderate–severe OSA in the general population ranges between 10% and 49% while in CKD patients, the prevalence is about 25%–57% with a higher prevalence with increased severity of kidney disease. Interestingly, severity of OSA symptoms also correlated with a 51% increase in incident CKD (Norman and Loredo, 2008; Pochetti et al., 2020). On the other hand, in a systematic review the prevalence of central sleep apnea in patients with CKD (n = 313) was lower at 9.6% with a global range varying widely between 0% and 75% (Nigam et al., 2016).

While the prevalence of OSA in CKD patients is much higher in older adults, there are other factors that are thought to have an impact, including geographical location, with the lowest prevalence of OSA being in Africa (31.0%) and the highest in South East Asia (51.7%), as well as CKD and the presence of renal replacement therapy. The prevalence of both moderate-to-severe and severe sleep-disordered breathing increased significantly with decreasing eGFR, with the highest prevalence being in predialysis CKD (54.0%) compared to hemodialysis (24.4%), peritoneal dialysis (35.3%), and post-kidney transplant (20.4%) (Zhang et al., 2024; Ogna et al., 2016; Full et al., 2020).

RLS and periodic limb movement disorder

RLS is defined as an unpleasant sensation in the legs, causing an urge to move or change position. It is often more common in the first part of the night and while sitting or resting.

RLS can be familial or idiopathic and has been associated with iron deficiency, chronic obstructive airway disease, hypertension, depression, pregnancy, and sleep apnea. Alcohol and tobacco use also increase the risk of RLS (Calviño et al., 2015).

The prevalence of RLS symptoms in the general population is around 5%. In patients with CKD, the prevalence is much higher, ranging from 15% to 30%, with increased rates in more advanced stages of CKD and ESKD (51%–84%) (Allen et al., 2005; Winkelman et al., 1996; Adam; Ogna et al., 2016; Safarpour et al., 2023). The heterogeneity noted in studies is thought to be related to the accuracy and method of RLS diagnosis. For instance, in a study comparing the diagnosis of RLS in nondialysis CKD patients using a probable RLS questionnaire versus a formal neurological examination, the RLS diagnostic rate with the questionnaire was 21%, while only 4.5% was confirmed by the neurological examination (Calviño et al., 2015).

Advanced sleep-wake phase disorder

Advanced sleep-wake phase disorder is a condition caused by a circadian rhythm abnormality in which individuals fall asleep and wake up earlier than intended, often experiencing a feeling of inadequate sleep. There is a significant direct relationship between circadian rhythm abnormalities and CKD, which is further accentuated by aging (Xiong et al., 2024). In recent studies on sleep duration, CKD patients were found to have 68.2% higher odds of long sleep duration (>10 h), and this was observed in up to a third of individuals with CKD (Okeke and Ugwuoke, 2024; Wang et al., 2024).

Evaluation and diagnosis

Insomnia

The diagnosis of insomnia is usually made clinically based on sleep complaints, which include difficulty initiating or maintaining sleep, along with associated daytime complaints such as somnolence or impairment in daily functioning. To aid in diagnosis, it is often necessary for the patient to complete a sleep diary, as this can help identify distinct factors that may adversely affect sleep. For example, taking excessive naps during the day or being sedentary may impact the ability to achieve 7 h of restful sleep at night (Feinsilver and Hernandez, 2017; Yaremchuk, 2018).

A detailed review of medications, as well as caffeine and alcohol intake, is also important, as these may adversely affect sleep patterns. Such medications include diuretics, corticosteroids, selective serotonin reuptake inhibitors, antiarrhythmics, and beta blockers. Caffeine and alcohol may disrupt nighttime sleep and increase wakefulness (Yaremchuk, 2018).

Obstructive sleep apnea (OSA)

OSA commonly presents symptoms of snoring, which occur as a result of upper airway muscle relaxation and obstruction during sleep, as well as daytime somnolence. In older adults, there may be associated cognitive deficits.

Obesity, male gender, age, and postmenopausal status are major risk factors for OSA. A body mass index of 30 kg/m^2 or greater, with a neck circumference of 17 inches or greater in a male and 14.5 inches or greater in a female, significantly increases the risk of OSA by up to 70%.

OSA is diagnosed with polysomnography (sleep study), which can be conducted in a certified sleep laboratory or as a home or portable sleep study. Sleep studies performed in the sleep laboratory are supervised with video recording, as well as monitoring of electroencephalography, electrocardiography, pulse oximetry, chest and abdominal sensors, limb movements, and extraocular movements (Yaremchuk, 2018). Home or portable sleep studies are more convenient to obtain, less expensive, and are increasingly used for the diagnosis of OSA. Heart rate, oximetry, and obstructive respiratory events are recorded by the portable sleep study device. The home sleep study is typically suitable for patients suspected of OSA with no significant comorbidities, while patients with significant pulmonary, cardiac, or neurologic disorders will likely require a supervised sleep study in a sleep laboratory for an appropriate diagnosis (Yaremchuk, 2018).

RLS and periodic limb movement disorder

RLS is diagnosed clinically with symptoms of an uncomfortable crawling or aching sensation in the legs, which is relieved with movement. Symptoms also usually return when at rest and often interfere with sleep. Iron deficiency is associated with RLS; as such, it is recommended to check iron stores and replenish iron as necessary in patients with symptoms of RLS (Yaremchuk, 2018).

With periodic limb movement disorder (PLMD), there are repeated lower or upper extremity jerking movements during sleep with associated sleep disruption. Oftentimes, patients are not aware of movements and the bed partner will complain about being hit or kicked at night. Both RLS and PMLD have significant clinical overlaps, with about 80% of patients with RLS also reporting PMLD symptoms. Both conditions are more common with aging (Yaremchuk, 2018).

Advanced sleep-wake phase disorder

Advanced sleep-wake phase disorder is common with aging and is diagnosed clinically. Patients often report sleeping earlier in the evening and then waking up early in the morning, with difficulty returning to sleep. As a result, there is a perceived poor quality of sleep, even though they may be getting an adequate amount of sleep overall (Yaremchuk, 2018).

Complications associated with poor sleep

Wang et al. showed that inadequate or excessive sleep was associated with increased cardiovascular (CV) diseases, mortality, and increased abdominal aortic calcification. Abdominal aortic calcification was noted to be more prevalent with long (>9 h) sleep duration compared to short (2–5 h) and intermediate (6–8 h) sleep durations. The prevalence of vascular calcification increases with aging (Wang et al., 2024). Impaired sleep quality also has adverse effects on the quality of life (QOL) in older adults, with associated decreases in mental component QOL scores (Sekercioglu et al., 2015).

Similarly, RLS was found to be associated with poor QOL and increased CV risks (Calviño et al., 2015). Age, however, has not been shown to be an independent factor for sleep quality in CKD patients (Sekercioglu et al., 2015).

OSA in patients with CKD is associated with the deterioration of renal function, leading to increased inflammation and oxidative stress, glucose metabolism abnormalities, and an elevated risk of cardiovascular events (Zhang et al., 2024).

Other poor outcomes associated with poor sleep in CKD patients include increased mortality, a higher risk of development and progression of CKD, a non-dipper pattern of hypertension, fatigue, decreased cognitive function, increased daytime sleepiness, and morning headaches (Lu et al., 2018; Zhang et al., 2017; Mehra et al., 2023; Norman and Loredo, 2008; Zhang et al., 2024). An older estimate assessed the total annual cost of insomnia alone to range between $92.5 billion and $107 billion (Stoller, 1994).

Similar poor outcomes of sleep disorders with CKD were noted in older adults with predialysis CKD and those on dialysis. Long and colleagues examined the United States Renal Data System (2008–2019) to assess the prevalence of dementia in older patients with CKD who were newly diagnosed with sleep disorders and showed that 26.3% of patients were diagnosed with sleep disorders, with a higher 5-year unadjusted cumulative incidence for any type of dementia (36.2% versus 32.3% with no sleep disorder; $P < .001$) (Long et al., 2024). Furthermore, poor sleep quality in older hemodialysis patients is associated with both depression and a lower QOL (Turkmen et al., 2012).

Treatment of sleep disorders

The first step in managing sleep disorders is to identify the cause, as well as modifiable risk factors. To identify the causes of sleep disturbances, an adequate history, including medication history, laboratory tests, polysomnography, and occasionally a referral to a sleep medicine specialist for expert assessment, may be required (Lindner et al., 2015).

Nonpharmacologic interventions

Trial of nonpharmacological interventions should initially be attempted before resorting to pharmacological management.

In a systematic review by Yang and colleagues, there was a demonstrated significant improvement in insomnia symptoms in dialysis patients using several nonpharmacologic approaches, including exercise, cognitive behavioral therapy (CBT), listening to music, acupuncture, and changes in dialysis modality (Yang et al., 2015).

Exercise may also improve sleep quality and reduce the use of sleep medications (Qiao et al., 2025).

Cognitive behavioral therapy for insomnia (CBT-I) may be helpful in managing insomnia, and it usually consists of five main components: stimulus control, sleep restriction, relaxation techniques, cognitive therapy, and education about sleep hygiene. In a metaanalysis, CBT-I resulted in significant improvement in several parameters of insomnia, including severity of insomnia, sleep onset latency, wakefulness after sleep onset, early morning awakening, and sleep efficiency (Takano et al., 2023).

The positive effects of CBT-I have also been demonstrated in patients with ESKD (Chen et al., 2008, 2011).

Other nonpharmacological approaches that may have some modest positive effects on sleep outcomes include acupuncture and music therapy (Döner et al., 2025; Burrai et al., 2019; Natale et al., 2019).

Patients with OSA should be counseled on weight loss if overweight (Peppard et al., 2000), as well as on avoiding supine positioning during sleep for those with positional OSA (Berger et al., 1997). Reducing alcohol consumption may also be helpful in the management of OSA (Peppard et al., 2007).

Pharmacologic treatment

The initial step in the pharmacological management of sleep disorders is to treat the comorbid conditions associated with the sleep disorder such as asthma, gastroesophageal reflux disease, pruritus, chronic pains, neurological diseases as parkinsonism and psychiatric illnesses as depression, anxiety and bipolar disease.

Insomnia

Benzodiazepines and non-benzodiazepine sedative-hypnotics act on gamma-aminobutyric acid neuroreceptors. While some have a rapid onset, others result in a long active half-life, making them high-risk for older adults (Xia et al., 2025).

Benzodiazepine and non-benzodiazepine sedative hypnotics may be effective in the short term for insomnia in older adults by shortening sleep latency, decreasing nighttime awakenings, and improving sleep efficiency. However, the long-term use of these agents in older adults is associated with significant side effects, including addictive potential, dependence, tolerance, cognitive impairment, and an increased risk of falls ("American Geriatrics Society 2023 updated AGS Beers Criteria® for potentially inappropriate medication use in older adults," 2023). As a result, benzodiazepines and non-benzodiazepine sedative hypnotics are included in the Beers list of potentially inappropriate medications for older adults, and the American Geriatrics Society strongly recommends against their use in this population of patients (Lindner et al., 2015). Melatonin receptor agonists and certain antidepressants may be effective in treating insomnia by shortening sleep latency and improving sleep efficiency, with a better safety profile and fewer adverse effects in older adults. Antidepressants such as trazodone, mirtazapine, and doxepin may be used in low doses, particularly in older adults who also have symptoms of depression. Even so, older adults still need to be carefully monitored when using these medications, as side effects such as dizziness and orthostatic hypotension may occur ("American Geriatrics Society 2023 updated AGS Beers Criteria® for potentially inappropriate medication use in older adults," 2023).

Patients with advanced CKD also require careful monitoring when using many of these agents, as they are at risk for adverse effects, including increased mortality, due to the longer half-life of medications associated with decreased kidney function (Lindner et al., 2015; Winkelmayer et al., 2007).

Obstructive sleep apnea (OSA)

Continuous positive airway pressure (CPAP) therapy remains the mainstay in managing OSA. Compliance with using CPAP, especially in older adults, remains a challenge. In a retrospective study of older adults ($n = 44$), it was noted that there was a stepwise decrease in compliance with CPAP with increasing age, dropping from 77% in the 55- to 59-year-olds to 58% in those >70 years (Russo-Magno et al., 2001).

Surgical procedures to help manage OSA include oro- and hypopharynx surgery, nasal reconstructive surgery, bariatric surgery, tracheostomy, and maxillary-mandibular advancement surgery. They are generally considered options of last resort in patients with symptoms refractory to other modalities. There is a paucity of data regarding the efficacy of surgical procedures in OSA, except for bariatric surgery in obese patients, which results in significant improvement in OSA symptoms (Norman and Loredo, 2008).

Restless leg syndrome (RLS)

Several medication groups have demonstrated effectiveness in managing RLS symptoms, including dopamine agonists and analogs, benzodiazepines, opiates, gabapentin, pregabalin, and iron. Exercise therapy may also be effective in reducing RLS symptoms in patients with ESKD (Giannaki et al., 2013).

Dopamine agonists used in managing RLS include ropinirole, pramipexole, rotigotine, cabergoline, and pergolide. They are associated with potential adverse effects, including worsening RLS symptoms, loss of efficacy, and rebound symptoms (Wijemanne and Jankovic, 2015; Safarpour et al., 2023).

Opioids, such as codeine, pentazocine, methadone, and meperidine, have been used effectively for patients with RLS, especially when other therapies have not achieved significant success. However, these medications are associated with significant adverse effects in older adults with kidney disease and should be used with caution or generally avoided.

Oral and parenteral iron have been shown to be effective in managing RLS in patients with low-normal serum ferritin. Iron therapy has demonstrated a similar benefit for RLS in patients with ESKD (Sloand et al., 2004).

Advanced sleep-wake phase disorder

Melatonin and melatonin analogs are effective in managing circadian rhythm abnormalities, resulting in a significant decrease in objective sleep onset latency, as well as an increase in sleep efficiency and total sleep time (Koch et al., 2009).

Bright light therapy may also help with sleep circadian rhythm disorders in older adults and those with kidney disease (Burkhalter et al., 2015).

Summary

Sleep disorders are common in older adults with kidney diseases. These sleep disorders are associated with significant morbidity and mortality, adding to the challenges faced by these patients. Several therapeutic options are available to manage these sleep disorders. Physicians, especially nephrologists, need to be aware of these challenges and familiarize themselves with the appropriate nonpharmacologic treatment modalities and medications used in managing sleep disorders in this patient population.

References

Agarwal, R., Light, R.P., 2011. Sleep and activity in chronic kidney disease: a longitudinal study. Clin. J. Am. Soc. Nephrol. 1555905X. 6 (6), 1258–1265. Available from: http://cjasn.asnjournals.org/content/6/6/1258.full.pdf+html. doi:10.2215/CJN.10581110.

Aggarwal, H.K., Jain, D., Dabas, G., Yadav, R.K., 2017. Prevalence of depression, anxiety and insomnia in chronic kidney disease patients and their co-relation with the demographic variables. PRILOZI. 1857-8985. 38 (2), 35–44. doi:10.1515/prilozi-2017-0020.

Allen, R.P., Walters, A.S., Montplaisir, J., Hening, W., Myers, A., Bell, T.J., Ferini-Strambi, L., 2005. Restless legs syndrome prevalence and impact: REST general population study. Arch. Intern. Med. 15383679. 165 (11), 1286–1292. Available from: http://archinte.ama-assn.org/cgi/reprint/165/11/1286.pdf. doi: 10.1001/archinte.165.11.1286.

American Geriatrics Society 2023 updated AGS Beers Criteria® for potentially inappropriate medication use in older adults. J. Am. Geriatr. Soc. 15325415. 71 (7) (2023), 2052–2081, Available from: http://onlinelibrary.wiley.com/journal/10.1111/(ISSN)1532-5415. doi:10.1111/jgs.18372.

Ayalon, L., Liu, L., Ancoli-Israel, S., 2004. Diagnosing and treating sleep disorders in the older adult. Med. Clin. North Am. 88 (3), 737–750. doi:10.1016/j.mcna.2004.01.005.

Berger, M., Oksenberg, A., Silverberg, D.S., Arons, E., Radwan, H., Iaina, A., 1997. Avoiding the supine position during sleep lowers 24 h blood pressure in obstructive sleep apnea (OSA) patients. J. Hum. Hypertens. 0950-9240. 11 (10), 657–664. doi:10.1038/sj.jhh.1000510.

Burkhalter, H., Wirz-Justice, A., Denhaerynck, K., Fehr, T., Steiger, J., Venzin, R.M., Cajochen, C., Weaver, T.E., De Geest, S., 2015. The effect of bright light therapy on sleep and circadian rhythms in renal transplant recipients: a pilot randomized, multicentre wait-list controlled trial. Transpl. Int. 14322277. 28 (1), 59–70. Available from: http://www.blackwellpublishing.com/journal.asp?ref=0934-0874&site=1. doi:10.1111/tri.12443.

Burrai, F., Lupi, R., Luppi, M., Micheluzzi, V., Donati, G., Manna, G.L., Raghavan, R., 2019. Effects of listening to live singing in patients undergoing hemodialysis: a randomized controlled crossover study. Biol. Res. Nurs. 15524175. 21 (1), 30–38. Available from: http://www.sagepub.com/journal.aspx?pid=114. doi:10.1177/1099800418802638.

Calviño, J., Cigarrán, S., Lopez, L.M., Martinez, A., Sobrido, M.J., 2015. Restless legs syndrome in non-dialysis renal patients: is it really that common? J. Clin. Sleep Med. 15509397. 11 (1), 57–60. Available from: http://www.aasmnet.org/jcsm/ViewAbstract.aspx?pid=29833. doi:10.5664/jcsm.4366.

Čengić, B., Resić, H., Spasovski, G., Avdić, E., Alajbegović, A., 2012. Quality of sleep in patients undergoing hemodialysis. Int. Urol. Nephrol. 0301-1623. 44 (2), 557–567. doi:10.1007/s11255-010-9881-x.

Chen, H.Y., Cheng, I.C., Pan, Y.J., Chiu, Y.L., Hsu, S.P., Pai, M.F., Yang, J.Y., Peng, Y.S., Tsai, T.J., Wu, K.D., 2011. Cognitive-behavioral therapy for sleep disturbance decreases inflammatory cytokines and oxidative stress in hemodialysis patients. Kidney Int. 15231755. 80 (4), 415–422. Available from: https://www.journals.elsevier.com/kidney-international. doi:10.1038/ki.2011.151.

Chen, H.Y., Chiang, C.K., Wang, H.H., Hung, K.Y., Lee, Y.J., Peng, Y.S., Wu, K.D., Tsai, T.J., 2008. Cognitive-behavioral therapy for sleep disturbance in patients undergoing peritoneal dialysis: a pilot randomized controlled trial. Am. J. Kidney Dis. 02726386. 52 (2), 314–323. doi:10.1053/j.ajkd.2008.03.012.

Chiu, Y.L., Chuang, Y.F., Fang, K.C., Liu, S.K., Chen, H.Y., Yang, J.Y., Pai, M.F., Peng, Y.S., Wu, K.D., Tsai, T.J., 2009. Higher systemic inflammation is associated with poorer sleep quality in stable haemodialysis patients. Nephrol. Dial. Transplant. 14602385. 24 (1), 247–251. doi:10.1093/ndt/gfn439.

Division, 2024. World Population Prospects. United Nations, Department of Economic and Social Affairs.

Döner, A., Taşci, S., Bilgin, A., 2025. The effect of massage, acupressure and reflexology on restless legs syndrome severity and sleep quality in patients receiving haemodialysis treatment: a systematic review and meta-analysis. Nurs. Open. 20541058. 12 (2). Available from: http://onlinelibrary.wiley.com/journal/10.1002/(ISSN)2054-1058. doi:10.1002/nop2.70135.

Erten, Y., Kokturk, O., Yuksel, A., Elbeg, S., Ciftci, T.U., Pasaoglu, H., Ozkan, S., Bali, M., Arinsoi, T., Sindel, S., 2005. Relationship between sleep complaints and proinflammatory cytokines in haemodialysis patients. Nephrology. 14401797. 10 (4), 330–335. doi:10.1111/j.1440-1797.2005.00418.x.

Feinsilver, S.H., 2021. Normal and abnormal sleep in the elderly. Clin. Geriatr. Med. 18798853. 37 (3), 377–386. Available from: http://www.elsevier.com/inca/publications/store/6/2/3/3/6/4/index.htt. doi:10.1016/j.cger.2021.04.001.

Feinsilver, S.H., Hernandez, A.B., 2017. Sleep in the elderly. Clin. Geriatr. Med. 07490690. 33 (4), 579–596. doi:10.1016/j.cger.2017.06.009.

Full, K.M., Jackson, C.L., Rebholz, C.M., Matsushita, K., Lutsey, P.L., 2020. Obstructive sleep apnea, other sleep characteristics, and risk of CKD in the atherosclerosis risk in communities sleep heart health study. J. Am. Soc. Nephrol. 15333450. 31 (8), 1859–1869. Available from: https://jasn.asnjournals.org/content/jnephrol/31/8/1859.full.pdf?with-ds=yes. doi:10.1681/ASN.2020010024.

Giannaki, C.D., Sakkas, G.K., Karatzaferi, C., Hadjigeorgiou, G.M., Lavdas, E., Kyriakides, T., Koutedakis, Y., Stefanidis, I., 2013. Effect of exercise training and dopamine agonists in patients with uremic restless legs syndrome: a six-month randomized, partially double-blind, placebo-controlled comparative study. BMC Nephrol. 14712369. 14 (1). doi:10.1186/1471-2369-14-194.

Jurado-Gamez, B., Martin-Malo, Alvarez-Lara, M.A., Cosano, A., Aljama, 2007. Sleep disorders are underdiagnosed in patients on maintenance hemodialysis. Nephron Clin. Pract. 105, c35–c42.

Koch, B.C.P., Nagtegaal, J.E., Hagen, E.C., Westerlaken, M.M.L.V.D., Boringa, J.B.S., Kerkhof, G.A., Wee, P.M.T., 2009. The effects of melatonin on sleep-wake rhythm of daytime haemodialysis patients: a randomized, placebo-controlled, cross-over study (EMSCAP study). Br. J. Clin. Pharmacol. 13652125. 67 (1), 68–75. doi:10.1111/j.1365-2125.2008.03320.x.

Koh, J.H., Lim, C.Y.J., Yam, K.J.M., Yeo, B.S.Y., Ng, A.C.W., Loh, S.R.H., Hsu, P.P., Gooley, J., Tan, C.S., Toh, S.T., 2024. Bidirectional association of sleep disorders with chronic kidney disease: a systematic review and meta-analysis. Clin. Kidney J. 20488513. 17 (11). Available from: http://ckj.oxfordjournals.org/. doi:10.1093/ckj/sfae279.

Krystal, A.D., Ashbrook, L.H., Prather, A.A., 2021. What is insomnia? JAMA. 15383598. 326 (23), 2444. Available from: http://jama.jamanetwork.com/journal.aspx. doi:10.1001/jama.2021.19283.

Lindner, A.V., Novak, M., Bohra, M., Mucsi, I., 2015. Insomnia in patients with chronic kidney disease. Semin. Nephrol. 15584488. 35 (4), 359–372. Available from: http://www.elsevier.com/inca/publications/store/6/2/3/3/3/5/index.htt. doi:10.1016/j.semnephrol.2015.06.007.

Long, J.J., Chen, Y., Kim, B., Bae, S., Li, Y., Orandi, B.J., Chu, N.M., Mathur, A., Segev, D.L., McAdams-DeMarco, M.A., 2024. Sleep disorders and dementia risk in older patients with kidney failure a retrospective cohort study. Clin. J. Am. Soc. Nephrol. 1555905X. 19 (10), 1301–1309. Available from: https://journals.lww.com/CJASN/Pages/default.aspx. doi:10.2215/CJN.0000000000000504.

Lu, J.L., Freire, A.X., Molnar, M.Z., Kalantar-Zadeh, K., Kovesdy, C.P., 2018. Association of chronic insomnia with mortality and adverse renal outcomes. Mayo Clin. Proc. 19425546. 93 (11), 1563–1570. Available from: http://www.journals.elsevier.com/mayo-clinic-proceedings. doi:10.1016/j.mayocp.2018.05.032.

Lyons, O.D., 2024. Sleep disorders in chronic kidney disease. Nat. Rev. Nephrol. 1759507X. 20 (10), 690–700. Available from: https://www.nature.com/nrneph/. doi:10.1038/s41581-024-00848-8.

Mehra, M., Yadav, R.K., Rajora, M.A.K., Dahiya, U., Agarwal, S.K., 2023. Factors affecting quality of daytime and nighttime sleep among dialysis patients: a single center experience. Semin. Dial. 1525139X. 36 (3), 231–239. Available from: http://onlinelibrary.wiley.com/journal/10.1111/(ISSN)1525-139X. doi:10.1111/sdi.13125.

Natale, P., Ruospo, M., Saglimbene, V.M., Palmer, S.C., Strippoli, G.F.M., 2019. Interventions for improving sleep quality in people with chronic kidney disease. Cochrane Database Syst. Rev. 1469493X. 2019 (5). Available from: https://www.cochranelibrary.com/cdsr/table-of-contents. doi:10.1002/14651858.CD012625.pub2.

Nigam, G., Pathak, C., Riaz, M., 2016. A systematic review of central sleep apnea in adult patients with chronic kidney disease. Sleep Breath. 15221709. 20 (3), 957–964. Available from: http://www.springeronline.com/sgw/cda/frontpage/0,11855,1-40109-70-39223762-0,00.html. doi:10.1007/s11325-016-1317-0.

Norman, D., Loredo, J.S., 2008. Obstructive sleep apnea in older adults. Clin. Geriatr. Med. 07490690. 24 (1), 151–165. doi:10.1016/j.cger.2007.08.006.

Ogna, A., Ogna, V.F., Rubio, J.H., Tobback, N., Andries, D., Preisig, M., Tafti, M., Vollenweider, P., Waeber, G., Marques-Vidal, P., Heinzer, R., 2016. Sleep characteristics in early stages of chronic kidney disease in the HypnoLaus cohort. Sleep. 15509109. 39 (4), 945–953. Available from: http://www.journalsleep.org/ViewAbstract.aspx?pid=30549. doi:10.5665/sleep.5660.

Okeke, F., Ugwuoke, U.T., 2024. Assessing the relationship between sleep duration and the prevalence of chronic kidney disease among veterans in the United States: a 2022 behavior risk factor surveillance system (BRFSS) cross-sectional study. Cureus. 2168-8184. 16 (9). doi:10.7759/cureus.68538.

Pai, M.F., Hsu, S.P., Yang, S.Y., Ho, T.I., Lai, C.F., Peng, Y.S., 2007. Sleep disturbance in chronic hemodialysis patients: the impact of depression and anemia. Ren. Fail. 15256049. 29 (6), 673–677. doi:10.1080/08860220701459642.

Peppard, P.E., Austin, D., Brown, R.L., 2007. Association of alcohol consumption and sleep disordered breathing in men and women. J. Clin. Sleep Med. 15509397. 3 (3), 265–270. Available from: http://jcsm.aasm.org. doi:10.5664/jcsm.26795.

Peppard, P.E., Young, T., Palta, M., Dempsey, J., Skatrud, J., 2000. Longitudinal study of moderate weight change and sleep-disordered breathing. JAMA. 00987484. 284 (23), 3015–3021. Available from: http://jama.jamanetwork.com/journal.aspx. doi:10.1001/jama.284.23.3015.

Pierratos, A., Hanly, P.J., 2011. Sleep disorders over the full range of chronic kidney disease. Blood Purif. 02535068. 31 (1–3), 146–150. doi:10.1159/000321859.

Pochetti, P., Azzolina, D., Ragnoli, B., Tillio, P.A., Cantaluppi, V., Malerba, M., 2020. Interrelationship among obstructive sleep apnea, renal function and survival: a cohort study. Int. J. Environ. Res. Public Health. 1660-4601. 17 (14), 4922. doi:10.3390/ijerph17144922.

Qiao, Y., Wang, C., Chen, Q., Zhang, P., 2025. Effects of exercise on sleep quality in women — a systematic review and meta-analysis. J. Sci. Med. Sport. 18781861. 28 (4), 274–281. Available from: https://www.sciencedirect.com/science/journal/14402440. doi:10.1016/j.jsams.2024.11.015.

Rosas, S.E., 2011. Sleep apnea in individuals with chronic kidney disease: a wake-up call. Clin. J. Am. Soc. Nephrol. 1555905X. 6 (5), 954–956. Available from: http://cjasn.asnjournals.org/content/6/5/954.full.pdf+html. doi:10.2215/CJN.02840311.

Russo-Magno, P., O'Brien, A., Panciera, T., 2001. Compliance with CPAP therapy in older men with obstructive sleep apnea. J. Am Geriatr Soc 49 (9), 1205–1211.

Safarpour, Y., Vaziri, N.D., Jabbari, B., 2023. Restless legs syndrome in chronic kidney disease-a systematic review. Tremor Other Hyperkinet. Mov. (N. Y.). 21608288. 13 (1). Available from: https://storage.googleapis.com/jnl-up-j-tohm-files/journals/1/articles/752/6424233a93752.pdf. doi:10.5334/tohm.752.

Sakaguchi, Y., Shoji, T., Kawabata, H., Niihata, K., Suzuki, A., Kaneko, T., Okada, N., Isaka, Y., Rakugi, H., Tsubakihara, Y., 2011. High prevalence of obstructive sleep apnea and its association with renal function among nondialysis chronic kidney disease patients in Japan: a cross-sectional study. Clin. J. Am. Soc. Nephrol. 1555905X. 6 (5), 995–1000. Available from: http://cjasn.asnjournals.org/content/6/5/995.full.pdf+html. doi:10.2215/CJN.08670910Japan.

Saran, R., Li, Y., Robinson, B., Ayanian, J., Balkrishnan, R., Bragg-Gresham, J., Chen, J.T.L., Cope, E., Gipson, D., He, K., Herman, W., Heung, M., Hirth, R.A., Jacobsen, S.S., Kalantar-Zadeh, K., Kovesdy, C.P., Leichtman, A.B., Lu, Y., Molnar, M.Z., Morgenstern, H., Nallamothu, B., O'Hare, A.M., Pisoni, R., Plattner, B., Port, F.K., Rao, P., Rhee, C.M., Schaubel, D.E., Selewski, D.T., Shahinian, V., Sim, J.J., Song, P., Streja, E., Tamura, M.K., Tentori. F., Eggers, P.W., Agodoa, L.Y.C., Abbott, K.C., 2015. US renal data system 2014 annual data report: epidemiology of kidney disease in the United States. Am. J. Kidney Dis. 15236838. 66 (1), A7. Available from: http://www.elsevier.com/inca/publications/store/6/2/3/2/7/6/index.htt. doi:10.1053/j.ajkd.2015.05.001.

Sekercioglu, N., Curtis, B., Murphy, S., Barrett, B., 2015. Sleep quality and its correlates in patients with chronic kidney disease: a cross-sectional design. Ren. Fail. 0886-022X. 37 (5), 757–762. doi:10.3109/0886022x.2015.1024555.

Sloand, J.A., Shelly, M.A., Feigin, A., Bernstein, P., Monk, R.D., Double-Blind, A., 2004. Placebo-controlled trial of intravenous iron dextran therapy in patients with ESRD and restless legs syndrome. Am. J. Kidney Dis. 02726386. 43 (4), 663–670. Available from: http://www.elsevier.com/inca/publications/store/6/2/3/2/7/6/index.htt. doi:10.1053/j.ajkd.2003.11.021.

Stoller, M.K., 1994. Economic effects of insomnia. Clin. Ther. 16 (5), 873–897.

Takano, Y., Ibata, R., Machida, N., Ubara, A., Okajima, I., 2023. Effect of cognitive behavioral therapy for insomnia in workers: a systematic review and meta-analysis of randomized controlled trials. Sleep Med. Rev. 15322955. 71. Available from: http://www.elsevier.com/inca/publications/store/6/2/3/0/7/4/index.htt. doi:10.1016/j.smrv.2023.101839.

Tan, L.H., Chen, P.S., Chiang, H.Y., King, E., Yeh, H.C., Hsiao, Y.L., Chang, D.R., Chen, S.H., Wu, M.Y., Kuo, C.C., 2022. Insomnia and poor sleep in CKD: a systematic review and meta-analysis. Kidney Med. 25900595. 4 (5). Available from: https://www.journals.elsevier.com/kidney-medicine. doi:10.1016/j.xkme.2022.100458.

Turkmen, K., Erdur, F.M., Guney, I., Gaipov, A., Turgut, F., Altintepe, L., Saglam, M., Tonbul, H.Z., Abdel-Rahman, E.M., 2012. Sleep quality, depression, and quality of life in elderly hemodialysis patients. Int. J. Nephrol. Renovasc. Dis. 11787058. 5, 135–142. Available from: http://www.dovepress.com/getfile.php?fileID=14169. doi:10.2147/ijnrd.s36493.

Unruh, M.L., 2007. Sleep apnea and dialysis therapies: things that go bump in the night? Hemodial. Int. 15424758. 11 (4), 369–378. doi:10.1111/j.1542-4758.2007.00203.x.

Unruh, M.L., Buysse, D.J., Dew, M.A., Evans, I.V., Wu, A.W., Fink, N.E., Powe, N.R., Meyer, K.B., 2006. Sleep quality and its correlates in the first year of dialysis. Clin. J. Am. Soc. Nephrol. 1555905X. 1 (4), 802–810. Available from: http://cjasn.asnjournals.org/content/1/4/802.full.pdf. doi:10.2215/CJN.00710206.

Virga, G., Stanic, L., Mastrosimone, S., Gastaldon, F., da Porto, A., Bonadonna, A., 2000. Hypercalcemia and insomnia in hemodialysis patients. Nephron. 1660-8151. 85 (1), 94–95. doi:10.1159/000045638.

Wang, Y., Liu, X., Zhang, J., Zhou, B., Yue, W., Hu, K., 2024. Long sleep duration is associated with abdominal aortic calcification among male adults with chronic kidney disease: NHANES 2013–2014. Sci. Rep. 2045-2322. 14 (1). doi:10.1038/s41598-024-72879-x.

Wijemanne, S., Jankovic, J., 2015. Restless legs syndrome: clinical presentation diagnosis and treatment. Sleep Med. 18785506. 16 (6), 678–690. Available from: www.elsevier.com/inca/publications/store/6/2/0/2/8/2. doi:10.1016/j.sleep.2015.03.002.

Winkelman, J.W., Chertow, G.M., Lazarus, J.M., 1996. Restless legs syndrome in end-stage renal disease. Am. J. Kidney Dis. 02726386. 28 (3), 372–378. Available from: http://www.elsevier.com/inca/publications/store/6/2/3/2/7/6/index.htt. doi:10.1016/S0272-6386(96)90494-1.

Winkelmayer, W.C., Mehta, J., Wang, P.S., 2007. Benzodiazepine use and mortality of incident dialysis patients in the United States. Kidney Int. 00852538. 72 (11), 1388–1393. doi:10.1038/sj.ki.5002548.

Xia, L., Liu, H., Ren, J., 2025. A review of symptom, pathogenesis and treatment characteristics of the elderly with chronic insomnia. Medicine. 1536-5964. 104 (5), e41346. doi:10.1097/md.0000000000041346.

Xiong, Y., Zhong, Q., Zhang, Y., Liu, Z., Wang, X., 2024. The association between circadian syndrome and chronic kidney disease in an aging population: a 4-year follow-up study. Front. Endocrinol. (Lausanne). 1664-2392. 15. doi:10.3389/fendo.2024.1338110.

Yang, B., Xu, J., Xue, Q., Wei, T., Xu, J., Ye, C., Mei, C., Mao, Z., 2015. Non-pharmacological interventions for improving sleep quality in patients on dialysis: systematic review and meta-analysis. Sleep Med. Rev. 15322955.

23, 68–82. Available from: http://www.elsevier.com/inca/publications/store/6/2/3/0/7/4/index.htt. doi:10.1016/j.smrv.2014.11.005.

Yaremchuk, K., 2018. Sleep disorders in the elderly. Clin. Geriatr. Med. 07490690. 34 (2), 205–216. doi:10.1016/j.cger.2018.01.008.

Yazıcı, R., Güney, İ., 2022. Prevalence and related factors of poor sleep quality in patients with pre-dialysis chronic kidney disease. Int. J. Artif. Organs. 17246040. 45 (11), 905–910. Available from: https://journals.sagepub.com/home/jao. doi:10.1177/03913988221118941.

Zhang, F., Huang, X., Wang, H., Bai, Y., Huang, L., Li, Y., Zhong, Y., 2024. Prevalence of obstructive sleep apnea in whole spectrum chronic kidney disease patients: a systematic review and meta-analysis. Sleep Med. 18785506. 119, 526–534. Available from: https://www.sciencedirect.com/science/journal/13899457. doi:10.1016/j.sleep.2024.05.047.

Zhang, J., Wang, C., Gong, W., Ye, Z., Tang, Y., Zhao, W., Peng, H., Lou, T., 2017. Poor sleep quality is responsible for the nondipper pattern in hypertensive but not in normotensive chronic kidney disease patients. Nephrology. 14401797. 22 (9), 690–698. Available from: http://onlinelibrary.wiley.com/journal/10.1111/(ISSN)1440-1797. doi:10.1111/nep.12839.

CHAPTER

11

Falls

Stephen Z. Fadem

Department of Medicine, Section of Nephrology, Baylor College of Medicine, Houston, TX, United States

Introduction—Definition of a fall

Falls are common in the chronic kidney disease (CKD) population, particularly among the elderly. They often lead to injuries that permanently impact the lifestyle of the patient and are associated with loss of independence and an inability to perform the usual activities of daily living. Falls can be defined as a sudden loss of balance control that results in unexpectedly dropping to a lower level or the ground, and they are the leading causes of hospitalization and the need for institutionalized care (Guralnik et al., 1995). In a study of dialysis patients, the fall rate was 47% over 190.5 person-years in 162 patients, with a fall incidence of 1.60 falls per person per year. The mean age of the patients was 74.7 years. Around a quarter of the patients experienced multiple falls, and 19.5% of falls were associated with injury (Cook et al., 2006).

Falls that cause injuries occur less frequently in the general population but are quite common in sports events like American football, wrestling, judo, and bull riding. In bull riding, a rodeo champion must stay on a bucking one-ton animal for at least 8 seconds before falling. The injury rate from a rodeo fall is 3.33 injuries per 100 events (3.32%), compared to 162 out of 2111 head injuries in elderly patients (7.674%). The incidence is higher in patients with CKD (adjusted odds ratio—aOR 2.80, 95% CI 1.25–5.75). Sports injuries among athletes are much less common than fall injuries in elderly and CKD patients. This population is healthier, fitter, and younger, but a significant factor is that athletes anticipate and even train to fall. This suggests that there are modifiable factors influencing fall injuries—fitness, health status, and especially the level of training. A study using judo-inspired exercises to teach falling techniques showed substantial improvement over a 10-week period. However, this limited study was conducted in a younger population (mean age 45) (Arkkukangas et al., 2021). The British Broadcasting Corporation has reported that judo lessons are now being taught to the elderly to prevent falls.

Falls present significant safety risks, particularly in the workplace. Many insights gained from other fields can be relevant to the CKD population, as there are many similarities.

Aging and the Kidney
https://doi.org/10.1016/B978-0-443-34069-7.00015-X

In the aging CKD population, impaired mobility is associated with functional impairment, particularly in strength and physical performance. Studies of 10-step climbing or one-quarter of a mile walking demonstrate a relationship between GFR and physical limitation, particularly when not adjusted for inflammatory factors, suggesting that inflammation is another modifiable risk factor (Fried et al., 2006). While falls can be categorized as either environmental (mechanical) or nonmechanical (stemming from underlying inherent conditions), there is significant overlap, since patients who are more prone to falling are often less aware of their surroundings and more likely to slip, stumble, misstep, or collide accidentally. Training efforts can improve awareness of fall risks and may reduce falls by up to 50%.

There are several predictors of falls, but no single tool meets all circumstances (Park, 2018). A simple predictor of falls is the Morse Fall Scale. Developed by Janice Morse, an anthropologist and nurse, and published in 1989 (Morse et al., 1989), it has been helpful in hospitals and other clinical settings for evaluating risks. The scale is simple, quick, widely used, and has been validated. It consists of the following six assessments:

- History of falling (yes = 25 points)
- Secondary diagnosis (yes = 15 points)
- Ambulatory aid (bed rest = 0; crutches, cane, walker = 15; furniture = 30)
- An intravenous line or heparin lock (yes = 20)
- Gait disorder (normal, bedridden, immobile = 0; weak = 10; impaired = 30).
- Mental status (forgets limitations = 15)

The sum of the risk points predicts patients at low risk (1–24), moderate risk (25–45), and high risk (>45). The scale has been a benchmark for validating other fall assessment tools. It is also adaptable to electronic medical records (Baek et al., 2014). More complex predictive tools that are superior to the Morse Scale are being developed. In Korea, a machine learning model to assess falls in hospital patients takes into account 83 known predictors grouped into seven categories. Validation of this tool shows a gradient boosting model receiver operating characteristic curve of 0.817 (CI 0.720–0.904) compared with 0.652 (CI 0.570–0.715) for the Morse scale (Shim et al., 2022). See Table 11.1.

Individual assessments of gait speed and stride, hand grip strength, or a timed up-and-go provide an added prediction. The timed up-and-go (TUG) assessment is a timed test that measures standing up from a chair, walking 10 feet, turning, returning, and sitting back

TABLE 11.1 Morse fall scale (https://www.ahrq.gov/patient-safety/settings/hospital/fall-prevention/toolkit/morse-fall-scale.html).

Assessment	Points
History of falling	25
Secondary diagnosis	15
Ambulatory aid	Bed rest = 0 Crutches, cane, walker = 15 Furniture = 30
An intravenous line or heparin lock	20

Assessment	Points
Gait disorder	Normal, bedridden, immobile = 0 Weak = 10 Impaired = 30
Mental status (forgets limitations)	15
Summation	
Low risk	1–24
Moderate risk	25–45
High risk	>45

From AHRQ, available at https://www.ahrq.gov/patient-safety/settings/hospital/fall-prevention/toolkit/morse-fall-scale.html.

down. Patients who take over 12 s are at risk for falling. The test is part of the CDC's STEADI assessment tools (http://www.cdc.gov/steadi).

Mechanics

To fully understand falls, with the expressed interest in trying to prevent them, one must review the mechanics of a fall and dissect the physical and environmental factors that relate to each phase. A fall occurs because the external force of gravity destabilizes the body's alignment, causing the center of gravity to move outside its support base. In the populations we are describing, the falls are unintentional and unexpected. When the center of gravity moves outside the base, the person becomes unstable and accelerates downward. Efforts to regain balance or compensate come into play, but if unsuccessful, the patient falls. Falls have classically been divided into four phases (Noury et al., 2016). Table 11.2 highlights the four phases in the mechanics of falling. Using these phases as a template, a fall video analysis questionnaire has been developed and validated to characterize falls based on video surveillance (Yang et al., 2013). A total of 221 falls from 136 residents in a long-term care facility were analyzed using 48 cameras strategically located around the facility. The mean age of the population was 82. Thirty-one percent were hypertensive, and 13% were diabetic. Nineteen percent had a previous stroke. Twenty-four percent had Alzheimer's disease, and 6% had Parkinson's disease. The study did not mention the incidence of patients with CKD.

Initiation

Some falls are initiated when an event leads to a loss of balance. These events occur when we lose control of our body position and include slipping on ice or water, tripping over an object (that probably should not have been there), a collision, or even a misstep. Mechanical falls result from these. Typically, tripping is an associated cause of falls in 34%, slipping in 25%, and being knocked over in 4% of cases. Men are more likely to slip, and women are

TABLE 11.2 Mechanics of a fall.

Initiation	Did the patient trip, slip, stumble, collide, or collapse?
Descent	What was the fall distance? Was the patient able to initiate fall prevention strategies?
Impact	What was the location, and what were the surface characteristics? What was the site? Common sites are wrist, hip, back, head, or side.
Recovery	Did the injury require hospitalization, and will rehabilitation be needed?

more likely to trip. Many people attribute their fall to hurrying (Berg et al., 1997). Neurosensory control of body position is centrally integrated with information from the surface (proprioception), the eyes, and the inner ear. Nonmechanical falls occur because of altered neurosensory function controlling balance, medication effects that adversely affect consciousness, gait or visual disorders, severe muscle weakness, neuropathy, sudden blood pressure loss, or syncope. The patient collapses in many types of nonmechanical falls, not because of a shift in the center of gravity but due to multifactorial causes that must be clinically assessed. Typically, legs giving way account for 4% of falls, loss of support in 35% of falls, and loss of balance in 95% of falls. Usually, during the initiation phase, the center of gravity shifts outside the support base, resulting in a fall. Evaluation of falls in the initiation phase includes identifying the cause of the imbalance, the activity at the time of the fall, whether any mobility aids were used, if the patient was holding any objects, the fall conditions (both wet/dry and transition), the distance of the fall, lighting status, the kind of footwear worn, and whether clutter contributed. In relating the video surveillance of falls to the questionnaire, studies by Yang's group demonstrate that walking, standing, and transferring to a sitting or lying position account for 89% of the responses (Yang et al., 2013).

Berg et al. report that falls occur in the home (58%) and in the afternoon (52%). In addition, 24% of falls occur when walking on uneven ground, and 14% involve stairs. Furthermore, 7% of falls occur during exercise (Berg et al., 1997).

Descent

During descent, if there is a loss of control, the body moves toward the ground. Since this involves the rapid accelerative force of gravity, it may be difficult or even impossible to regain balance. The body's position may vary, affecting impact. Being able to rapidly shift weight and realign the center of gravity with the base of support may help prevent the fall. In addition, grabbing onto something may help reduce fall risk. When there is a high risk of falling, one may minimize chances by using handrails in stairwells or grab bars in the shower. Training programs designed to help regain the center of gravity can also help prevent descent. Balance training, resistance exercises, and martial arts programs can help maintain control during descent (Fadem, 2023). During the descent phase, the evaluation of falls includes the fall direction (forward, backward, or sideways), whether steps were involved, and if the patient attempted a reach-to-grasp maneuver. The most commonly selected responses in the Yang study were falling backward or sideways. Forty-two percent of patients reported attempting a recovery step. The reach-to-grasp response did have good inter-rater reliability and, thus, was given a low probability confidence value (Yang et al., 2013).

The time of descent is the square root of (−2 × distance/gravity). From 1 m, it would be the square root of −2/−9.8 m/s^2, or 0.45 s. The human reaction time is around 0.4 s in a healthy individual but slower in an elderly or CKD patient, lessening the chance of grabbing a bar. Most head injuries that lead to hospitalization happen on stairs at home.

Impact

Impact is the phase where the body makes contact with a surface or the ground. The height of the fall (acceleration) and the surface's hardness can affect the severity of the impact. The area of the body impacted also influences the injury. The landing configuration, type of flooring, site of maximum energy absorption, and injury risk (head, pelvis, torso, hand or wrist, elbow or forearm, knee, shoulder) are all factors to consider. In the Yang questionnaire, most patients reported falling backward with impact to the head in 42% of cases and to the hands in 71% of cases. Most of the falls involved multiple body sites (Yang et al., 2013).

Head injury related to falls can be mild to severe, ranging from minor pain to a hemorrhage. 64.2% of falls that lead to head injury are mechanical. Although motor vehicle accidents are the most common cause of the 1.9 million annual admissions for traumatic brain injury (TBI), the fall is the most common reason for admission in the elderly. 13% of hospitalized patients admitted with a head injury die. A concussion is the most common cause of TBI requiring hospitalization and accounts for 24% of admissions. Its symptoms can include confusion, disorientation, dizziness, nausea, memory lapse, and a headache. The prognosis from a single concussion is generally good, but multiple concussions can lead to traumatic encephalopathy. A brain contusion is more severe than a concussion and can result in hemorrhage, particularly in elderly patients on blood thinners or dialysis patients who have just been heparinized. Blood is very toxic to brain tissue, and contusions can lead to permanent injury or death. A skull fracture can be serious as the head can hit the pavement or furniture with a hard impact. Fractures to the base of the skull can result in clear fluid running from the ears and nose and bruising around the eyes. The patient may be dizzy, nauseated with vomiting, and have loss of consciousness. Severe head injuries can result in hematomas, and their symptoms depend on their location. They are frightening because they may initially present with mild symptoms that progress to unconsciousness and brain herniation as the hematoma expands. Epidural hematomas are less common, but bleeding beneath the dura—subdural hematomas make up 42.95 of head injuries in patients over 85 years old who are admitted. Subarachnoid hematoma is a collection of blood between the pia mater and the brain. It is most likely associated with a ruptured aneurysm and can lead to a nonmechanical fall (Harvey and Close, 2012).

Hip injuries—A fracture of the femoral neck, or a "hip fracture," is the result of a fall in the elderly 95% of the time. Fortunately, among the millions of falls annually, hip fractures occur in only 1%–2% of the time. This is probably because, in most falls, an upper limb precedes the hip when hitting the ground. The hip is the first body part to hit the ground in 17% of falls. However, in 60% of hip fractures, the first area to hit the ground is the knee. The hip fracture that results from direct impact of the hip area with enough force to break the bone depends on the state of the bone. Osteoporosis and metabolic bone disease associated with kidney disease decrease bone mass, leading to less ability to withstand force and increasing the fracture risk. Bone-strengthening exercises can reduce the fall risk in both the elderly and the CKD population. Also, efforts to reduce vascular calcification and bone demineralization in kidney patients positively impact general health (Yang et al., 2020).

Vertebral fractures related to falls are common in the elderly and are also independent risk factors for a subsequent hip fracture caused by a subsequent fall. Just over 50% of fractures are in the lower back, while around one in three fractures (29.5% in males and 35.6% in females) occur in the thoracic spine. A fractured spine occurs more frequently from a mechanical fall when indoors and is associated with toileting, a misstep, or falling backward or sideways. Women are more likely to fall when walking, rising from a chair, or stepping down, while men are most likely to fall forward, either slipping, tripping, or falling on an uneven floor (Yu et al., 2021).

Recovery

The recovery phase is the immediate aftermath of the impact. The amount of shock absorbed, and whether the person rolls or slides, determines the severity of the injury. Programs to improve conditioning and fall skills have been developed; they include judo and recovery step training.

A judo-inspired 10-week exercise program was conducted in 79 middle-aged adults. It focused on physical exercise to develop strength, balance, and falling strategies (breakfall techniques). Physical function, activity level, fall-related self-efficacy, and safe landing techniques were evaluated. The patients served as their own controls with a pre test and a posttest. At the end of the testing period, forward and backward falling techniques and tests for physical activity significantly improved. The Falls Efficacy Test, which was designed to test confidence in the ability to perform activities without falling, did not improve during the course (Arkkukangas et al., 2020).

Thirteen studies have characterized falls based on falling direction, examining impact load in seven landing strategies: squatting, elbow flexion, forward rotation, martial arts rolling, martial arts slapping, relaxed muscle, and recovery steps. The only strategy that does not reduce load is martial arts slapping. Squatting helps reduce the impact of backward falling, while elbow flexion with outstretched arms effectively reduces the impact of forward falling. Forward rotation and martial arts rolling are most effective when falling sideways. The review suggests that learning martial arts and landing strategies might reduce injuries in falls among the elderly, but further investigation is necessary (Moon and Sosnoff, 2017).

Underlying reasons for a fall

Falls can be either environmental (mechanical) or nonmechanical—related to medical conditions. Medical conditions can be attributed to CNS abnormalities such as stroke and cognitive decline, medications such as sedatives or antihypertensives, and medical changes, including age, frailty, CKD, muscle weakness, balance and gait issues, vision and sensorium disorders, diabetes, and circulatory and cardiac diseases. Although environmental events are

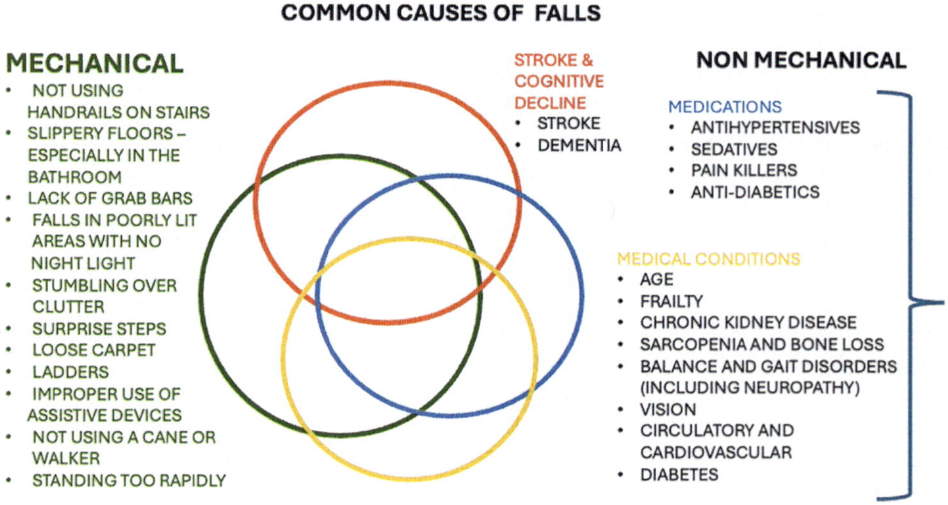

FIG. 11.1 Common causes of falls. While falls are categorized as either mechanical or nonmechanical, their etiologies are multifactorial and overlapping. *Modified from Fadem, S., 2023. Understanding and Preventing Falls. Springer Nature, Cham, Switzerland. Used with permission of the author.*

more likely to initiate mechanical falls, considerable overlap exists between the main falling spheres (Fig. 11.1).

Stroke and cognitive decline

It is estimated that between 37% and 73% of stroke victims fall during the first 6 months posthospital discharge, and the high risk continues. Stroke patients are also more likely to fall repeatedly. Patients who experience a fall related to their initial stroke have a fear of falling that usually decreases over a 6-month period. Falls are likely to occur during transition periods, i.e., from the hospital to the rehabilitation center or from the rehabilitation center to home. Falls in stroke patients likely occur in the mornings between 10 and 11 AM and in the evenings between 5 and 6 PM. They occur most frequently in the patient's bedroom or bathroom. They can occur while walking, transferring, or sitting in a wheelchair. Most often, falls are to the affected side and result from a loss of balance or a misstep where the step or surface height is incorrectly judged. Obstacle crossing and turning to avoid the obstacle may be impaired in 50% of people with a stroke, so it is incumbent to ensure clutter (clothes, towels, shoes, pillows) is not present in the walking path. The most common injury from a fall in a stroke patient is soft tissue injury, but hip fractures and head injuries can also occur. The risk of a stroke-related fall increases with a loss of ability to perform activities of daily living or to maintain balance. Age, gender, or type of stroke are not risk factors for a fall.

Efforts to reduce the risk of falling include using vitamin D to increase muscle and bone strength, removing clutter, monitoring medications that could potentiate a fall or injury (like anticoagulants), and supervised exercise. Environmental assistive devices, such as sensors or voice-activated alert systems, are also emerging (Batchelor et al., 2012).

A metaanalysis of exercise interventions to prevent falls in neurodegenerative diseases and aging identified 64 studies, encompassing 13,241 participants. In stroke survivors, exercises targeting muscle strength, bone mass, balance, posture, and gait reduced falls by a rate ratio of 0.4 (95% CI: 0.27–0.57) (Feng et al., 2023).

Cognitive dysfunction is 8–10 times more likely to result in a fall when compared with people without dementia (Casey et al., 2020). Falls in dementia are more likely to cause injury and are the leading cause of hospital readmission among those discharged to home or home health care (Hoffman et al., 2019). Risk factors for falls in dementia parallel those in the elderly population and include chronic disease, visual and spatial deficits, depression, gait and balance limitations, sensory deficits, and environmental factors such as home safety issues. Other risks include the use of alcohol, poor footwear, frailty, depression, and a fear of falling. Improper use of assistive devices also contributes to falls. Dementia causes a lack of independence and is also associated with wandering. In dementia, the onset of visuospatial changes may precede dementia by three years. Exercise, gait retraining, physical therapy, and occupational therapy have a clear place in preventing falls in patients with dementia (Casey et al., 2020).

An alternative training approach for conceptual rehabilitation is errorless learning. With this technique, a task is designed to reduce any opportunity for guessing or mistakes and is practiced using a consistent structure until mastered. The cues preempt mistakes and thus enhance learning and performance. The cues can then be removed. This highly structured learning technique may be valuable in improving independence through physical therapy tasks such as sitting to standing (Kessels, 2018).

Medications

About 65%–95% of fall-related injuries occur in patients who are using either sleeping pills or antidepressant drugs. Opioids also increase the risk of falls. Reducing the use of fall-related injury drugs (FRIDs) lowers the fall risk but often must be combined with other interventions. When possible, patients using opioids should be transitioned to other medications. Selective antidepressants and medications like gabapentin or pregabalin may be more useful in treating neuropathy. Nonsteroidal antiinflammatory drugs, while nephrotoxic when ingested by persons with impaired kidney function, are available as ointments, which, when directly applied to the joints, can offer some relief. Drugs that contain ketamine are risky to use in patients prone to falls.

Diuretics are associated with a threefold risk of falls and can cause postural hypotension. Although the treatment of hypertension has more benefits than risks, intense treatment is associated with a risk of hospital readmission, particularly in those who are frail. Elderly CKD patients on antihypertensive therapy should be monitored closely by healthcare providers. The use of remote patient monitoring for blood pressure is encouraging for identifying both peaks and lows in home BP management.

Treatment with antidiabetic medication can be associated with falls. One must consider that many diabetic patients have multiple comorbidities and are more prone to falling regardless of care. The use of continuous glucose monitoring can help patients self-regulate their diabetes management and minimize hypoglycemia. Current guidelines for managing diabetes in CKD patients recommend measuring the HbA1C quarterly and targeting <6.5% in mild diabetics. However, in elderly patients, those who are less independent, may live alone, and lack the resources to seek immediate attention, the HbA1C should be kept at <8.0% (Fadem, 2023).

Medical conditions

Age

Falls are now the main cause of injury leading to emergency room visits and account for 70% of accidental deaths in persons 75 years old (Fuller, 2000). Irrespective of kidney disease, it has been reported that over 14 million people aged ≥65 years and living in the United States fall each year. When kidney patients fall, particularly those on hemodialysis, the incidence of hip fractures is three to four times that of the general population, and kidney patients have a higher mortality rate (Papakonstantinopoulou and Sofianos, 2017). It is recommended that fall-prevention interventions be implemented in persons with a history of falls, slow gait speed (<0.8 m/s), or a fear of falling. A review of 59 randomized trials confirmed that exercise to improve balance and muscle mass lowered the fall incidence from 850 to 655 falls per 1000 patient-years compared with those not exercising. This amounts to a relative risk (RR) of 0.77 (95% CI, 0.71–0.83). There are multiple risk factors for fall victims. Interocular lens replacement surgery, podiatry intervention, and environmental modification reduced the risk from 2317 to 1785 falls per 1000 patient-years (RR, 0.77; 95% CI, 0.67–0.87) (Colón-Emeric et al., 2024). Other interventions include dance-based therapy. A metaanalysis of 29 randomized clinical trials showed a 37% reduced risk of falling in 8 trials (n = 1579, RR 0.63; 95% CI, 0.49–0.80) and a significantly reduced risk of 31% in 7 trials (n = 2012, RR 0.69; 95% CI, 0.53–0.89). Dance therapy also significantly improved balance, mobility, and lower body strength (Mattle et al., 2020).

Frailty

Frailty is the body's response to aging and chronic illness. It is associated with immobility, extreme fatigue, and poor nutrition. It represents the intermediate step between a loss in the performance of activities of daily living and death. It is characterized by a weight loss of more than 5% over the past year, an inability to perform five sit-to-stand repetitions, decreased grip strength and walking speed, and a lack of energy. Studies demonstrate that the fall rate in frail individuals is 31.8%; frail patients have a 97% higher risk of falling than robust patients (Lu et al., 2021). Intrinsic capacity evaluations combine assessments of mental status, physical performance, nutrition, hearing, and vision. A decline in intrinsic capacity is associated with frailty and an increased fall risk (Shen et al., 2023).

Oxidative stress in diabetes and kidney disease shortens telomeres and impacts DNA survival. It also damages mitochondria. As DNA damage worsens, cells cannot make the enzymes needed for survival and die. As mitochondria numbers dwindle, the production of ATP, vital for the phosphorylation of enzymes, decreases, potentiating further cell damage and even death. The energy loss contributes to frailty, a marker of advancing chronic disease and a strong risk factor for falls. The accumulation of uremic toxins is related to the mechanisms that cause frailty. Phosphate, indoxyl sulfate, and p-cresyl sulfate are known contributors to organ dysfunction. Peroxisome proliferator-activated receptor γ (PPAR γ) and its coactivator (coactivator 1α) bind DNA to increase insulin sensitization, reduce inflammation, and regulate lipid metabolism. It targets Klotho and blocks the angiotensin II receptor. Thus it has a role in maintaining glomerular endothelial cells, mesangial cells, podocytes, and tubular cells. Free fatty acids, hyperglycemia, insulin resistance, glomerular hypertension, and reactive oxygen species suppress PPAR γ and result in inflammation, as well as TGF-β, SMAD, and subsequently, JAK-STAT signaling pathways that lead to fibrosis and renal damage.

Serum phosphorus increases Runt-related transcription factor 2 (RUNX2), resulting in vascular calcification. mTOR/Raptor signaling is crucial for this bone formation. The stiff matrix associated with CKD also regulates inflammasomes. The skeletonization of blood vessels potentiates vascular stiffness and exacerbates cardiac failure, fibrosis, and arrhythmias (Li et al., 2025). Uremic toxins impact several organ systems involved in frailty, particularly the muscles, brain, bone, vasculature, and heart (Chao and Lin, 2021).

Metabolic acidosis leads to muscle breakdown through the ubiquitin-proteasome system, and the immobility associated with early frailty reduces bone density and muscle mass (Chao and Lin, 2021).

As we more fully understand the mechanisms associated with frailty, we can design therapies that mitigate its impact on quality of life and survival. Approaches for kidney patients include adequate dialysis, better control of metabolic acidosis and mineral-bone disorders, inflammation reduction strategies, the avoidance of immobility, and exercise (Jadczak et al., 2018).

CKD

Uremic toxins, hypertension, metabolic acidosis, increased inflammation, increased oxidative stress, metabolic bone disease, muscle weakness, and poor nutrition are all factors associated with progressive kidney disease. Each of these interferes with motor function and ultimately leads to a fall risk.

One of the side effects of CKD is metabolic acidosis, which is associated with the ubiquitination of muscle protein and sarcopenia. Sarcopenia results in less activity, further stimulating the proteasomal breakdown of muscle. Immobility also causes bone loss, increasing the risk of fractures (Fadem et al., 2023a).

Kidney patients generally take several medications. The number of drugs, particularly those that cause sedation or hypotension, is associated with a higher risk of falls. A previous history of falls, fear of falling, and poor education also increase the risk of falling.

Fall predictors can be easily assessed in CKD patients. A straightforward screening is the timed up-and-go (TUG), a sit-to-stand maneuver accompanied by walking a short distance, then returning and sitting down. A time of 13.5 s indicates a high risk. Serum folic acid level and frailty are both independent predictors. Age, education, and vitamin D levels can also indicate a fall risk in CKD (Heybeli et al., 2022).

Patients with CKD exhibit fall patterns similar to those of the elderly; however, CKD heightens specific fall risks, increasing the likelihood of falls and related injuries. As CKD patients age, their risk of falling also escalates. By age 75, 70% of these patients have experienced at least one fall.

The dialysis patient presents a unique case. An analysis of fall-related studies among dialysis patients found that 28.4% of patients aged 20–92 experienced falls. Frail dialysis patients fell at a rate of 4.82 (CI 2.85–8.17). The Center for Epidemiologic Studies-Depression Scale (CES-D), when administered to dialysis patients, showed that a score of ≥18 while on antidepressants was linked to an unadjusted odds ratio (OR) of 4.03 (CI 2.12–7.66) for falling in the prior 12 months. Other factors within the dialysis population that raise the risk of falls include diabetes, heart failure, coronary artery disease, a history of stroke, chronic obstructive pulmonary disease, and peripheral vascular disease. A study adjusting for age and comorbidities indicated a higher fall risk in hemodialysis patients than those on peritoneal dialysis (HR 1.27, CI 1.06–1.52) (Wang et al., 2020).

Dialysis patients risk falling after the end of dialysis due to volume shifts and low blood pressure. Dialysis teammates are generally aware of this and provide appropriate assistance.

Muscle weakness

In normal individuals, there is a balance between the synthesis of muscle proteins and the breakdown of proteins. Sarcopenia, a condition where the breakdown of proteins exceeds their production, is observed in CKD and also in space travel, immobility, and other microgravity environments. This phenomenon occurs across all species. Inflammation also accelerates muscle breakdown and is associated with CKD, as well as with HIV, neoplasia, advancing age, and diabetes. It is characterized by a loss of muscle mass, particularly low grip strength and low gait speed. Muscle breakdown is further aggravated by angiotensin II and diabetes. Sarcopenia is estimated to occur in 10%–16% of the global population but is more prevalent in patients with chronic diseases (Yuan and Larsson, 2023). Low muscle mass and low muscle strength are associated with increased mortality in the dialysis population (OR 1.71; CI 1.20–2.44, OR 2.15; CI 1.51–2.07, respectively) (Wathanavasin et al., 2022).

An extensive review of 52,838 elderly (≥65) patients with sarcopenia demonstrated that falling and sustaining an injury was higher in patients with sarcopenia (OR 1.89, CI 1.33–2.68). Fractures were more likely in sarcopenia patients (OR 1.84, CI 1.30–2.62) (Yeung et al., 2019). Muscle synthesis can be induced through amino acid intake and resistance exercise. Properly designed exercise programs that target fall prevention may be beneficial in reducing the fall incidence in the elderly (Rodrigues et al., 2022).

Balance and gait

Lower extremity function is recognized as a predictor of subsequent disability in elderly patients. Those performing poorly on tests, such as being able to move from a sitting to a standing position five times, balancing on one foot, or walking at a normal pace, are 4.2–4.9 times more likely to have a disability in four years.

The gait cycle is divided into two phases: the swing phase and the stance phase. The swing phase measures the time between a foot leaving and returning to the ground, while the stance phase measures the time the foot is on the ground. The double support phase, a subset of the stance phase, occurs when both feet are on the ground simultaneously. Gait criteria include how slowly one walks (gait speed), stride length, and the double support phase time. A walkway mat fitted with sensors can reliably and accurately measure gait abnormalities and has been validated in numerous studies (Menz et al., 2004).

Cognitive abnormalities, peripheral neuropathy—even when mild and subclinical—balance abnormalities, and sarcopenia can affect the normal gait cycle. Lower extremity abnormalities are markers of overall physical function. A slow gait speed in the elderly indicates a poor prognosis, the onset of dementia, and a risk for falls. Likewise, a slow gait is also associated with worse outcomes in CKD patients.

Quantitative gait assessments also provide subtle indicators of a gait abnormality. Of 330 patients aged 65 years, 134 had CKD. All patients were assessed for gait abnormalities, and among those with CKD, a lower GFR was independently associated with abnormal gait, as measured by a shorter stride length, less time in the swing phase, and greater time in the double support phase. The patients with abnormal gait were at increased risk for a fall (95% CI 1.06–2.81) (Tran et al., 2019).

Gait assessment has been useful in helping to predict fall risk in patients with CKD. Gait speed and step length are part of the Short Physical Performance Battery. In two prospective studies of 82 patients with advanced disease (Stage 4 and 5) low step length and slow gait speed were associated with lower handgrip strength and poor physical performance. Low step length predicted falls with an odds ratio (OR) of 3.90 (CI 1.05–14.60), and slow gait speeds were predictive with an OR of 4.25 (CI 1.24–14.58). CKD patients scoring poorly on both tests had a 6.55 times higher OR of falling (CI 1.40–30.71) (Kimura et al., 2022).

Vision

Eye disease is common with age, CKD, and diabetes. In diabetes, background diabetic retinopathy can lead to blindness. Macular degeneration leads to a loss of central vision, while glaucoma decreases peripheral vision. Cataracts are common in the elderly and can be repaired by implanting an intraocular lens, improving or restoring vision.

Since vision contributes to balance control, impaired vision and depth perception make it no surprise that the National Health and Aging Trends Study demonstrated that 27.6% of people with vision impairment had a higher prevalence of falls (Jin et al., 2024). Falls are not associated with visual acuity and may depend on depth perception. Multifocal lenses impair depth perception, and when monofocal lenses are used instead, the incidence of falls decreases (Campbell et al., 2010). Combined exercise training and vision correction can reduce the odds of falling in older individuals (0.17, CI 0.07–0.38) (Tricco et al., 2017).

Circulatory and cardiac diseases (Denfeld et al., 2022)

Cardiovascular disease is a major cause of fall-related injuries and may occur in 40%–60% of patients. The multiple causes include coronary heart disease, peripheral artery disease, polypharmacy, frailty, postural hypotension, disorders in gait and balance, and sensory impairment. The American Heart Association has outlined recommendations to mitigate falls in patients with cardiac disease, and this would be even more relevant in patients with combined heart disease and CKD (Denfeld et al., 2022).

CKD is a well-recognized risk factor for atherosclerosis and subsequent coronary artery disease. The uremic environment is directly linked to oxidative stress, endothelial dysfunction, and inflammation (Cai et al., 2013). Coronary artery disease potentiates arrhythmias, hypotension, heart failure, and subsequently, falls. Altered circulation due to peripheral vascular disease leads to limb weakness, which raises the risk of nonmechanical falls and makes mechanical falls more likely. It also complicates recovery options because of the challenges associated with restoring or maintaining balance. Amputations further heighten the risk of falls. Although often overlooked, peripheral vascular disease that affects the hands limits mobility and contributes to falls.

Vascular calcification is common in patients with kidney disease, especially those with diabetes. Calcium deposits not only form as plaques inside endothelial cells but also as a bone-like substance in vascular smooth muscle. In CKD, this is related to mineral bone disease associated with impaired phosphorus excretion, increased parathyroid hormone, FGF23, and impaired vitamin D absorption. This process is coupled with elevated serum phosphorus and is dependent on mTOR. The osteopenia, which is worsened by metabolic acidosis, leaves bones more fragile and likely to sustain fractures. In addition, the elevated phosphorus enables DNA transcription factors like RUNX-2 to increase bone-like matrix in blood vessel walls, giving the freed calcium a place to deposit. This skeletonization stiffens blood vessels, making them less compliant and worsening target organ damage, resulting in muscle hypertrophy without accompanying capillary growth. This can lead to cardiac fibrosis, and since fibrotic tissues cannot propagate the sinoatrial conduction mechanism, aberrant arrhythmias, even ventricular fibrillation, may develop.

Postural hypotension is common in the elderly and is associated with injury-related falls. It is defined as a systolic blood pressure (BP) drop of >20 mm Hg and a diastolic BP drop of >10 mm Hg. It occurs when plasma volume redistributed in the abdomen and legs is slow to return to the heart upon standing, leading to a reduced stroke volume. Patients at the end of dialysis or on antihypertensive medications are at risk of experiencing a drop in blood pressure. Although baroreceptors send signals to the brain, the resultant sympathetic outflow may be ineffective in elderly or diabetic patients with autonomic insufficiency. The hypotension that results may lead to syncope. In patients with hypotension related to standing, medications should be reviewed, particularly long-acting antihypertensives and sedatives. Patients should be educated on positions that exacerbate hypotension and should be closely monitored at the end of dialysis treatment. Midodrine may help support blood pressure during dialysis (Dani et al., 2021).

Atrial fibrillation is common in CKD for a multitude of reasons. It is estimated that as many as 27% of dialysis patients have atrial fibrillation (Genovesi et al., 2005). Uremic toxins potentiate oxidative injury and activation of the inflammasome. This is further augmented by mitochondrial damage and endothelial dysfunction. The activated inflammasome triggers NF- KB, a trigger for inflammatory cytokines that induce fibrosis. Although fibroblasts are not excitable, they allow electrical currents to pass through and depolarize neighboring myocytes, which can cause atrial fibrillation (Gadde et al., 2022). The pulmonary veins in CKD become laden with calcium, prolonging calcium release from the sarcoplasmic reticulum, and potentiate arrhythmias such as atrial fibrillation (Huang et al., 2017). Apixaban has a favorable safety profile and is clinically effective in reducing emboli and stroke in nonvalvular patients with atrial fibrillation (Mandt et al., 2024).

Diabetes

CKD occurs in 14% of the population, and 11.3% of the population is diabetic. Both conditions independently increase tissue aging, but when combined, they have a synergy that accelerates the aging process. Sugar alone is toxic to both glomeruli and pancreatic beta cells. It also increases insulin resistance by blocking the metabolic pathway whereby insulin controls glucose absorption. The consequent effects of insulin turn off mTOR and autophagy, interfering with cellular function. Both diseases are associated with inflammation and oxidative stress. Inflammation controls TGF-β and SMAD and increases transcription factors that cause fibrosis. Since diabetes interferes with endothelial cell function, systemic damage to not just blood vessels but also target organs like the brain, eye, kidney, extremities, and nerves leads to comorbidities that are recognized in CKD patients with diabetes. Damage to each organ independently can cause a fall risk, but when many organs are damaged, the chances of a serious fall worsen.

Metabolic syndrome: The metabolic imbalance between eating and insulin release potentiates hunger and obesity. A high BMI (>30 kg/m^2) defines obesity. In obesity, adiponectin is reduced, decreasing subcutaneous fat absorption while increasing visceral fat absorption. Visceral fat accumulation causes inflammation and atherosclerosis. Heart disease is a nonmechanical fall risk through atrial fibrillation, decreased ejection fraction, arrhythmias, and hypotension. Metabolic syndrome can be associated with insulin resistance and result in type 2 diabetes.

A longitudinal study of diabetics aged 70–79 revealed that those with poor glycemic control have a high risk of fall-related injuries requiring hospitalization (HR 1.48, CI 1.12–1.95) (Yau et al., 2013). Yet, 81% of diabetics did not believe that diabetes increased the risk of falls, and 68% did not realize its association with falls. In addition, 90% reported that their physicians did not discuss fracture risks with them. Fifty-four percent of patients participated in moderate aerobic exercises, and those not exercising reported a lack of motivation as the most common barrier (Drummond et al., 2022). Osteoporotic fractures are one of the most important causes of mortality in older diabetics. Inflammation, advanced glycosylation end products, and microangiopathy accompany CKD as significant factors leading to this comorbidity (Montagnani et al., 2011).

Therapy

One approach to tailoring prevention strategies is categorizing the fall as either mechanical (based on mechanical factors) or nonmechanical (based on medical disorders). Next, it is best to focus on modifiable preventative factors. The CDC has developed STEADI (http://cdc.gov/steadi), a comprehensive web-based program for fall prevention. It is easily adaptable to kidney patients and dialysis unit care. The program focuses on tips that can be useful to prevent falls, screen for fall risks, and assess risk factors. It then offers strategies and tools that can be used to educate patients and provide follow-up.

Preventing nonmechanical falls

There is an overlap between therapy for nonmechanical falls and mechanical falls because, to achieve the aim of reducing falls, one must take a multifactorial approach.

The CDC program emphasizes that less than half of older patients will inform their doctor, partly due to fears of losing independence and the acceptance that falls are a natural occurrence. Many patients do not recognize that there are validated maneuvers designed to prevent falls and mitigate injuries associated with them. The STEADI program developed a screening tool to identify patients at high risk. Practically all advanced-stage CKD patients, especially those on dialysis, would fail the screening, particularly due to comorbidities associated with CKD, such as cardiovascular disease and diabetes. Patients who fail the screening complete a questionnaire that helps them and their providers identify eight modifiable risk factors:

(1) Gait, strength, and balance—assessment and follow-up physical therapy. The assessment encompasses tests that identify muscle strength, inability to walk, and poor balance. Exercises and physical therapy tailored to the individual can help with gait, balance, and muscle strength. Encouraging dialysis patients to become more mobile may help preserve these motor skills.
(2) Identify medications and medication combinations that could precipitate a fall. These include sedatives, sleeping medications, painkillers, and antihypertensives. Diabetic medications can also increase the risk of falls. It is challenging to avoid polypharmacy in dialysis patients, but efforts to reduce excess painkillers or sedatives can be rewarding.
(3) Help the patient fall-proof the home environment by checking for loose carpeting, installing night lights and grab bars where appropriate, and changing habits to avoid cluttering the walking pathway.
(4) Monitor for orthostatic hypotension: This is particularly true in diabetic patients with autonomic insufficiency and in patients who are at or below their dry weight at the end of hemodialysis treatment. The dialysis patient is highly vulnerable at the end of treatment, and fall-risk patients should be accompanied to the scales and closely observed, particularly if they are unsteady.
(5) Visual acuity: This, too, is particularly important in diabetic patients on dialysis because diabetic retinopathy can cause blindness. Cataracts, macular degeneration, and glaucoma are common disorders that can increase the risk of falls. Regular eye checkups are helpful in elderly kidney patients and can help preserve vision.
(6) Assessment of footwear: Peripheral neuropathy is associated with diabetes, and in dialysis patients, it may present as burning in the foot area. However, numbness and a loss of proprioception can also occur. Proprioception is a key component of balance. Diabetic ulcers that do not heal are a source of amputation. Footwear designed for diabetics and regular foot checks are key tools in preventing this comorbidity.
(7) Vitamin D deficiency is associated with bone pathology. In CKD, vitamin D activation is impaired, interfering with calcium absorption. Also, phosphorus excretion is impaired, leading to an accumulation of phosphorus and the release of the phosphate regulator, fibroblast growth factor 23 (FGF23). The release of parathyroid hormone to preserve serum calcium levels causes bone demineralization. Acidosis requires bone as a buffer and also reduces bone mass. Combined with this is inflammation and the increased production of RUNX2. RUNX2 is essential to maintain bones. However, it binds to DNA when activated in vascular smooth muscle cells (VSMC). It promotes bone deposition in the medial layer of the VSMC, leading to vascular calcification, stiff and noncompliant blood vessels, and worsening cardiac function (Lin et al., 2015). Vitamin D management can reduce the risk of falling.
(8) Comorbidities associated with CKD include hyperkalemia, metabolic acidosis, hypoalbuminemia, inflammation, access-related problems, mineral and bone disorders, heart failure, stroke, and cognitive decline.

The identification of risk factors led to interventions that were associated with reduced fall-related hospitalizations compared to those who received no intervention. A metaanalysis of 53 studies from 20 countries demonstrated that, while patients could identify some fall risk factors, they did not perceive themselves as being at risk. Patients also have mixed feelings—that falls are both inevitable and preventable. There is potential to educate, inform, and motivate patients to understand that falls are preventable. The studies cited that senior adults look to their healthcare providers as trusted sources of prevention information (Alfaro Hudak et al., 2023; Fadem et al., 2023b).

Preventing mechanical falls

Preventing mechanical falls in the home is designed to minimize slipping, tripping, taking a misstep, or avoiding a collision. Patients with impaired balance lose their footing quickly and have difficulty regaining balance once they fall. Since many accidents occur on stairs, using handrails is essential. Fall-risk patients should not attempt to carry objects in their hands when ascending or descending stairs. Stairs should be well lit and even. Heavily worn and slippery stairs are dangerous. Vulnerable individuals should also avoid wet surfaces, especially in the bathroom. Grab bars by the toilet, tub, and shower are essential to the fall prevention strategy. The Americans with Disabilities Act website has guidelines for bathroom design standards (http://www.ada.gov). Uneven surfaces can easily throw a vulnerable person off balance. Snow, ice, leaves, uneven pavement, and tree roots are common causes of serious injuries. A person falling from an upright position should try to lean into it, protect their head, and land on a soft body part. Wearing a hat when walking will offer some protection and buffering. In addition to falls, many elderly patients easily bump into open cabinet doors. This may cause serious injury to patients on blood thinners. Awareness of the surroundings can be challenging for those with cognitive impairments, but training can sometimes make a difference. Clutter is usually the clothing, bedding, or other items left on the floor in the pathway of the fall victim. Retraining to learn new habits to keep items off the floor may reduce this type of fall. Older patients often get up at night to urinate. Walking to the restroom can be treacherous in the dark. Automatic nightlights are inexpensive and should be installed along the pathways that potential fall patients take.

In many patients who are cognitively impaired, have had a stroke, are frail, or have balance issues, either a walker, rollator, cane, or wheelchair may be necessary and can often prevent falls. The cane is often used but should not be used for weight-bearing. The rollator has front and back wheels, and while it is helpful for weight-bearing, it can be a hazard regarding balance. Devices must be used correctly and kept in good working order. Trip hazards and accidents are common with walkers or rollators. Often, patients resist using devices but relent once they realize these devices increase mobility and independence (Fadem, 2023).

Illustrative cases

Case 1

A 76-year-old man with a history of a previous fall has advanced kidney disease, hypertension, and diabetes. He is not on dialysis. He is experiencing some cognitive decline and lives alone. He has struggled with balance and has fallen twice in the past six months. He did not sustain any severe injuries that required hospitalization but did fall on his knee. Since then, he has required pain medications and has become less active. He is taking medications to control hypertension and is on antidepressants. He has noticed that his muscles are weaker.

This case demonstrates that the risks of falling are additive. Factors such as age, kidney disease, hypertension, and diabetes increase the likelihood of falls. In addition, the absence of a support system, timely assistance, and a balance disorder contribute to this risk. Following his most recent fall, the patient is on medications that may exacerbate kidney disease and increase the risk of further falls. Furthermore, inactivity can aggravate sarcopenia, another contributing factor to falls.

Without a support system and a responsible caregiver, he is at serious risk of continued falls. Interventions should begin with a social evaluation to determine eligibility for placement in an assisted living center, where he can undergo an assessment, rehabilitative exercises, balance training, medication review, and diet planning.

Case 2

A 74-year-old woman experienced a drop in blood pressure twice during her dialysis treatment and walked unassisted to the scale for her post-weight measurement. She fainted while approaching the scale, hitting her head and briefly losing consciousness. Upon waking, she told the nurse that she felt fine. Her ride picked her up, but during the trip home, she became unresponsive in the van. She was taken to a nearby emergency room, where she suffered a severe episode of subdural bleeding and herniation. She passed away later that day.

This case emphasizes a significant risk associated with dialysis therapy. At the conclusion of the treatment, the process of fluid removal may result in hypovolemia. Fluid shifts to compensate for extracellular fluid removal require several minutes; during this interval, the patient is at increased risk of developing postural hypotension upon standing. A considerable number of patients may have diabetes accompanied by autonomic insufficiency and could also be receiving antihypertensive therapy that inhibits the sympathetic and renin-angiotensin systems. In certain patients, volume restoration is frequently the sole means to maintain blood pressure. Patients are typically anticoagulated during dialysis treatment, and heparin-induced anticoagulation persists into the postdialysis period. The act of standing and walking unassisted to the scale may represent a precarious moment, and a fall resulting in the patient striking their head could potentially lead to a brain contusion and a delayed, expanding intracranial hemorrhage, which may not be immediately apparent. Individuals who experience an acute blow to the head may display a clouded sensorium and impaired judgment. Staff in the dialysis unit should exercise heightened caution and diligently monitor patients following dialysis. Should a fall with head impact occur, it is imperative that the patient be transported to the hospital via ambulance for an immediate CT scan of the head, irrespective of whether they appear entirely alert.

Conclusion

Aging can reduce kidney function and accelerate the risk of a nonmechanical fall. While cognitive impairment, stroke, frailty, and medication use can cause falls, there are many underlying mechanisms related to kidney disease and its associated morbidities that also predispose the patient to become fall-prone. Kidney disease is associated with cardiovascular disease, resulting in hypotension, arrhythmias, and heart failure. It is also associated with sarcopenia, which interferes with gait. The diabetes commonly seen with CKD leads to postural hypotension, peripheral neuropathy, imbalance, and gait disturbances. Visual and auditory disturbances are among other associated harbingers of a fall. Mechanical falls are environmental and may be induced by the patient either slipping on a wet surface, missing a grab bar, stumbling and losing balance, colliding and being thrown off balance, or having a misstep. Mechanical falls occur more often in patients with debilitating diseases and, as a consequence of osteopenia and decreased reflex times, are more likely to result in an injury.

The steps to prevent a fall start with an assessment and identification of risk factors, followed by the creation of a program around each factor. Fall prevention requires the collaboration of the patient's supportive caregivers and medical personnel. Patients who live alone and have no one to assist them are at a disadvantage.

AI disclosure

During the preparation of this work, the author(s) used Grammarly to aid in readability and help correct typographical errors. After using this tool/service, the author(s) reviewed and edited the content as needed and take(s) full responsibility for the content of the publication.

References

Alfaro Hudak, K.M., Adibah, N., Cutroneo, E., Liotta, M., Sanghera, A., Weeks-Gariepy, T., Strunz, E., Rein, D.B., 2023. Older adults' knowledge and perception of fall risk and prevention: a scoping review. Age Ageing. 14682834. 52 (11). Available from: http://ageing.oxfordjournals.org/. doi:10.1093/ageing/afad220.

Arkkukangas, M., Bååthe, K.S., Ekholm, A., Tonkonogi, M., 2021. A 10-week judo-based exercise programme improves physical functions such as balance, strength and falling techniques in working age adults. BMC Public Health 21 (1), 744. doi:10.1186/s12889-021-10775-z.

Arkkukangas, M., Strömqvist Bååthe, K., Ekholm, A., Tonkonogi, M., 2020. Health promotion and prevention: the impact of specifically adapted judo-inspired training program on risk factors for falls among adults. Prev. Med. Rep. 22113355. 19, 101126. doi:10.1016/j.pmedr.2020.101126.

Baek, S., Piao, J., Jin, Y., Lee, S.M., 2014. Validity of the Morse fall scale implemented in an electronic medical record system. J. Clin. Nurs. 13652702. 23 (17–18), 2434–2441. Available from: www.blackwellpublishing.com/journal.asp?ref=0962-1067. doi:10.1111/jocn.12359.

Batchelor, F.A., Mackintosh, S.F., Said, C.M., Hill, K.D., 2012. Falls after stroke. Int. J. Stroke. 17474949. 7 (6), 482–490. doi:10.1111/j.1747-4949.2012.00796.x.

Berg, W.P., Alessio, H.M., Mills, E.M., Tong, C., 1997. Circumstances and consequences of falls in independent community-dwelling older adults. Age Ageing. 00020729. 26 (4), 261–268. doi:10.1093/ageing/26.4.261.

Cai, Q., Mukku, V.K., Ahmad, M., 2013. Coronary artery disease in patients with chronic kidney disease: a clinical update. Curr. Cardiol. Rev. 18756557. 9 (4), 331–339. doi:10.2174/1573403X10666140214122234.

Campbell, A.J., Sanderson, G., Robertson, M.C., 2010. Poor vision and falls. BMJ. 0959-8138. 340, c2456. doi:10.1136/bmj.c2456.

Casey, C.M., Caulley, J., Phelan, E.A., 2020. The intersection of falls and dementia in primary care: evaluation and management considerations. Med. Clin. North Am. 15579859. 104 (5), 791–806. Available from: http://www.medical.theclinics.com/. doi:10.1016/j.mcna.2020.06.003.

Chao, C.T., Lin, S.H., 2021. Uremic toxins and frailty in patients with chronic kidney disease: a molecular insight. Int. J. Mol. Sci. 14220067. 22 (12). Available from: https://www.mdpi.com/1422-0067/22/12/6270/pdf. doi:10.3390/ijms22126270.

Colón-Emeric, C.S., McDermott, C.L., Lee, D.S., Berry, S.D., 2024. Risk assessment and prevention of falls in older community-dwelling adults: a review. JAMA. 15383598. 331 (16), 1397–1406. Available from: http://jama.jamanetwork.com/journal.aspx. doi:10.1001/jama.2024.1416.

Cook, W.L., Tomlinson, G., Donaldson, M., Markowitz, S.N., Naglie, G., Sobolev, B., Jassal, S.V., 2006. Falls and fall-related injuries in older dialysis patients. Clin. J. Am. Soc. Nephrol. 1555905X. 1 (6), 1197–1204. doi:10.2215/CJN.01650506.

Dani, M., Dirksen, A., Taraborrelli, P., Panagopolous, D., Torocastro, M., Sutton, R., Lim, P.B., 2021. Orthostatic hypotension in older people: considerations, diagnosis and management. Clin. Med. (Lond.). 14734893. 21 (3), E275. Available from: https://www.rcpjournals.org/lookup/doi/10.7861/clinmed.2020-1044. doi:10.7861/CLINMED.2020-1044.

Denfeld, Q.E., Turrise, S., MacLaughlin, E.J., Chang, P.S., Clair, W.K., Lewis, E.F., Forman, D.E., Goodlin, S.J., 2022. Preventing and managing falls in adults with cardiovascular disease: a scientific statement from the American Heart Association. Circ. Cardiovasc. Qual. Outcomes. 19417705. 15 (6), E000108. Available from: http://circoutcomes.ahajournals.org/. doi:10.1161/HCQ.0000000000000108.

Drummond, K., Bennett, R., Gibbs, J., Wei, R., Hu, W., Tardio, V., Gagnon, C., Berger, C., Morin, S.N., 2022. Perceptions of fracture and fall risk and of the benefits and barriers to exercise in adults with diabetes. Osteoporos. Int. 14332965. 33 (12), 2563–2573. Available from: https://www.springer.com/journal/198. doi:10.1007/s00198-022-06524-6.

Fadem, S., 2023. Understanding and Preventing Falls. Springer Nature, Cham, Switzerland.

Fadem, S., Moura-Neto, J., Golper, T. (Eds.), 2023a. Complications in Dialysis. Springer-Nature, New York.

Fadem, S., Moura-Neto, Golper, T., 2023b. Complications in Dialysis. Springer-Nature, Houston.

Feng, F., Xu, H., Sun, Y., Zhang, X., Nan, L., Sun, X., Tian, X., Zhao, R., 2023. Exercise for prevention of falls and fall-related injuries in neurodegenerative diseases and aging-related risk conditions: a meta-analysis. Front. Endocrinol. (Lausanne). 1664-2392. 14. doi:10.3389/fendo.2023.1187325.

Fried, L.F., Jung, S.L., Shlipak, M., Chertow, G.M., Green, C., Ding, J., Harris, T., Newman, A.B., 2006. Chronic kidney disease and functional limitation in older people: health, aging and body composition study. J. Am. Geriatr. Soc. 15325415. 54 (5), 750–756. doi:10.1111/j.1532-5415.2006.00727.x.

Fuller, G.F., 2000. Falls in the elderly. Am. Fam. Physician 61 (7), 2159–2168.

Gadde, S., Kalluru, R., Cherukuri, S.P., Chikatimalla, R., Dasaradhan, T., Koneti, J., 2022. Atrial fibrillation in chronic kidney disease: an overview. Cureus. 2168-8184. 14 (8). doi:10.7759/cureus.27753.

Genovesi, S., Pogliani, D., Faini, A., Valsecchi, M.G., Riva, A., Stefani, F., Acquistapace, I., Stella, A., Bonforte, G., DeVecchi, A., DeCristofaro, V., Buccianti, G., Vincenti, A., 2005. Prevalence of atrial fibrillation and associated factors in a population of long-term hemodialysis patients. Am. J. Kidney Dis. 02726386. 46 (5), 897–902. doi:10.1053/j.ajkd.2005.07.044.

Guralnik, J.M., Ferrucci, L., Simonsick, E.M., Salive, M.E., Wallace, R.B., 1995. Lower-extremity function in persons over the age of 70 years as a predictor of subsequent disability. N. Engl. J. Med. 15334406. 332 (9), 556–562. doi:10.1056/NEJM199503023320902.

Harvey, L.A., Close, J.C.T., 2012. Traumatic brain injury in older adults: characteristics, causes and consequences. Injury. 18790267. 43 (11), 1821–1826. doi:10.1016/j.injury.2012.07.188.

Heybeli, C., Kazancioglu, R., Smith, L., Veronese, N., Soysal, P., 2022. Risk factors for high fall risk in elderly patients with chronic kidney disease. Int. Urol. Nephrol. 0301-1623. 54 (2), 349–356. doi:10.1007/s11255-021-02884-w.

Hoffman, G.J., Liu, H., Alexander, N.B., Tinetti, M., Braun, T.M., Min, L.C., 2019. Posthospital fall injuries and 30-day readmissions in adults 65 years and older. JAMA Netw. Open. 25743805. 2 (5). Available from: https://jamanetwork.com/journals/jamanetworkopen. doi:10.1001/jamanetworkopen.2019.4276.

Huang, S.Y., Chen, Y.C., Kao, Y.H., Hsieh, M.H., Lin, Y.K., Chen, S.A., Chen, Y.J., 2017. Redox and activation of protein kinase A dysregulates calcium homeostasis in pulmonary vein cardiomyocytes of chronic kidney disease. J. Am. Heart Assoc. 20479980. 6 (7). Available from: http://jaha.ahajournals.org/content/ahaoa/6/7/e005701full.pdf?download=true. doi:10.1161/JAHA.117.005701.

Jadczak, A.D., Makwana, N., Luscombe-Marsh, N., Visvanathan, R., Schultz, T.J., 2018. Effectiveness of exercise interventions on physical function in community-dwelling frail older people: an umbrella review of systematic reviews. JBI Database Syst. Rev. Implement. Rep. 22024433. 16 (3), 752–775. doi:10.11124/JBISRIR-2017-003551.

Jin, H., Zhou, Y., Stagg, B.C., Ehrlich, J.R., 2024. Association between vision impairment and increased prevalence of falls in older US adults. J. Am. Geriatr. Soc. 15325415. 72 (5), 1373–1383. Available from: http://onlinelibrary.wiley.com/journal/10.1111/(ISSN)1532-5415. doi:10.1111/jgs.18879.

Kessels, R.P.C., 2018. Application of Errorless Learning in Dementia Errorless Learning in Neuropsychological Rehabilitation: Mechanisms, Efficacy and Application. Taylor and Francis, Netherlands, pp. 82–100. Available from http://www.tandfebooks.com/doi/book/10.4324/9781315660738. doi:10.4324/9781315660738.

Kimura, A., Paredes, W., Pai, R., Farooq, H., Buttar, R.S., Custodio, M., Munugoti, S., Kotwani, S., Randhawa, L.S., Dalezman, S., Elters, A.C., Nam, K., Ibarra, J.S., Venkataraman, S., Abramowitz, M.K., 2022. Step length and fall risk in adults with chronic kidney disease: a pilot study. BMC Nephrol. 14712369. 23 (1). Available from: https://bmcnephrol.biomedcentral.com/. doi:10.1186/s12882-022-02706-w.

Li, Z., Wu, H., Yao, F., Li, Y., Li, Y., Xie, S.-A., Yu, F., Fu, Y., Wang, L., Zhou, J., Kong, W., 2025. Runx2-NLRP3 axis orchestrates matrix stiffness-evoked vascular smooth muscle cell inflammation. Am. J. Physiol. Cell Physiol. 0363-6143. 328 (2), C467. doi:10.1152/ajpcell.00448.2024.

Lin, M.E., Chen, T., Leaf, E.M., Speer, M.Y., Giachelli, C.M., 2015. Runx2 expression in smooth muscle cells is required for arterial medial calcification in mice. Am. J. Pathol. 15252191. 185 (7), 1958–1969. Available from: http://ajp.amjpathol.org/. doi:10.1016/j.ajpath.2015.03.020.

Lu, Z., Er, Y., Zhan, Y., Deng, X., Jin, Y., Pengpeng, Y., Duan, L., 2021. Association of frailty status with risk of fall among middle-aged and older adults in China: a nationally representative cohort study. J. Nutr. Health Aging. 12797707. 25 (8), 985–992. doi:10.1007/s12603-021-1655-x.

Mandt, S.R., Thadathil, N., Klem, C., Russ, C., McNamee, P.L., Stigge, K., Cheng, D., 2024. Apixaban use in patients with kidney impairment: a review of pharmacokinetic, interventional, and observational study data. Am. J. Cardiovasc. Drugs. 1179187X. 24 (5), 603–624. Available from: https://www.springer.com/journal/40256. doi:10.1007/s40256-024-00664-2.

Mattle, M., Chocano-Bedoya, P.O., Fischbacher, M., Meyer, U., Abderhalden, L.A., Lang, W., Mansky, R., Kressig, R.W., Steurer, J., Orav, E.J., Bischoff-Ferrari, H.A., 2020. Association of dance-based mind-motor activities with falls and physical function among healthy older adults: a systematic review and meta-analysis. JAMA Netw. Open. 25743805. 3 (9). Available from: https://jamanetwork.com/journals/jamanetworkopen. doi:10.1001/jamanetworkopen.2020.17688.

Menz, H.B., Latt, M.D., Tiedemann, A., Kwan, M.M.S., Lord, S.R., 2004. Reliability of the GAITRite® walkway system for the quantification of temporo-spatial parameters of gait in young and older people. Gait Posture 20 (1), 20–25. doi:10.1016/S0966-6362(03)00068-7.

Montagnani, A., Gonnelli, S., Alessandri, M., Nuti, R., 2011. Osteoporosis and risk of fracture in patients with diabetes: an update. Aging Clin. Exp. Res. 1594-0667. 23 (2), 84–90. doi:10.1007/bf03351073.

Moon, Y., Sosnoff, J.J., 2017. Safe landing strategies during a fall: systematic review and meta-analysis. Arch. Phys. Med. Rehabil. 1532821X. 98 (4), 783–794. Available from: http://www.elsevier.com/inca/publications/store/6/2/3/3/5/4/index.htt. doi:10.1016/j.apmr.2016.08.460.

Morse, J.M., Black, C., Oberle, K., Donahue, P., 1989. A prospective study to identify the fall-prone patient. Soc. Sci. Med. 02779536. 28 (1), 81–86. doi:10.1016/0277-9536(89)90309-2.

Noury, N., Poujaud, J., Cousin, P., Poujaud, N., 2016. Biomechanical analysis of a fall: velocities at impact. In: Proceedings of the Annual International Conference of the IEEE Engineering in Medicine and Biology Society, EMBS. Institute of Electrical and Electronics Engineers Inc., France, pp. 561–565. 9781457702204. doi:10.1109/EMBC.2016.7590764.

Papakonstantinopoulou, K., Sofianos, I., 2017. Risk of falls in chronic kidney disease. J. Frailty Sarcopenia Falls. 24594148. 02 (2), 33–38. doi:10.22540/JFSF-02-033.

Park, S.-H., 2018. Tools for assessing fall risk in the elderly: a systematic review and meta-analysis. Aging Clin. Exp. Res. 1720-8319. 30 (1), 1–16. doi:10.1007/s40520-017-0749-0.

Rodrigues, F., Domingos, C., Monteiro, D., Morouço, P., 2022. A review on aging, sarcopenia, falls, and resistance training in community-dwelling older adults. Int. J. Environ. Res. Public Health. 1660-4601. 19 (2), 874. doi:10.3390/ijerph19020874.

Shen, S., Xie, Y., Zeng, X., Chen, L., Guan, H., Yang, Y., Xiushao, W., Chen, X., 2023. Associations of intrinsic capacity, fall risk and frailty in old inpatients. Front. Public Health. 2296-2565. 11. doi:10.3389/fpubh.2023.1177812.

Shim, S., Yu, J.Y., Jekal, S., Song, Y.J., Moon, K.T., Lee, J.H., Yeom, K.M., Park, S.H., Cho, I.S., Song, M.R., Heo, S., Hong, J.H., 2022. Development and validation of interpretable machine learning models for inpatient fall events and electronic medical record integration. Clin. Exp. Emerg. Med. 23834625. 9 (4), 345–353. Available from: https://www.ceemjournal.org/upload/pdf/ceem-22-354.pdf. doi:10.15441/ceem.22.354.

Tran, J., Ayers, E., Verghese, J., Abramowitz, M.K., 2019. Gait abnormalities and the risk of falls in CKD. Clin. J. Am. Soc. Nephrol. 1555905X. 14 (7), 983–993. Available from: https://cjasn.asnjournals.org/content/14/7/983.full.pdf. doi:10.2215/CJN.13871118.

Tricco, A.C., Thomas, S.M., Veroniki, A.A., Hamid, J.S., Cogo, E., Strifler, L., Khan, P.A., Robson, R., Sibley, K.M., MacDonald, H., Riva, J.J., Thavorn, K., Wilson, C., Holroyd-Leduc, J., Kerr, G.D., Feldman, F., Majumdar, S.R., Jaglal, S.B., Hui, W., Straus, S.E., 2017. Comparisons of interventions for preventing falls in older adults: a systematic review and meta-analysis. JAMA. 15383598. 318 (17), 1687–1699. Available from: https://jamanetwork.com/journals/jama/articlepdf/2661578/jama_tricco_2017_oi_170119.pdf. doi:10.1001/jama.2017.15006.

Wang, H.H., Wu, J.L., Lee, Y.C., Ho, L.C., Chang, M.Y., Liou, H.H., Hung, S.Y., 2020. Risk of serious falls between hemodialysis and peritoneal dialysis patients: a nationwide population-based cohort study. Sci. Rep. 20452322. 10 (1). Available from: www.nature.com/srep/index.html. doi:10.1038/s41598-020-64698-7.

Wathanavasin, W., Banjongjit, A., Avihingsanon, Y., Praditpornsilpa, K., Tungsanga, K., Eiam-Ong, S., Susantitaphong, P., 2022. Prevalence of sarcopenia and its impact on cardiovascular events and mortality among dialysis patients: a systematic review and meta-analysis. Nutrients. 20726643. 14 (19). Available from: http://www.mdpi.com/journal/nutrients/. doi:10.3390/nu14194077.

Yang, Y., Schonnop, R., Feldman, F., Robinovitch, S.N., 2013. Development and validation of a questionnaire for analyzing real-life falls in long-term care captured on video. BMC Geriatr. 14712318. 13 (1). doi:10.1186/1471-2318-13-40.

Yang, Y., Komisar, V., Shishov, N., Lo, B., Korall, A.M.B., Feldman, F., Robinovitch, S.N., 2020. The effect of fall biomechanics on risk for hip fracture in older adults: a cohort study of video-captured falls in long-term care. J. Bone Miner. Res. 15234681. 35 (10), 1914–1922. Available from: http://onlinelibrary.wiley.com/journal/10.1002/(ISSN)1523-4681. doi:10.1002/jbmr.4048.

Yau, R.K., Strotmeyer, E.S., Resnick, H.E., Sellmeyer, D.E., Feingold, K.R., Cauley, J.A., Vittinghoff, E., De Rekeneire, N., Harris, T.B., Nevitt, M.C., Cummings, S.R., Shorr, R.I., Schwartz, A.V., 2013. Diabetes and risk of hospitalized fall injury among older adults. Diabetes Care. 0149-5992. 36 (12), 3985–3991. doi:10.2337/dc13-0429.

Yeung, S.S.Y., Reijnierse, E.M., Pham, V.K., Trappenburg, M.C., Lim, W.K., Meskers, C.G.M., Maier, A.B., 2019. Sarcopenia and its association with falls and fractures in older adults: a systematic review and meta-analysis. J. Cachexia Sarcopenia Muscle. 21906009. 10 (3), 485–500. Available from: http://onlinelibrary.wiley.com/journal/10.1007/13539.2190-6009. doi:10.1002/jcsm.12411.

Yu, W.-Y., Hwang, H.-F., Chen, C.-Y., Lin, M.-R., 2021. Situational risk factors for fall-related vertebral fractures in older men and women. Osteoporos. Int. 0937-941X. 32 (6), 1061–1070. doi:10.1007/s00198-020-05799-x.

Yuan, S., Larsson, S.C., 2023. Epidemiology of sarcopenia: prevalence, risk factors, and consequences. Metabolism. 15328600. 144. Available from: http://www.elsevier.com/inca/publications/store/6/2/3/3/1/9/index.htt. doi:10.1016/j.metabol.2023.155533.

CHAPTER

12

Fatigue and frailty in kidney disease

Totini Sagorika Chatterjee[a,b] *and Lucile Parker Gregg*[c,d]

[a]Division of Geriatrics, Department of Medicine, University of Texas Medical Branch, Galveston, TX, United States

[b]Division of Nephrology, Department of Medicine, University of Texas Medical Branch, Galveston, TX, United States

[c]Medicine, Selzman Institute for Kidney Health, Baylor College of Medicine, Houston, TX, United States

[d]Center for Innovations in Quality, Effectiveness and Safety, Michael E. DeBakey VA Medical Center, Houston, TX, United States

Introduction

Understanding fatigue and frailty is crucial for providing patient-centered, comprehensive care for older adults with kidney diseases. Fatigue is a heterogeneous symptom complex that can occur in clusters with other symptoms and profoundly impact life participation. It can be severe in quality, duration, or intensity and is typically one of the patients' chief concerns. Among older adults, frailty is a key fatigue syndrome to recognize, as this has implications for patients' long-term outcomes. Kidney disease itself has several direct effects that can contribute to fatigue and frailty. This chapter discusses frailty in people with kidney diseases and management strategies for fatigue and frailty that may help improve quality of life.

Epidemiology

Frailty is a common clinical syndrome in older adults that carries an increased risk for poor health outcomes, including falls, incident disability, hospitalization, and mortality (Xue, 2011). It is a multisystem syndrome manifesting as a decline in physiologic reserve and an increased risk for adverse clinical outcomes (Nair et al., 2025; Fried et al., 2001; Rockwood et al., 2005). Several factors are associated with frailty, including decreased glomerular filtration rate, older age, female sex, higher waist circumference, increased multimorbidity, depressive symptoms, and diabetes mellitus (Lorenz et al., 2021; Chang et al., 2022).

This clinical syndrome is highly prevalent in both the older adult population and the population with kidney disease, with kidney disease itself serving as a potent driver of frailty

Aging and the Kidney
https://doi.org/10.1016/B978-0-443-34069-7.00016-1

starting even at younger chronological ages. Although studies have used different measurement criteria to define frailty, generally the prevalence ranges from 14% to 40% among people with nondialysis chronic kidney disease (CKD), 31%–82% of people with kidney failure on hemodialysis (HD), and 14%–69% of people with kidney failure on peritoneal dialysis (PD) (Nair et al., 2025; Lorenz et al., 2021).

Frailty has important clinical implications for people with kidney disease, including an increased risk of mortality, atherosclerotic cardiovascular disease events, and incident heart failure (Hannan et al., 2024). Among individuals with kidney failure on HD, frailty is associated with complications, including elevated inflammatory biomarkers, intradialytic hypotension, increased time to arteriovenous fistula (AVF) use, delayed AVF maturation, and AVF thrombosis (Nair et al., 2025; Joseph et al., 2023; Chan et al., 2024; Woo et al., 2022; Luo et al., 2022; Chao et al., 2017). When experiencing vascular access-related complications, these patients often require temporary dialysis catheters, which put them at risk for bacteremia. Among kidney transplant recipients, frailty is associated with an increased risk of delayed graft function, longer hospital stays, 30-day rehospitalization, and infections (Quint et al., 2021; Chen et al., 2025; Lorenz et al., 2024c).

Diagnosis

Although many instruments exist to identify frailty, there is currently no consensus on which instrument is best to use among people with kidney disease. One of the tools most frequently used in geriatrics to assess a patient in a holistic manner is the comprehensive geriatric assessment (Parker et al., 2018; Turner and Clegg, 2014). This framework involves a multidisciplinary team to first determine impairments in a variety of domains, including medical, psychosocial, and functional. This approach emphasizes the 4 Ms: Medications, Mobility, Mind, and what Matters most to the patient (Molnar and Frank, 2019). A fifth M, included by many, is Multicomplexity, which is pertinent to people with kidney disease who often have multiple medical comorbidities (Molnar and Frank, 2019). The comprehensive geriatric assessment focuses on detecting and managing impairments in each of these domains that lead to frailty (Pilotto et al., 2020). An ongoing clinical trial, Comprehensive Geriatric Assessment for Frail Older People with CKD (GOAL), is examining whether incorporating the comprehensive geriatric assessment in an older adult population with CKD and frailty improves patients' ability to achieve their self-identified goals at 3 months (clinicaltrials.gov NCT04538157) (Logan et al., 2023). In general, this is a more comprehensive way to recognize frailty and is considered relevant to integrate into CKD care (Voorend et al., 2024).

However, a comprehensive geriatric assessment requires time and additional training and may be challenging to incorporate into a nephrology practice. Many other instruments are available, each with unique advantages and disadvantages (Table 12.1) (Nair et al., 2025). There is significant variability between available instruments in terms of what data are required (e.g., self-report, medical record review, objective measurements, or some combination of these) and in the identification of frailty. Some instruments include physical performance tests, such as grip strength measurement or gait speed, which may require additional training, space, or equipment to perform. It is important to standardize measures within a clinical setting, as there is high variability between instruments, and consistency is important to monitor patients' progress over time.

TABLE 12.1 Advantages and disadvantages of frailty instruments that have been used for people with CKD or kidney failure on dialysis.

Instrument	No. of items	Advantages	Disadvantages
Clinical Frailty Scale (Rockwood et al., 2005)	7	Brief, incorporates ADLs	Subjective assessment
Edmonton Frail Scale (Rolfson et al., 2006)	11	Incorporates multiple domains	Based entirely on self-report
FRAIL scale (Abellan van Kan et al., 2008)	5	Brief, can be administered by MSA or RN prior to the clinic visit	Based entirely on self-report
Frailty Index (Rockwood et al., 2017)	70	More comprehensive, extensively validated, and incorporates patient-reported and clinical conditions	Long
Frailty Index—CKD (Hubbard et al., 2015)	58	Specifically developed for people with CKD	Long, based on self-reports and medical record reviews
Frailty Index for Dialysis (Hall et al., 2022)	53	Specifically developed for people with kidney failure on dialysis	Based on medical record review
Hospital Frailty Risk Score (Gilbert et al., 2018)	99	Potentially automatable in the electronic health record	Based on ICD-10 codes
Laboratory Index for Dialysis (Chao et al., 2020)	34	Developed for people with kidney failure on dialysis, it incorporates blood tests and vital signs	Longer
Physical frailty phenotype (Fried et al., 2001)	5	Brief, extensively validated, incorporates patient-reported symptoms and objective measurements	Requires some specialized equipment
PRISMA-7 (Raîche et al., 2008)	7	Brief, incorporates ADLs	Based entirely on self-report
Study of Osteoporotic Fractures Index (Ensrud et al., 2008)	3	Brief, can be administered by MSA or RN prior to the clinic visit	Based entirely on self-report
Tilburg Frailty Indicator (Gobbens et al., 2010)	10	Brief, incorporates multiple domains	Based entirely on self-report

Abbreviations: *ADLs*, activities of daily living; *FRAIL*, fatigue, resistance, ambulation, illnesses, loss of weight; *ICD-10*, International Classification of Diseases, 10th Revision; *PRISMA-7*, Program on Research for Integrating Services for the Maintenance of Autonomy-7.

Pathophysiology

People with kidney disease have high rates of factors known to be associated with frailty, such as older chronological age, cognitive impairment, multimorbidity, and depressive symptoms. However, the pathophysiology of frailty also includes reduced energy intake and protein-energy wasting, decreased physical activity, and the direct effects of kidney disease (Fig. 12.1).

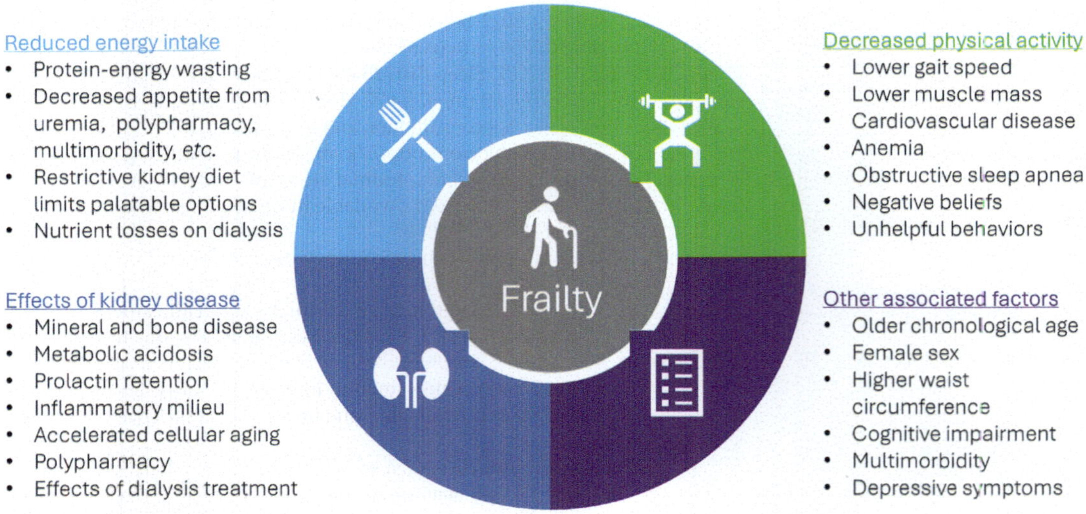

FIG. 12.1 Factors contributing to frailty in people with kidney diseases.

Reduced energy intake and protein-energy wasting

As kidney function worsens, a natural decline in food intake occurs. Medications, uremic toxins, inflammation, metabolic acidosis, and comorbid illnesses contribute to anorexia, which is prevalent in approximately 44% of people with kidney failure on dialysis (Rhee et al., 2020; Tseng et al., 2024; Kalantar-Zadeh et al., 2004). The restrictive diet prescribed to people with advanced CKD or kidney failure may leave them with few options they enjoy, particularly options that limit phosphorus intake while maintaining adequate protein intake. Among older adults with CKD, higher intake of total, animal, and plant-based protein was associated with lower mortality but not with estimated glomerular filtration rate (eGFR) decline (Carballo-Casla et al., 2024; Sekiguchi et al., 2022). Other causes of protein-energy wasting include catabolic stress and chronic nutrient loss from the dialysis procedure (Kim et al., 2013). About 6–12 g of amino acids and 7–8 g of protein are lost during each HD session, contributing to hypoalbuminemia, which is a strong predictor of malnutrition and mortality (Sahathevan et al., 2020).

Decreased physical activity

Physical activity decreases with both aging and kidney disease, attributed in part to muscle atrophy and other physiological processes of natural aging. This can contribute to worsening frailty *via* reduced lean body mass and sarcopenia (Nixon et al., 2018; Johansen et al., 2000, 2010; Bowlby et al., 2016; Beddhu et al., 2009; Majchrzak et al., 2007). People with CKD are more likely to have a reduced exercise capacity, at least in part due to anemia, mineral bone disease, cardiovascular disease, obstructive sleep apnea, and polypharmacy (Gregg et al., 2021b; Odden et al., 2004). There is also a psychological component to physical activity, such that depression, stress, negative beliefs about fatigue, and unhelpful behaviors may also contribute to low physical activity (Picariello et al., 2018). The severity of CKD is associated with quantitative gait abnormalities, such as shorter stride length, less time in the swing phase, and more time in double support, which may lead to a higher fall risk and decreases in physical activity (Tran et al., 2019). Clinicians can incorporate a visual gait assessment when walking patients in and out of the office. The timed up-and-go test is another quick screen that can easily be employed in an office visit to assess mobility.

Effects of kidney disease

Complications of CKD and kidney failure also contribute to accelerated aging, fatigue, and frailty. CKD mineral and bone disease causes increased skeletal remodeling (Hruska et al., 2008). Bone resorption exceeding new bone formation has implications for bone strength and mass, and ultimately, mobility. Vitamin D insufficiency is associated with frailty and poorer physical performance among adults with CKD and may affect contractile muscle function and muscle size (Gordon et al., 2012). However, this relationship may be less pronounced among older adults, in whom the association between vitamin D or parathyroid hormone levels with muscle mass or strength is not consistent (Marantes et al., 2011).

Metabolic acidosis is associated with poorer physical functioning in older adults (Yenchek et al., 2014). Chronic metabolic acidosis activates ubiquitin protein ligases, which inhibit intracellular signaling of insulin and insulin-like growth factor-1 (Reaich et al., 1995; Raphael, 2019). This process increases muscle protein breakdown, adrenal gland glucocorticoid production, and protein catabolism, contributing to sarcopenia (Zhang et al., 2010).

Hypogonadism is another consequence of kidney disease that may contribute to frailty. Prolactin retention in the setting of kidney disease can impair the production of gonadotropic hormones such as testosterone, which is an anabolic hormone essential in muscle protein synthesis. Testosterone deficiency is present in up to 77% of men with kidney failure on dialysis and is independently associated with lower muscle mass and strength (Nixon et al., 2018; Cigarrán et al., 2013).

Changes associated with premature aging are observed at the biochemical level, including cellular senescence, loss of telomeric structures, mitochondrial dysfunction, increased free radical production, and poor DNA repair capability, and these occur prematurely in people with CKD (Lorenz et al., 2023a, 2024a). Uremic toxins, including advanced glycation end products, accumulate in the setting of CKD due to increased generation and decreased clearance (Zhao et al., 2022). This contributes to increased production of reactive oxygen species, which damage cells and affect tissue function. Senescent cells secrete cytokines, chemokines, growth factors, and other proteins, which are associated with age, frailty, and adverse health outcomes in people with chronic disease (Lorenz et al., 2021).

Iatrogenic treatments can also directly contribute to frailty through multiple mechanisms. Multimorbidity and polypharmacy are common in people with kidney disease and are associated with frailty, possibly due in part to an increased absolute risk of drug-related adverse effects (Mayne et al., 2024). The time commitment and fatigue associated with HD may be potent barriers to physical activity. The cardiovascular effects of dialysis treatments, such as intradialytic hypotension, are associated with frailty among older adults (Joseph et al., 2023). PD contributes to the accumulation of advanced glycated end-products in blood vessels, muscles, tendons, and cartilage, resulting in endothelial dysfunction and muscle and joint stiffness (Chan et al., 2024). Exposure to glucose-containing dialyzate can lead to adverse metabolic effects, including obesity and insulin resistance, further worsening frailty (Chan et al., 2024).

Management

Few studies have assessed management strategies for frailty among people with kidney disease, but key concepts of management can be extrapolated from studies in the general population (Nair et al., 2025). The management of frailty focuses on a comprehensive, individualized approach that addresses multiple contributing factors. Because frailty is multifactorial, management requires attention to multiple domains, including medical, cognitive, physical, and psychosocial. Given that frailty and its risk factors are dynamic conditions, they need to be repeatedly assessed. Treatment strategies for frailty and fatigue in people with kidney disease are summarized in Fig. 12.2.

Kidney transplantation

Frailty is considered part of a comprehensive assessment of a patient's candidacy for kidney transplantation. In one study, up to 50% of kidney transplant recipients had a degree

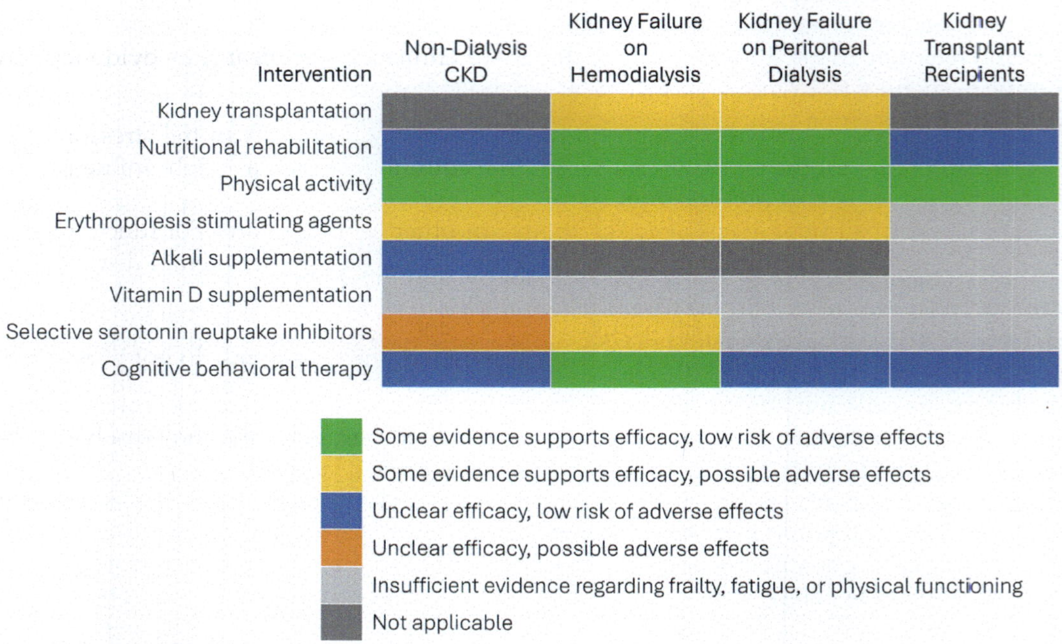

FIG. 12.2 Evidence supporting the management of fatigue and frailty in people with kidney diseases. This figure highlights areas where there is evidence-based therapy for fatigue and frailty management in predialysis CKD, hemodialysis, peritoneal dialysis, and transplantation.

of frailty, and 20% were overtly frail (McAdams-DeMarco et al., 2015). Despite a risk of worsening frailty in the immediate posttransplant period, this generally improves by 3 months posttransplant (McAdams-DeMarco et al., 2015; Bevan et al., 2025). Some proposed mechanisms include the restoration of kidney function, improved appetite, and increased physical activity due to the termination of dialysis and improved quality of life (McAdams-DeMarco et al., 2015). Some people may benefit from comprehensive geriatric assessment-based recommendations to improve their frailty status prior to transplantation (Alfieri et al., 2022).

Nutritional rehabilitation

Nutritional rehabilitation programs focusing on increased calorie or protein intake are another potential way to modify frailty and protein-energy wasting (Ikizler et al., 2013). Kidney Disease: Improving Global Outcomes (KDIGO) guidelines reflect that older adults with frailty may benefit from higher protein and calorie targets and generally emphasize plant-based, as opposed to animal-based, sources of protein, as higher plant-based protein intake has been associated with slower decline in eGFR and lower risk of death in observational studies (**Kidney Disease: Improving Global Outcomes work Group, 2024**). Dietary recommendations should be individualized whenever possible; for example, if a patient has hypoalbuminemia or sarcopenia but no hyperkalemia or hyperphosphatemia, a more liberalized diet aimed toward overall nutrition and higher protein intake may be reasonable. Dietary protein supplements may also help people with frailty (Ikizler et al., 2020). In one study of people with kidney failure on HD with hypoalbuminemia, oral nutritional supplementation was associated with higher albumin at 6 months and an approximately 20 percentage point lower rate of hospitalization within 1 year, but no difference in all-cause mortality (Cheu et al., 2013).

Physical activity

Lower physical activity and higher sedentary time are important, potentially modifiable mechanisms of frailty among people with kidney disease, with many studies showing the benefit of exercise on frailty, fatigue scores, or measures of physical functioning such as the 6-min walk test (Anding et al., 2015; Bennett et al., 2016; Chen et al., 2010; Greenwood et al., 2019; Heiwe and Jacobson, 2014; Hellberg et al., 2019; Koh et al., 2010; Lorenz et al., 2020; Mallamaci et al., 2020; Manfredini et al., 2017; Rossi et al., 2014; Sheshadri et al., 2020; Nixon et al., 2021). For example, one pilot randomized trial in 35 older adults with CKD and frailty showed that home-based exercise led to a perception of improved fitness, balance, strength, and energy levels, among other qualitative benefits (Nixon et al., 2021). Another trial of 50 individuals with kidney failure on HD showed that intra-dialytic low-intensity strength training improved physical performance compared to an attention control group focused on stretching (Chen et al., 2010). Prehabilitation in anticipation of receiving a kidney transplant may improve frailty (Lorenz et al., 2020; 2023b). Physical activity has been shown to be safe and beneficial for fatigue and frailty compared to baseline measures (Lorenz et al., 2023b, 2024b). Despite these promising data, larger trials are needed to demonstrate a definitive impact of physical activity on frailty scores.

Studies have used variable exercise regimens, including home-based, intra-dialytic, and supervised interventions, as well as aerobic exercise and strength training, and there is currently no consensus about the best or most effective recommendations. A focus on activities that are sustainable, individualized, and enjoyable to the patient may help increase adherence. While physical activity should be recommended routinely, special attention should be paid to feasibility. Individualized recommendations should be made to increase physical activity, particularly when a structured exercise regimen is unavailable.

Management of kidney disease complications

Sodium-glucose co-transporter 2 inhibitors have become the standard of care for most people with CKD. These agents decrease the risk of kidney disease progression and cardiovascular events, with the greatest benefits observed in those at the highest risk of frailty (Mayne et al., 2024). Kidney disease also has many modifiable complications that can contribute directly to decreased physical activity and fatigue, and thus likely frailty. Although data on the direct impact of managing these conditions on frailty are not well established, they may generally contribute to a person's overall energy level or physical functioning. The treatment of metabolic acidosis with alkali supplementation may improve muscle strength (Abramowitz et al., 2013; De Brito-Ashurst et al., 2009; Dubey et al., 2020). The management of CKD mineral and bone disease with vitamin D supplementation has less clear effects on muscle strength, physical functioning, or fatigue (Westerberg et al., 2018; Taskapan et al., 2011). Treating anemia with erythropoiesis-stimulating agents may have small effects on fatigue, although potential benefits to fatigue must be weighed against the risk of adverse cardiovascular effects (Drüeke et al., 2006; Pfeffer et al., 2009).

Management of comorbidities

Blood pressure goals for frail older adults may be adjusted based on factors such as orthostatic hypotension, the ability to complete activities of daily living, and life expectancy (Benetos et al., 2019). Depressive symptoms may contribute to fatigue and can be managed with cognitive behavioral therapy, with or without a cautious trial of a selective serotonin reuptake inhibitor (Gregg et al., 2021a). Polypharmacy is also a key consideration in the management of comorbidities in people with kidney diseases. The benefits and risks of each treatment should be weighed, and clinicians may consider deprescribing agents that are no longer necessary. This can be tailored to a patient's expected lifespan; for example, statins have important long-term benefits, but these may not outweigh polypharmacy concerns in a person with a limited expected lifespan (Triantafylidis et al., 2018).

Conclusions

Fatigue and frailty are primary concerns for older adults with kidney diseases, including those with nondialysis CKD, kidney failure on dialysis, and kidney transplant recipients. Effectively addressing this requires a holistic and comprehensive approach to the patient's care, including attentiveness to nutrition, complications of kidney diseases, and management of comorbidities. Physical activity should be recommended through shared decision-making with the patient to tailor a unique plan that will be feasible, enjoyable, and sustainable for the patient.

Acknowledgments

The opinions expressed reflect those of the authors and not necessarily those of the Department of Veterans Affairs or the US government.

Funding

LPG is supported by a VA Clinical Sciences Research and Development Career Development Award (IK2CX002368). This work was supported, in part, by the Houston VA Health Services Research and Development Center for Innovations grant (CIN13-413).

Disclosures

LPG served as an editorial fellow for the Journal of the American Society of Nephrology and receives research funding from Calliditas Therapeutics and the Texas Health Resources Foundation outside of this work. TSC has nothing to disclose.

References

Abellan van Kan, G.A., Rolland, Y.M., Morley, J.E., Vellas, B., 2008. Frailty: toward a clinical definition. J. Am. Med. Dir. Assoc. 9 (2), 71–72. doi:10.1016/j.jamda.2007.11.005.

Abramowitz, M.K., Melamed, M.L., Bauer, C., Raff, A.C., Hostetter, T.H., 2013. Effects of oral sodium bicarbonate in patients with CKD. Clin. J. Am. Soc. Nephrol. 1555905X. 8 (5), 714–720. Available from: http://cjasn.asnjournals.org/content/8/5/714.full.pdf+html. doi:10.2215/CJN.08340812.

Alfieri, C., Malvica, S., Cesari, M., Vettoretti, S., Benedetti, M., Cicero, E., Miglio, R., Caldiroli, L., Perna, A., Cervesato, A., Castellano, G., 2022. Frailty in kidney transplantation: a review on its evaluation, variation and long-term impact. Clin. Kidney J. 2048-8505. 15 (11), 2020–2026. doi:10.1093/ckj/sfac149.

Anding, K., Bär, T., Trojniak-Hennig, J., Kuchinke, S., Krause, R., Rost, J.M., Halle, M., 2015. A structured exercise programme during haemodialysis for patients with chronic kidney disease: clinical benefit and long-term adherence. BMJ Open. 20446055. 5 (8). Available from: http://bmjopen.bmj.com/content/5/8/e008709full.pdf+html. doi:10.1136/bmjopen-2015-008709.

Beddhu, S., Baird, B.C., Zitterkoph, J., Neilson, J., Greene, T., 2009. Physical activity and mortality in chronic kidney disease (NHANES III). Clin. J. Am. Soc. Nephrol. 1555905X. 4 (12), 1901–1906. Available from: http://cjasn.asnjournals.org/cgi/reprint/4/12/1901. doi:10.2215/CJN.01970309.

Benetos, A., Petrovic, M., Strandberg, T., 2019. Hypertension management in older and frail older patients. Circ. Res. 0009-7330. 124 (7), 1045–1060. doi:10.1161/circresaha.118.313236.

Bennett, P.N., Fraser, S., Barnard, R., Haines, T., Ockerby, C., Street, M., Wang, W.C., Daly, R., 2016. Effects of an intradialytic resistance training programme on physical function: a prospective stepped-wedge randomized controlled trial. Nephrol. Dial. Transplant. 14602385. 31 (8), 1302–1309. Available from: http://ndt.oxfordjournals.org/. doi:10.1093/ndt/gfv416.

Bevan, A., Avery, J., Cheah, H.L., Carter, B., Hewitt, J., 2025. Change in frailty status in the 12 months following solid organ transplantation: a systematic review and meta-analysis. Age Ageing. 14682834. 54 (1). Available from: http://ageing.oxfordjournals.org/. doi:10.1093/ageing/afae283.

Bowlby, W., Zelnick, L.R., Henry, C., Himmelfarb, J., Kahn, S.E., Kestenbaum, B., Robinson-Cohen, C., Utzschneider, K.M., De Boer, I.H., 2016. Physical activity and metabolic health in chronic kidney disease: a cross-sectional study.

BMC Nephrol. 14712369. 17 (1), 1–9. Available from: http://www.biomedcentral.com/bmcnephrol/. doi:10.1186/s12882-016-0400-x.

Carballo-Casla, A., Avesani, C.M., Beridze, G., Ortolá, R., García-Esquinas, E., Lopez-Garcia, E., Dai, L., Dunk, M.M., Stenvinkel, P., Lindholm, B., Carrero, J.J., Rodríguez-Artalejo, F., Vetrano, D.L., Calderón-Larrañaga, A., 2024. Protein intake and mortality in older adults with chronic kidney disease. JAMA Netw. Open. 25743805. 7 (8), e2426577. Available from: https://jamanetwork.com/journals/jamanetworkopen. doi:10.1001/jamanetworkopen.2024.26577.

Chan, G.C.K., Kalantar-Zadeh, K., Ng, J.K.C., Tian, N., Burns, A., Chow, K.M., Szeto, C.C., Li, P.K.T., 2024. Frailty in patients on dialysis. Kidney Int. 15231755. 106 (1), 35–49. Available from: https://www.sciencedirect.com/science/journal/00852538. doi:10.1016/j.kint.2024.02.026.

Chang, J., Hou, W., Yanchun, L., Shujuan, L., Zhao, K., Wang, Y., Hou, Y., Sun, Q., 2022. Prevalence and associated factors of cognitive frailty in older patients with chronic kidney disease: a cross-sectional study. BMC Geriatr. 1471-2318. 22 (1). doi:10.1186/s12877-022-03366-z.

Chao, C.T., Chiang, C.K., Huang, J.W., Hung, K.Y., 2017. Self-reported frailty among end-stage renal disease patients: a potential predictor of dialysis access outcomes. Nephrology. 14401797. 22 (4), 333–334. Available from: http://onlinelibrary.wiley.com/journal/10.1111/(ISSN)1440-1797. doi:10.1111/nep.12961.

Chao, C.T., Huang, J.W., Chiang, C.K., Hung, K.Y., 2020. Applicability of laboratory deficit-based frailty index in predominantly older patients with end-stage renal disease under chronic dialysis: a pilot test of its correlation with survival and self-reported instruments. Nephrology. 14401797. 25 (1), 73–81. Available from: http://onlinelibrary.wiley.com/journal/10.1111/(ISSN)1440-1797. doi:10.1111/nep.13583.

Chen, J.L.T., Godfrey, S., Ng, T.T., Moorthi, R., Liangos, O., Ruthazer, R., Jaber, B.L., Levey, A.S., Castaneda-Sceppa, C., 2010. Effect of intra-dialytic, low-intensity strength training on functional capacity in adult haemodialysis patients: a randomized pilot trial. Nephrol. Dial. Transplant. 14602385. 25 (6), 1936–1943. doi:10.1093/ndt/gfp739.

Chen, L., Chu, F., Hangbin, M., Chen, Z., Yuning, M., Qiwei, J., Zhou, H., 2025. Hospital frailty risk score predicts graft failure severe infection and mortality in hospitalized kidney transplant recipients from 2010 to 2018 US data. Sci. Rep. 2045-2322. 15 (1). doi:10.1038/s41598-025-85482-5.

Cheu, C., Pearson, J., Dahlerus, C., Lantz, B., Chowdhury, T., Sauer, P.F., Farrell, R.E., Port, F.K., Ramirez, S.P.B., 2013. Association between oral nutritional supplementation and clinical outcomes among patients with ESRD. Clin. J. Am. Soc. Nephrol. 1555905X. 8 (1), 100–107. Available from: http://cjasn.asnjournals.org/content/8/1/100.full.pdf+html. doi:10.2215/CJN.13091211.

Cigarrán, S., Pousa, M., Castro, M.J., González, B., Martínez, A., Barril, G., Aguilera, A., Coronel, F., Stenvinkel, P., Carrero, J.J., 2013. Endogenous testosterone, muscle strength, and fat-free mass in men with chronic kidney disease. J. Ren. Nutr. 10512276. 23 (5), e89. doi:10.1053/j.jrn.2012.08.007.

De Brito-Ashurst, I., Varagunam, M., Raftery, M.J., Yaqoob, M.M., 2009. Bicarbonate supplementation slows progression of CKD and improves nutritional status. J. Am. Soc. Nephrol. 15333450. 20 (9), 2075–2084. Available from: http://jasn.asnjournals.org/cgi/reprint/20/9/2075. doi:10.1681/ASN.2008111205.

Drüeke, T.B., Locatelli, F., Clyne, N., Eckardt, K.U., Macdougall, I.C., Tsakiris, D., Burger, H.U., Scherhag, A., 2006. Normalization of hemoglobin level in patients with chronic kidney disease and anemia. N. Engl. J. Med. 15334406. 355 (20), 2071–2084. Available from: http://content.nejm.org/cgi/reprint/355/20/2071.pdf. doi:10.1056/NEJMoa062276France.

Dubey, A.K., Sahoo, J., Vairappan, B., Haridasan, S., Parameswaran, S., Priyamvada, P.S., 2020. Correction of metabolic acidosis improves muscle mass and renal function in chronic kidney disease stages 3 and 4: a randomized controlled trial. Nephrol. Dial. Transplant. 14602385. 35 (1), 121–129. Available from: http://ndt.oxfordjournals.org/. doi:10.1093/ndt/gfy214.

Ensrud, K.E., Ewing, S.K., Taylor, B.C., Fink, H.A., Cawthon, P.M., Stone, K.L., Hillier, T.A., Cauley, J.A., Hochberg, M.C., Rodondi, N., Tracy, J.K., Cummings, S.R., 2008. Comparison of 2 frailty indexes for prediction of falls, disability, fractures, and death in older women. Arch. Intern. Med. 15383679. 168 (4), 382–389. Available from: http://archinte.ama-assn.org/cgi/reprint/168/4/382. doi:10.1001/archinternmed.2007.113.

Fried, L.P., Tangen, C.M., Walston, J., Newman, A.B., Hirsch, C., Gottdiener, J., Seeman, T., Tracy, R., Kop, W.J., Burke, G., McBurnie, M.A., 2001. Frailty in older adults: evidence for a phenotype. J. Gerontol. A Biol. Sci. Med. Sci. 10795006. 56 (3), M146. Available from: http://biomedgerontology.oxfordjournals.org/. doi:10.1093/gerona/56.3.m146.

Gilbert, T., Neuburger, J., Kraindler, J., Keeble, E., Smith, P., Ariti, C., Arora, S., Street, A., Parker, S., Roberts, H.C., Bardsley, M., Conroy, S., 2018. Development and validation of a hospital frailty risk score focusing on older people in acute care settings using electronic hospital records: an observational study. Lancet. 1474547X.

391 (10132), 1775–1782. Available from: http://www.journals.elsevier.com/the-lancet/. doi:10.1016/S0140-6736(18)30668-8.

Gobbens, R.J.J., van Assen, M.A.L.M., Luijkx, K.G., Wijnen-Sponselee, M.T., Schols, J.M.G.A., 2010. The tilburg frailty indicator: psychometric properties. J. Am. Med. Dir. Assoc. 15389375. 11 (5), 344–355. doi:10.1016/j.jamda.2009.11.003.

Gordon, P.L., Doyle, J.W., Johansen, K.L., 2012. Association of 1,25-dihydroxyvitamin D levels with physical performance and thigh muscle cross-sectional area in chronic kidney disease stage 3 and 4. J. Ren. Nutr. 22 (4), 423–433. doi:10.1053/j.jrn.2011.10.006.

Greenwood, S.A., Castle, E., Lindup, H., Mayes, J., Waite, I., Grant, D., Mangahis, E., Crabb, O., Shevket, K., Macdougall, I.C., Maclaughlin, H.L., 2019. Mortality and morbidity following exercise-based renal rehabilitation in patients with chronic kidney disease: the effect of programme completion and change in exercise capacity. Nephrol. Dial. Transplant. 14602385. 34 (4), 618–625. Available from: http://ndt.oxfordjournals.org/. doi:10.1093/ndt/gfy351.

Gregg, L.P., Bossola, M., Mauricio Ostrosky-Frid, S.S.H., 2021b. Fatigue in CKD: epidemiology, pathophysiology, and treatment. Clin. J. Am. Soc. Nephrol. 16 (9), 1445–1455. doi:10.2215/CJN.19891220.

Gregg, L.P., Trombello, J.M., Meredith Mcadams, S.S.H., 2021a. Diagnosis and management of depression in patients with kidney disease. Semin. Nephrol. 41 (6), 505–515.

Hall, R.K., Morton, S., Wilson, J., Kim, D.H., Colón-Emeric, C., Scialla, J.J., Platt, A., Ephraim, P.L., Boulware, L.E., 2022. Development of an administrative data-based frailty index for older adults receiving dialysis. Kidney360. 26417650. 3 (9), 1566–1577. Available from: https://kidney360.asnjournals.org/. doi:10.34067/KID.0000032022.

Hannan, M., Chen, J., Hsu, J., Zhang, X., Saunders, M.R., Brown, J., McAdams-DeMarco, M., Mohanty, M.J., Vyas, R., Hajjiri, Z., Carmona-Powell, E., Meza, N., Porter, A.C., Ricardo, A.C., Lash, J.P., Chen, J., Cohen, D.L., Feldman, H.I., Go, A.S., Nelson, R.G., Rahman, M., Rao, P.S., Shah, V.O., Unruh, M.L., 2024. Frailty and cardiovascular outcomes in adults with CKD: findings from the chronic renal insufficiency cohort (CRIC) study. Am. J. Kidney Dis. 15236838. 83 (2), 208–215. Available from: https://www.sciencedirect.com/science/journal/02726386. doi:10.1053/j.ajkd.2023.06.009.

Heiwe, S., Jacobson, S.H., 2014. Exercise training in adults with CKD: a systematic review and meta-analysis. Am. J. Kidney Dis. 15236838. 64 (3), 383–393. Available from: http://www.elsevier.com/inca/publications/store/6/2/3/2/7/6/index.htt. doi:10.1053/j.ajkd.2014.03.020.

Hellberg, M., Höglund, P., Svensson, P., Clyne, N., 2019. Randomized controlled trial of exercise in CKD—the RENEXC study. Kidney Int. Rep. 24680249. 4 (7), 963–976. Available from: http://www.journals.elsevier.com/kidney-international-reports. doi:10.1016/j.ekir.2019.04.001.

Hruska, K.A., Mathew, S., Lund, R., Qiu, P., Pratt, R., 2008. Hyperphosphatemia of chronic kidney disease. Kidney Int. 15231755. 74 (2), 148–157. Available from: https://www.journals.elsevier.com/kidney-international. doi:10.1038/ki.2008.130.

Hubbard, R.E., Peel, N.M., Smith, M., Dawson, B., Lambat, Z., Bak, M., Best, J., Johnson, D.W., 2015. Feasibility and construct validity of a Frailty index for patients with chronic kidney disease. Australas. J. Ageing. 17416612. 34 (3), E9. Available from: http://onlinelibrary.wiley.com/journal/10.1111/(ISSN)1741-6612. doi:10.1111/ajag.12231Australia.

Ikizler, T.A., Burrowes, J.D., Byham-Gray, L.D., Campbell, K.L., Carrero, J.J., Chan, W., Fouque, D., Friedman, A.N., Ghaddar, S., Goldstein-Fuchs, D.J., Kaysen, G.A., Kopple, J.D., Teta, D., Wang, A.Y.-M., Cuppari, L., 2020. KDOQI clinical practice guideline for nutrition in CKD: 2020 update. Am. J. Kidney Dis. 15236838. 76 (3), S1. Available from: http://www.elsevier.com/inca/publications/store/6/2/3/2/7/6/index.htt. doi:10.1053/j.ajkd.2020.05.006.

Ikizler, T.A., Cano, N.J., Franch, H., Fouque, D., Himmelfarb, J., Kalantar-Zadeh, K., Kuhlmann, M.K., Stenvinkel, P., TerWee, P., Teta, D., Wang, A.Y.-M., Wanner, C., 2013. Prevention and treatment of protein energy wasting in chronic kidney disease patients: a consensus statement by the International Society of Renal Nutrition and Metabolism. Kidney Int. 84 (6), 1096–1107. doi:10.1038/ki.2013.147.

Johansen, K.L., Chertow, G.M., Kutner, N.G., Dalrymple, L.S., Grimes, B.A., Kaysen, G.A., 2010. Low level of self-reported physical activity in ambulatory patients new to dialysis. Kidney Int. 15231755. 78 (11), 1164–1170. Available from: https://www.journals.elsevier.com/kidney-international. doi:10.1038/ki.2010.312.

Johansen, K.L., Chertow, G.M., Ng, A.V., Mulligan, K., Carey, S., Schoenfeld, P.Y., Kent-Braun, J.A., 2000. Physical activity levels in patients on hemodialysis and healthy sedentary controls. Kidney Int. 00852538. 57 (6), 2564–2570. Available from: https://www.journals.elsevier.com/kidney-international. doi:10.1046/j.1523-1755.2000.00116.x.

Joseph, J., Vellaisamy, M., Subramanian, T., Fernando, E., Kaliaperumal, T., Srinivasaprasad, N.D., Surendran, S., Annadurai, P., Haridas, N., 2023. Frailty in patients with chronic kidney disease stage five. Cureus. 2168-8184. 15 (8). doi:10.7759/cureus.43787.

Kalantar-Zadeh, K., Block, G., McAllister, C.J., Humphreys, M.H., Kopple, J.D., 2004. Appetite and inflammation, nutrition, anemia, and clinical outcome in hemodialysis patients. Am. J. Clin. Nutr. 00029165. 80 (2), 299–307. http://www.ajcn.org/contents-by-date.2005.shtml. doi:10.1093/ajcn/80.2.299.

KDIGO, 2024. Clinical practice guideline for the evaluation and management of chronic kidney disease. Kidney Int. 105 (4S), S117–S314.

Kim, J.C., Kalantar-Zadeh, K., Kopple, J.D., 2013. Frailty and protein-energy wasting in elderly patients with end stage kidney disease. J. Am. Soc. Nephrol. 15333450. 24 (3), 337–351. Available from: http://jasn.asnjournals.org/content/24/3/337.full.pdf+html. doi:10.1681/ASN.2012010047.

Koh, K.P., Fassett, R.G., Sharman, J.E., Coombes, J.S., Williams, A.D., 2010. Effect of intradialytic versus home-based aerobic exercise training on physical function and vascular parameters in hemodialysis patients: a randomized pilot study. Am. J. Kidney Dis. 02726386. 55 (1), 88–99. doi:10.1053/j.ajkd.2009.09.025.

Logan, B., Viecelli, A., Johnson, D., Aquino, E., Bailey, J., Comans, T., Gray, L., Hawley, C., Hickey, L., Janda, M., Jaure, A., Jose, M., Kalaw, E., Kiriwandeniya, C., Matsuyama, M., Mihala, G., Nguyen, K., Pascoe, E., Pole, J., Polkinghorne, K., Pond, D., Raj, R., Reidlinger, D., Scholes-Robertson, N., Varghese, J., Wong, G., Hubbard, R., Buckle, G., Carswell, P., Cerni, J., Collins, M.G., Elms, A., Fanning, J., Fischer, K., Flavell, A., Gordon, E.H., Grainer, N., Green, S., Guha, C., Hand, S., Hibbs, M., Hockley, B., Irvine, R., Ismail, I., Jesudason, S., Kan, G., Kennedy, D., Khelgi, V., Kokoszka, S., Krishnan, A., Leadbitter, J., Leary, D., Makris, A., Marquez, K.K., McIntyre, D., Murie, P., Murphy, K., Peel, N., Qiu, X., Rapisardi, M., Roberts, M.A., Roger, S.D., Saade, M., Sen, S., Tataro, G., Weaver, B., Yates, P.A., Yip, B., 2023. Study protocol for The GOAL Trial: comprehensive geriatric assessment for frail older people with chronic kidney disease to increase attainment of patient-identified goals—a cluster randomised controlled trial. Trials. 17456215. 24 (1). Available from: https://trialsjournal.biomedcentral.com/. doi:10.1186/s13063-023-07363-4.

Lorenz, E.C., Bonikowske, A.R., Ashley, C., Meter, D.-V., Munson, C.L., Roschen, C.A., Salstrand, R.M., Wolter, A.D., Murthy, B.V., Davis, L.A., Choi, N.G., Kennedy, C.C., 2024b. A multicenter home-based prehabilitation intervention in kidney transplant candidates. Transplant. Direct 10 (12). doi:10.1097/TXD.0000000000001731.

Lorenz, E.C., Hickson, L.J., Hogan, M.C., Kennedy, C.C., 2023b. Examining the safety and effectiveness of a 4-week supervised exercise intervention in the treatment of frailty in patients with chronic kidney disease. Clin. Kidney J. 16 (11), 2003–2010. doi:10.1093/ckj/sfad192.

Lorenz, E.C., Hickson, L.T.J., Khairallah, P., Najafi, B., Kennedy, C.C., 2023a. Cellular senescence and frailty in transplantation. Curr. Transplant. Rep. 21963029. 10 (2), 51–59. Available from: https://www.springer.com/journal/40472. doi:10.1007/s40472-023-00393-6.

Lorenz, E.C., Hickson, L.T.J., Weatherly, R.M., Thompson, K.L., Walker, H.A., Rasmussen, J.M., Stewart, T.L., Garrett, J.K., Amer, H., Kennedy, C.C., 2020. Protocolized exercise improves frailty parameters and lower extremity impairment: a promising prehabilitation strategy for kidney transplant candidates. Clin. Transplant. 13990012. 34 (9). Available from: http://onlinelibrary.wiley.com/journal/10.1111/(ISSN)1399-0012. doi:10.1111/ctr.14017.

Lorenz, E.C., Kennedy, C.C., Rule, A.D., LeBrasseur, N.K., Kirkland, J.L., Hickson, L.T.J., 2021. Frailty in CKD and transplantation. Kidney Int. Rep. 24680249. 6 (9), 2270–2280. Available from: http://www.journals.elsevier.com/kidney-international-reports. doi:10.1016/j.ekir.2021.05.025.

Lorenz, E.C., Smith, B.H., Mour, G., Wadei, H.M., Kennedy, C.C., Schinstock, C.A., Kremers, W.K., Cheville, A.L., LeBrasseur, N.K., Rule, A.D., 2024c. Prospective cohort study examining the ability of performance-based and self-reported frailty measures to predict 30-day rehospitalizations after kidney transplantation. Clin. Transplant. 38 (8). doi:10.1111/ctr.15433.

Lorenz, E.C., Smith, B.H., Wadei, H.M., Mour, G., Kennedy, C.C., Schinstock, C.A., Kremers, W.K., Cheville, A.L., Hickson, L.T.J., Atkinson, E.J., White, T.A., Rule, A.D., LeBrasseur, N.K., 2024a. Senescence biomarkers and trajectories of frailty and physical function after kidney transplantation. Clin. Transplant. 13990012. 38 (11). Available from: http://onlinelibrary.wiley.com/journal/10.1111/(ISSN)1399-0012. doi:10.1111/ctr.70022.

Luo, C.M., Hsieh, M.Y., Cheng, C.H., Chen, C.H., Liao, M.T., Chuang, S.Y., Wu, C.C., 2022. Association of frailty with thrombosis of hemodialysis vascular access: a prospective taiwanese cohort study. Am. J. Kidney Dis. 15236838. 80 (3), 353. Available from: http://www.elsevier.com/inca/publications/store/6/2/3/2/7/6/index.htt. doi:10.1053/j.ajkd.2021.12.017.

Majchrzak, K.M., Pupim, L.B., Sundell, M., Ikizler, T.A., 2007. Body composition and physical activity in end-stage renal disease. J. Ren. Nutr. 10512276. 17 (3), 196–204. doi:10.1053/j.jrn.2007.01.003.

Mallamaci, F., Pisano, A., Tripepi, G., 2020. Physical activity in chronic kidney disease and the EXerCise Introduction To Enhance trial. Nephrol. Dial. Transplant. 0931-0509. 35 (Supplement_2), ii18. doi:10.1093/ndt/gfaa012.

Manfredini, F., Mallamaci, F., D'Arrigo, G., Baggetta, R., Bolignano, D., Torino, C., Lamberti, N., Bertoli, S., Ciurlino, D., Rocca-Rey, L., Barillà, A., Battaglia, Y., Rapanà, R.M., Zuccalà, A., Bonanno, G., Fatuzzo, P., Rapisarda, F., Rastelli, S., Fabrizi, F., Messa, P., Paola, L.D., Lombardi, L., Cupisti, A., Fuiano, G., Lucisano, G., Summaria, C., Felisatti, M., Pozzato, E., Malagoni, A.M., Castellino, P., Aucella, F., Elhafeez, S.A., Provenzano, P.F., Tripepi, G., Catizone, L., Zoccali, C., 2017. Exercise in patients on dialysis: a multicenter, randomized clinical trial. J. Am. Soc. Nephrol. 15333450. 28 (4), 1259–1268. Available from: http://jasn.asnjournals.org/content/28/4/1259.full.pdf+html. doi:10.1681/ASN.2016030378.

Marantes, I., Achenbach, S.J., Atkinson, E.J., Khosla, S., Melton, L.J., 3rd, Amin, S., 2011. Is vitamin D a determinant of muscle mass and strength? J. Bone Miner. Res. 26 (12), 2860–2871. doi:10.1002/jbmr.510.

Mayne, K.J., Sardell, R.J., Staplin, N., Judge, P.K., Zhu, D., Sammons, E., Cherney, D.Z.I., Cheung, A.K., Maggioni, A.P., Nangaku, M., Rossello, X., Tuttle, K.R., Ihara, K., Iwata, T., Wanner, C., Emberson, J., Preiss, D., Landray, M.J., Baigent, C., Haynes, R., Herrington, W.G., 2024. Frailty, Multimorbidity, and polypharmacy: exploratory analyses of the effects of empagliflozin from the EMPA-KIDNEY trial. Clin. J. Am. Soc. Nephrol. 1555905X. 19 (9), 1119–1129. Available from: https://journals.lww.com/CJASN/Pages/default.aspx. doi:10.2215/CJN.0000000000000498.

McAdams-DeMarco, M.A., Isaacs, K., Darko, L., Salter, M.L., Gupta, N., King, E.A., Walston, J., Segev, D.L., 2015. Changes in frailty after kidney transplantation. J. Am. Geriatr. Soc. 15325415. 63 (10), 2152–2157. Available from: http://www.blackwellpublishing.com/journal.asp?ref=0002-8614&site=1. doi:10.1111/jgs.13657.

Molnar, F., Frank, C.C., 2019. Optimizing geriatric care with the GERIATRIC 5Ms. College of Family Physicians of Canada. Can. Fam. Physician 0008350X. 65 (1), 39. Available from http://www.cfp.ca/content/65/1/39.

Nair, D., Liu, C.K., Raslan, R., McAdams-DeMarco, M., Hall, R.K., 2025. Frailty in kidney disease: a comprehensive review to advance its clinical and research applications. Am. J. Kidney Dis. 15236838. 85 (1), 89–103. Available from: https://www.sciencedirect.com/science/journal/02726386. doi:10.1053/j.ajkd.2024.04.018.

Nixon, A.C., Bampouras, T.M., Gooch, H.J., Young, H.M.L., Finlayson, K.W., Pendleton, N., Mitra, S., Brady, M.E., Dhaygude, A.P., 2021. Home-based exercise for people living with frailty and chronic kidney disease: a mixed-methods pilot randomised controlled trial. PLoS ONE. 19326203. 16 (7). Available from: https://journals.plos.org/plosone/article/file?id=10.1371/journal.pone.0251652&type=printable. doi:10.1371/journal.pone.0251652.

Nixon, A.C., Bampouras, T.M., Pendleton, N., Woywodt, A., Mitra, S., Dhaygude, A., 2018. Frailty and chronic kidney disease: current evidence and continuing uncertainties. Clin. Kidney J. 20488513. 11 (2), 236–245. Available from: http://ckj.oxfordjournals.org/. doi:10.1093/ckj/sfx134.

Odden, M.C., Whooley, M.A., Shlipak, M.G., 2004. Association of chronic kidney disease and anemia with physical capacity: the heart and soul study. J. Am. Soc. Nephrol. 10466673. 15 (11), 2908–2915. Available from: https://journals.lww.com/jasn/pages/default.aspx. doi:10.1097/01.ASN.0000143743.78092.E3.

Parker, S.G., McCue, P., Phelps, K., McCleod, A., Arora, S., Nockels, K., Kennedy, S., Roberts, H., Conroy, S., 2018. What is comprehensive geriatric assessment (CGA)? An umbrella review. Age Ageing. 0002-0729. 47 (1), 149–155. doi:10.1093/ageing/afx166.

Pfeffer, M.A., Burdmann, E.A., Chen, C.Y., Cooper, M.E., De Zeeuw, D., Eckardt, K.U., Feyzi, J.M., Ivanovich, P., Kewalramani, R., Levey, A.S., Lewis, E.F., McGill, J.B., McMurray, J.J.V., Parfrey, P., Parving, H.H., Remuzzi, G., Singh, A.K., Solomon, S.D., Toto, R., 2009. A trial of darbepoetin alfa in type 2 diabetes and chronic kidney disease. N. Engl. J. Med. 15334406. 361 (21), 2019–2032. Available from: http://content.nejm.org/cgi/reprint/361/21/2019.pdf. doi:10.1056/NEJMoa0907845.

Picariello, F., Moss-Morris, R., Macdougall, I.C., Chilcot, J., 2018. 'It's when you're not doing too much you feel tired': a qualitative exploration of fatigue in end-stage kidney disease. Br. J. Health Psychol. 20448287. 23 (2), 311–333. Available from: http://onlinelibrary.wiley.com/journal/10.1111/(ISSN)2044-8287. doi:10.1111/bjhp.12289.

Pilotto, A., Custodero, C., Maggi, S., Polidori, M.C., Veronese, N., Ferrucci, L., 2020. A multidimensional approach to frailty in older people. Ageing Res. Rev. 15681637. 60, 101047. doi:10.1016/j.arr.2020.101047.

Quint, E.E., Zogaj, D., Banning, L.B.D., Benjamens, S., Annema, C., Bakker, S.J.L., Nieuwenhuijs-Moeke, G.J., Segev, D.L., Mcadams-Demarco, M.A., Pol, R.A., 2021. Frailty and kidney transplantation: a systematic review and meta-analysis. Transplant. Direct. 23738731. 7 (6), E701. Available from: https://journals.lww.com/transplantationdirect/pages/default.aspx. doi:10.1097/TXD.0000000000001156.

Raîche, M., Hébert, R., Dubois, M.F., 2008. PRISMA-7: a case-finding tool to identify older adults with moderate to severe disabilities. Arch. Gerontol. Geriatr. 01674943. 47 (1), 9–18. Available from: www.elsevier.com/locate/archger. doi:10.1016/j.archger.2007.06.004.

Raphael, K.L., 2019. Metabolic acidosis in CKD: core curriculum 2019. Am. J. Kidney Dis. 15236838. 74 (2), 263–275. Available from: http://www.elsevier.com/inca/publications/store/6/2/3/2/7/6/index.htt. doi:10.1053/j.ajkd.2019.01.036.

Reaich, D., Price, S.R., England, B.K., Mitch, W.E., 1995. Mechanisms causing muscle loss in chronic renal failure. Am. J. Kidney Dis. 02726386. 26 (1), 242–247. doi:10.1016/0272-6386(95)90179-5.

Rhee, E.P., Guallar, E., Hwang, S., Kim, N., Tonelli, M., Moe, S.M., Himmelfarb, J., Thadhani, R.I., Powe, N.R., Shafi, T., 2020. Prevalence and persistence of uremic symptoms in incident dialysis patients. Kidney360. 26417650. 1 (2), 86–92. Available from: https://kidney360.asnjournals.org/. doi:10.34067/KID.0000072019.

Rockwood, K., Blodgett, J.M., Theou, O., Sun, M.H., Feridooni, H.A., Mitnitski, A., Rose, R.A., Godin, J., Gregson, E., Howlett, S.E., 2017. A frailty index based on deficit accumulation quantifies mortality risk in humans and in mice. Sci. Rep. 2045-2322. 7 (1). doi:10.1038/srep43068.

Rockwood, K., Song, X., MacKnight, C., Bergman, H., Hogan, D.B., McDowell, I., Mitnitski, A., 2005. A global clinical measure of fitness and frailty in elderly people. CMAJ. 14882329. 173 (5), 489–495. Available from: http://www.cmaj.ca/. doi:10.1503/cmaj.050051.

Rolfson, D.B., Majumdar, S.R., Tsuyuki, R.T., Tahir, A., Rockwood, K., 2006. Validity and reliability of the edmonton frail scale [4]. Age Ageing. 14682834. 35 (5), 526–529. doi:10.1093/ageing/afl041.

Rossi, A.P., Burris, D.D., Lucas, F.L., Crocker, G.A., Wasserman, J.C., 2014. Effects of a renal rehabilitation exercise program in patients with CKD: a randomized, controlled trial. Clin. J. Am. Soc. Nephrol. 1555905X. 9 (12), 2052–2058. Available from: http://cjasn.asnjournals.org/content/9/12/2052.full.pdf. doi:10.2215/CJN.11791113.

Sahathevan, S., Khor, B.H., Ng, H.M., Gafor, A.H.A., Daud, Z.A.M., Mafra, D., Karupaiah, T., 2020. Understanding development of malnutrition in hemodialysis patients: a narrative review. Nutrients. 20726643. 12 (10), 1–30. Available from: https://www.mdpi.com/2072-6643/12/10/3147/pdf. doi:10.3390/nu12103147.

Sekiguchi, T., Kabayama, M., Ryuno, H., Tanaka, K., Kiyoshige, E., Akagi, Y., Godai, K., Sugimoto, K., Akasaka, H., Takami, Y., Takeya, Y., Yamamoto, K., Yasumoto, S., Masui, Y., Ikebe, K., Gondo, Y., Arai, Y., Ishizaki, T., Rakugi, H., Kamide, K., 2022. Association between protein intake and changes in renal function among Japanese community-dwelling older people: the SONIC study. Geriatr. Gerontol. Int. 1444-1586. 22 (4), 286–291. doi:10.1111/ggi.14355.

Sheshadri, A., Kittiskulnam, P., Lazar, A.A., Johansen, K.L., 2020. A walking intervention to increase weekly steps in dialysis patients: a pilot randomized controlled trial. Am. J. Kidney Dis. 15236838. 75 (4), 488–496. Available from: http://www.elsevier.com/inca/publications/store/6/2/3/2/7/6/index.htt. doi:10.1053/j.ajkd.2019.07.026.

Taskapan, H., Baysal, O., Karahan, D., Durmus, B., Altay, Z., Ulutas, O., 2011. Vitamin D and muscle strength, functional ability and balance in peritoneal dialysis patients with vitamin D deficiency. Clin. Nephrol. 0301-0430. 76 (08), 110–116. doi:10.5414/CN107160.

Tran, J., Ayers, E., Verghese, J., Abramowitz, M.K., 2019. Gait abnormalities and the risk of falls in CKD. Clin. J. Am. Soc. Nephrol. 1555905X. 14 (7), 983–993. Available from: https://cjasn.asnjournals.org/content/14/7/983.full.pdf. doi:10.2215/CJN.13871118.

Triantafylidis, L.K., Hawley, C.E., Perry, L.P., Paik, J.M., 2018. The role of deprescribing in older adults with chronic kidney disease. Drugs Aging. 11791969. 35 (11), 973–984. Available from: http://rd.springer.com/journal/40266. doi:10.1007/s40266-018-0593-8.

Tseng, P.W., Lin, T.Y., Hung, S.C., 2024. Association of frailty with nutritional status in patients with chronic kidney disease. J. Ren. Nutr. 10512276. 34 (2), 133–140. Available from: https://www.sciencedirect.com/science/journal/10512276. doi:10.1053/j.jrn.2023.09.003.

Turner, G., Clegg, A., 2014. Best practice guidelines for the management of frailty: a British geriatrics society, age UK and royal college of general practitioners report. Age Ageing. 14682834. 43 (6), 744–747. Available from: http://ageing.oxfordjournals.org/. doi:10.1093/ageing/afu138.

Voorend, C.G.N., Berkhout-Byrne, N.C., van Bodegom-vos, L., Diepenbroek, A., Franssen, C.F.M., Joosten, H., Mooijaart, S.P., Bos, W.J.W., van Buren, M., van Alphen, A., Berkhout-Byrne, N., van Breda, F., Boom, H., Bos, W.J., Emmelot-Vonk, M., Franssen, C., Gaillard, C., Groeneweg-Peeters, N., Hoekstra, B., Hommes, N., Hoornaar, F., Lagro, J., Litjens, E., Molenaar, F., Mooijaart, S., Neradova, A., Peters, M., Troost, M., Veldman, W., Voorend,

C., Westerbos, L., Westerman-van der Wijden, C., Wierdsma, J., 2024. Geriatric assessment in CKD care: an implementation study. Kidney Med. 25900595. 6 (5). Available from: https://www.sciencedirect.com/science/journal/25900595. doi:10.1016/j.xkme.2024.100809.

Westerberg, P.A., Sterner, G., Ljunggren, Ö., Isaksson, E., Elvarson, F., Dezfoolian, H., Linde, T., 2018. High doses of cholecalciferol alleviate the progression of hyperparathyroidism in patients with CKD Stages 3-4: results of a 12-week double-blind, randomized, controlled study. Nephrol. Dial. Transplant. 14602385. 33 (3), 466–471. Available from: http://ndt.oxfordjournals.org/. doi:10.1093/ndt/gfx059.

Woo, K., Gascue, L., Norris, K., Lin, E., 2022. Patient frailty and functional use of hemodialysis vascular access: a retrospective study of the US renal data system. Am. J. Kidney Dis. 02726386. 80 (1), 30–45. doi:10.1053/j.ajkd.2021.10.011.

Xue, Q.L., 2011. The frailty syndrome: definition and natural history. Clin. Geriatr. Med. 07490690. 27 (1), 1–15. doi:10.1016/j.cger.2010.08.009.

Yenchek, R., Ix, J.H., Rifkin, D.E., Shlipak, M.G., Sarnak, M.J., Garcia, M., Patel, K.V., Satterfield, S., Harris, T.B., Newman, A.B., Fried, L.F., 2014. Association of serum bicarbonate with incident functional limitation in older adults. Clin. J. Am. Soc. Nephrol. 1555905X. 9 (12), 2111–2116. Available from: http://cjasn.asnjournals.org/content/9/12/2111.full.pdf. doi:10.2215/CJN.05480614.

Zhang, L., Wang, X.H., Wang, H., Du, J., Mitch, W.E., 2010. Satellite cell dysfunction and impaired IGF-1 signaling cause CKD-induced muscle atrophy. J. Am. Soc. Nephrol. 15333450. 21 (3), 419–427. Available from: http://jasn.asnjournals.org/cgi/reprint/21/3/419. doi:10.1681/ASN.2009060571.

Zhao, J.L., Qiao, X.H., Mao, J.H., Liu, F., Fu, H.D., 2022. The interaction between cellular senescence and chronic kidney disease as a therapeutic opportunity. Front. Pharmacol. 16639812. 13. Available from: http://www.frontiersin.org/Pharmacology. doi:10.3389/fphar.2022.974361.

CHAPTER

13

Hospitalizations

Neha Siddiqui and Samaya Anumudu

Baylor College of Medicine, Houston, TX, United States

Introduction

Patients with chronic kidney disease (CKD) often have multiple health complications, especially hospitalizations. Coupled with advancing age, the impact of hospitalizations in this population has significant implications for their overall health and healthcare systems. The percentage of the elderly population (over the age of 60) worldwide is expected to nearly double from 11% to 22% by 2050 (Kanasi et al., 2016). Although individuals older than 65 years of age make up approximately 16% of the total population, they are responsible for more than 40% of hospitalizations in the United States. They also have a significant impact on healthcare expenses, contributing to approximately half of all hospital-related costs (Adamowicz and Lee, 2021: Shreya et al., 2025). These figures are not just numbers; they emphasize the need for a change in health systems all over the world to adapt and prepare for the increased healthcare needs of a growing elderly population with CKD.

CKD poses a significant burden on the aging population, with approximately 40% of individuals aged 65 and older affected worldwide. Recently, there has been an increase in the number of patients older than 75 years of age starting dialysis, reflecting both the growing aging population and the rising prevalence of severe kidney impairment in this age group (Merchant and Ling, 2023).

Etiology

The etiology of hospitalizations in older patients with CKD is multifactorial, including aging, declining physiologic function and frailty, renal impairment, and other comorbid conditions. While some hospitalizations are planned, such as for the surgical placement of dialysis access or the initiation of dialysis, many visits are often unplanned. Below, we have listed various conditions among elderly patients with CKD that lead to hospitalizations and discuss potential mitigation strategies:

Aging and the Kidney
https://doi.org/10.1016/B978-0-443-34069-7.00014-8

1. Cardiovascular disease and associated complications are among the leading causes of hospitalizations in the United States among individuals with CKD (Schrauben et al., 2020). The increased risk of these hospitalizations can be attributed to a higher incidence of fluid overload, vascular calcification, hypertension (often uncontrolled), and electrolyte abnormalities in this specific patient population. In the United States, individuals 65 years of age and older account for more than half of all cardiovascular-related hospitalizations and procedures, and nearly 80% of all cardiovascular-related deaths (Rich et al., 2016). The prevalence of heart failure, myocardial infarction, valvular heart disease, and arrhythmias, including atrial fibrillation, is known to increase with age (Yazdanyar and Newman, 2009). The United States Preventive Services Task Force reports that the age-adjusted prevalence of coronary artery disease is approximately 16% among individuals aged 65–74 and rises to nearly 23% in those aged 75 and older, demonstrating an increase in risk with advancing age (Curry et al., 2018).
2. Infectious causes, in the context of the potential immunosuppressive effects of advanced kidney disease, coupled with a gradual decline in the immune system in some older adults, place elderly CKD patients at an increased risk for severe infections. In a study conducted from 1998 to 2004, infection-related hospitalizations accounted for approximately 13% of all hospital charges for older adults in the United States (Curns et al., 2008). Respiratory tract infections, urinary tract infections, and sepsis are frequent causes of hospitalizations in this age group (Curns et al., 2005). In addition, some hospitalizations are prolonged due to the need for an extended course of intravenous (IV) antibiotics.
3. Falls and bone fractures can be related to mineral bone disorders of CKD, sarcopenia, inadequate nutrition, and orthostatic hypotension in elderly patients. In the United States, approximately 800,000 patients are hospitalized each year due to fall-related injuries, and about 300,000 receive treatment for hip fractures (Vaishya and Vaish, 2020).
4. Stroke is another significant cause of hospitalization among the elderly. It stands as the third leading cause of death and plays a major role in contributing to long-term disabilities. Studies have shown a high prevalence of stroke in the elderly population, which can be attributed to several risk factors, including being overweight, stress, smoking, physical inactivity, hypertension, diet, sleep disorders or disturbances, and other underlying health conditions such as diabetes and kidney disease (Rajati et al., 2023).
5. Electrolyte and acid–base abnormalities, such as dysnatremias, hyperkalemia, and metabolic acidosis, are common in patients with CKD and can be associated with high morbidity and mortality in the elderly population. Due to their potential rapid onset and possible life-threatening consequences, patients are often hospitalized for close monitoring and further management. Hyponatremia is a common electrolyte abnormality, and the prevalence in one emergency department population was 3%, with the most common causes being thiazide diuretics (17%), syndrome of inappropriate antidiuretic hormone (14%), and other diuretics (14%) (Olsson et al., 2013).
6. Fluid overload is another major cause of hospitalizations in this subset of the population. It can be a precipitating factor for hospitalizations related to heart failure. Impaired sodium and water excretion can lead to pulmonary edema and acute

respiratory compromise, particularly in patients with concurrent diagnoses of heart failure or fluid retention syndromes. In the United States, hospitalizations associated with heart failure have increased in adults since 2014, particularly in individuals over 80 years of age (Bozkurt et al., 2023).

7. Acute kidney injury (AKI) is also not surprising in this population and is often precipitated by factors such as hypovolemia, nephrotoxic medications, or hemodynamic instability. It is associated with an increased risk of CKD/end stage idney disease (ESKD) and short- and long-term death. AKI may also be related to a decline in functional status and quality of life (Coca, 2010).
8. Anemia and associated complications, such as fatigue, frailty, and the need for transfusions, are common among older patients and patients with CKD. Anemia in the elderly can result from renal dysfunction, chronic diseases, nutritional deficiencies, and hematologic problems and is associated with frequent hospitalizations and mortality. These patients may need to be hospitalized for blood transfusions and/or intravenous iron therapy. In addition, there are noted higher healthcare costs in patients with CKD and anemia (Girelli et al., 2018).
9. Renal replacement therapy: Patients on dialysis are frequently admitted to the hospital as a result of dialysis-related complications, such as vascular access-related infections or malfunction. In addition, patients may experience electrolyte disturbances, hypotension during or after dialysis, uncontrolled hypertension, volume overload, missed dialysis sessions, or the need for placement at a new dialysis center.

Interventions

Elderly patients with CKD are particularly vulnerable to multiple hospitalizations due to a combination of progressive renal dysfunction, age-related decline in physiological function, and an increased burden of comorbidities, subsequently leading to an increased disease burden. Successful interventions, therefore, need to go beyond just kidney function and address systemic causes of disease progression. A proactive, patient-centered, and multidisciplinary approach is pivotal in reducing the risk of hospital admissions in this vulnerable population (Table 13.1).

The optimal management of comorbidities is a key element in preventing hospitalization. Improved control of chronic conditions, such as hypertension, diabetes mellitus, and heart failure, is essential to prevent not only cardiovascular complications but also to slow the progression and/or reduce the incidence and prevalence of CKD. The appropriate use of renin–angiotensin–aldosterone system (RAAS) inhibitors is crucial for the management of proteinuria and blood pressure when appropriate (Lewis et al., 1993). However, they should be prescribed with caution, especially in the elderly, as they can sometimes increase the risk of hyperkalemia and kidney injury, along with hypotension, in a population inherently at risk of falls. In addition, all pharmacologic therapies should be dosed appropriately per kidney function to prevent potential accumulation of metabolites and toxicity (Matzke et al., 2011).

Appropriately timed assessments, including frequent laboratory analyses to monitor kidney function, electrolytes, and hemoglobin levels, facilitate early identification of potential

TABLE 13.1 Drivers of unplanned hospitalizations. This table highlights some of the common causes of hospital admissions in patients with CKD and older adults, and offers strategies to mitigate them.

Hospitalization driver	Risk factors in older adults with chronic kidney disease	Mitigation
Cardiovascular disease	Excess body fluid, vascular calcification, uncontrolled high blood pressure, and electrolyte disturbances increase the risk. Older adults account for a large share of cardiovascular hospitalizations and deaths (Rich et al., 2016).	Optimize the management of high blood pressure, diabetes mellitus, and heart failure; use renin–angiotensin–aldosterone system inhibitors when appropriate, with careful monitoring. Manage volume status and electrolytes closely, and schedule frequent follow-ups.
Infections	Chronic kidney disease and age are associated with reduced immune function, increasing the likelihood of respiratory and urinary tract infections and sepsis (Curns et al., 2005, Curns et al., 2008).	Ensure recommended vaccinations; provide early evaluation of fever and symptoms; start timely treatment when indicated; reinforce hand hygiene and, for dialysis patients, access-care hygiene; and use outpatient intravenous and/or oral medications when safe and appropriate.
Falls and fractures	Mineral and bone disorders related to chronic kidney disease, loss of muscle mass, inadequate nutrition, and low blood pressure upon standing raise fall risk; hip fractures and other fall injuries frequently require hospitalization (Vaishya and Vaish, 2020).	Perform a comprehensive fall-risk assessment; identify patients at risk of falling; initiate physical and occupational therapy when possible; address nutrition and bone health; implement home safety modifications; and review and adjust medications that may lower blood pressure or cause dizziness.
Stroke	Stroke is a major cause of hospitalization, death, and long-term disability. The risk increases with a higher body mass index, chronic stress, tobacco use, physical inactivity, high blood pressure, an unhealthy diet, sleep disorders, diabetes mellitus, and kidney disease (Rajati et al., 2023).	Control blood pressure and blood lipids; detect and manage arrhythmias; optimize diabetes care; support smoking cessation; prescribe structured physical activity; evaluate and treat sleep disorders; and provide dietary counseling.
Electrolyte and acid–base disorders	Low or high sodium, high potassium, and metabolic acidosis occur more often as kidney function declines and may present suddenly with life-threatening symptoms (Olsson et al., 2013).	Use standardized laboratory monitoring, adjust medication doses according to kidney function, provide counseling by a renal dietitian, and create same-day outpatient treatment pathways for severe sodium disorders or high potassium when safe.
Fluid overload and heart failure	Reduced ability to excrete sodium and water, pulmonary edema, and breathing difficulty may contribute to hospitalizations (Bozkurt et al., 2023).	Optimize diuretic therapy; counsel on sodium and fluid intake; encourage daily weight tracking; provide rapid-access clinic appointments for early decompensation; consider remote monitoring when available.

Hospitalization driver	Risk factors in older adults with chronic kidney disease	Mitigation
Acute kidney injury	Often triggered by low blood volume, kidney-toxic medications, or unstable blood flow; it is associated with progression to more severe chronic kidney disease, higher short- and long-term mortality, functional decline, and reduced quality of life (Ferenbach and Bonventre, 2015; Coca, 2010).	Avoid kidney-toxic agents when possible; provide "sick-day" instructions to pause angiotensin-converting enzyme inhibitors, angiotensin receptor blockers, diuretics, and certain diabetic medications during dehydrating illnesse when appropriates; promptly recheck laboratory results after illnesses or procedures; and carefully assess volume status.
Anemia and related complications	Due to reduced erythropoietin production, chronic inflammation, nutrient deficiencies, and hematologic conditions, which contribute to fatigue, frailty, the need for blood transfusions or intravenous iron, frequent admissions, mortality, and higher costs (Zhang et al., 2023; Girelli et al., 2018; Stauffer et al., 2014).	Order iron studies and replenish iron as needed; use erythropoiesis-stimulating agents according to guidelines; evaluate for bleeding and nutritional deficiencies; and coordinate outpatient transfusion or intravenous iron when appropriate.
Dialysis-related complications	Vascular access infection or malfunction; electrolyte disturbances; low blood pressure during or after dialysis; uncontrolled high blood pressure; volume overload; missed treatments; transfers between dialysis centers (Ng et al., 2011; 2022).	Plan permanent arteriovenous fistula placement early when appropriate for patients on hemodialysis; teach meticulous access care and hygiene; optimize target (dry) weight; provide transportation and adherence support; and arrange backup scheduling and coordinated transfer when relocating.

adverse events and the prevention of acute decompensation leading to hospitalizations. Multidisciplinary coordination between primary care providers, nephrologists, dialysis centers, and other health professionals in the care team is critical for continuity of care.

Preventive care is another crucial aspect. Encouraging patients to stay up to date with their routine health maintenance visits, health screenings, medications, and vaccinations can have a positive impact on infection-related hospitalizations (Dalrymple and Go, 2008). In addition, timely social and mental health support, such as depression screenings among patients with advanced kidney disease and/or end-stage kidney disease, may be associated with better outcomes regarding lower mortality and hospitalization rates (Fischer et al., 2021).

For patients on dialysis or nearing dialysis, establishing pathways and encouraging nephrologists to create more permanent vascular access modalities, such as arteriovenous fistulas, as early as safely possible is important. Patients should also be educated and trained in proper access care and hygiene practices to minimize possible infections and identify potential issues early (Ng et al., 2011).

Nutritional management is also of paramount importance. Tailored dietary interventions, with the help of a trusted dietitian, can help optimize electrolytes and promote adequate nutrition for patients with CKD.

Implementation Checklist for Clinic or Health System

1.Risk registry: Flag adults, especially the elderly with CKD Stages 3-5, and patients with heart failure, atrial fibrillation, or diabetes.
2.Nurse-pharmacist pathway: Monthly medication review, preferably with a clinical pharmacist, to adjust medications for CKD. Laboratory triggers for potassium, sodium, bicarbonate, hemoglobin, blood sugar, platelet count, white blood count, and hemoglobin.
3.Rapid access slots: Same-week clinic appointments for patients with dyspnea/weight gain, hyperkalemia, urinary tract infections, or rising creatinine.
4.Vaccination & infection bundle: Standing Orders and Reminders for Influenza, Pneumococcal, Shingles, and RSV Vaccines.
5.Falls program: Orthostatic vital signs, home safety referral, physical therapy exercises, balance assessment and therapy, and bone health assessment.
6.Dialysis Readiness: Early education. Optimal and urgent starts. Early vascular access and peritoneal access planning. Access-care education and contingency plans for missed treatments.
7.Psychosocial screening: Includes depression screening, social work referrals, and caregiver engagement.
8.Goals of care: Routine advanced care planning, palliative care access for advanced CKD.

FIG. 13.1 **Implementation items to share with your clinic or healthcare system.** A checklist of implementation strategies that can be useful to help reduce hospitalization.

Achieving optimal mobility through balance and strength training, as well as promoting fall and fracture prevention and recovery, can be essential for elderly patients with CKD (Kutner and Bowling, 2019). Polypharmacy is also a significant concern in this population and can negatively affect overall health. Therefore regular review of patient medications and the discontinuation of unnecessary or duplicate drugs can help prevent potential adverse drug events (Kurczewska-Michalak et al., 2021).

Patient and caregiver education is encouraged and essential to the overall care plan for elderly patients with CKD. Patient education, in particular, is associated with better outcomes, and including caregivers may help them better support the individuals they assist in caring for (Narva et al., 2016).

Finally, palliative care support and advance care planning are essential components for the holistic management of elderly patients, particularly those with advanced CKD. Such approaches not only make treatment more congruent with the goals and needs of the patient but could also decrease unnecessary hospitalizations. In addition, they can improve patient and family/caregiver satisfaction and quality of life, along with a reduction in healthcare expenses (Holley and Davison, 2015) (Fig. 13.1).

Conclusion

Hospitalizations in elderly patients with CKD often encompass more than kidney care alone. Cardiovascular disease, infections, falls, electrolyte abnormalities, and anemia all contribute to patient vulnerability. The strategies mentioned above include addressing the underlying primary cause of kidney disease, providing optimal comorbidity management, nutritional support, monitoring kidney function and medications, and fall prevention. Where and when appropriate, palliative care should be introduced and utilized. These strategies form the foundation of a comprehensive, integrated care model aimed at minimizing avoidable hospitalizations and, hopefully, improving overall outcomes and quality of life for elderly patients living with CKD.

AI disclosure

During the preparation of this work, the author(s) used Open Evidence and ChatGPT to get started but conducted their own literature review and content composition. After using these tools/services, the author(s) reviewed and edited the content as needed and take full responsibility for the content of the publication.

References

Adamowicz, D.H., Lee, E.E., 2021. Predicting and improving hospital outcomes for older adults. Int. Psychogeriatr. 1741203X. 33 (3), 205–207. Available from: https://www.sciencedirect.com/journal/international-psychogeriatrics. doi:10.1017/S1041610220003580.

Bozkurt, B., Ahmad, T., Alexander, K.M., Baker, W.L., Bosak, K., Breathett, K., Fonarow, G.C., Heidenreich, P., Ho, J.E., Hsich, E., Ibrahim, N.E., Jones, L.M., Khan, S.S., Khazanie, P., Koelling, T., Krumholz, H.M., Khush, K.K., Lee, C., Morris, A.A., Page, R.L., Pandey, A., Piano, M.R., Stehlik, J., Stevenson, L.W., Teerlink, J.R., Vaduganathan, M., Ziaeian, B., 2023. Heart failure epidemiology and outcomes statistics: a report of the Heart Failure Society of America. J. Card. Fail. 15328414. 29 (10), 1412–1451. Available from: https://www.journals.elsevier.com/journal-of-cardiac-failure. doi:10.1016/j.cardfail.2023.07.006.

Coca, S.G., 2010. Acute kidney injury in elderly persons. Am. J. Kidney Dis. 02726386. 56 (1), 122–131. doi:10.1053/j.ajkd.2009.12.034.

Curns, A.T., Holman, R.C., Sejvar, J.J., Owings, M.F., Schonberger, L.B., 2005. Infectious disease hospitalizations among older adults in the United States from 1990 through 2002. Arch. Intern. Med. 15383679. 165 (21), 2514–2520. Available from: http://archinte.ama-assn.org/cgi/reprint/165/21/2514. doi: 10.1001/archinte.165.21.2514

Curns, A.T., Steiner, C.A., Sejvar, J.J., Schonberger, L.B., 2008. Hospital charges attributable to a primary diagnosis of infectious diseases in older adults in the United States, 1998 to 2004. J. Am. Geriatr. Soc. 15325415. 56 (6), 969–975. doi:10.1111/j.1532-5415.2008.01712.x.

Curry, S.J., Krist, A.H., Owens, D.K., Barry, M.J., Caughey, A.B., Davidson, K.W., Doubeni, C.A., Epling, J.W., Kemper, A.R., Kubik, M., Landefeld, C.S., Mangione, C.M., Silverstein, M., Simon, M.A., Tseng, C.W., Wong, J.B., 2018. Risk assessment for cardiovascular disease with nontraditional risk factors: US preventive services task force recommendation statement. JAMA. 15383598. 320 (3), 272–280. Available from: https://jamanetwork.com/journals/jama/articlepdf/2687225/jama_curry_2018_us_180016.pdf. doi:10.1001/jama.2018.8359.

Dalrymple, L.S., Go, A.S., 2008. Epidemiology of acute infections among patients with chronic kidney disease. Clin. J. Am. Soc. Nephrol. 1555905X. 3 (5), 1487–1493. doi:10.2215/CJN.01290308.

Ferenbach, D.A., Bonventre, J.V., 2015. Mechanisms of maladaptive repair after AKI leading to accelerated kidney ageing and CKD. Nat. Rev. Nephrol. 1759507X. 11 (5), 264–276. Available from: http://www.nature.com/nrneph/archive/index.html. doi:10.1038/nrneph.2015.3.

Fischer, M.J., Streja, E., Hsiung, J.T., Crowley, S.T., Kovesdy, C.P., Kalantar-Zadeh, K., Kourany, W.M., 2021. Depression screening and clinical outcomes among adults initiating maintenance hemodialysis. Clin. Kidney J. 20488513. 14 (12), 2548–2555. Available from: http://ckj.oxfordjournals.org/. doi:10.1093/ckj/sfab097.

Girelli, D., Marchi, G., Camaschella, C., 2018. Anemia in the elderly. HemaSphere. 2572-9241. 2 (3). doi:10.1097/hs9.0000000000000040.

Holley, J.L., Davison, S.N., 2015. Advance care planning for patients with advanced CKD: a need to move forward. J. Am. Soc. Nephrol. 1555905X. 10 (3), 344–346. Available from: http://cjasn.asnjournals.org/content/10/3/344.full.pdf. doi:10.2215/CJN.00290115.

Kanasi, E., Ayilavarapu, S., Jones, J., 2016. The aging population: demographics and the biology of aging. Periodontol. 2000. 0906-6713. 72 (1), 13–18. doi:10.1111/prd.12126.

Kurczewska-Michalak, M., Lewek, P., Jankowska-Polańska, B., Giardini, A., Granata, N., Maffoni, M., Costa, E., Midão, L., Kardas, P., 2021. Polypharmacy management in the older adults: a scoping review of available interventions. Front. Pharmacol. 1663-9812. 12. doi:10.3389/fphar.2021.734045.

Kutner, N.G., Bowling, C.B., 2019. Targeting fall risk in CKD. Clin. J. Am. Soc. Nephrol. 1555905X. 14 (7), 965–966. Available from: https://cjasn.asnjournals.org/content/14/7/965.full.pdf. doi:10.2215/CJN.06040519.

Lewis, E.J., Hunsicker, L.G., Bain, R.P., Rohde, R.D., 1993. The effect of angiotensin-converting-enzyme inhibition on diabetic nephropathy. N. Engl. J. Med. 15334406. 329 (20), 1456–1462. doi:10.1056/NEJM199311113292004.

Matzke, G.R., Aronoff, G.R., Atkinson, A.J., Bennett, W.M., Decker, B.S., Eckardt, K.U., Golper, T., Grabe, D.W., Kasiske, B., Keller, F., Kielstein, J.T., Mehta, R., Mueller, B.A., Pasko, D.A., Schaefer, F., Sica, D.A., Inker, L.A., Umans, J.G., Murray, P., 2011. Drug dosing consideration in patients with acute and chronic kidney diseasea clinical update from kidney disease: improving Global Outcomes (KDIGO). Kidney Int. 15231755. 80 (11), 1122–1137. Available from: https://www.journals.elsevier.com/kidney-international. doi:10.1038/ki.2011.322.

Merchant, A.A., Ling, E., 2023. An approach to treating older adults with chronic kidney disease. CMAJ. 14882329. 195 (17), E612. Available from: https://www.cmaj.ca/content/195/17/E612. doi:10.1503/cmaj.221427.

Narva, A.S., Norton, J.M., Boulware, L.E., 2016. Educating patients about CKD: the path to self-management and patient-centered care. Clin. J. Am. Soc. Nephrol. 1555905X. 11 (4), 694–703. Available from: http://cjasn.asnjournals.org/content/11/4/694.full.pdf. doi:10.2215/CJN.07680715.

Ng, L.J., Chen, F., Pisoni, R.L., Krishnan, M., Mapes, D., Keen, M., Bradbury, B.D., 2011. Hospitalization risks related to vascular access type among incident US hemodialysis patients. Nephrol. Dial. Transplant. 0931-0509. 26 (11), 3659–3666. doi:10.1093/ndt/gfr063.

Ng, M., Mark, L.K.F., Fatimah, L., 2022. Management of difficult intravenous access: a qualitative review. World J. Emerg. Med. 19208642. 13 (6), 467–478. Available from: http://wjem.com.cn/EN/10.5847/wjem.j.1920-8642.2022.104. doi:10.5847/wjem.j.1920-8642.2022.104.

Olsson, K., Öhlin, B., Melander, O., 2013. Epidemiology and characteristics of hyponatremia in the emergency department. Eur. J. Intern. Med. 18790828. 24 (2), 110–116. doi:10.1016/j.ejim.2012.10.014.

Rajati, F., Rajati, M., Rasulehvandi, R., Kazeminia, M., 2023. Prevalence of stroke in the elderly: a systematic review and meta-analysis. Interdiscip. Neurosurg. 22147519. 32, 101746. doi:10.1016/j.inat.2023.101746.

Rich, M.W., Chyun, D.A., Skolnick, A.H., Alexander, K.P., Forman, D.E., Kitzman, D.W., Maurer, M.S., McClurken, J.B., Resnick, B.M., Shen, W.K., Tirschwell, D.L., 2016. Knowledge gaps in cardiovascular care of older adults: a scientific statement from the American Heart Association, American College of Cardiology, and American Geriatrics Society: executive summary. J. Am. Geriatr. Soc. 15325415. 64 (11), 2185–2192. Available from: http://www.blackwellpublishing.com/journal.asp?ref=0002-8614&site=1. doi:10.1111/jgs.14576.

Schrauben, S.J., Chen, H.Y., Lin, E., Jepson, C., Yang, W., Scialla, J.J., Fischer, M.J., Lash, J.P., Fink, J.C., Hamm, L.L., Kanthety, R., Rahman, M., Feldman, H.I., Anderson, A.H., 2020. Hospitalizations among adults with chronic kidney disease in the United States: a cohort study. PLoS Med. 15491676. 17 (12). Available from: https://storage.googleapis.com/plos-corpus-prod/10.1371/journal.pmed.1003470/1/pmed.1003470.pdf. doi:10.1371/journal.pmed.1003470.

Shreya, D., Fish, P.N., Du, D., 2025. Navigating the future of elderly healthcare: a comprehensive analysis of aging populations and mortality trends using national inpatient sample (NIS) data (2010-2024). Cureus. 2168-8184. 17 (3). doi:10.7759/cureus.80442.

Stauffer, M.E., Fan, T., Moura, I.C., 2014. Prevalence of anemia in chronic kidney disease in the United States. PLoS One. 1932-6203. 9 (1), e84943. doi:10.1371/journal.pone.0084943.

Vaishya, R., Vaish, A., 2020. Falls in older adults are serious. Indian J. Orthop. 19983727. 54 (1), 69–74. Available from: https://www.springer.com/journal/43465. doi:10.1007/s43465-019-00037-x.

Yazdanyar, A., Newman, A.B., 2009. The burden of cardiovascular disease in the elderly: morbidity, mortality, and costs. Clin. Geriatr. Med. 07490690. 25 (4), 563–577. doi:10.1016/j.cger.2009.07.007.

Zhang, J., Diwan, V., Wang, Z., Healy, H.G., Venuthurupalli, S.K., Abeysekera, R., Hoy, W.E., 2023. The impact of anaemia on outcomes, admissions, and costs in patients with chronic kidney disease in two public nephrology practices in queensland: a CKD.QLD Registry Study. Int. J. Nephrol. 20902158. 2023. Available from: http://www.hindawi.com/journals/ijn/. doi:10.1155/2023/8720293.

CHAPTER

14

Depression

Jessica Lowe[a] *and Angelina Edwards*[b]

[a]Internal Medicine Resident, Department of Medicine, Houston Methodist Hospital, Houston, TX, United States

[b]Department of Medicine, Division of Nephrology, Houston Methodist Academic Institute, Houston Methodist Hospital, Weill Cornell Medical College, Houston, Texas, United States

Epidemiology

Prevalence

Unipolar depressive disorders were ranked as the third highest in the global burden of disease by the World Health Organization, causing 65.5 million disability-adjusted life-years globally, with projections to become the highest by 2030 (World Health Organization, 2004). Major depressive disorder (MDD) and dysthymic disorder, now categorized as persistent depressive disorder per DSM-V, have lifetime prevalence rates of 6.7% and 3.6%, respectively (Waraich et al., 2004).

One in seven adults in the United States is estimated to have chronic kidney disease (CKD), approximately 14% of the US population. According to the most current estimates from 2024, CKD is more prevalent in older cohorts (age 65 and older) at 34%, compared to younger cohorts at 16% for those aged 45–64 and 6% for those aged 18–44. CKD is also slightly more prevalent in women than in men, 14% vs. 12%, respectively. In the United States, CKD prevalence was highest among Black individuals (18.8%) and lowest among Hispanic individuals (12%) (United States Renal Data System, 2024).

The prevalence of depression in people with CKD and ESRD has been demonstrated to be higher than in the general population. Overall, up to 25% of patients with CKD meet the criteria for interview-defined depression. Rates of depression were higher in ESRD patients on dialysis (39%) than their CKD (21%) and transplant counterparts (26%) (Palmer et al., 2013).

https://doi.org/10.1016/B978-0-443-34069-7.00020-3

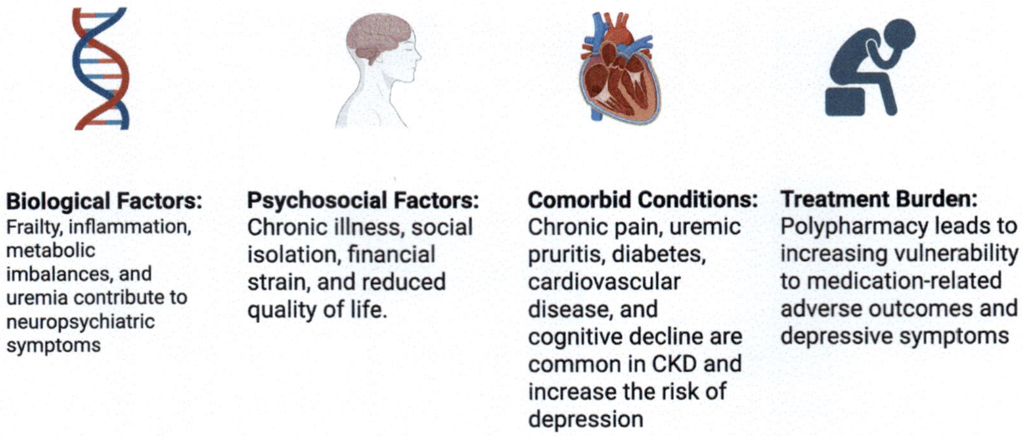

FIG. 14.1 Risk factors for depression. This figure shows the four major risk factors for depression: biological causes, psychosocial factors, comorbidities, and treatment burden. Made with https://biorender.com.

Risk factors for depression

Several risk factors contribute to the high prevalence of depression in CKD patients, particularly in the elderly. One significant risk factor is self-perceived poor health. Studies show that elderly patients who rate their health poorly have nearly three times the mortality risk, even when controlling for objective health status, age, sex, life satisfaction, income, and urban versus rural residence (Lefrère et al., 2025; Mossey and Shapiro, 1982) (Fig. 14.1).

Biological factors, psychosocial factors, comorbid conditions, and treatment burden predict an additional risk for depression in CKD.

Biological factors

Inflammation, metabolic imbalances, and uremia contribute to neuropsychiatric symptoms. Symptom burden is high in kidney disease and includes fatigue and frailty. Fatigue is one of the main criteria for MDD and commonly coexists in CKD, with fatigue severity and the need for antidepressant therapy mirroring CKD severity (Gregg et al., 2019). Fatigue is a complex, multifaceted experience of both psychological and physical symptoms. Psychological symptoms include a perception of increased effort and decreased cognitive fortitude, while physical symptoms include muscle weakness with diminished endurance. Approximately 70% of patients with CKD report fatigue, which carries a high risk of death, dialysis initiation, and hospitalization (Gregg et al., 2021). Equally debilitating is the prevalence of frailty. Frailty is defined as a clinical syndrome characterized by immobility, inactivity, reduced strength, sarcopenia, accelerated end-organ impairments, and decreased physiological reserve (Fried et al., 2001). Frailty, both measured and self-reported, is two times more prevalent among those with kidney disease compared to community-dwelling older adults and increases with CKD progression. Among patients with advanced CKD, frailty ranges from 42% to 74% in patients with CKD stage 4 and is as high as 82% in the predialysis population (Chowdhury et al., 2017). Frailty portends a high risk of loss of independence, reduced quality of life, accelerated aging, and is associated with higher rates of healthcare utilization, dialysis initiation, and all-cause mortality. When considering the pathophysiology of frailty, chronic-inflammatory states, hypercortisolism, and oxidative stress lead to an imbalance of immune regulatory factors, ultimately resulting in hypercatabolic states, muscle sarcopenia, neuronal deterioration, and enhanced vulnerability to environmental stressors (Kennard et al., 2024). CKD is an intense inflammatory state, marked by metabolic derangements, uremia, metabolic acidosis, bone demineralization, vascular calcification, anemia, and impaired oxygen delivery, and dysregulation of the renin-angiotensin system. Uremia contributes to dysgeusia, cognitive dysfunction, progressive impairment, and symptom burden, which carries a high risk of depression and fatigue. Chronic metabolic acidosis contributes to exertional muscle fatigue. In addition, patients with CKD develop lactic acidosis with minimal activity at a higher rate than healthy controls, further contributing to muscle fatigue (Gregg et al., 2021).

Psychosocial factors

Chronic illness, social isolation, financial strain, and reduced quality of life are highly prevalent in individuals with depression and CKD. When compared to chronic disease populations with primary heart or lung conditions, those with primary kidney disease experience greater functional disability. In the elderly, preserving functional ability is closely linked to social and family support. The lack of social engagement, or social isolation, is associated with frailty, falls, disability, and mortality. Social isolation has also been linked to chronic inflammatory states. Individuals with nondialysis-dependent CKD have lower social contact compared to those with higher eGFR. Social isolation may exacerbate the chronic inflammatory state of CKD (Moorthi and Latham-Mintus, 2019). Furthermore, caregiver support for elderly individuals with advanced CKD may strain existing social and family connections. The burden of responsibilities and tasks, including medication administration, travel to medical appointments, and providing psychosocial and emotional support, is well established among caregivers of individuals with advanced kidney disease (Shankar et al., 2024). In addition, nondialysis-dependent CKD is associated with financial burdens (Small et al., 2017). These factors are linked to low health-related quality of life, with a significant decline in mental and physical health domains, particularly in the year prior to dialysis initiation (de Rooij et al., 2022).

Comorbid symptoms and conditions

Chronic pain, uremic pruritus, diabetes, cardiovascular disease, and cognitive decline are common in CKD and increase the risk of depression.

Chronic pain is common in patients with advanced CKD. In the elderly, the etiology of pain is predominantly musculoskeletal, specifically from the effects of arthritis and osteoporosis, but it can also be neuropathic in nature. Chronic pain carries significant disability, lower health-related quality of life, higher health care utilization, and increased depressive symptoms (Davison et al., 2021).

Uremic pruritus is a debilitating and burdensome symptom that affects over 40% of patients with advanced CKD but is often underreported and undertreated. Itching is non-dermatomal, generalized, and involves large areas of distribution. Symptoms can occur day or night, impacting sleep quality, mood, and overall quality of life. Patients often express a sense of obsession with their itching and often feel hopeless as therapies may not prove effective (Metzger et al., 2021).

The prevalence of comorbid conditions, such as diabetes and cardiovascular disease, is high in those with advanced CKD. Both conditions predispose individuals to the development of a loss of cognitive resilience. Cognitive impairment, including dementia, increases with declining renal function and manifests as deficiencies in executive function, orientation, and attention. Cognitive impairment and depression are closely linked, with depression in later life often manifesting as a symptom of dementia rather than its cause. In those with advanced CKD, non-kidney-specific factors for cognitive decline include age and cardiovascular disease. Patients with renal impairment carry a disproportionately high burden of cardiovascular disease due to a high prevalence of comorbidities, including diabetes, hypertension, and hyperlipidemia. Small vessel disease causes cardiovascular disease and vascular dementia. Kidney-specific factors for cognitive decline include chronic inflammation, hypercoagulable states, oxidative stress, and hyper-homocysteinemia. Retention of uremic metabolites, specifically 4-hydroxyphenylacetate, phenylacetylglutamine, hippurate, and prolyl-hydroxyproline, is independently associated with cognitive impairment (Murtaza and Dasgupta, 2021). Lastly, microalbuminuria is a risk factor for poor cognitive testing, lower executive function and memory, and higher magnetic resonance imaging (MRI) white matter volume abnormalities, with subsequent cerebral atrophy (Tamura et al., 2020; Bikbov et al., 2022).

Treatment burden

Polypharmacy, defined as the regular intake of > 5 medications, is common in the elderly and highly prevalent in people with CKD (Letts et al., 2024). This is due to the need for complex management of CKD-related disorders, such as bone mineral metabolism, anemia of chronic disease, and symptom burden, along with comorbidities (Van Oosten et al., 2021). Those living with long-term health conditions, including CKD, have a greater number of healthcare interactions, individual prescribers, and lower rates of deprescribing. Polypharmacy is associated with treatment burden, medication nonadherence, drug-drug interactions, hospitalizations, falls, and decreased quality of life, all of which lead to increased vulnerability to depressive symptoms (Ma et al., 2023).

Screening and assessment

Mandatory screening (KDIGO and USPSTF guidelines)

The Kidney Disease Improving Global Outcomes (KDIGO) CKD workgroup recommends screening for depression when considering management strategies for the common symptom burden in CKD patients (Stevens et al., 2024). Depression may be related to the patient's perception of CKD, the perceived loss of control, medication side effects, and/or be associated with other CKD symptoms, including chronic pain, uremic pruritus, restless legs with sleep deprivation, and poor appetite with anorexia. Screening for depression is often captured when assessing the mental health domain in various patient-reported health-related quality of life screens. These assessments often involve structured interviews and validated tools such as the PHQ-9. KDIGO also highlights the importance of recognizing cognitive symptoms, which may otherwise be overlooked in standard depression screening but are critical for comprehensive care in the CKD population. Furthermore, those with identified psychological issues should be treated appropriately to improve patient outcomes.

The U.S. Preventive Services Task Force (USPSTF) recommends routine depression screening in adults, including older populations and pregnant/postpartum patients. This Grade B recommendation reflects high-certainty evidence that screening provides a moderate to substantial net benefit (Barry et al., 2023). However, routine suicide risk screening in adults remains a Grade I recommendation, indicating insufficient evidence to support its efficacy.

USPSTF does not mandate a specific screening tool, but it suggests the use of standardized, validated instruments such as the Patient Health Questionnaire Two-Item or Nine-Item (PHQ-2 or PHQ-9).

Patient health questionnaire—Two item (PHQ-2)

1. *"Over the past two weeks, have you felt down, depressed, or hopeless?"*
2. *"Over the past two weeks, have you felt little interest or pleasure in doing things?"*

If a patient answers "yes" to one or both questions, the full PHQ-9 is typically administered. This two-step process is intended to maximize screening efficiency while minimizing patient burden. The USPSTF also emphasizes that screening should only be implemented when there are systems in place to ensure accurate diagnosis, effective treatment, and appropriate follow-up (Barry et al., 2023).

Patient health questionnaire—Nine item (PHQ-9)

For patients with CKD, the PHQ-9 offers a structured method to identify depressive symptoms that may otherwise be misattributed to the underlying medical condition. Because many CKD-related symptoms—such as fatigue, appetite changes, and sleep disturbances—overlap with depressive symptoms, a formal tool like the PHQ-9 can help clinicians differentiate between physical and psychological causes. Regular use of the PHQ-9 in nephrology clinics may enhance early detection and facilitate timely referral to mental health services, thereby improving quality of life and treatment adherence in this high-risk population. The PHQ-9 is a validated tool for screening and diagnosing depression. It consists of nine questions that assess key depressive symptoms over the past 2 weeks, including mood, anhedonia, sleep disturbances, energy levels, appetite, and suicidal ideation. Each item is scored from 0 (not at all) to 3 (nearly every day), giving a total score ranging from 0 to 27. A score of 10 or higher typically indicates moderate to severe depression, warranting further evaluation and intervention.

Nine questions of the PHQ-9

The nine questions of the PHQ-9 are as follows:

1. Little interest or pleasure in doing things?
2. Feeling down, depressed, or hopeless?
3. Trouble falling asleep, staying asleep, or sleeping too much?
4. Feeling tired or having little energy?
5. Poor appetite or overeating?
6. Feeling bad about yourself—or feeling like you are a failure or have let yourself or your family down?
7. Trouble concentrating on things such as reading the newspaper or watching television?
8. Moving or speaking so slowly that other people could have noticed? Or the opposite—being so fidgety or restless that you have been moving around much more than usual?
9. Thoughts that you would be better off dead, or of hurting yourself in some way?

The Beck Depression Inventory (BDI)

The Beck Depression Inventory (BDI) is another widely used screening tool for assessing depressive symptoms in patients with CKD. Hedayati et al. evaluated several depression screening instruments in patients with CKD and found the BDI to have acceptable sensitivity and specificity for identifying MDD, making it a practical tool for routine clinical use. The authors concluded that the BDI could effectively identify depressive symptoms in both predialysis and dialysis populations (Hedayati et al., 2009). It has also been validated in several CKD populations, including racially and ethnically diverse cohorts. Ricardo et al. validated the BDI among US Hispanic patients with CKD, demonstrating its reliability and internal consistency in this underserved group. The study emphasized the importance of culturally sensitive screening tools that account for language and literacy barriers in assessing depression (Ricardo et al., 2025). These findings support the incorporation of the BDI alongside other tools, like the PHQ-9, in nephrology settings, particularly when tailoring screening strategies for diverse patient populations.

Types of depression

Major depressive disorder

According to the DSM-V, MDD is diagnosed when five (or more) of the following symptoms are present during the same 2-week period, representing a change from previous functioning. At least one of the symptoms must be either (1) depressed mood or (2) loss of interest or pleasure:

1. Depressed mood most of the day, nearly every day.
2. Markedly diminished interest or pleasure in all, or almost all, activities for most of the day.
3. Significant weight loss when not dieting, or weight gain, or a decrease or increase in appetite.
4. Insomnia or hypersomnia nearly every day.
5. Psychomotor agitation or retardation occurs nearly every day.
6. Fatigue or loss of energy.
7. Feelings of worthlessness or excessive or inappropriate guilt.
8. Diminished ability to think or concentrate, or indecisiveness.
9 Recurrent thoughts of death, suicidal ideation, suicide attempt, or a specific plan for committing suicide.

Symptoms must cause clinically significant distress or impairment and not be attributable to a substance or another medical condition (Sarmiento and Lau, 2020).

In the United States, the yearly prevalence of MDD is approximately 7%, with gender and age differences. Younger adults, 18–29 years old, have threefold higher rates of MDD than their older counterparts, 60 years or older. Women also have a 1.5- to 3-fold higher prevalence than men.

In CKD patients, MDD often presents with overlapping symptoms such as fatigue and sleep issues. MDD is characterized by persistent low mood, anhedonia, cognitive dysfunction, and somatic symptoms lasting at least two weeks. In CKD patients, MDD often manifests as fatigue, sleep disturbances, and hopelessness, which may overlap with symptoms of renal disease (Palmer et al., 2013).

Persistent depressive disorder

Persistent depressive disorder (PDD), as defined by the DSM-V (American Psychiatric Association, 2022), is characterized by a depressed mood for most of the day, for more days than not, for at least two years (or one year in children and adolescents).

In addition, at least two of the following symptoms must be present:

1. Poor appetite or overeating.
2. Insomnia or hypersomnia.
3. Low energy or fatigue.
4. Low self-esteem.
5. Poor concentration or difficulty in making decisions.
6. Feelings of hopelessness.

During the 2-year period, the individual has never been without symptoms for more than 2 months at a time. The disorder causes clinically significant distress or impairment in social, occupational, or other important areas of functioning (Sarmiento and Lau, 2020).

PDD symptoms in CKD patients are often chronic and may be mistaken for somatic complaints. Previously termed "dysthymia," PDD is a chronic form of depression lasting 2 years or longer. Symptoms are generally less severe than MDD but contribute significantly to decreased quality of life and increased morbidity in CKD patients.

Depressive disorder due to another medical condition

According to the DSM-V, the diagnostic criteria for depressive disorder due to other medical conditions include (Sarmiento and Lau, 2020):

1. *A prominent and persistent period of depressed mood or markedly diminished interest or pleasure in all, or almost all, activities that predominates in the clinical picture.*
2. *There is evidence from the history, physical examination, or laboratory findings that the disturbance is a direct pathophysiological consequence of another medical condition.*
3. *The disturbance is not better explained by another mental disorder* (e.g., *adjustment disorder with depressed mood, where the stressor is a serious medical condition).*
4. *The disturbance does not occur exclusively during the course of delirium.*
5. *The disturbance causes clinically significant distress or impairment in social, occupational, or other important areas of functioning (APA, 2013). A prominent and persistent period of depressed mood or markedly diminished interest or pleasure in all, or almost all, activities predominates in the clinical picture.*
6. *There is evidence from history, physical examination, or laboratory findings that the disturbance is a direct pathophysiological consequence of another medical condition.*
7. *The disturbance is not better explained by another mental disorder* (e.g., *adjustment disorder with depressed mood, where the stressor is a serious medical condition).*
8. *The disturbance does not occur exclusively during the course of a delirium.*
9. *The disturbance causes clinically significant distress or impairment in social, occupational, or other important areas of functioning.*

In the context of CKD, this diagnosis is particularly relevant because depressive symptoms may arise directly from physiological changes related to renal dysfunction. Uremic toxins, anemia, hyperparathyroidism, and electrolyte disturbances can affect the central nervous system and disrupt neurotransmitter function, contributing to mood disorders. A study published in *Frontiers in Pharmacology* highlights that inflammation and oxidative stress, common in CKD, play key roles in the pathophysiology of depression in these patients (Silva et al., 2019). Therefore CKD itself can be the medical condition precipitating depressive symptoms, especially in patients who do not have a prior history of mental illness.

Adjustment disorder with depressed mood

In CKD patients, adjustment disorder with depressed mood often arises as a reaction to the diagnosis of kidney disease, changes in physical ability, or the demands of treatment, such as dialysis or dietary restrictions. Research has shown that approximately 30% of CKD patients experience significant psychological distress following diagnosis or initiation of dialysis, with many cases meeting the criteria for adjustment disorders (Kimmel et al., 2019). Unlike MDD, which is more persistent and less tied to specific external events, adjustment disorder involves the development of emotional or behavioral symptoms in response to an identifiable stressor(s) within 3 months of the onset of the stressor(s). These symptoms or behaviors are clinically significant, as evidenced by one or both of the following:

1. Marked distress that is out of proportion to the severity or intensity of the stressor, taking into account the external context and the cultural factors that might influence symptom severity and presentation.
2. Significant impairment in social, occupational, or other important areas of functioning.
3. The stress-related disturbance does not meet the criteria for another mental disorder and is not merely an exacerbation of a preexisting mental disorder.
4. The symptoms do not represent normal bereavement.
5. Once the stressor or its consequences have terminated, the symptoms do not persist for more than an additional 6 months.

Adjustment disorder symptoms are closely related to life stressors and may resolve as the individual adapts to their condition or receives psychological support.

Common mood and cognitive symptoms of depression

Dysphoria

In the context of CKD, dysphoria can result from both physiological and psychosocial stressors. CKD patients experience a wide range of life disruptions—from dietary restrictions and fluid management to dependence on dialysis—that can contribute to a chronic sense of dissatisfaction or unease. In addition, biochemical imbalances may disrupt neurochemical pathways involved in mood regulation, exacerbating feelings of sadness or emotional discomfort. Studies have shown that dysphoric mood in CKD patients correlates with lower quality of life and poorer treatment adherence, making it a critical symptom to identify and manage early (Wang et al., 2019; Cukor et al., 2007).

Anhedonia

In CKD patients, anhedonia often stems from the chronicity of the illness and the limitations imposed by treatment regimens, such as dietary restrictions, dialysis schedules, and frequent hospital visits. This loss of control over daily life can dull interest in previously enjoyable activities. Neurochemical changes due to uremic toxins and inflammatory cytokines may also contribute to dysfunction in reward pathways in the brain, further reducing motivation and pleasure (Wang et al., 2019).

Worthlessness or excessive guilt

Chronic illnesses like CKD can lead patients to perceive themselves as burdens to family and caregivers, particularly if they are no longer able to work or maintain previous social roles. These feelings are compounded by a sense of dependency and diminished autonomy. Studies show that CKD patients often report low self-esteem and internalized guilt, especially if they believe their condition resulted from poor lifestyle choices (Cukor et al., 2007).

Suicidal ideation or behavior

The emotional burden of living with CKD, especially at advanced stages, can result in hopelessness and suicidal ideation. The constant management of a life-altering illness, financial stress, and loss of independence are significant risk factors. Research indicates that suicidal ideation is more prevalent in dialysis patients than in the general population, with a higher risk observed in those with untreated depression and limited psychosocial support (Cukor et al., 2007; Kimmel et al., 2000).

Epidemiological studies show that the suicide rate in the general population of the United States is approximately 14 per 100,000 individuals annually. In contrast, individuals undergoing dialysis for ESRD face a substantially increased risk, with suicide rates ranging from 40 to 100 per 100,000, depending on comorbid factors and the duration of dialysis (Hedayati et al., 2010). This elevated risk highlights the urgent need for proactive mental health screening and support in CKD populations.

Cognitive dysfunction

Cognitive dysfunction is common in CKD due to both structural and metabolic brain changes caused by reduced kidney function. Impaired clearance of neurotoxic substances, such as urea and homocysteine, can alter cognitive processing. Furthermore, anemia and fluctuations in blood pressure, common in CKD, reduce cerebral perfusion, contributing to issues like forgetfulness, poor attention span, and executive dysfunction (Wang et al., 2019).

Adverse effects of depression

All-cause mortality

Depression significantly increases mortality in CKD and ESRD patients. Multiple studies have shown that depressed CKD patients have a 1.5- to 2-fold increased risk of death compared to their nondepressed counterparts, even after adjusting for demographics, comorbidities, and dialysis modality (Hedayati et al., 2008; Speyer et al., 2024).

A prospective cohort study by Hedayati et al. (2008), involving patients with stage 5 CKD, found that those with MDD had a 2.95-fold higher risk of all-cause mortality and initiation of dialysis compared to nondepressed patients. Similarly, the Dialysis Outcomes and Practice Patterns Study (DOPPS) reported that hemodialysis patients with depressive symptoms had a significantly higher risk of death and hospitalization over a 1-year period (Lopes et al., 2002).

These findings underscore the need for early identification and treatment of depression in the CKD population, as it directly influences survival outcomes. Routine mental health screening and timely intervention may reduce the burden of premature mortality among these patients.

Hospitalization

Hospitalization due to mental disorders was 1.5–3 times higher in CKD patients compared to other chronically ill patients with comorbidities, such as diabetes, ischemic heart disease, cerebrovascular disease, or peptic ulcer disease. Particularly for those aged 65 and older, rates of hospitalization for a primary diagnosis of depression were higher in CKD patients than in those with other chronic illnesses, except diabetes. Among ESRD patients, those on peritoneal dialysis had overall fewer hospitalizations from depression compared to those on hemodialysis. Underlying causes of ESRD were not associated with differing rates of hospitalization from mental disorders (Kimmel et al., 1998).

Withdrawal from dialysis

Depression is a leading cause of voluntary dialysis withdrawal. Studies indicate that dialysis patients with depressive symptoms are up to four times more likely to discontinue treatment compared to their nondepressed counterparts (Weisbord et al., 2003). Withdrawal from dialysis is often preceded by a period of poor treatment adherence, decreased appetite, social isolation, and expressed hopelessness.

In one large cohort study, 20% of dialysis patients who died had previously elected to discontinue treatment, and depression was frequently cited as a significant contributing factor (El-Magd et al., 2023). This decision is associated with high short-term mortality and is often made without adequate psychological evaluation or intervention. The presence of untreated depression can impair decision-making capacity, raising ethical concerns about patient autonomy and informed consent.

From an ethical standpoint, voluntary withdrawal from dialysis by a depressed patient poses several challenges. Central to the ethical dilemma is the distinction between a competent, informed refusal of treatment and a decision influenced by a potentially treatable psychiatric condition. Depression can distort cognition and impair judgment, thereby undermining true autonomy. Clinicians must assess whether the patient's decision reflects an informed, rational choice or stems from untreated psychological suffering. If the latter, efforts should focus on treating the underlying depression and revisiting the patient's decision once mental health has improved.

From a legal and policy standpoint, dialysis withdrawal by a patient with untreated depression raises questions about capacity, consent, and healthcare provider obligations. In many jurisdictions, a patient's right to refuse medical treatment is protected under legal principles of autonomy and bodily integrity. However, if a patient's decision-making is significantly impaired by a psychiatric disorder such as depression, providers may be ethically and legally required to assess and address mental health issues before honoring such a decision.

Policies in many healthcare institutions mandate a formal psychiatric evaluation before a dialysis withdrawal request can be considered valid, especially if the patient has exhibited symptoms of depression or suicidal ideation. Legal frameworks may also require documentation of mental status, interdisciplinary case review, and engagement with ethics committees.

These procedures are designed to ensure that the decision to withdraw is informed, voluntary, and not driven by a potentially reversible mental health condition.

Furthermore, palliative care consultations are increasingly recommended or required as part of the withdrawal process to ensure comprehensive symptom management and emotional support. Ensuring access to mental health professionals and legal safeguards helps protect vulnerable patients from premature or unrecognized suicidal behavior under the guise of treatment refusal.

Equitable access to mental health care must be ensured to support informed end-of-life decision-making. Involving mental health professionals, ethicists, and the patient's family in a shared decision-making process is essential to safeguard patient rights while minimizing preventable loss of life. Timely recognition and treatment of depression in ESRD patients are critical not only for improving quality of life but also for potentially preventing premature withdrawal from life-sustaining dialysis therapy.

Management and treatment

When to refer

Referral to mental health specialists is important for CKD patients with moderate to severe depression, suicidal ideation, or an inadequate response to initial treatment. Nephrologists should work closely with psychiatrists, psychologists, and primary care providers to optimize mental health care.

This collaborative approach is essential because CKD patients often present with complex physical and psychological symptoms that can complicate diagnosis and treatment. Mental health professionals can provide comprehensive psychiatric evaluations to distinguish between overlapping somatic symptoms and clinical depression. They are also better equipped to manage coexisting psychiatric conditions, such as anxiety or cognitive impairment, which frequently occur in CKD.

Specialists can initiate psychotherapeutic interventions like cognitive behavioral therapy or prescribe psychotropic medications, with consideration for renal dosing and drug-drug interactions. Referral is particularly critical in cases of suicidality, psychosis, or when there is a need for multidisciplinary care involving social work, behavioral counseling, and long-term psychiatric monitoring.

Evidence suggests that integrated care models—where mental health support is embedded into nephrology services—improve patient adherence to CKD treatment, reduce hospitalizations, and enhance the overall quality of life for CKD patients with moderate to severe depression, suicidal ideation, or inadequate response to initial treatment. Nephrologists should work closely with psychiatrists, psychologists, and primary care providers to optimize mental health care.

Pharmacotherapy

Pharmacologic management of depression in CKD patients requires careful consideration of drug metabolism, renal clearance, and side effect profiles. The selection of antidepressants

TABLE 14.1 Key considerations for antidepressants in CKD patients.

Antidepressant class	Common agents	Pros	Cons	CKD considerations
SSRIs	Sertraline, Citalopram	Well tolerated, first-line treatment	GI upset, sexual dysfunction	Dosage adjustments may be needed in advanced CKD
SNRIs	Venlafaxine, Duloxetine	Effective for anxiety and pain	Hypertension, nausea, withdrawal symptoms	Duloxetine is contraindicated if eGFR < 30 mL/min/1.73m^2
Atypical Antidepressants	Mirtazapine, Bupropion	Weight/appetite gain (mirtazapine); energizing (bupropion)	Sedation (mirtazapine), insomnia (bupropion)	Dosage adjustments are recommended in moderate to severe CKD
TCAs	Nortriptyline, Desipramine	May be helpful in treatment-resistant cases	Anticholinergic effects, cardiotoxicity	Use with caution; avoid in elderly or cardiac patients
MAOIs	Phenelzine, Tranylcypromine	Rarely used; for resistant depression	Drug and food interactions, hypertensive crisis	Generally not recommended in CKD
Serotonin modulators	Trazodone, Vilazodone	Useful for insomnia (trazodone)	Sedation, dizziness	Monitor for hypotension and sedation

should be guided by symptom severity, patient comorbidities, and the potential for drug interactions (see Table 14.1).

- **Selective serotonin reuptake inhibitors (SSRIs)**: SSRIs are generally first-line agents due to their safety and tolerability. Sertraline and citalopram are commonly used in CKD and ESRD populations. Dose adjustments may be necessary in advanced stages of kidney disease. The CAST (Chronic Kidney Disease Antidepressant Sertraline Trial) found no significant difference in depressive symptom improvement with sertraline compared to placebo in nondialysis CKD patients, though sertraline was well tolerated. Secondary analyses of this trial data did find that patients with higher inflammatory markers, such as C-reactive protein, were associated with somatic depressive symptoms and did show benefit from the initiation of sertraline (Gregg and Hedayati, 2020). However, a large retrospective study by Vangala et al. found that SSRI use in patients on hemodialysis was associated with significantly higher rates of hip fractures, underscoring the need to weigh the benefits of symptom relief against potential musculoskeletal risks in this vulnerable population (Vangala et al., 2020). One study did find that renally adjusted SSRIs had lower hazards of short-term outcomes, such as upper gastrointestinal bleeding, compared to standard dosing. Interestingly, the lower dose was associated with higher rates of cardiac arrest, which the study notes is likely due to confounding by contraindication (Zhu et al., 2023). Nevertheless, the general consensus is that the initiation of low-dose, newer-generation SSRIs with lower cardiovascular side effect profiles, such as sertraline, is safe to initiate for CKD patients with careful monitoring.

- **Serotonin-norepinephrine reuptake inhibitors (SNRIs)**: SNRIs, such as venlafaxine and duloxetine, can be effective but may require cautious use in CKD due to renal elimination and the risk of hypertension or an increased bleeding tendency. Duloxetine is contraindicated in patients with an eGFR < 30 mL/min/1.73m^2.
- **Atypical Antidepressants**:
- **Mirtazapine**: Generally believed to be beneficial for patients with insomnia or poor appetite due to its sedating and appetite-stimulating properties, with dose reduction required in renal impairment. However, a 2023 nationwide comparative effectiveness study by Zhu et al. examined outcomes associated with Selective Serotonin Reuptake Inhibitors (SSRIs) versus mirtazapine in patients with CKD and depression. Using a large Swedish database of over 240,000 CKD patients newly prescribed either SSRIs or mirtazapine, the study evaluated the risks of all-cause mortality, hospitalization, and progression to ESRD. After propensity score matching and adjusting for covariates, results showed that patients initiated on mirtazapine had a higher risk of all-cause mortality (HR 1.11) compared to those started on SSRIs. There was no significant difference in progression to ESRD or other long-term outcomes between the groups. These findings suggest that SSRIs may offer a more favorable safety profile than mirtazapine in CKD populations, particularly in terms of mortality and hospitalization (Zhu et al., 2023). While mirtazapine may be useful for specific indications like insomnia or appetite stimulation, this study underscores the importance of individualized risk-benefit assessments, especially in patients with advanced renal impairment.
- **Bupropion**: A norepinephrine-dopamine reuptake inhibitor (NDRI) that is stimulating and may be useful for patients with anhedonia or fatigue. It is cleared renally and requires dose adjustment in moderate to severe CKD.
- **Tricyclic antidepressants (TCAs)**: Generally avoided in CKD due to anticholinergic effects, orthostatic hypotension, and the risk of cardiotoxicity. If used, agents like nortriptyline and desipramine may be preferred for their relatively better tolerability.
- **Monoamine oxidase inhibitors (MAOIs)**: Rarely used due to dietary restrictions and a high risk of drug interactions. Their use in CKD patients is limited and generally discouraged.
- **Serotonin modulators**: Agents like trazodone and vilazodone may be considered. Trazodone is frequently used off-label for sleep disturbances in CKD patients, and it requires careful monitoring for hypotension and sedation.

Coordination with nephrology and pharmacy is recommended when initiating or adjusting antidepressant therapy in this population, particularly for CKD patients, due to their favorable side-effect profile. However, dose adjustments may be required for patients with advanced kidney disease. TCAs and MAOIs are generally avoided due to their potential nephrotoxicity and cardiovascular side effects.

Comparison of antidepressant classes in CKD patients

Cognitive behavioral therapy

Cognitive behavioral therapy (CBT) is an effective nonpharmacological treatment for depression in CKD patients. It targets maladaptive thought patterns and behaviors, improving coping skills and emotional regulation. CBT helps patients develop practical strategies for managing stress, illness-related anxiety, and depressive symptoms that commonly arise with chronic illness (Table 14.2).

Evidence supports its efficacy in the CKD population. A randomized controlled trial by Cukor et al. demonstrated that CBT significantly reduced depressive symptoms in patients undergoing hemodialysis compared to usual care. Participants receiving CBT also reported improvements in quality of life and treatment adherence (Cukor et al., 2014). Another study found that a telehealth-delivered CBT intervention was feasible and associated with sustained reductions in depression scores among CKD patients (Hedayati et al., 2016).

In addition, the ASCEND trial, a multicenter randomized trial, tested both pharmacologic (sertraline) and behavioral (CBT) interventions for depression in CKD patients (Mehrotra et al., 2019). The trial found that while sertraline did not significantly outperform placebo, CBT demonstrated clinically meaningful reductions in depressive symptoms. Notably, CBT was associated with fewer side effects and had a lower dropout rate

TABLE 14.2 Comparison of cognitive behavioral therapy and pharmacologic treatment modalities in CKD patients.

Feature	CBT	Pharmacotherapy (e.g., SSRIs)
Efficacy	Shown to effectively reduce depressive symptoms	Mixed results: the CAST trial showed no superiority over placebo
Side effects	Minimal, primarily fatigue or emotional discomfort	Common (e.g., GI upset, sexual dysfunction)
Dropout rate	Lower	Higher due to side effects or lack of perceived benefit
Delivery format	In-person or via telehealth	Oral medication, often requiring monitoring
Suitability in CKD	Well tolerated; no renal dose adjustment needed	Requires careful dose adjustment and monitoring
ASCEND Trial findings	Fewer side effects, lower dropout, sustained benefit	No significant difference vs. placebo

Modified from Mehrotra, R., Cukor, D., Unruh, M., Rue, T., Heagerty, P., Cohen, S.D., Dember, L.M., Diaz-Linhart, Y., Dubovsky, A., Greene, T., Grote, N., Kutner, N., Trivedi, M.H., Quinn, D.K., Halen, N., Weisbord, S.D., Young, B.A., Kimmel, P.L., Hedayati, S.S. (2019). Comparative efficacy of therapies for treatment of depression for patients undergoing maintenance hemodialysis. Ann. Intern. Med. 15393704. 170 (6), 369–379. https://annals.org/aim/fullarticle/2726666/comparative-efficacy-therapies-treatment-depression-patients-undergoing-maintenance-hemodialysis-randomized.

compared to pharmacologic treatment, underscoring its value as a well tolerated and effective therapeutic option. These results support the prioritization of CBT, particularly for patients who may be at risk for medication-related adverse effects or who prefer nonpharmacologic approaches. The trial found that while sertraline did not significantly outperform placebo, CBT demonstrated clinically meaningful reductions in depressive symptoms, supporting its value as a primary therapeutic approach. These findings highlight CBT's adaptability and effectiveness in diverse CKD populations, including those with limited access to in-person care. Integration of CBT into nephrology services, particularly via telemedicine platforms, can enhance access to mental health support and improve overall patient outcomes for depression in CKD patients.

Adjunctive therapy

Additional strategies for managing depression include (see Table 14.3).

- **Exercise therapy**: Compared with older individuals with normal kidney function, older patients with CKD exhibit greater frailty and reduced lower extremity function. It is well established that low physical activity levels lead to adverse clinical events, including cardiovascular events, declining kidney function, and increased mortality in nondialysis CKD patients (Nakamura et al., 2020). Therefore incorporating exercise training into a multidisciplinary lifestyle modification program can yield substantial benefits in activities of daily living and quality of life, as well as increased muscle strength, without detrimental effects on kidney function. The Lifestyle Interventions and Independence for Elders (LIFE) clinical trial, a randomized controlled trial across eight academic centers in the United States, aimed to assess the impact of exercise on CKD progression among community-dwelling, sedentary adults aged 70–89 years old (Shlipak et al., 2022). Participants were randomized to the intervention group, consisting

TABLE 14.3 Comparison of adjunctive interventions in CKD patients with depression.

Intervention	Benefits	Limitations	CKD Considerations
Exercise therapy	Improves mood, physical function, and energy	May be limited by physical disability or fatigue	Should be tailored to individual ability and CKD stage
Mindfulness-based stress reduction (MBSR)	Reduces anxiety and depressive symptoms	Requires training and consistent practice	Safe and non-pharmacologic
Support groups	Enhances emotional support and social connections	Availability and stigma may limit participation	Especially beneficial for dialysis patients
Nutritional counseling	Supports dietary management, reduces anxiety	Requires collaboration with renal dietitian	Addresses diet-related mood symptoms and energy levels
Psychoeducational interventions	Delays dialysis initiation; improves coping	Effectiveness varies with individual engagement	Effective in early CKD and with ongoing follow-up

of a moderate-intensity, supervised exercise program for 2 years, or the control group, who received health education workshops that addressed a variety of health topics relevant to older adults but did not specifically address physical activity. Those in the intervention group exhibited a slower decline in eGFR than participants in the control group. In a situation where patients with CKD often feel helpless and hopeless to change their disease course, improvement in the trajectory of kidney disease with exercise can empower patients to embrace lifestyle change.
- **Mindfulness-based stress reduction (MBSR)**: While large randomized controlled trials in CKD patients are lacking, the use of meditation and mindfulness has shown meaningful improvement in the reduction of anxiety, stress, and depression in those with chronic disease states, as well as improved mental health-related quality of life in those with CKD awaiting a kidney transplant (Gross et al., 2017; Keng et al., 2011).
- **Support groups**: Provide emotional support and enhance social connectedness. Empowering patients through education allows them to participate in care decisions and engage in self-management support (Narva et al., 2016).
- **Nutritional counseling**: Addresses dietary concerns and promotes overall well-being. Both animal models and clinical studies have associated very low dietary protein intake with the preservation of renal function. However, low-protein diets lead to sarcopenia and protein-energy wasting, particularly in the elderly. Adequate protein intake is important to counteract age-related muscle catabolism (Chewcharat et al., 2020). Of note, several studies have shown that the risk of death is a more important concern than the risk of progression of kidney failure in older patients, particularly in those over the age of 85. In a recent cohort of Canadian adults with CKD stage IV, the risk of death was 24-fold higher than the risk of kidney failure among those aged 85–94 years (Ravani et al., 2020). Therefore a more nuanced approach to protein restriction, plant-based proteins, and supplementation with keto acid analogs would support the health needs of the patient, minimize protein-energy wasting, and delay the progression of kidney disease.

Comparison of adjunctive interventions in CKD patients with depression

In conclusion, the relationship between CKD and depression is complex and exacerbated by common geriatric syndromes in the elderly. Given its high prevalence and significant impact on morbidity and mortality, aggressive screening and therapeutic intervention are paramount. Physicians must be mindful of drug pharmacokinetics with reduced kidney capacity and should encourage the use of non-pharmacologic interventions that will yield substantial benefits.

References

American Psychiatric Association, 2022. Diagnostic and statistical manual of mental disorders (5th ed., text rev.). doi:10.1176/appi.books.9780890425787.

Barry, M.J., Nicholson, W.K., Silverstein, M., Chelmow, D., Coker, T.R., Davidson, K.W., Davis, E.M., Donahue, K.E., Jaén, C.R., Li, L., Ogedegbe, G., Pbert, L., Rao, G., Ruiz, J.M., Stevermer, J.J., Tsevat, J., Underwood, S.M., Wong,

J.B., 2023. Screening for depression and suicide risk in adults: US preventive services task force recommendation statement. JAMA. 15383598. 329 (23), 2057–2067. Available from: http://jama.jamanetwork.com/journal.aspx. doi:10.1001/jama.2023.9297.

Bikbov, B., Soler, M.J., Pešić, V., Capasso, G., Unwin, R., Endres, M., Remuzzi, G., Perico, N., Gansevoort, R., Mattace-Raso, F., Bruchfeld, A., Figurek, A., Hafez, G., 2022. Albuminuria as a risk factor for mild cognitive impairment and dementia—what is the evidence? Nephrol. Dial. Transplant. 14602385. 37, II55. Available from http://ndt.oxfordjournals.org/. doi:10.1093/ndt/gfab261.

Chewcharat, A., Takkavatakarn, K., Wongrattanagorn, S., Panrong, K., Kittiskulnam, P., Eiam-Ong, S., Susantitaphong, P., 2020. The effects of restricted protein diet supplemented with ketoanalogue on renal function, blood pressure, nutritional status, and chronic kidney disease-mineral and bone disorder in chronic kidney disease patients: a systematic review and meta-analysis. J. Ren. Nutr. 10512276. 30 (3), 189–199. doi:10.1053/j.jrn.2019.07.005.

Chowdhury, R., Peel, N.M., Krosch, M., Hubbard, R.E., 2017. Frailty and chronic kidney disease: a systematic review. Arch. Gerontol. Geriatr. 18726976. 68, 135–142. Available from: www.elsevier.com/locate/archger. doi:10.1016/j.archger.2016.10.007.

Cukor, D., Coplan, J., Brown, C., Friedman, S., Cromwell-Smith, A., Peterson, R.A., Kimmel, P.L., 2007. Depression and anxiety in urban hemodialysis patients. Clin. J. Am. Soc. Nephrol. 2 (3), 484–490. doi:10.2215/CJN.00040107.

Cukor, D., Halen, N.V., Asher, D.R., Coplan, J.D., Weedon, J., Wyka, K.E., Saggi, S.J., Kimmel, P.L., 2014. Psychosocial intervention improves depression, quality of life, and fluid adherence in hemodialysis. J. Am. Soc. Nephrol. 15333450. 25 (1), 196–206. Available from: http://jasn.asnjournals.org/content/25/1/196.full.pdf+html. doi:10.1681/ASN.2012111134.

Davison, S.N., Rathwell, S., Ghosh, S., George, C., Pfister, T., Dennett, L., 2021. The prevalence and severity of chronic pain in patients with chronic kidney disease: a systematic review and meta-analysis. Can. J. Kidney Health Dis. 20543581. 8. Available from: http://www.cjkhd.org/. doi:10.1177/2054358121993995.

de Rooij, E.N.M., Meuleman, Y., de Fijter, J.W., Le Cessie, S., Jager, K.J., Chesnaye, N.C., Evans, M., Pagels, A.A., Caskey, F.J., Torino, C., Porto, G., Szymczak, M., Drechsler, C., Wanner, C., Dekker, F.W., Hoogeveen, E.K., 2022. Quality of life before and after the start of dialysis in older patients. Clin. J. Am. Soc. Nephrol. 1555905X. 17 (8), 1159–1167. Available from: https://cjasn.asnjournals.org/content/17/8/1159/full-text.pdf?with-ds=yes. doi:10.2215/CJN.16371221.

El-Magd, E.S., Schouten, R.W., Nadort, E., Shaw, P.K.C., Smets, Y.F.C., Vleming, L.J., Dekker, F.W., Broekman, B.F.P., Honig, A., Siegert, C.E.H., 2023. Dialysis withdrawal and symptoms of anxiety and depression: a prospective cohort study. BMC Nephrol. 24 (1), 219. doi: 10.1186/s12882-023-03267-2.

Fried, L.P., Tangen, C.M., Walston, J., Newman, A.B., Hirsch, C., Gottdiener, J., Seeman, T., Tracy, R., Kop, W.J., Burke, G., McBurnie, M.A., 2001. Frailty in older adults: evidence for a phenotype. J. Gerontol. A Biol. Sci. Med. Sci. 1079-5006. 56 (3), M146. doi:10.1093/gerona/56.3.m146.

Gregg, L.P., Bossola, M., Ostrosky-Frid, M., Hedayati, S.S., 2021. Fatigue in CKD. Clin. J. Am. Soc. Nephrol. 1555-9041. 16 (9), 1445–1455. doi:10.2215/cjn.19891220.

Gregg, L.P., Hedayati, S.S., 2020. Pharmacologic and psychological interventions for depression treatment in patients with kidney disease. Curr. Opin. Nephrol. Hypertens. 14736543. 29 (5), 457–464. Available from: http://journals.lww.com/co-nephrolhypertens/pages/default.aspx. doi:10.1097/MNH.0000000000000629.

Gregg, L.P., Jain, N., Carmody, T., Minhajuddin, A.T., Rush, A.J., Trivedi, M.H., Hedayati, S.S., 2019. Fatigue in nondialysis chronic kidney disease: correlates and association with kidney outcomes. Am. J. Nephrol. 14219670. 50 (1), 37–47. Available from: www.karger.ch/journals/ajn/ajn_jh.htm. doi:10.1159/000500668.

Gross, C.R., Reilly-Spong, M., Park, T., Zhao, R., Gurvich, O.V., Ibrahim, H.N., 2017. Telephone-adapted mindfulness-based stress reduction (tMBSR) for patients awaiting kidney transplantation. Contemp. Clin. Trials. 15592030. 57, 37–43. Available from: http://www.elsevier.com/wps/find/journaldescription.cws_home/704636/description#description. doi:10.1016/j.cct.2017.03.014.

Hedayati, S.S., Bosworth, H.B., Briley, L.P., Sloane, R.J., Pieper, C.F., Kimmel, P.L., Szczech, L.A., 2008. Death or hospitalization of patients on chronic hemodialysis is associated with a physician-based diagnosis of depression. Kidney Int. 74 (7), 930–936. doi:10.1038/ki.2008.311.

Hedayati, S.S., Daniel, D.M., Cohen, S., Comstock, B., Cukor, D., Diaz-Linhart, Y., Dember, L.M., Dubovsky, A., Greene, T., Grote, N., Heagerty, P., Katon, W., Kimmel, P.L., Kutner, N., Linke, L., Quinn, D., Rue, T., Trivedi, M.H., Unruh, M., Weisbord, S., Young, B.A., Mehrotra, R., 2016. Rationale and design of a trial of sertraline vs. cognitive behavioral therapy for end-stage renal disease patients with depression (ASCEND). Contemp. Clin.

Trials. 15592030. 47, 1–11. Available from: http://www.elsevier.com/wps/find/journaldescription.cws_home/704636/description#description. doi:10.1016/j.cct.2015.11.020.

Hedayati, S.S., Minhajuddin, A.T., Afshar, M., Toto, R.D., Trivedi, M.H., Rush, A.J., 2010. Association between major depressive episodes in patients with chronic kidney disease and initiation of dialysis, hospitalization, or death. JAMA 303 (19), 1946-53. doi: 10.1001/jama.2010.619.

Hedayati, S.S., Minhajuddin, A.T., Toto, R.D., Morris, D.W., Rush, A.J., 2009. Validation of depression screening scales in patients with CKD. Am. J. Kidney Dis. 02726386. 54 (3), 433–439. doi:10.1053/j.ajkd.2009.03.016.

Keng, S.L., Smoski, M.J., Robins, C.J., 2011. Effects of mindfulness on psychological health: a review of empirical studies. Clin. Psychol. Rev. 18737811. 31 (6), 1041–1056. doi:10.1016/j.cpr.2011.04.006.

Kennard, A.L., Glasgow, N.J., Rainsford, S.E., Talaulikar, G.S., 2024. Narrative review: clinical implications and assessment of frailty in patients with advanced CKD. Kidney Int. Rep. 24680249. 9 (4), 791–806. Available from: https://www.sciencedirect.com/science/journal/24680249. doi:10.1016/j.ekir.2023.12.022.

Kimmel, P.L., Fwu, C.W., Abbott, K.C., Moxey-Mims, M.M., Mendley, S., Norton, J.M., Eggers, P.W., 2019. Psychiatric illness and mortality in hospitalized ESKD dialysis patients. Clin. J. Am. Soc. Nephrol. 1555905X. 14 (9), 1363–1371. Available from: https://cjasn.asnjournals.org/content/clinjasn/14/9/1363.full.pdf. doi:10.2215/CJN.14191218.

Kimmel, P.L., Peterson, R.A., Weihs, K.L., 2000. Multiple measurements of depression predict mortality in a longitudinal study of chronic hemodialysis outpatients. Kidney Int. 57, 2098. doi:10.1046/j.1523-1755.2000.00059.x.

Kimmel, P.L., Thamer, M., Richard, C.M., Ray, N.F., 1998. Psychiatric illness in patients with end-stage renal disease. Am. J. Med. 00029343. 105 (3), 214–221. doi:10.1016/S0002-9343(98)00245-9.

Lefrère, A., Burtey, S., Bobot, S., Belzeaux, R., Bobot, M., 2025. Depression in chronic kidney disease: particularities, specific mechanisms and therapeutic considerations, a narrative review. Behav. Brain Res. 01664328. 483, 115467. doi:10.1016/j.bbr.2025.115467.

Letts, M., Chesnaye, N.C., Pippias, M., Caskey, F., Jager, K.J., Dekker, F.W., Van Diepen, M., Evans, M., Torino, C., Vilasi, A., Szymczak, M., Drechsler, C., Wanner, C., Hole, B., Hayward, S., Schneider, A., Torp, A., Iwig, B., Perras, B., Marx, C., Drechsler, C., Blaser, C., Wanner, C., Emde, C., Krieter, D., Fuchs, D., Irmler, E., Platen, E., Schmidt-Gürtler, H., Schlee, H., Naujoks, H., Schlee, I., Cäsar, S., Beige, J., Röthele, J., Mazur, J., Hahn, K., Blouin, K., Neumeier, K., Anding-Rost, K., Schramm, L., Hopf, M., Wuttke, N., Frischmuth, N., Ichtiaris, P., Kirste, P., Schulz, P., Aign, S., Biribauer, S., Manan, S., Röser, S., Heidenreich, S., Palm, S., Schwedler, S., Delrieux, S., Renker, S., Schättel, S., Stephan, T., Schmiedeke, T., Weinreich, T., Leimbach, T., Stövesand, T., Bahner, U., Seeger, W., Cupisti, A., Sagliocca, A., Ferraro, A., Mele, A., Naticchia, A., Còsaro, A., Ranghino, A., Stucchi, A., Pignataro, A., De Blasio, A., Pani, A., Tsalouichos, A., Antonio, B., Iorio, B.R.D., Alessandra, B., Abaterusso, C., Somma, C., D'Alessandro, C., Torino, C., Zullo, C., Pozzi, C., Bergamo, D., Ciurlino, D., Motta, D., Russo, D., Favaro, E., Vigotti, F., Ansali, F., Conte, F., Cianciotta, F., Giacchino, F., Cappellaio, F., Pizzarelli, F., Greco, G., Porto, G., Bigatti, G., Marinangeli, G., Cabiddu, G., Fumagalli, G., Caloro, G., Piccoli, G., Capasso, G., Gambaro, G., Tognarelli, G., Bonforte, G., Conte, G., Toscano, G., Rosso, G.D., Capizzi, I., Baragetti, I., Oldrizzi, L., Gesualdo, L., Biancone, L., Magnano, M., Ricardi, M., Bari, M.D., Laudato, M., Sirico, M.L., Ferraresi, M., Provenzano, M., Malaguti, M., Palmieri, N., Murrone, P., Cirillo, P., Dattolo, P., Acampora, P., Nigro, R., Boero, R., Scarpioni, R., Sicoli, R., Malandra, R., Savoldi, S., Bertoli, S., Borrelli, S., Maxia, S., Maffei, S., Mangano, S., Cicchetti, T., Rappa, T., Palazzo, V., De Simone, W., Schrander, A., Van Dam, B., Siegert, C., Gaillard, C., Beerenhout, C., Verburgh, C., Janmaat, C., Hoogeveen, E., Hoorn, E., Dekker, F., Boots, J., Boom, H., Eijgenraam, J.W., Kooman, J., Rotmans, J., Jager, K., Vogt, L., Raasveld, M., Vervloet, M., Van Buren, M., Van Diepen, M., Chesnaye, N., Leurs, P., Voskamp, P., Blankestijn, P., Van Esch, S., Boorsma, S., Berger, S., Konings, C., Aydin, Z., Musiała, A., Szymczak, A., Olczyk, E., Augustyniak-Bartosik, H., Miśkowiec-Wiśniewska, I., Manitius, J., Pondel, J., Jędrzejak, K., Nowańska, K., Nowak, Ł., Szymczak, M., Durlik, M., Dorota, S., Nieszporek, T., Heleniak, Z., Jonsson, A., Blom, A.L., Rogland, B., Wallquist, C., Vargas, D., DimCrossed, E., Sign©ny, D., Sundelin, F., Uhlin, F., Welander, G., Hernandez, I.B., Gröntoft, K.C., Stendahl, M., Svensson, M., Evans, M., Heimburger, O., Kashioulis, P., Melander, S., Almquist, T., Jensen, U., Woodman, A., McKeever, A., Ullah, A., McLaren, B., Harron, C., Barrett, C., O'Toole, C., Summersgill, C., Geddes, C., Glowski, D., McGlynn, D., Sands, D., Caskey, F., Roy, G., Hirst, G., King, H., McNally, H., Masri-Senghor, H., Murtagh, H., Rayner, H., Turner, J., Wilcox, J., Berdeprado, J., Wong, J., Banda, J., Jones, K., Haydock, L., Wilkinson, L., Carmody, M., Weetman, M., Joinson, M., Dutton, M., Matthews, M., Morgan, N., Bleakley, N., Cockwell, P., Roderick, P., Mason, P., Kalra, P., Sajith, R., Chapman, S., Navjee, S., Crosbie, S., Brown, S., Tickle, S., Mathavakkannan, S., Kuan, Y., 2024. Prescribing patterns in older people with advanced chronic kidney disease towards the end of life. Clin. Kidney J. 20488513. 17 (11). Available from: http://ckj.oxfordjournals.org/. doi:10.1093/ckj/sfae301.

Ma, J.E., Berkowitz, T.S.Z., Olsen, M.K., Smith, B., Lorenz, K.A., Bowling, C.B., 2023. Phenotypes of symptom, function, and medication burden in older adults with nondialysis advanced kidney disease. Kidney360. 26417650. 4 (10), 1430–1436. Available from: https://kidney360.asnjournals.org/. doi:10.34067/KID.0000000000000241.

Mehrotra, R., Cukor, D., Unruh, M., Rue, T., Heagerty, P., Cohen, S.D., Dember, L.M., Diaz-Linhart, Y., Dubovsky, A., Greene, T., Grote, N., Kutner, N., Trivedi, M.H., Quinn, D.K., Halen, N., Weisbord, S.D., Young, B.A., Kimmel, P.L., Hedayati, S.S., 2019. Comparative efficacy of therapies for treatment of depression for patients undergoing maintenance hemodialysis. Ann. Intern. Med. 15393704. 170 (6), 369–379. Available from: https://annals.org/aim/fullarticle/2726666/comparative-efficacy-therapies-treatment-depression-patients-undergoing -maintenance-hemodialysis-randomized. doi:10.7326/M18-2229.

Metzger, M., Abdel-Rahman, E.M., Boykin, H., Song, M.K., 2021. A narrative review of management strategies for common symptoms in advanced CKD. Kidney Int. Rep. 24680249. 6 (4), 894–904. Available from: http://www.journals.elsevier.com/kidney-international-reports. doi:10.1016/j.ekir.2021.01.038.

Moorthi, R.N., Latham-Mintus, K., 2019. Social isolation in chronic kidney disease and the role of mobility limitation. Clin. Kidney J. 20488513. 12 (4), 602–610. Available from: http://ckj.oxfordjournals.org/. doi:10.1093/ckj/sfy134.

Mossey, J.M., Shapiro, E., 1982. Self-rated health: a predictor of mortality among the elderly. Am. J. Public Health. 00900036. 72 (8), 800–808. doi:10.2105/AJPH.72.8.800.

Murtaza, A., Dasgupta, I., 2021. Chronic kidney disease and cognitive impairment. J. Stroke Cerebrovasc. Dis. 10523057. 30 (9), 105529. doi:10.1016/j.jstrokecerebrovasdis.2020.105529.

Nakamura, K., Sasaki, T., Yamamoto, S., Hayashi, H., Ako, S., Tanaka, Y., 2020. Effects of exercise on kidney and physical function in patients with non-dialysis chronic kidney disease: a systematic review and meta-analysis. Sci. Rep. 2045-2322. 10 (1). doi:10.1038/s41598-020-75405-x.

Narva, A.S., Norton, J.M., Boulware, L.E., 2016. Educating patients about CKD. Clin. J. Am. Soc. Nephrol. 1555-9041. 11 (4), 694–703. doi:10.2215/cjn.07680715.

Palmer, S., Vecchio, M., Craig, J.C., Tonelli, M., Johnson, D.W., Nicolucci, A., Pellegrini, F., Saglimbene, V., Logroscino, G., Fishbane, S., Strippoli, G.F.M., 2013. Prevalence of depression in chronic kidney disease: systematic review and meta-analysis of observational studies. Kidney Int. 15231755. 84 (1), 179–191. Available from: https://www.journals.elsevier.com/kidney-international. doi:10.1038/ki.2013.77.

Ravani, P., Quinn, R., Fiocco, M., Liu, P., Al-Wahsh, H., Lam, N., Hemmelgarn, B.R., Manns, B.J., James, M.T., Joanette, Y., Tonelli, M., 2020. Association of age with risk of kidney failure in adults with stage IV chronic kidney disease in Canada. JAMA Netw. Open. 25743805. 3 (9). Available from: https://jamanetwork.com/journals/jamanetworkopen. doi:10.1001/jamanetworkopen.2020.17150.

Ricardo, A.C., Park, S., Carmona-Powell, E., Larkin, C., Quiroga, A., Fischer, M.J., Lora, C.M., Chen, J., Missikpode, C., Pineda, M., Zhang, X., Hsu, J.Y., Shankman, S., Lash, J., Anderson, A.H., Appel, L.J., Chen, J., Cohen, D.L., Dember, L.M., Go, A.S., Lash, J.P., Rahman, M., Rao, P.S., Shah, V.O., Unruh, M.L., 2025. Validation of the beck depression inventory in US hispanic patients with CKD. Clin. J. Am. Soc. Nephrol. 1555905X. 20 (4), 495–501. Available from: https://journals.lww.com/CJASN/Pages/default.aspx. doi:10.2215/CJN.0000000655.

Sarmiento, C., Lau, C., 2020. Diagnostic and Statistical Manual of Mental Disorders, 5th Ed. The Wiley Encyclopedia of Personality and Individual Differences: Model and Theories: Measurement and Assessment: Personality Processes and Individual Differences: Clinical, Applied, and Cross-Cultural Research: Vol. 1-4. 125–129. Available from: https://onlinelibrary.wiley.com/doi/book/10.1002/9781118970843. doi:10.1002/9781118970843.ch198.

Shankar, R., Luo, N., Lim, Y.W., Khatri, P., Leong, L., Teo, G.Y.X., Mukhopadhyay, A., Choo, J., Chua, H.R., Teng, G.G., Phua, J., Hong, W.Z., 2024. Assessing caregiver burden in advanced kidney disease: protocol for a systematic review of the measurement properties of instruments and tools. BMJ Open. 20446055. 14 (2). Available from: http://bmjopen.bmj.com/content/early/by/section. doi:10.1136/bmjopen-2023-078767.

Shlipak, M.G., Sheshadri, A., Hsu, F.C., Chen, S.H., Jotwani, V., Tranah, G., Fielding, R.A., Liu, C.K., Ix, J., Coca, S.G., 2022. Effect of structured, moderate exercise on kidney function decline in sedentary older adults: an ancillary analysis of the life study randomized clinical trial. JAMA Intern. Med. 21686114. 182 (6), 650–659. Available from: http://archinte.jamanetwork.com/issues.aspx. doi:10.1001/jamainternmed.2022.1449.

Silva, A.C.S., Miranda, A.S., Rocha, N.P., Teixeira, A.L., 2019. Neuropsychiatric disorders in chronic kidney disease. Front. Pharmacol. 16639812. 10 (JULY). Available from: http://www.frontiersin.org/Pharmacology. doi:10.3389/fphar.2019.00932.

Small, C., Kramer, H.J., Griffin, K.A., Vellanki, K., Leehey, D.J., Bansal, V.K., Markossian, T.W., 2017. Non-dialysis dependent chronic kidney disease is associated with high total and out-of-pocket healthcare expenditures. BMC

Nephrol. 14712369. 18 (1). Available from: http://www.biomedcentral.com/bmcnephrol/. doi:10.1186/s12882-016-0432-2.

Speyer, E., Tu, C., Zee, J., Sesso, R., Lopes, A.A., Moutard, E., Omorou, A.Y., Stengel, B., Finkelstein, F.O., Pecoits-Filho, R., de Pinho, N.A., Pisoni, R.L., Lopes, A., Pecoits-Filho, R., Combe, C., Jacquelinet, C., Massy, Z., Stengel, B., Alencar de Pinho, N., Zee, J., 2024. Symptom burden and its impact on quality of life in patients with moderate to severe CKD: The International Chronic Kidney Disease Outcomes and Practice Patterns Study (CKDopps). Am. J. Kidney Dis. 84 (6), 696–707.e1. doi:10.1053/j.ajkd.2024.06.011.

Stevens, P.E., Ahmed, S.B., Carrero, J.J., Foster, B., Francis, A., Hall, R.K., Herrington, W.G., Hill, G., Inker, L.A., Kazancıoğlu, R., Lamb, E., Lin, P., Madero, M., McIntyre, N., Morrow, K., Roberts, G., Sabanayagam, D., Schaeffner, E., Shlipak, M., Shroff, R., Tangri, N., Thanachayanont, T., Ulasi, I., Wong, G., Yang, C.W., Zhang, L., Levin, A., 2024. KDIGO 2024 Clinical Practice Guideline for the Evaluation and Management of Chronic Kidney Disease. Kidney Int. 15231755. 105 (4), S117. Available from: https://www.sciencedirect.com/science/journal/00852538. doi:10.1016/j.kint.2023.10.018.

Tamura, M.K., Gaussoin, S.A., Pajewski, N.M., Chelune, G.J., Freedman, B.I., Gure, T.R., Haley, W.E., Killeen, A.A., Oparil, S., Rapp, S.R., Rifkin, D.E., Supiano, M., Williamson, J.D., Weiner, D.E., 2020. Kidney disease, intensive hypertension treatment, and risk for dementia and mild cognitive impairment: the systolic blood pressure intervention trial. J. Am. Soc. Nephrol. 15333450. 31 (9), 2122–2132. Available from: https://jasn.asnjournals.org/content/31/9/2122. doi:10.1681/ASN.2020010038.

United States Renal Data System, 2024. 2024 USRDS Annual Data Report: Epidemiology of Kidney Disease in the United States. National Institutes of Health, National Institute of Diabetes and Digestive and Kidney Diseases. Bethesda, MD.

Van Oosten, M.J.M., Logtenberg, S.J.J., Hemmelder, M.H., Leegte, M.J.H., Bilo, H.J.G., Jager, K.J., Stel, V.S., 2021. Polypharmacy and medication use in patients with chronic kidney disease with and without kidney replacement therapy compared to matched controls. Clin. Kidney J. 20488513. 14 (12), 2497–2523. Available from: http://ckj.oxfordjournals.org/. doi:10.1093/ckj/sfab120.

Vangala, C., Niu, J., Montez-Rath, M.E., Yan, J., Navaneethan, S.D., Winkelmayer, W.C., 2020. Selective serotonin reuptake inhibitor use and Hip fracture risk among patients on hemodialysis. Am. J. Kidney Dis. 15236838. 75 (3), 351–360. Available from: http://www.elsevier.com/inca/publications/store/6/2/3/2/7/6/index.htt. doi:10.1053/j.ajkd.2019.07.015.

Wang, W.L., Liang, S., Zhu, F.L., Liu, J.Q., Wang, S.Y., Chen, X.M., Cai, G.Y., 2019. The prevalence of depression and the association between depression and kidney function and health-related quality of life in elderly patients with chronic kidney disease: a multicenter cross-sectional study. Clin Interv Aging. 14, 905–913. doi:10.2147/CIA.S203186.

Waraich, P., Goldner, E.M., Somers, J.M., Hsu, L., 2004. Prevalence and incidence studies of mood disorders: a systematic review of the literature. Can. J. Psychiatry. 07067437. 49 (2), 124–138. doi:10.1177/070674370404900208.

Weisbord, S.D., Carmody, S.S., Bruns, F.J., Rotondi, A.J., Cohen, L.M., Zeidel, M.L., Arnold, R.M. 2003. Symptom burden, quality of life, advance care planning and the potential value of palliative care in severely ill hemodialysis patients. Nephrol. Dial. Transplant. 18 (7), 1345–1352. doi: 10.1093/ndt/gfg105.

World Health Organization, 2004. The global burden of disease: 2004 update. WHO, Geneva.

Zhu, N., Hong, X., Lagerberg, T., Johnell, K., Jesús Carrero, J., Chang, Z., 2023. Comparative safety of antidepressants in adults with CKD. Clin. J. Am. Soc. Nephrol. 1555-9041. 19 (2). doi:10.2215/cjn.0000000000000348.

CHAPTER

15

Sarcopenia

Sheryl Cababat Caberto[a], *Lynn Schlanger*[a], *and Stephen Z. Fadem*[b]

[a]Division of Renal Medicine, Emory University School of Medicine, Atlanta, GA, United States

[b]Department of Medicine, Section of Nephrology, Baylor College of Medicine, Houston, TX, United States

Introduction

The physiological processes in muscle involve the kidney in maintaining protein balance and metabolic homeostasis, both of which are essential for muscle growth and function. With aging, there is a decrease in muscle protein synthesis and a physiological decline in renal function, contributing to decreased muscle mass and strength—a condition known as sarcopenia. Sarcopenia is defined as the age-related loss of skeletal muscle mass and function. While commonly associated with aging, it is also linked to chronic diseases, low protein intake, and physical inactivity (Moorthi and Avin, 2017). The interplay between aging, renal dysfunction, and muscle metabolism has a significant impact on the development of sarcopenia, accelerating muscle wasting. Sarcopenia is a major contributor to disability in older adults and individuals with chronic kidney disease (CKD).

Muscle stasis

Muscle production and the kidney and aging

Lack of activity—decreased mTOR activity

Progressive muscle wasting is observed with aging (Morley, 2012). The loss of muscle mass in CKD is associated with protein wasting and metabolic derangements due to uremia, causing decreased muscle synthesis. In CKD, the persistence of muscle protein catabolism results in the loss of muscle proteins due to protein turnover and imbalances between protein synthesis and degradation (Wang and Mitch, 2014). Muscle protein synthesis is controlled by the insulin-like

https://doi.org/10.1016/B978-0-443-34069-7.00021-5

growth factor (IGF)—AKT—mTOR pathway. The mechanistic target of rapamycin (mTOR) is a protein kinase involved in cellular growth and metabolism that plays a pivotal role in muscle homeostasis (Zhang et al., 2019). mTOR signaling is known to be involved in muscle growth, although it is not absolutely understood (Bodine et al., 2001). mTOR nucleates into mTORC1, a rapamycin- and nutrient-sensitive multiprotein complex, and it is associated with muscle hypertrophy when acutely activated and with muscle atrophy when chronically activated in vivo (Guertin and Sabatini, 2007; Castets et al., 2013; Baar and Esser, 1999). Muscle contraction activates mTORC1 because of the anabolic process that occurs when muscles are used (Deutz et al., 2014). Therefore physical inactivity decreases mTORC1 activation, resulting in reduced muscle growth and potentially muscle atrophy. Understanding this cascade of muscle production is essential for potential therapeutic approaches in the treatment of muscle wasting in aging and functional impairment. The mainstay of promoting muscle synthesis in health, disease, and aging is resistance exercise. Compound lifts with overload directly stimulate mTORC1.

Inadequate nutrition—amino acids

Another component of muscle growth is dietary protein (Martinho et al., 2022). The protein derived from diet provides amino acids that are required for muscle protein synthesis. These amino acids, which are commonly called the essential amino acids (EAAs), are histidine, isoleucine, leucine, lysine, methionine, phenylalanine, threonine, tryptophan, and valine. A large and rapid increase in peripheral concentrations of EAAs improves protein synthesis in muscles (Church et al., 2020). Muscle protein synthesis can be augmented by branched-chain amino acids (BCAAs)—leucine, valine, and isoleucine. BCAA powder is popular among weightlifters; however, no human studies have shown increased muscle protein synthesis from oral BCAA intake alone. The potential for BCAAs alone to stimulate muscle protein synthesis is limited because other EAAs must come from muscle breakdown, and some EAAs are inevitably lost to oxidation (Wolfe, 2017). In a 14-week controlled diet study with leucine infusion in older people aged 55–77 years, the whole-body leucine metabolism and composition may adapt to the protein RDA; however, metabolic compromise was evident with the reduction in mid-thigh muscle and urinary nitrogen excretion. Therefore the current protein RDA may be insufficient to completely support the metabolic and physiological needs of the elderly (Campbell et al., 2001). The recommended dietary allowance (RDA) of protein is 0.8 g/kg/day. Data obtained from NHANES 2005–2006 showed inadequate protein intake in individuals over 70 years old, with 24% of women and 12% of men not meeting the requirement (Berner et al., 2013). The European Society for Clinical Nutrition and Metabolism (ESPEN) workshop in 2013 provided guidance for maintaining muscle strength and function in older adults: Healthy older adults should consume 1.0–1.2 g of protein per kg of body weight per day; older adults with illness or at risk of malnutrition should aim for 1.2–1.5 g/kg/day, or more in cases of severe illness or injury (Deutz et al., 2014). Elderly individuals with low protein intake are at higher risk for developing sarcopenia; therefore adequate protein is necessary in the treatment of age-related loss in muscle mass, strength, and function.

Inflammation and aging

Aging results from an imbalance between cellular damage and repair, in which the immune system plays a central role in resilience. However, the immune system is persistently activated with aging, causing chronic inflammation known as inflammaging. This condition is associated with chronic disease, frailty, and death. Inflammation is considered a clinical biomarker of aging and a major risk factor for many age-related diseases, including sarcopenia and increased mortality in older adults (Singh et al., 2024; Franceschi and Campisi, 2014). Aging is commonly linked to low-grade inflammation (LGI), characterized by elevated levels of pro-inflammatory mediators like TNFα, IL-6, and CRP, due to the accumulation of senescent cells. These inflammatory markers are commonly observed with increased levels in sarcopenic individuals (Dalle et al., 2017). The senescence biomarker is a potential risk factor for physical dysfunction in older adults, indicating that inflammation at the cellular level may have functional consequences (Justice et al., 2018). In a meta-analysis of over 11,249 individuals, 3072 sarcopenic patients had an elevated inflammatory profile with significantly higher levels of CRP (Bano et al., 2017). Several mechanisms explain how chronic inflammation may contribute to sarcopenia. It disrupts muscle homeostasis through proteolysis, impairs muscle regeneration, and exacerbates oxidative stress (Franceschi and Campisi, 2014; Dalle et al., 2017).

Chronic disease

Sarcopenia can be primary, which is age-related, or secondary, which is disease-related. Chronic diseases associated with muscle wasting include malignant cancer, chronic obstructive pulmonary disease (COPD), heart failure, and renal failure (Bauer et al., 2019). Sarcopenia is common in CKD, especially in patients with end-stage kidney disease on hemodialysis, where it results from accelerated protein catabolism and inadequate nutritional intake rather than aging alone (Sabatino et al., 2021). In a study of patients with end-stage kidney disease on hemodialysis, using ultrasonography to evaluate muscle mass, it was found that end-stage kidney disease patients had significantly lower muscle measurements than healthy and hospitalized controls, with the lowest values observed in those with poor nutritional status (Sabatino et al., 2019). Sarcopenia is more prevalent in advanced stages of CKD and is associated with poorer physical function (De Souza et al., 2017). Sarcopenia in elderly patients with chronic disease is a multifactorial condition that significantly worsens physical function and overall prognosis.

Muscle breakdown, the kidney, and aging

Factors influencing myostatin and ubiquitin

Myostatin

Myostatin is a member of the TGF-β family. It is governed by the MSTN gene and inhibits protein synthesis by binding to its TGF receptor, activin receptor 2 (ACVR2B). This activates ALK4/5 kinases (Loomans and Andl, 2016) that promote the phosphorylation of SMAD2 and SMAD3, and their translocation to the nucleus, promoting transcription factors that interfere with the IGF1-AKT-mTOR signaling system, decreasing muscle protein synthesis. SMAD activation is independent of satellite cells and of muscle RING-finger protein 1 (MuRF1) (Sartori et al., 2009). Myostatin is a negative regulator of skeletal muscle mass. It is an inhibitor of muscle growth by blocking satellite cell activation and promoting protein degradation pathways (Lee, 2004). Myostatin expression is upregulated in elderly individuals with CKD due to systemic inflammation, oxidative stress, and metabolic acidosis. Glucocorticoids also upregulate myostatin. Elderly CKD patients have reduced physical activity, and this further stimulates the production of myostatin, resulting in muscle loss (Gonzalez-Cadavid et al., 1998; Zhang et al., 2011) (Fig. 15.1). A rare disorder characterized by mutations in MSTN results in muscle hypertrophy (Schuelke et al., 2004). Piedmontese cattle, known for their skeletal mass bulk, have a C313Y myostatin mutation that removes a disulfide bond essential for ligand binding (Starck and Sutherland-Smith, 2011). The following illustration shows some of the drivers of increased myostatin.

Ubiquitin

The ubiquitin-proteasome system (UPS) is a critical molecular pathway implicated in muscle protein breakdown. Muscle wasting in CKD is driven by complex mechanisms involving the activation of mediators that trigger the ATP-dependent UPS (Workeneh and Mitch, 2010). These pathways are influenced by a range of physiological and pathological factors that contribute to muscle atrophy, functional decline, and increased mortality. E3 ligases are the enzymes in the ubiquitin-proteasome pathway that recognize the myosins, actins, and structural muscle proteins to be degraded and then target them. The major muscle-specific enzymes are muscle RING finger 1 (MuRF1) and muscle atrophy F-box (MAFbx)/Atrogin-1. They are controlled by genes that are upregulated during interleukin-1 cachexia, inactivity, and corticosteroid use. The MuRF1 and MAFbx genes are also upregulated with fasting, denervation, immobilization, CKD, diabetes, sepsis, cachexia, HIV, COPD, aging, alcohol use, heart failure, and space flight (Bodine and Baehr, 2014). Transcription mediators

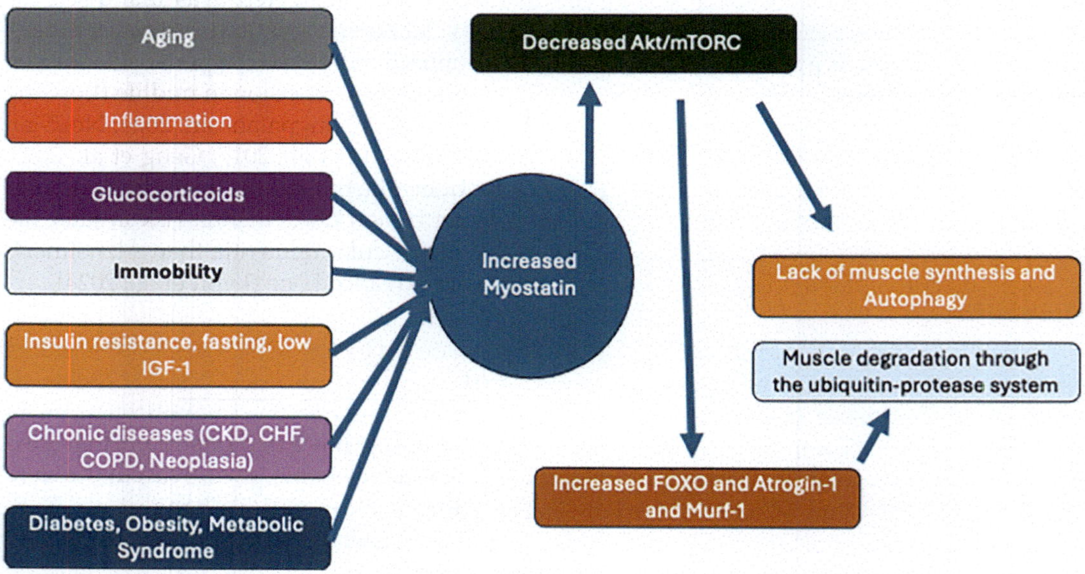

FIG. 15.1 **Factors increasing myostatin.** Some of the factors that increase myostatin and thereby induce sarcopenia.

include FOXO1 and FOXO3a, NF-κB, Smad 3, Glucocorticoid receptor, C/EBPβ, and KLF 15. MuRF1 targets myofibrils, while Atrogin (MAFbx) regulates protein synthesis. Metabolic acidosis also works through the E3 ligase system (Mitch et al., 1994). In addition to the E3 ligases, there are E1 enzymes that activate ubiquitin and E2 enzymes that act as carriers. The E3 is a ubiquitin-protein ligase that ties the carrier protein to ubiquitin. Ubiquitin consists of 76 amino acids and can be chain-linked to the ill-fated protein. The ligases can also mark a protein for repair by linking only one ubiquitin. The long-chain ubiquitin complexes are most likely to be associated with proteasomal degradation.

The UPS is the primary mechanism for the selective degradation of intracellular proteins by tagging damaged or unnecessary proteins with ubiquitin for subsequent degradation by the 26S proteasome (Lecker et al., 2006). In sarcopenia, skeletal muscles show increased activity of the UPS. Since muscle loss in aging differs from loss due to disuse, disease, or fasting, these mechanisms may combine in older adults, worsening muscle decline and function (Altun et al., 2010).

Myostatin signaling may interact with the UPS, causing increased UPS activity that results in muscle wasting. The enhanced activity of the UPS breaks down important muscle components, which are essential for muscle growth and function, such as sarcomeric proteins, nuclear proteins, protein synthesis machinery, and mitochondrial proteins (Lokireddy et al., 2012). The crosstalk between all these components establishes a direct regulatory pathway where myostatin not only inhibits muscle growth but also promotes protein breakdown through the UPS, which accelerates muscle breakdown and functional decline in the elderly.

A picture of muscle synthesis and breakdown

IGF-1 binds IGF1R (insulin-like growth factor 1 receptor), signaling through IRS-1 (insulin receptor substrate-1) to activate PI3K (phosphoinositide 3-kinase) and phosphorylate Akt (protein kinase B) (Fig. 15.2). Active Akt phosphorylates and inhibits FOXO (Forkhead box O) transcription factors, preventing their nuclear entry and the transcription of Atrogin-1 (F-box only protein 32; FBXO32) and MuRF1 (muscle RING finger 1), two E3 ubiquitin ligases that target myofibrillar proteins for degradation. Akt also phosphorylates and inhibits TSC2 (tuberous sclerosis complex 2; tuberin), thereby releasing RHEB (Ras homolog enriched in brain) to activate mTORC1 (mechanistic target of rapamycin complex 1). Active mTORC1 stimulates translation by activating S6K1 (ribosomal protein S6 kinase beta-1; RPS6KB1) and inhibiting 4E-BP1 (eukaryotic translation initiation factor 4E-binding protein 1; EIF4EBP1), thereby promoting muscle protein synthesis. In contrast, energy stress activates AMPK (AMP-activated protein kinase), which stimulates TSC2 and thereby restrains RHEB and mTORC1. When mTORC1 activity is low or inactive, autophagy proceeds. When mTORC1 is active, autophagy is suppressed. Myostatin (growth differentiation factor 8; GDF-8) binds to ActRIIB (activin A receptor type IIB; ACVR2B) (often with ActRIIA/ACVR2A). The ligand-bound type II receptor then recruits a type I receptor—ALK4 (activin receptor-like kinase 4; ACVR1B, also called ActRI-B) or ALK5 (activin receptor-like kinase 5; TGFBR1)—to form the signaling complex. The type I receptor phosphorylates SMAD2 (SMAD family member 2) and SMAD3 (SMAD family member 3), which complex with SMAD4 (SMAD family member 4) and translocate to the nucleus to drive the transcription of Atrogin-1 (FBXO32) and MuRF1

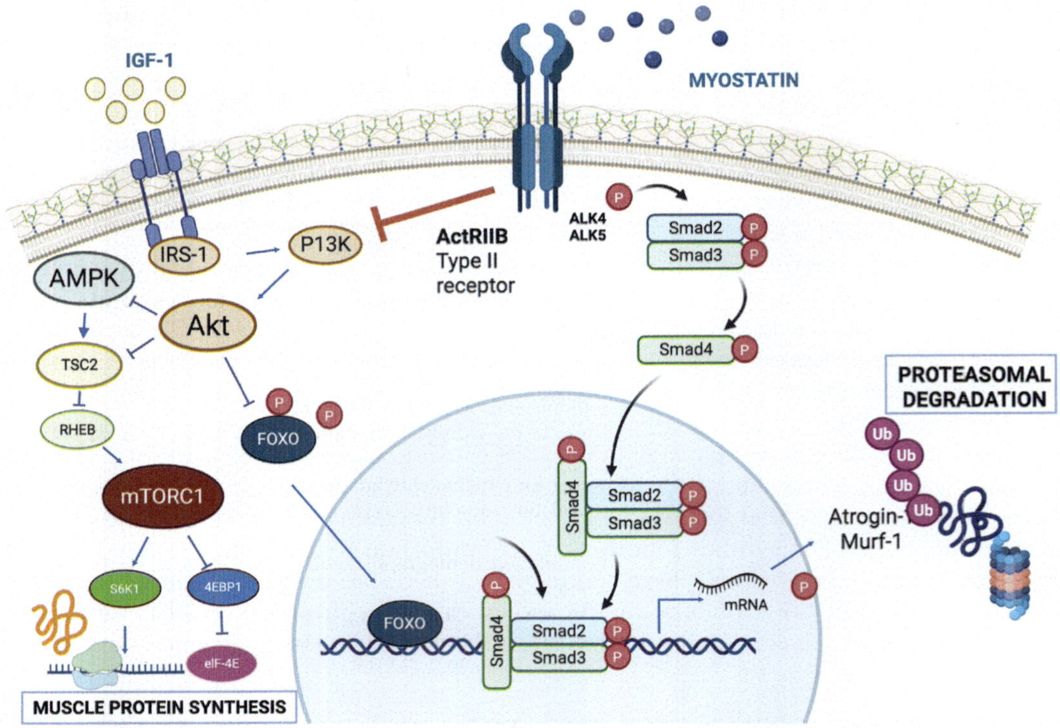

FIG. 15.2 **Muscle synthesis and breakdown.** Myostatin mechanism for muscle breakdown occurs through the transcription of E3 ligases, activating the ubiquitin pathway and impairing protein muscle synthesis. Without myostatin, mTORC promotes muscle synthesis. See text for explanation. *Created in BioRender. (Fadem, S. (2023)).*

(TRIM63). Myostatin/SMAD signaling thereby promotes ubiquitin-mediated proteolysis and functionally antagonizes the PI3K–Akt–mTORC1 anabolic pathway. Created in BioRender. Fadem, S. (2025).

Muscle synthesis and breakdown

mTOR and inflammation

The mTOR pathway plays a central role in the regulation of muscle protein synthesis, cell growth, and metabolism, which is essential for the maintenance of muscle mass. In patients with CKD, dysregulation of mTOR signaling causes a progressive loss of muscle mass and strength. Chronic inflammation in CKD disrupts the anabolic signaling of mTOR. Elevated levels of pro-inflammatory cytokines, such as tumor necrosis factor-alpha (TNF-α) and interleukin-6 (IL-6), inhibit mTOR complex 1 (mTORC1) activity, leading to a reduction in protein synthesis and an increase in protein degradation (Workeneh and Mitch, 2010). The persistent suppression of mTOR activity and the dominance of catabolic pathways result in a chronic imbalance between protein synthesis and degradation, contributing to accelerated sarcopenia and physical decline in CKD patients.

Insulin resistance

Insulin resistance is present in both aging and CKD-related sarcopenia; thus insulin resistance in elderly patients with CKD significantly contributes to the development of sarcopenia. Protein breakdown and Akt–protein kinase B activation, which are increased by insulin, are reduced in aging (Wilkes et al., 2009). Insulin is essential for stimulating muscle protein synthesis via the PI3K/Akt/mTOR pathway, but its anabolic effects are diminished in CKD due to chronic inflammation, oxidative stress, and hormonal imbalances (Wang and Mitch, 2014). In CKD, insulin resistance and reduced amino acid sensitivity are common, which further impair mTOR signaling, leading to anabolic resistance even in the presence of adequate nutrition (Zhang et al., 2019).

Decreased mitochondrial function

Muscle contraction requires large amounts of ATP, and thus any damage to mitochondria limits ATP production. When less ATP is generated, excess reactive oxygen species (ROS) and inflammation result in damage to proteins and DNA. The excess ROS results in increased activation of NF-κB and inflammation, further impairing protein synthesis. The decrease in oxidative phosphorylation shifts dependence to anaerobic glycolysis. This is less efficient, leading to increased lactate production. The increased lactate results in a burning pain and fatigue. The inability to fully manufacture ATP results in an increase in AMP production, and AMP is quickly metabolized to uric acid. The decreased mitochondrial function is also tied to the other hallmarks of aging (Chen et al., 2022).

Decreased enzymes

The mitochondrial enzymes are downregulated as early as stage 3 CKD, especially those involved in electron transport chain complexes. These include NADH dehydrogenase and cytochrome *c* oxidase, resulting in impaired oxidative phosphorylation. These changes can also occur in aging and result in decreased ATP production. This also results in increased reactive oxygen species production, further damaging cell structures. Enzyme production is also decreased. Decreased production of pyruvate dehydrogenase and citrate synthase disrupts citric acid cycle function, leading to anaerobic metabolism and increased lactate production. When fatty acid oxidation enzymes are also impaired, there is a further decline in energy production and oxidative stress. The result of decreased enzyme production is an impairment in P13 K/Akt phosphorylation and increased FOXO3a signaling, resulting in upregulation of MAFbx and MuRF-1, E3 ubiquitin ligases that bind ubiquitin to muscle fibrils, leading to their degradation (Gungor et al., 2023; Ying et al., 2023). Although enzyme decline occurs in both aging and CKD, age-related enzymatic decline results from mitochondrial dysfunction, while the driving factors in CKD are uremic toxins, metabolic acidosis, and inflammation (Fig. 15.3).

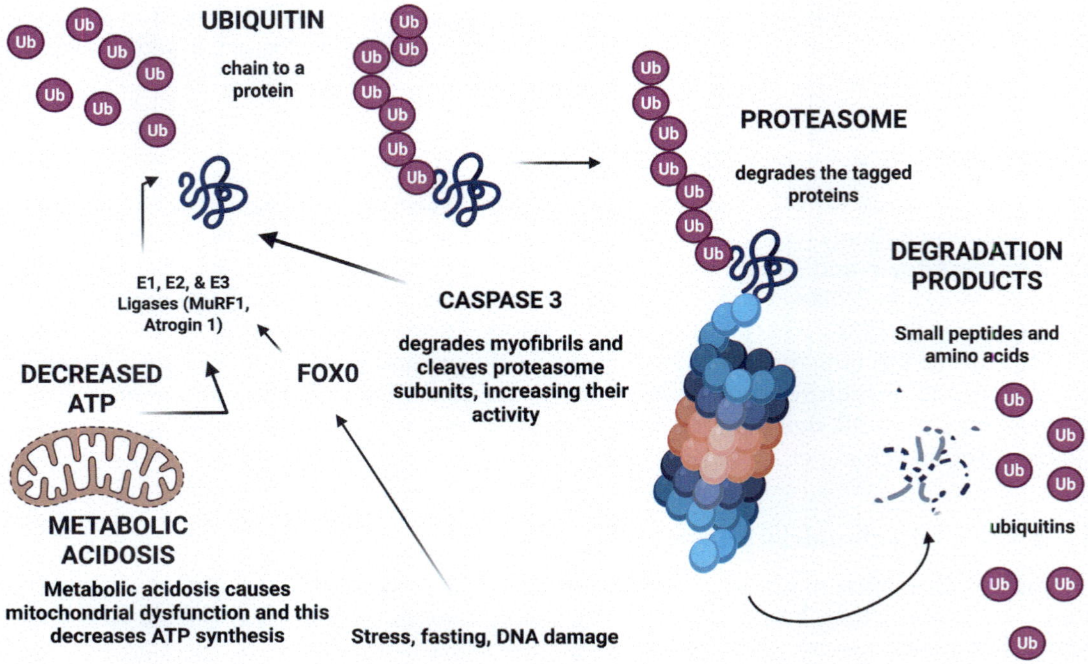

FIG. 15.3 How metabolic acidosis causes muscle protein degradation. Metabolic acidosis causes mitochondrial dysfunction, decreasing ATP production. This upregulates the E3 ligases Atrogin – 1 and MuRF1, resulting in the conjugation of ubiquitins to the myofibril. The myofibril is then ferried to the 26S ubiquitin proteasome, where it is degraded. *Created in BioRender. Fadem, S. (2025).*

Decreased epigenetic mechanisms

Epigenetic mechanisms interact to control cellular processes, and the occurrence of dysregulation contributes to functional decline in multiple organs, including the kidney, brain, heart, and skeletal muscle. These mechanisms are increasingly recognized as key regulators of aging and age-related diseases and include DNA methylation, histone modifications, and noncoding RNAs (Sen et al., 2016). A review of epigenetic mechanisms is presented in Chapter 5. These epigenetic changes establish a mechanistic interconnection between kidney aging and sarcopenia, where compromised gene regulation exacerbates systemic aging and functional decline.

Epigenesis plays a role in muscle damage as it involves modifications to DNA, as well as to RNA and histones, that are independent of the underlying genetic sequence. DNA methylation is catalyzed by members of the DNA methyltransferase family (DNMT). DNMT3 methylates DNA at CpG sites, essentially deactivating it. CpG sites on a region of DNA are where a cytosine nucleotide is followed by a guanine. Normally, skeletal muscle is hypomethylated, but with age, methylation increases. DNA hypermethylation is associated with age-related muscle atrophy. The uremic toxins indoxyl sulfate and p-cresyl sulfate also cause the dysregulation of DNA methylation, resulting in catabolism and epimutations that induce muscle wasting beyond the level of CKD (Ding et al., 2021). DNA demethylation in the promoter regions of atrophy-related genes (atrogenes), such as MuRF1 and MAFbx, can lead to their upregulation and consequent muscle atrophy. It also plays a role in the muscle atrophy of bedridden and critically ill patients. DNMT3 also activates NF-κB, increasing the E3 ligase MuRF1. Genome-wide analyses reveal that aging kidneys undergo substantial DNA methylation changes that result in renal aging and damage.

With histone acetylation, acetyl groups are added to the lysine amino acid on histone proteins. The combination of the DNA and its histone is known as chromatin. DNA is tightly wrapped around histones under normal conditions, protecting it and making it less accessible. Acetylation loosens the chromatin, facilitating DNA transcription. Histone acetylation is regulated by histone acetyltransferases (HATs) and histone deacetylases (HDACs). HDAC activation contributes to kidney aging. Sirtuins, which depend upon NAD+, include SIRT1, SIRT3, and SIRT6. Sirtuins also deacetylate histones, removing acetyl groups and causing the chromatin structure to tighten. With sirtuin reduction, acetylation of histones occurs. Histone acetylation, as a result of decreased sirtuins, exacerbates age-related glomerulosclerosis, nephrosclerosis, and renal fibrosis through activated transcription involving TGF-β1, NF-κB signaling, and the hyperacetylation of key proteins. Decreased sirtuins are also implicated in renal fibrosis, with HATs causing fibrosis and inflammation. Histone methylation, regulated by lysine methyltransferases (KMTs) and demethylases (KDMs), also plays a critical role in kidney aging through age-related gene regulation. Histone modification also shifts as a result of aging. This may be due to a decrease in histone acetylation enzymes and sirtuins.

The noncoding RNAs (ncRNAs), including microRNAs (miRNAs) and long noncoding RNAs (lncRNAs), are key epigenetic regulators in kidney aging. MicroRNA noncoding RNA fragments bind to the 3′UTR region of mRNA and thus halt mRNA activity. In aging kidneys, upregulation of miRNAs promotes collagen I and III deposition, while lncRNAs modulate inflammation, apoptosis, senescence, and cell cycle regulators to influence renal aging. The expressions of several microRNAs, including miR-1, miR-143, miR-181, and miR-378, are critical for muscle homeostasis but become altered in aging. miR-1 has been shown in computer simulation models to downregulate Pax3, a factor that blocks muscle synthesis. Thus miR-1 is a key miRNA switching on myogenesis and is downregulated with aging. The inflammatory cytokine IL-6 downregulates miR-143, another myogenic stimulator, demonstrating a pathway for inflammation to interfere with muscle production. miR-181 maintains myogenesis by inhibiting Hox-A11, releasing MyoD. miR-378 inhibits musculin and releases MyoD, increasing myogenesis. They are both suppressed with aging (Proctor and Goljanek-Whysall, 2017). miR-29 suppresses fibrosis but becomes downregulated in CKD, leading to increased collagen deposition in muscle. The downregulation of miR-29 increases the mammalian transcription factor Yin-Yang1's (YY1) mRNA activity, negatively regulating muscle cell differentiation (Wang et al., 2011; Kalan et al., 2025). Decreased miR-29 increases the expression of the E3 MuRF1 and Arogin-1. CKD downregulates miR-23a, miR-27a, and miR-486. Each of these activates Ak1 and blocks SMAD signaling, thus improving muscle mass (Tsai et al., 2025a).

After exercise, young men were found to have a reduction in specific pri-miRNAs and miR-1, while older men were found to have a blunted or dysregulated miRNA response. Both groups increased Rheb protein (associated with protein synthesis) expression post-stimulus. These findings suggest an association between aging and elevated basal miRNA expression, as well as impaired miRNA adaptability to anabolic stimuli. A study on the role of muscle-specific microRNAs (miRNAs) in response to an anabolic stimulus—resistance exercise plus leucine-enriched EAAs—in young and older men found that older men had higher expression of several primary miRNAs compared with younger men at baseline (Drummond and Rasmussen, 2008).

miR-181a is a regulator of SIRT1 gene expression, and its target microRNA is disrupted with age, leading to sarcopenia (Soriano-Arroquia et al., 2016). SIRT1 is an NAD + dependent histone deacetylase, an epigenetic regulator of aging. It can be induced by caloric restriction but normally declines with age. NAD + is a cofactor that works with sirtuins, and its reduction decreases mitochondrial function. SIRT1 blocks mitochondrial impairment, inflammation, and oxidative stress—three factors that lead to sarcopenia (Anwar et al., 2023). A study showed that SIRT1 plays a role in FoxO transcription factors, and when activated, it may result in muscle atrophy. The decreased levels of SIRT1 in type II skeletal muscle caused atrophy, while overexpression prevented muscle wasting due to the protective effects of its deacetylase activity, which suppresses FoxO activation and the expression of atrogenes and autophagy genes (Lee and Goldberg, 2013).

It has been demonstrated that adipose cells can communicate with muscle cells through epigenetic signals. Sarcopenia responds to epigenetic signals from miR-146a-5 fragments that are ferried by exosomes from adipose tissue to muscle cells. The microRNAs signal the IGF/Akt/MTOR pathway to promote muscle synthesis. In knockout studies where miR-146a-5 is absent, the animals become wasted and lose their ability to exercise. This is quickly reversed when the microRNA is restored (Qin et al., 2024).

Impaired autophagy

Autophagy entails the capture of damaged proteins or organelles and encasing them as "cargo" that joins with a lysosome, which breaks them into recyclable particles. It is turned on by MTOR inhibition. It is critical for muscle development and remodeling but must remain in balance. The multiple catabolic stresses caused by CKD, inactivity, acidosis, insulin resistance, the uremic toxins indoxyl sulfate and p-cresyl sulfate, and inflammation result in mitochondrial dysfunction, ATP decline, and oxidative stress. AMPK-FOXO3 and a decrease in IGF/Akt/mTORC1 induce autophagy. Myostatin signaling may also interact with UPS, causing increased UPS activity that results in muscle wasting by the targeted removal of muscle proteins through the ubiquitin-proteasome.

In aging, satellite cell autophagy is downregulated, and the cells become senescent. Restoring satellite cell autophagy can reverse this process (García-Prat et al., 2016). While aging is characterized by inefficient autophagy, the loss of autophagy leads to the accumulation of damaged proteins and fibers. The substrate for new muscle synthesis declines. This is accompanied by dysregulation of mitochondrial autophagy, or mitophagy, which results in mitochondrial dysfunction, reactive oxygen species, and sarcopenia.

Consequences and relationships between sarcopenia and aging in kidney disease

Falls

Falls have been discussed in Chapter 11 of this book. CKD contributes to metabolic and hormonal disturbances that damage multiple organs, including skeletal muscle. Sarcopenia leads to impaired mobility and reduced physical performance, which, in older adults, is strongly linked to disability, falls, fractures, hospitalization, and mortality (Roshanravan et al., 2013). Sarcopenia increases the risk of falls. Polypharmacy, comorbidity, cognitive function, and nutritional status are also moderators of fall risk (Coelho-Júnior et al., 2025). Both mechanical and nonmechanical falls can occur as a result of muscle dysfunction. As a consequence of CKD-related muscle breakdown, falls are common when the kidneys fail. Not only is muscle function decreased, but the associated muscle memory that helps regulate balance is also lost. In a systematic review of 52,838 persons over 65, sarcopenia was significantly associated with falls (OR 1.60; 95% CI 1.37–1.86, $P < 0.001$) and fractures (OR 1.84; 95% CI 1.30–2.62, $P = 0.001$) (Yeung et al., 2019). Chronic illness, age, and renal function decline are associated with gait disorders, immobility, inflammation, hypovolemia, and vision and hearing loss. Each of these factors is associated with falling. Furthermore, CKD patients are often on multiple medication regimens. Polypharmacy, particularly when sedatives or opioids are involved, is associated with falls. Preventing falls first involves assessing the patient's risk and trying to minimize the disease characteristics associated with that risk. This often includes physical therapy, balance training, adjusting medications, evaluating vision and hearing, and assessing cardiac status. Increased aerobic exercise and resistance training are associated with improved muscle function and a reduction in falls, particularly in dialysis patients (Clarkson et al., 2019; Fadem, 2023).

Inactivity

Astronauts, nematodes, and bedridden patients share the genetic mechanisms that cause muscle unloading secondary to antigravity. Skeletal muscle preservation depends on the dystrophin-associated glycoprotein complex. This stabilizes muscle membranes during contraction and relaxation, enables muscles to endure mechanical force, and serves as a sensor to detect mechanical stress and signal the nucleus. In the nucleus, genes are regulated to modulate protein synthesis. The molecular mechanisms were further analyzed by exposing nematodes (*Caenorhabditis elegans*) to spaceflight conditions aboard the International Space Station. Gene expression, protein synthesis and breakdown, and physiological characteristics were evaluated. As force on muscles in a reduced gravity environment decreases, there is a general downregulation in mitochondrial proteins, reduced ATP production, and decreased protein synthesis. This is accompanied by increased oxidative stress, triggering the mitochondrial unfolded protein response and further stress. *C. elegans* has muscle cells that are analogous to human skeletal muscle. In the nematodes, spaceflight triggered a reduction in myosin heavy chain expression and decreased expression of genes associated with locomotion. Troponin and tropomyosin genes were also downregulated. The loss of protein muscle fibers results from muscle-specific E3 ubiquitin ligases—atrogenes that govern MuRF1 and MAFbx are upregulated, leading to ubiquitination of targeted muscle fibers and proteasomal degradation. This process is mitigated by resistance exercise (Beckett et al., 2024).

Metabolic acidosis

Sulfur-containing amino acids in meat are a major source of dietary acids, and it is well known that acidosis increases protein degradation. Metabolic acidosis also impairs protein synthesis and disrupts mitochondrial function. Since aging is associated with declining kidney function and impaired renal acid secretion, the chronic acidosis often accompanying aging contributes to muscle protein breakdown. Dietary proteins are broken down to either be stored in the amino acid pool, oxidized to be used as an energy source, or to synthesize new proteins. However, instead of protein synthesis, CKD and metabolic acidosis stimulate protein degradation and muscle loss (Dawson-Hughes et al., 2008).

The protein degradation in metabolic acidosis works through signal transduction. The ATP-dependent ubiquitin-proteasome pathway plays the predominant role in acidosis-induced protein degradation. In 1994, William Mitch demonstrated that metabolic acidosis upregulated ubiquitin mRNA in muscle cells (Mitch et al., 1994). Since then, it has been demonstrated that the E3 ligase system is upregulated, and the ligases MuRF1, MAFbx, and Atrogin-1 conjugate ubiquitin with targeted muscle fragments. These fragments are then recognized, catalyzed, and cleaved into peptides by the 19S, 20S, and 26S proteasomes, respectively (Workeneh and Mitch, 2010) (Fig. 15.3).

Bone disease

Bone disease is a consequence of sarcopenia in both aging and CKD. The disruption of muscle–bone interaction leads to the development of bone disease. Sarcopenia is critically involved in bone disease as it is an age-related and disease-associated loss of skeletal muscle mass, strength, and function. Research has highlighted that vitamin D deficiency disrupts bone and mineral metabolism, which is common in patients with CKD. A study on the effects of 1,25-dihydroxyvitamin D (1,25-D3) on myoblasts showed that it enhanced vitamin D receptor activity, reduced myoblast proliferation and IGF-I expression, and promoted myogenic differentiation while downregulating myostatin. Vitamin D deficiency, altered parathyroid hormone levels, and hormonal dysregulation contribute to secondary hyperparathyroidism, which further exacerbates the deterioration of muscle and bone (Cuppari and Garcia-Lopes, 2009). Patients with CKD are at high risk of bone loss and fractures with hyperparathyroidism and elevated bone turnover (Nickolas et al., 2013). Osteosarcopenia, the coexistence of osteoporosis and sarcopenia in older adults, impairs mobility, independence, and quality of life. The combination of sarcopenia and bone disease in the aging population increases the risk of falls and fractures and negatively impacts overall musculoskeletal health (Kirk et al., 2020).

Inflammation due to lack of exercise

Physical inactivity, a common consequence of sarcopenia in aging and CKD, contributes significantly to systemic inflammation. Chronic inflammation has been reported in studies as the underlying mechanism driving physical function decline in older adults. Elevated inflammatory markers such as IL-6, CRP, and IL-1RA are strongly associated with reduced physical performance and muscle strength, which may further be aggravated in CKD by the accumulation of uremic toxins (Carrero et al., 2013; Cesari et al., 2004). Thus the lack of exercise exacerbates systemic inflammation, which in turn promotes further muscle wasting and worsens outcomes in CKD.

Therapy in kidney disease and aging

1. Bicarbonate—decreases myostatin/ubiquitin (Table 15.1). The strategy to treat patients with CKD using bicarbonate has remained unchanged since 1917, when sodium bicarbonate was first used as a treatment for uremia (Alexander Aiken, 2013). While exercise has been demonstrated to prevent muscle loss and its consequences in both the elderly and CKD patients, blood lactate accumulation during exercise creates an acidic environment that activates MuRF1-E3 ligase conjugation of ubiquitin to targeted muscle proteins, resulting in their proteasomal degradation. Lactic acid can accumulate during exercise, and marathon runners claim it enhances performance. In a study of CKD patients over a period of 6 months involving walking exercise with additional bicarbonate supplementation (serum bicarbonate raised to 29), E3 ligase expression significantly dropped, suggesting bicarbonate might be helpful in countering exercise-induced acidosis (Watson et al., 2013). As insulin resistance is a contributor to sarcopenia, sodium bicarbonate correction for just two weeks has been shown to improve insulin sensitivity in patients undergoing maintenance dialysis (Mak, 1998). An alkaline diet rich in fruits and vegetables may help elderly patients preserve muscle function (Dawson-Hughes et al., 2008).

TABLE 15.1 Managing sarcopenia in CKD and aging. Here is a snapshot of recommended measures to reduce sarcopenia in the elderly and individuals with CKD.

Intervention	CKD/ aging	Target	Suggestion	Resource
Exercise	CKD, Aging	Lowers myostatin Increases mTORC, enhances mitochondrial function, and decreases inflammation	Resistance, aerobic, and flexibility exercises Otago program or Tai Chi Mechanical stress lowers myostatin and increases mTORC	(Aguirre and Villareal, 2015; Tsai et al., 2025; Radley et al., 2024)
Nutrition	CKD	mTORC to enable protein synthesis	Ample protein, essential amino acids, ketoanalogues Sirt foods	(Yoon, 2017; Clarkson et al., 2019)
Metabolic Acidosis	CKD	Down regulate E3 ligases and proteolysis	Bicarbonate and/or alkali diet	(Watson et al., 2013; Dawson-Hughes et al., 2008)
Dialysis	CKD (ESKD)	Reduces inflammation and acidosis	Adequate dialysis therapy	(Brightwell et al., 2021; Murashima et al., 2024)
Vitamin D	CKD, aging	Downregulates myostatin	Supplementation—bone strength and fall prevention	(Cuppari and Garcia-Lopes, 2009; Nickolas et al., 2013)
Fall prevention	CKD, aging	Muscle strength and memory, coordination	Balance exercises, strength training, Otago exercises	(Landi et al., 2012; Fadem, 2023)

Adequate dialysis—rescues muscle

Adequate dialysis is the mainstay therapy for advanced CKD, which effectively removes uremic toxins and maintains the homeostasis of fluid and electrolytes. The uremic milieu, characterized by toxin accumulation, chronic inflammation, and metabolic dysregulation, accelerates muscle breakdown. CKD leads to the disruption of muscle integrity—muscle fibrosis and maladaptation—but the initiation of dialysis in advanced CKD improves muscle strength and structural integrity, suggesting that the clearance of uremic toxins with adequate dialysis drives maladaptive muscle remodeling (Brightwell et al., 2021). However, dialysis in older patients often follows a more tolerant management approach, prioritizing quality of life by lessening the treatment burden and focusing on overall well-being (Kurella et al., 2007). Thus dialysis treatment must be tailored to older individuals' goals of care.

Exercise

The average person experiences a 30% reduction in muscle strength between the ages of 50 and 70, with the decline worsening after 70. Elderly patients, particularly those with CKD, are often poorly mobile, have lost significant muscle mass—particularly type II fibers—and are weak. They exhibit low physical activity, slowed motor function, and poor tolerance for exercise. Yet, it is this population that benefits most from resistance and aerobic exercise. In a study of 10,000 older adults, the likelihood of not being disabled at the time of death was twofold higher among those who were physically active. After the age of 30, the decline in working muscle parallels an increase in fat mass. Thus obese patients can paradoxically become frail. Oxidative capacity and resistance to fatigue increase with training. Although peak VO_2 declines with age, it can be improved through endurance training. In a 9-month study of frail older men, walking therapy increased VO_2 max by 14%. Among 77–87 year olds, the increase in VO_2 max was 15%, though not as significant as the exercise program performed by 60–71 year olds, who experienced a 24–30% increase in VO_2 max. In healthy elderly patients, resistance training can increase muscle mass by 16% to 23%. Although frail patients have an attenuated response to resistance training, their muscle mass can still increase by 2.0%–9%. Gait speed in the elderly and frail also improves with exercise. The combination of aerobic and resistance exercise is synergistic (Aguirre and Villareal, 2015).

Resistance training involves the use of weights or elastic bands and increases muscle mass and strength in patients with sarcopenia or frailty. Improved bone density also follows. Gait speed and sit-to-stand performance improve with lower-body and core exercises. Upper body training also enhances functional performance. Aerobic training can be performed on an elliptical machine, treadmill, or bicycle. However, the ideal therapy is walking. It is associated with better exercise performance, as described above. It also decreases oxidative stress, improves inflammation, and helps control blood pressure, lipid, and glucose profiles. Dialysis patients have been shown to benefit from aerobic exercise (Tsai et al., 2025; Radley et al., 2024).

Since balance and coordination decrease in the elderly, especially the frail, and in an accelerated fashion in dialysis patients, balance and flexibility exercise programs such as Otago exercises, yoga, Tai Chi, and stretching with a trainer are helpful to increase balance and coordination. This is critical to help avoid falls, improve posture, and mobility (Radley et al., 2024).

Vitamin D—bones and muscles work in tandem

Vitamin D is essential for regulating mineral metabolism and maintaining bone integrity, which is particularly relevant in older adults who are at risk of osteoporosis and in CKD patients who have bone mineral metabolism disorders. In the bone, vitamin D regulates calcium absorption and mineralization, while it influences protein synthesis and mitochondrial function through vitamin D receptor (VDR) activation in the muscle. When bone-muscle crosstalk is disrupted, it results in low bone mineral density, sarcopenia, and an increased risk of falls and fractures, particularly in aging and CKD populations (Garcia et al., 2011; Cuppari and Garcia-Lopes, 2009). Vitamin D deficiency in CKD leads to secondary hyperparathyroidism by reducing intestinal calcium absorption, causing low serum calcium levels. The parathyroid glands respond by increasing parathyroid hormone (PTH) secretion to maintain calcium homeostasis. In chronic CKD, there is impaired renal activation of vitamin D, and chronically elevated PTH due to secondary hyperparathyroidism accelerates bone turnover and reduces bone mineral density, contributing to bone disease (Nickolas et al., 2013; Kirk et al., 2020). Supplementation with ergocalciferol or cholecalciferol is necessary to prevent any bone complications. Vitamin D deficiency contributes to impaired muscle performance, reduced bone strength, and a higher risk of falls. Vitamin D receptor activators and calcimimetics might be beneficial among dialysis patients who are less active (Murashima et al., 2024).

Protein or ketoanalogues—required for muscle growth

IGF-1 is a hormone similar to insulin. When it binds to its receptor, it recruits insulin receptor substrate-1 (IRS-1), which transmits signals that activate the downstream kinase Akt, also known as protein kinase B. Through a series of reactions, Akt activates mTORC1. In fed conditions after exercise, mTORC1 activates ribosomal biogenesis and protein translation through the activation of S6K1 (ribosomal protein S6 kinase 1) and inactivation of the translation repressor 4EBP1 (eukaryotic translation initiation factor 4E-binding protein 1), releasing the translational factor eIF4E (eukaryotic initiation factor 4E). Muscle breakdown results from decreased mTOR activity because of the deactivation of Akt by myostatin. Myostatin binds to the Type II activin receptor (ActRIIB), activating kinases and interacting with ALK4/ALK5, which phosphorylate Smads2/3. This leads to the pairing of Smad4 with Smads2/3. The Smad complex translocates to the nucleus, blocking Akt activation and inhibiting mTORC1. Chronic mTOR activation leads to the paradox of muscle atrophy because autophagy is impaired, reducing substrate availability (Yoon, 2017).

This mechanism helps explain the relationship between exercise, feeding, and muscle protein synthesis. Nutrition in the elderly and in CKD is discussed in Chapter 7, and although there is controversy as to whether a very low-protein diet reduces kidney disease progression, protein intake in the elderly is associated with improved body mass (Farsijani et al., 2016). A plant-based diet that allows but limits animal protein and balances it with healthier fruits and vegetables is ideal. In patients with advanced kidney disease, ketoanalogues—a comprehensive literature review supports that supplementing a low-protein diet with ketoanalogues can be useful to increase muscle mass—but treating patients with a restricted protein diet alone can result in malnutrition. In a randomized trial of 79 nondiabetic stage 3b-4 CKD patients on a low-protein diet (0.6 g/kg/day) or a group receiving supplemental ketoanalogues, the group receiving ketoanalogues preserved body mass indices and had higher sKlotho and lower FGF-23 levels than the group treated with a low-protein diet alone (Milovanova et al., 2018).

Frailty avoidance

Frailty has been discussed in Chapter 12. It generally accompanies advanced disease and, in many cases, can be mitigated through proactive management of the underlying morbidities. Immobility sets into play many of the factors that cause muscle and bone degradation. Thus efforts to keep the patient as active as possible can be helpful. Resistance exercises, along with sufficient nutrition, can upregulate protein synthesis. Since falls can accompany frailty with sarcopenia, balance training can help restore muscle memory and retrain the patient on maneuvers that can minimize their consequences (Landi et al., 2012). Older adults with poor mobility can potentially benefit from outdoor walking exercises (Su et al., 2025).

Sacral decubiti are common with immobility and are a source of inflammation. Inflammation increases insulin resistance and decreases muscle protein synthesis. Immobility in frail persons is to be discouraged. Pressure ulcers are predictable, and early indicators give caregivers a chance to identify those at risk and intervene early.

Diet plays a role in worsening frailty and sarcopenia and is a modifiable risk factor. Sirt foods may be particularly helpful. Controlling metabolic acidosis can also promote protein synthesis. A diet high in ultraprocessed foods that is low in protein and essential nutrients but high in additives and preservatives is associated with frailty, inflammation, and sarcopenia. This is based on a systematic review of 43 studies. Markers included C-reactive protein, IL-6, TNF-α, gait speed, grip strength, and muscle mass (Kanbay et al., 2025).

Conclusion

Both the aging process and CKD are associated with muscle wasting. This occurs through mechanisms that both block muscle protein synthesis and accelerate muscle breakdown. Since there are modifiable factors, these mechanisms are worth studying and understanding.

Protein synthesis is regulated through the IGF-1/Akt/IRS/mTORC1 signaling pathway. mTORC1 drives ribosome biogenesis and translation through the activation of S6K1, inhibiting 4EBP1, which releases eIF4E to activate synthesis. Feeding, particularly the amino acid leucine, and resistance exercise potentiate the signals that promote synthesis.

Muscle breakdown occurs when myostatin is stimulated and binds to its receptor, recruiting ALK4/5 and activating the Smad system, enabling it to translocate to the nucleus, both switching on factors that suppress Akt and mTORC1, blocking muscle synthesis, and also potentiating autophagy, which recycles muscle fibers and creates new substrate. In CKD, this autophagy is less effective.

The Smad translocation also upregulates atrogenes such as the E3ligases, MAFbx and MuRF1. These lead to the conjugation of ubiquitins with muscle proteins, targeting them for degradation by the 26S proteasome. This, too, leads to recycling and is thus essential for muscle recovery.

Inflammation and metabolic acidosis are associated with CKD. Inflammation is associated with insulin resistance, mainly by attenuating the insulin receptor substrate (IRS) and blocking mTORC1. Metabolic acidosis both upregulates Smad and atrogenes. Aging is strongly associated with mitochondrial dysfunction, epigenetic changes, and enzyme decline.

Both aging and CKD are associated with decreased activity, which signals muscle breakdown and results in reduced strength and performance, loss of balance, impaired or slower gait, and frailty. The loss of muscle function and coordination results in falls and debilitating fractures. These changes are aggravated by polypharmacy and poor nutrition. Resistance training substantially increases muscle synthesis. Treating metabolic acidosis with bicarbonate supplements and an alkali diet rich in fruits and vegetables downregulates E3 ligases and the Smads. Healthy protein consumption aligned with resistance exercise, as well as stretching, drives protein synthesis, and when balanced to potentiate AMPK, inhibits mTORC1 to drive autophagy.

Aging, in many ways, mirrors CKD and may be stalled through lifestyle changes that limit smoking and increase activity. Cigarettes are a powerful potentiator of inflammation and a major factor in aging. The Mediterranean diet encompasses many of the dietary factors that promote good health and may be worthwhile to consider.

AI disclosure

During the preparation of this work, the author(s) used Perplexity, ChatGPT, and Grammarly to get started and select references. The reference review and content development were created by the authors. After using this tool/service, the author(s) reviewed and edited the content as needed and take(s) full responsibility for the content of the publication.

References

Aguirre, L.E., Villareal, D.T., 2015. Physical exercise as therapy for frailty. Nestle Nutr. Inst. Workshop Ser. 16642155. 83, 83–92. Available from: http://www.karger.com/BookSeries/Home/229022. doi:10.1159/000382065.

Alexander Aiken, C.G., 2013. History of medical understanding and misunderstanding of acid base balance. J. Clin. Diagn. Res. 7 (9), 2038–2041. Available from: http://www.jcdr.net/articles/PDF/3400/65-%205230_E(C)_F(T)_PF1(P.r_P)_PFA(P).pdf. doi:10.7860/JCDR/2013/5230.3400.

Altun, M., Besche, H.C., Overkleeft, H.S., Piccirillo, R., Edelmann, M.J., Kessler, B.M., Goldberg, A.L., Ulfhake, B., 2010. Muscle wasting in aged, sarcopenic rats is associated with enhanced activity of the ubiquitin proteasome pathway. J. Biol. Chem. 1083351X. 285 (51), 39597–39608. Available from: http://www.jbc.org/content/285/51/39597.full.pdf+html. doi:10.1074/jbc.M110.129718.

Anwar, M., Pradhan, R., Dey, S., Kumar, R., 2023. The role of sirtuins in sarcopenia and frailty. Aging Dis. 21525250. 14 (1), 25–32. Available from: https://www.aginganddisease.org/EN/10.14336/AD.2022.0622. doi:10.14336/AD.2022.0622.

Baar, K., Esser, K., 1999. Phosphorylation of p70(S6k) correlates with increased skeletal muscle mass following resistance exercise. Am. J. Physiol. Cell Physiol. 03636143. 276 (1), C120. Available from: https://www.physiology.org/toc/ajpcell/current. doi:10.1152/ajpcell.1999.276.1.c120.

Bano, G., Trevisan, C., Carraro, S., Solmi, M., Luchini, C., Stubbs, B., Manzato, E., Sergi, G., Veronese, N., 2017. Inflammation and sarcopenia: a systematic review and meta-analysis. Maturitas. 03785122. 96, 10–15. doi:10.1016/j.maturitas.2016.11.006.

Bauer, J., Morley, J.E., Schols, A.M.W.J., Ferrucci, L., Cruz-Jentoft, A.J., Dent, E., Baracos, V.E., Crawford, J.A., Doehner, W., Heymsfield, S.B., Jatoi, A., Kalantar-Zadeh, K., Lainscak, M., Landi, F., Laviano, A., Mancuso, M., Muscaritoli, M., Prado, C.M., Strasser, F., von Haehling, S., Coats, A.J.S., Anker, S.D., 2019. Sarcopenia: a time for action. An SCWD position paper. J. Cachexia Sarcopenia Muscle. 21906009. 10 (5), 956–961. Available from: http://onlinelibrary.wiley.com/journal/10.1007/13539.2190-6009. doi:10.1002/jcsm.12483.

Beckett, L.J., Williams, P.M., Toh, L.S., Hessel, V., Gerstweiler, L., Fisk, I., Toronjo-Urquiza, L., Chauhan, V.M., 2024. Advancing insights into microgravity induced muscle changes using *Caenorhabditis elegans* as a model organism. Npj Microgravity. 23738065. 10 (1). Available from: https://www.nature.com/npjmgrav/. doi:10.1038/s41526-024-00418-z.

Berner, L.A., Becker, G., Wise, M., Doi, J., 2013. Characterization of dietary protein among older adults in the United States: amount, animal sources, and meal patterns. J. Acad. Nutr. Diet. 22122672. 113 (6), 809–815. doi:10.1016/j.jand.2013.01.014.

Bodine, S.C., Stitt, T.N., Gonzalez, M., Kline, W.O., Stover, G.L., Bauerlein, R., Zlotchenko, E., Scrimgeour, A., Lawrence, J.C., Glass, D.J., Yancopoulos, G.D., 2001. Akt/mTOR pathway is a crucial regulator of skeletal muscle hypertrophy and can prevent muscle atrophy in vivo. Nat. Cell Biol. 14657392. 3 (11), 1014–1019. doi:10.1038/ncb1101-1014.

Bodine, S.C., Baehr, L.M., 2014. Skeletal muscle atrophy and theE3ubiquitin ligases MuRF1 and MAFbx/atrogin-1. Am. J. Physiol. Endocrinol. Metab. 15221555. 307 (6), E469. Available from: http://ajpendo.physiology.org/content/ajpendo/307/6/E469full.pdf. doi:10.1152/ajpendo.00204.2014.

Brightwell, C.R., Kulkarni, A.S., Paredes, W., Zhang, K., Perkins, J.B., Gatlin, K.J., Custodio, M., Farocq, H., Zaidi, B., Pai, R., Buttar, R.S., Tang, Y., Melamed, M.L., Hostetter, T.H., Pessin, J.E., Hawkins, M., Fry, C.S., Abramowitz, M.K., 2021. Muscle fibrosis and maladaptation occur progressively in CKD and are rescued by dialysis. JCI Insight. 23793708. 6 (24). Available from: https://insight.jci.org/articles/view/150112/pdf. doi:10.1172/jci.insight.150112.

Campbell, W.W., Trappe, T.A., Wolfe, R.R., Evans, W.J., 2001. The recommended dietary allowance for protein may not be adequate for older people to maintain skeletal muscle. J. Gerontol. Ser. A Biol. Sci. Med. Sci. 10795006. 56 (6), M373. doi:10.1093/gerona/56.6.M373.

Carrero, J.J., Stenvinkel, P., Cuppari, L., Ikizler, T.A., Kalantar-Zadeh, K., Kaysen, G., Mitch, W.E., Price, S.R., Wanner, C., Wang, A.Y.M., Wee, P.T., Franch, H.A., 2013. Etiology of the protein-energy wasting syndrome in chronic kidney disease: a consensus statement from the International Society of Renal Nutrition and Metabolism (ISRNM). J. Ren. Nutr. 10512276. 23 (2), 77–90. doi:10.1053/j.jrn.2013.01.001.

Castets, P., Lin, S., Rion, N., Di Fulvio, S., Romanino, K., Guridi, M., Frank, S., Tintignac, L.A., Sinnreich, M., Rüegg, M.A., 2013. Sustained activation of mTORC1 in skeletal muscle inhibits constitutive and starvation-induced autophagy and causes a severe, late-onset myopathy. Cell Metab. 19327420. 17 (5), 731–744. doi:10.1016/j.cmet.2013.03.015.

Cesari, M., Penninx, B.W.J.H., Pahor, M., Lauretani, F., Corsi, A.M., Williams, G.R., Guralnik, J.M., Ferrucci, L., 2004. Inflammatory markers and physical performance in older persons: the InCHIANTI study. J. Gerontol. Ser. A Biol. Sci. Med. Sci. 1079-5006. 59 (3), M242. doi:10.1093/gerona/59.3.m242.

Chen, T.-H., Koh, K.-Y., Lin, K.M.-C., Chou, C.-K., 2022. Mitochondrial dysfunction as an underlying cause of skeletal muscle disorders. Int. J. Mol. Sci. 1422-0067. 23 (21), 12926. doi:10.3390/ijms232112926.

Church, D.D., Hirsch, K.R., Park, S., Kim, I.Y., Gwin, J.A., Pasiakos, S.M., Wolfe, R.R., Ferrando, A.A., 2020. Essential amino acids and protein synthesis: insights into maximizing the muscle and whole-body response to feeding. Nutrients. 20726643. 12 (12), 1–14. Available from: https://www.mdpi.com/2072-6643/12/12/3717/pdf. doi:10.3390/nu12123717.

Clarkson, M.J., Bennett, P.N., Fraser, S.F., Warmington, S.A., 2019. Exercise interventions for improving objective physical function in patients with end-stage kidney disease on dialysis: a systematic review and meta-analysis. Am. J. Physiol. Renal Physiol. 15221466. 316 (5), F856. Available from: https://www.physiology.org/doi/pdf/10.1152/ajprenal.00317.2018. doi:10.1152/ajprenal.00317.2018.

Coelho-Júnior, H.J., Calvani, R., Picca, A., Russo, A., Landi, F., Marzetti, E., 2025. Exploring the role of intrinsic and extrinsic factors on the associations between sarcopenia and falls in older adults. Sci. Rep. 20452322. 15 (1). Available from: https://www.nature.com/srep/. doi:10.1038/s41598-025-15259-3.

Cuppari, L., Garcia-Lopes, M.G., 2009. Hypovitaminosis D in chronic kidney disease patients: prevalence and treatment. J. Ren. Nutr. 10512276. 19 (1), 38–43. doi:10.1053/j.jrn.2008.10.005.

Dalle, S., Rossmeislova, L., Koppo, K., 2017. The role of inflammation in age-related sarcopenia. Front. Physiol. 1664-042X. 8. doi:10.3389/fphys.2017.01045.

Dawson-Hughes, B., Harris, S.S., Ceglia, L., 2008. Alkaline diets favor lean tissue mass in older adults. Am. J. Clin. Nutr. 00029165. 87 (3), 662–665. Available from: http://www.ajcn.org/cgi/reprint/87/3/662. doi:10.1093/ajcn/87.3.662.

De Souza, V.A., Oliveira, D., Barbosa, S.R., Corrêa, J.O.D.A., Colugnati, F.A.B., Mansur, H.N., Fernandes, N.M.D.S., Bastos, M.G., 2017. Sarcopenia in patients with chronic kidney disease not yet on dialysis: analysis of the prevalence and associated factors. PLoS One. 19326203. 12 (4). Available from: http://journals.plos.org/plosone/article/file?id=10.1371/journal.pone.0176230&type=printable. doi:10.1371/journal.pone.0176230.

Deutz, N.E.P., Bauer, J.M., Barazzoni, R., Biolo, G., Boirie, Y., Bosy-Westphal, A., Cederholm, T., Cruz-Jentoft, A., Krznariç, Z., Nair, K.S., Singer, P., Teta, D., Tipton, K., Calder, P.C., 2014. Protein intake and exercise for optimal muscle function with aging: recommendations from the ESPEN expert group. Clin. Nutr. 15321983. 33 (6), 929–936. Available from: http://www.elsevier-international.com/journals/clnu/. doi:10.1016/j.clnu.2014.04.007.

Ding, H., Zhang, L., Yang, Q., Zhang, X., Li, X., 2021. Epigenetics in kidney diseases. Adv. Clin. Chem. 104, 233–297. Available from: http://www.elsevier.com/wps/find/bookdescription.cws_home/705213/description#description. doi:10.1016/bs.acc.2020.09.005.

Drummond, M.J., Rasmussen, B.B., 2008. Leucine-enriched nutrients and the regulation of mammalian target of rapamycin signalling and human skeletal muscle protein synthesis. Curr. Opin. Clin. Nutr. Metab. Care. 15353885. 11 (3), 222–226. doi:10.1097/MCO.0b013e3282fa17fb.

Fadem, S., 2023. Understanding and Preventing Falls. Springer-Nature, New York.

Farsijani, S., Morais, J.A., Payette, H., Gaudreau, P., Shatenstein, B., Gray-Donald, K., Chevalier, S., 2016. Relation between mealtime distribution of protein intake and lean mass loss in free-living older adults of the NuAge study. Am. J. Clin. Nutr. 19383207. 104 (3), 694–703. Available from: http://ajcn.nutrition.org/content/104/3/694.full.pdf. doi:10.3945/ajcn.116.130716.

Franceschi, C., Campisi, J., 2014. Chronic inflammation (Inflammaging) and its potential contribution to age-associated diseases. J. Gerontol. – Ser. A Biol. Sci. Med. Sci. 1758535X. 69, S4. Available from: http://biomedgerontology.oxfordjournals.org/. doi:10.1093/gerona/glu057.

Garcia, L.A., King, K.K., Ferrini, M.G., Norris, K.C., Artaza, J.N., 2011. 1,25(OH)2vitamin D3 stimulates myogenic differentiation by inhibiting cell proliferation and modulating the expression of promyogenic growth factors and myostatin in C2C12 skeletal muscle cells. Endocrinology. 19457170. 152 (8), 2976–2986. Available from: http://endo.endojournals.org/content/152/8/2976.full.pdf+html. doi: 10.1210/en.2011-0159.

García-Prat, L., Martínez-Vicente, M., Perdiguero, E., Ortet, L., Rodríguez-Ubreva, J., Rebollo, E., Ruiz-Bonilla, V., Gutarra, S., Ballestar, E., Serrano, A.L., Sandri, M., Muñoz-Cánoves, P., 2016. Autophagy maintains stemness by preventing senescence. Nature. 14764687. 529 (7584), 37–42. Available from: http://www.nature.com/nature/index.html. doi:10.1038/nature16187.

Gonzalez-Cadavid, N.F., Taylor, W.E., Yarasheski, K., Sinha-Hikim, I., Ma, K., Ezzat, S., Shen, R., Lalani, R., Asa, S., Mamita, M., Nair, G., Arver, S., Bhasin, S., 1998. Organization of the human myostatin gene and expression in healthy men and HIV-infected men with muscle wasting. Proc. Natl. Acad. Sci. U. S. A. 95 (25), 14938–14943. doi:10.1073/pnas.95.25.14938.

Guertin, D.A., Sabatini, D.M., 2007. Defining the role of mTOR in cancer. Cancer Cell. 15356108. 12 (1), 9–22. doi:10.1016/j.ccr.2007.05.008.

Gungor, O., Kara, A.V., Hasbal, N.B., Kalantar-Zadeh, K., 2023. Dietary protein and muscle wasting in chronic kidney disease: new insights. Curr. Opin. Clin. Nutr. Metab. Care. 14736519. 26 (3), 226–234. Available from: http://journals.lww.com/co-clinicalnutrition/pages/default.aspx. doi:10.1097/MCO.0000000000000903.

Justice, J.N., Gregory, H., Tchkonia, T., Lebrasseur, N.K., Kirkland, J.L., Kritchevsky, S.B., Nicklas, B.J., 2018. Cellular senescence biomarker p16 INK4a + cell burden in thigh adipose is associated with poor physical function in older women. J. Gerontol. A Biol. Sci. Med. Sci. 1758535X. 73 (7), 939–945. Available from: http://biomedgerontology.oxfordjournals.org/. doi:10.1093/gerona/glx134.

Kalan, J.J., Varghese, L.N., Katare, R., 2025. Molecular pathogenesis of sarcopenia: regulatory networks involving MicroRNAs in age-related skeletal muscle decline. Front. Biosci. (Landmark Ed.) 30 (8). doi:10.31083/fbl38106.

Kanbay, M., Abdel-Rahman, S.M., Guldan, M., Ozbek, L., Covic, A., Mallamaci, F., Zoccali, C., 2025. The impact of ultra-processed food consumption on frailty and sarcopenia: a systematic review. J. Hum. Nutr. Diet. 1365277X. 38 (4). Available from: http://onlinelibrary.wiley.com/journal/10.1111/(ISSN)1365-277X. doi:10.1111/jhn.70096.

Kirk, B., Miller, S., Zanker, J., Duque, G., 2020. A clinical guide to the pathophysiology, diagnosis and treatment of osteosarcopenia. Maturitas. 18734111. 140, 27–33. Available from: www.elsevier.com/locate/maturitas. doi:10.1016/j.maturitas.2020.05.012.

Kurella, M., Covinsky, K.E., Collins, A.J., Chertow, G.M., 2007. Octogenarians and nonagenarians starting dialysis in the United States. Ann. Intern. Med. 00034819. 146 (3), 177–183. Available from: http://www.annals.org/cgi/reprint/146/3/177.pdf. doi:10.7326/0003-4819-146-3-200702060-00006.

Landi, F., Liperoti, R., Russo, A., Giovannini, S., Tosato, M., Capoluongo, E., Bernabei, R., Onder, G., 2012. Sarcopenia as a risk factor for falls in elderly individuals: results from the ilSIRENTE study. Clin. Nutr. 15321983. 31 (5), 652–658. doi:10.1016/j.clnu.2012.02.007.

Lecker, S.H., Goldberg, A.L., Mitch, W.E., 2006. Protein degradation by the ubiquitin-proteasome pathway in normal and disease states. J. Am. Soc. Nephrol. 10466673. 17 (7), 1807–1819. Available from: https://journals.lww.com/jasn/pages/default.aspx. doi:10.1681/ASN.2006010083.

Lee, D., Goldberg, A.L., 2013. SIRT1 protein, by blocking the activities of transcription factors FoxO1 and FoxO3, inhibits muscle atrophy and promotes muscle growth. J. Biol. Chem. 1083351X. 288 (42), 30515–30526. Available from: http://www.jbc.org/content/288/42/30515.full.pdf+html. doi: 10.1074/jbc.M113.489716.

Lee, S.J., 2004. Regulation of muscle mass by myostatin. Annu. Rev. Cell Dev. Biol. 10810706. 20, 61–86. doi:10.1146/annurev.cellbio.20.012103.135836.

Lokireddy, S., Wijesoma, I.W., Sze, S.K., McFarlane, C., Kambadur, R., Sharma, M., 2012. Identification of atrogin-1-targeted proteins$\theta\delta$ during the myostatin-induced skeletal muscle wasting. Am. J. Physiol. Cell Physiol. 15221563. 303 (5), C512. Available from: http://ajpcell.physiology.org/content/303/5/C512.full.pdf+html. doi:10.1152/ajpcell.00402.2011.

Loomans, H.A., Andl, C.D., 2016. Activin receptor-like kinases: a diverse family playing an important role in cancer. Am. J. Cancer Res. 21566976. 6 (11), 2431–2447. Available from: http://www.ajcr.us/files/ajcr0041138.pdf.

Mak, R.H.K., 1998. Effect of metabolic acidosis on insulin action and secretion in uremia. Kidney Int. 0085-2538. 54 (2), 603–607. doi:10.1046/j.1523-1755.1998.00023.x.

Martinho, D.V., Nobari, H., Faria, A., Field, A., Duarte, D., Sarmento, H., 2022. Oral branched-chain amino acids supplementation in athletes: a systematic review. Nutrients. 2072-6643. 14 (19), 4002. doi:10.3390/nu14194002.

Milovanova, L., Fomin, V., Moiseev, S., Taranova, M., Milovanov, Y., Lysenko (Kozlovskaya), L., Kozlov, V., Kozevnikova, E., Milovanova, S., Lebedeva, M., Reshetnikov, V., 2018. Effect of essential amino acid кetoanalogues and protein restriction diet on morphogenetic proteins (FGF-23 and Klotho) in 3b–4 stages chronic кidney disease patients: a randomized pilot study. Clin. Exp. Nephrol. 14377799. 22 (6), 1351–1359. Available from: https://link.springer.de/link/service/journals/10157/index.htm. doi:10.1007/s10157-018-1591-1.

Mitch, W.E., Medina, R., Grieber, S., May, R.C., England, B.K., Price, S.R., Bailey, J.L., Goldberg, A.L., 1994. Metabolic acidosis stimulates muscle protein degradation by activating the adenosine triphosphate-dependent pathway involving ubiquitin and proteasomes. J. Clin. Invest. 0021-9738. 93 (5), 2127–2133. doi:10.1172/JCI117208.

Moorthi, R.N., Avin, K.G., 2017. Clinical relevance of sarcopenia in chronic kidney disease. Curr. Opin. Nephrol. Hypertens. 14736543. 26 (3), 219–228. Available from: http://journals.lww.com/co-nephrolhypertens/pages/default.aspx. doi:10.1097/MNH.0000000000000318.

Morley, J.E., 2012. Sarcopenia in the elderly. Fam. Pract. 0263-2136. 29 (suppl 1), i44. doi:10.1093/fampra/cmr063.

Murashima, M., Yamamoto, R., Kanda, E., Kurita, N., Noma, H., Hamano, T., Fukagawa, M., 2024. Associations of vitamin D receptor activators and calcimimetics with falls and effect modifications by physical activity: a prospective cohort study on the Japan Dialysis Outcomes and Practice Patterns Study. Ther. Apher. Dial. 17449987. 28 (4), 547–556. Available from: http://onlinelibrary.wiley.com/journal/10.1111/(ISSN)1744-9987. doi:10.1111/1744-9987.14122.

Nickolas, T.L., Stein, E.M., Dworakowski, E., Nishiyama, K.K., Komandah-Kosseh, M., Zhang, C.A., McMahon, D.J., Liu, X.S., Boutroy, S., Cremers, S., Shane, E., 2013. Rapid cortical bone loss in patients with chronic kidney disease. J. Bone Miner. Res. 15234681. 28 (8), 1811–1820. Available from: http://onlinelibrary.wiley.com/journal/10.1002/(ISSN)1523-4681. doi:10.1002/jbmr.1916.

Proctor, C.J., Goljanek-Whysall, K., 2017. Using computer simulation models to investigate the most promising microRNAs to improve muscle regeneration during ageing. Sci. Rep. 20452322. 7 (1). Available from: https://www.nature.com/srep/. doi:10.1038/s41598-017-12538-6.

Qin, M., Zhu, J., Xing, L., Fan, Y., Luo, J., Sun, J., Chen, T., Zhang, Y., Qianyun, X., 2024. Adipose-derived exosomes ameliorate skeletal muscle atrophy via miR-146a-5p/IGF-1R signaling. J. Nanobiotechnol. 1477-3155. 22 (1). doi:10.1186/s12951-024-02983-7.

Radley, A., Van Craenenbroeck, A.H., Stevens, K.I., 2024. Can exercise improve outcomes for frail haemodialysis patients? Clin. Kidney J. 20488513. 17 (5). Available from: http://ckj.oxfordjournals.org/. doi:10.1093/ckj/sfae138.

Roshanravan, B., Robinson-Cohen, C., Patel, K.V., Ayers, E., Littman, A.J., De Boer, I.H., Ikizler, T.A., Himmelfarb, J., Katzel, L.I., Kestenbaum, B., Seliger, S., 2013. Association between physical performance and all-cause mortality in CKD. J. Am. Soc. Nephrol. 15333450. 24 (5), 822–830. Available from: http://jasn.asnjournals.org/content/24/5/822.full.pdf+html. doi:10.1681/ASN.2012070702.

Sabatino, A., Cuppari, L., Stenvinkel, P., Lindholm, B., Avesani, C.M., 2021. Sarcopenia in chronic kidney disease: what have we learned so far? J. Nephrol. 17246059. 34 (4), 1347–1372. Available from: http://www.springer.com/medicine/nephrology/journal/40620. doi:10.1007/s40620-020-00840-y.

Sabatino, A., Regolisti, G., Delsante, M., Di Motta, T., Cantarelli, C., Pioli, S., Grassi, G., Batini, V., Gregorini, M., Fiaccadori, E., 2019. Noninvasive evaluation of muscle mass by ultrasonography of quadriceps femoris muscle in End-Stage Renal Disease patients on hemodialysis. Clin. Nutr. 02615614. 38 (3), 1232–1239. doi:10.1016/j.clnu.2018.05.004.

Sartori, R., Milan, G., Patron, M., Mammucari, C., Blaauw, B., Abraham, R., Sandri, M., 2009. Smad2 and 3 transcription factors control muscle mass in adulthood. Am. J. Physiol. Cell Physiol. 15221563. 296 (6), C1248. Available from: http://ajpcell.physiology.org/cgi/reprint/296/6/C1248. doi:10.1152/ajpcell.00104.2009.

Schuelke, M., Wagner, K.R., Stolz, L.E., Hübner, C., Riebel, T., Kömen, W., Braun, T., Tobin, J.F., Lee, S.J., 2004. Myostatin mutation associated with gross muscle hypertrophy in a child. N. Engl. J. Med. 350 (26), 2682–2688. doi:10.1056/NEJMoa040933.

Sen, P., Shah, P.P., Nativio, R., Berger, S.L., 2016. Epigenetic mechanisms of longevity and aging. Cell. 10974172. 166 (4), 822–839. Available from: https://www.sciencedirect.com/journal/cell. doi:10.1016/j.cell.2016.07.050.

Singh, A., Schurman, S.H., Bektas, A., Kaileh, M., Roy, R., Wilson, D.M., Sen, R., Ferrucci, L., 2024. Aging and Inflammation. Cold Spring Harb. Perspect. Med. 2157-1422. 14 (6), a041197. doi:10.1101/cshperspect.a041197.

Soriano-Arroquia, A., House, L., Tregilgas, L., Canty-Laird, E., Goljanek-Whysall, K., 2016. The functional consequences of age-related changes in microRNA expression in skeletal muscle. Biogerontology. 1389-5729. 17 (3), 641–654. doi:10.1007/s10522-016-9638-8.

Starck, C.S., Sutherland-Smith, A.J., 2011. The C313Y Piedmontese mutation decreases myostatin covalent dimerisation and stability. BMC Res. Notes. 17560500. 4. doi:10.1186/1756-0500-4-442.

Su, T.-T., Barclay, R., Moineddin, R., Salbach, N.M., Pilleron, S., 2025. The impact of outdoor walking interventions on frailty among older adults with mobility limitations: findings from the getting older adults outdoors (GO-OUT) study. PLoS One. 1932-6203. 20 (9), e0323923. doi:10.1371/journal.pone.0323923.

Tsai, C.C., Wang, P.C., Hsiung, T., Fan, Y.H., Wu, J.T., Kan, W.C., Shiao, C.C., 2025. Sarcopenia in chronic kidney disease: a narrative review from pathophysiology to therapeutic approaches. Biomedicines. 22279059. 13 (2). Available from: www.mdpi.com/journal/biomedicines. doi:10.3390/biomedicines13020352.

Wang, X.H., Hu, Z., Klein, J.D., Zhang, L., Fang, F., Mitch, W.E., 2011. Decreased miR-29 suppresses myogenesis in CKD. J. Am. Soc. Nephrol. 15333450. 22 (11), 2068–2076. Available from: http://jasn.asnjournals.org/content/22/11/2068.full.pdf+html. doi:10.1681/ASN.2010121278.

Wang, X.H., Mitch, W.E., 2014. Mechanisms of muscle wasting in chronic kidney disease. Nat. Rev. Nephrol. 1759507X. 10 (9), 504–516. Available from: http://www.nature.com/nrneph/archive/index.html. doi:10.1038/nrneph.2014.112.

Watson, E.L., Kosmadakis, G.C., Smith, A.C., Viana, J.L., Brown, J.R., Molyneux, K., Pawluczyk, I.Z.A., Mulheran, M., Bishop, N.C., Shirreffs, S., Maughan, R.J., Owen, P.J., John, S.G., McIntyre, C.W., Feehally, J., Bevington, A., 2013. Combined walking exercise and alkali therapy in patients with CKD4-5 regulates intramuscular free amino acid pools and ubiquitinE3ligase expression. Eur. J. Appl. Physiol. 14396319. 113 (8), 2111–2124. doi:10.1007/s00421-013-2628-5.

Wilkes, E.A., Selby, A.L., Atherton, P.J., Patel, R., Rankin, D., Smith, K., Rennie, M.J., 2009. Blunting of insulin inhibition of proteolysis in legs of older subjects may contribute to age-related sarcopenia. Am. J. Clin. Nutr. 00029165. 90 (5), 1343–1350. Available from: http://www.ajcn.org/cgi/reprint/90/5/1343. doi:10.3945/ajcn.2009.27543.

Wolfe, R.R., 2017. Branched-chain amino acids and muscle protein synthesis in humans: myth or reality? J. Int. Soc. Sports Nutr. 15502783. 14 (1). Available from: http://www.jissn.com/. doi:10.1186/s12970-017-0184-9.

Workeneh, B.T., Mitch, W.E., 2010. Review of muscle wasting associated with chronic kidney disease. Am. J. Clin. Nutr. 00029165. 91 (4), 1128S. doi:10.3945/ajcn.2010.28608b.

Yeung, S.S.Y., Reijnierse, E.M., Pham, V.K., Trappenburg, M.C., Lim, W.K., Meskers, C.G.M., Maier, A.B., 2019. Sarcopenia and its association with falls and fractures in older adults: a systematic review and meta-analysis. J. Cachexia Sarcopenia Muscle. 21906009. 10 (3), 485–500. Available from: http://onlinelibrary.wiley.com/journal/10.1007/13539.2190-6009. doi:10.1002/jcsm.12411.

Ying, L., Yeping, J., Hui, W., Nan, Z., FuQian, S.Y., 2023. Screening of key genes in the pathogenesis of muscle atrophy in CKD-PEW children based on RNA sequencing. BMC Med. Genomics. 1755-8794. 16 (1). doi:10.1186/s12920-023-01718-1.

Yoon, M.S., 2017. mTOR as a key regulator in maintaining skeletal muscle mass. Front. Physiol. 1664042X. 8. Available from: https://www.frontiersin.org/articles/10.3389/fphys.2017.00788/full. doi:10.3389/fphys.2017.00788.

Zhang, L., Rajan, V., Lin, E., Hu, Z., Han, H.Q., Zhou, X., Song, Y., Min, H., Wang, X., Du, J., Mitch, W.E., 2011. Pharmacological inhibition of myostatin suppresses systemic inflammation and muscle atrophy in mice with chronic kidney disease. FASEB J. 15306860. 25 (5), 1653–1663. Available from: http://www.fasebj.org/content/25/5/1653.full.pdf+html. doi:10.1096/fj.10-176917.

Zhang, Q., Duplany, A., Moncollin, V., Mouradian, S., Goillot, E., Mazelin, L., Gauthier, K., Streichenberger, N., Angleraux, C., Chen, J., Ding, S., Schaeffer, L., Gangloff, Y.G., 2019. Lack of muscle mTOR kinase activity causes early onset myopathy and compromises whole-body homeostasis. J. Cachexia Sarcopenia Muscle. 21906009. 10 (1), 35–53. Available from: http://onlinelibrary.wiley.com/journal/10.1007/13539.2190-6009. doi:10.1002/jcsm.12336.

PART 3

Aging in specific diseases

CHAPTER

16

Hypertension

Faruk Hilmi Turgut[a] *and Emaad M. Abdel-Rahman*[b]

[a]Department of Internal Medicine, Division of Nephrology, Hatay Mustafa Kemal University, Hatay, Turkey

[b]Division of Nephrology, University of Virginia, Charlottesville, VA, United States

Introduction

Arterial hypertension is one of the modifiable risk factors for cardiovascular disease, contributing to increasing morbidity and mortality rates (Fuchs and Whelton, 2020; Zhou et al., 2018). Most of the older adult population suffers from arterial hypertension. Numerous aspects differentiate arterial hypertension in older adults from that in younger patients. Older adults are more likely to exhibit isolated systolic hypertension, widened pulse pressure, and orthostatic hypotension due to arterial stiffening and reduced baroreceptor sensitivity (Whelton et al., 2017; Mancia et al., 2023). Older adults are more prone to hypertension complications and uncontrolled blood pressure (BP). Managing hypertension in older adults presents several unique and complex challenges that require careful consideration and a tailored approach.

Definition and classification of hypertension

The optimal diagnostic threshold for primary hypertension is not well defined, with significant differences in BP classification and treatment goals among the different guidelines (Table 16.1). This could be related to the substantial discrepancies in the definition of hypertension across the various guidelines.

The American College of Cardiology/American Heart Association (ACC/AHA) hypertension guidelines use lower values to define hypertension (systolic BP ≥ 130 and/or diastolic BP ≥ 80 mmHg). These guidelines were based primarily on the results from the Systolic Blood Pressure Intervention Trial (SPRINT) (Whelton et al., 2017; Williamson et al., 2016).

However, the European Society of Cardiology/European Society of Hypertension (ESC/ESH) and the International Society of Hypertension BP guidelines define hypertension as systolic BP ≥140 and/or diastolic BP ≥90 mmHg, as measured in the office (Mancia et al.,

Aging and the Kidney
https://doi.org/10.1016/B978-0-443-34069-7.00017-3

TABLE 16.1 The definition and classification of hypertension across various guidelines.

BP Category	2020 ISH SBP/DBP (mmHg)	2023 ESH/ESC SBP/DBP (mmHg)	2025 ACC/AHA SBP/DBP (mmHg)
Threshold	≥140 and/or ≥ 90	≥140 and/or ≥ 90	≥130 and/or ≥ 80
Optimal		<120/80	N/A
Normal	<130 and < 85	120–129/80–84	<120/80
Elevated (High-normal)	130–139 and/or 85–89	130–139 and/or 85–89	120–129/ < 80
Stage (Grade) 1	140–159 and/or 90–99	140–159 and/or 90–99	130–139 or 80–89
Stage (Grade) 2	≥160 and/or ≥ 100	160–179 and/or 100–109	≥140 or ≥ 90
Stage (Grade) 3	N/A	≥180 and/or ≥ 110	N/A
ISH	N/A	≥140 (and DBP < 90)	≥160
IDH	N/A	DBP ≥ 90 (and SBP < 140)	N/A
Treatment goals			
65–79 years	<130/80	<140/80[a]	<130/80
≥80 years	<140/80	140–150/ < 80	<130/80

ACC/AHA, the American College of Cardiology/American Heart Association; BP, blood pressure; DBP, diastolic blood pressure; ESH/ESC, the European Society of Cardiology/European Society of Hypertension; IDH, isolated diastolic hypertension; ISH, isolated systolic hypertension; ISH, the International Society of Hypertension; SBP, systolic blood pressure; WHO, World Health Organization.
[a]*Target < 130/80 if tolerated.*

2023). For those 80 years and older, the ESC/ESH guidelines recommend a higher BP threshold of 160 mmHg before beginning treatment (Mancia et al., 2023).

Prevalence and characteristics of hypertension in older adults

Prevalence: Hypertension is highly prevalent and associated with a higher morbidity in older adults. Studies have shown that the frequency of development of hypertension progressively increases with aging (Vasan et al., 2001) with the prevalence of hypertension being as high as 70% to >80% (Oliveros et al., 2020) in the older adult population.

According to the National Health and Nutrition Examination Survey (NHANES), 76% of adults aged 65 to 74 years and 82% of adults aged 75 years or older have hypertension, based on the definition of ACC/AHA thresholds (Muntner et al., 2018). At younger ages, hypertension is more prevalent in men, but the prevalence reverses to be greater in women among older adults (Mancia et al., 2023). It has also been noted that the prevalence of both masked and white coat hypertension increases in geriatric patients with varying prognostic outcomes (Pierdomenico et al., 2017). This increased prevalence of hypertension in the older adult population may be attributed to a variety of etiological factors, often in combination, including primary or secondary autonomic dysfunction, polypharmacy, a tendency for volume depletion, vascular aging (characterized by increased arterial stiffness), and greater BP variability (Mancia et al., 2023).

Characteristics: Several noted characteristics of hypertension in the older adult population are observed. BP variability is more common in the older adult population, contributing to organ damage and increasing the risk of adverse events (Saren et al., 2024; Bencivenga et al., 2022). This variability in BP in this age group could be related to arterial stiffness and autonomic dysfunction. Specific BP phenotypes, such as reverse-dipping, extreme-dipping, and postural or postprandial hypotension, are also more commonly observed in older adults compared to younger individuals.

Pathophysiology and risk factors of hypertension in older adults

The development of arterial hypertension is influenced by a complex and multifactorial interaction involving genetic predisposition, aging-related physiological changes, and environmental factors. Normal physiological aging is a gradual and regulated process; however, it poses a significant and independent risk for hypertension and subsequent cardiovascular events.

Age-related changes in the cardiovascular system

Age-related alterations in the cardiovascular system have been extensively studied and demonstrated to significantly contribute to the age-related increase in BP. Changes in the vascular structure and physiology, sympathetic nervous system, and kidney function are key determinants in the pathophysiology of increased BP in older adults.

Aging is associated with functional, structural, and mechanical changes in arteries that closely resemble the vascular alterations in hypertension (Fig. 16.1). The arterial changes observed in hypertension accelerate and augment age-related vascular changes, indicating a strong interaction between aging and BP elevation. The functional and structural changes in arteries that occur with normal aging, such as endothelial dysfunction, myocardial fibrosis, vascular remodeling, increased stiffness, and inflammation, are also characteristic features of hypertension (Harvey et al., 2015).

Endothelial dysfunction, increased extracellular fibrosis, and cellular senescence are well-established causes of vascular stiffness. In aging, alterations in the levels of angiotensin II, angiotensin-converting enzyme, and mineralocorticoid receptors are observed. These factors stimulate extracellular matrix production and result in the development of inflammation, oxidative stress, and fibrosis, contributing to the arterial stiffness observed with aging (Krug et al., 2010). In general, vascular stiffness increases with age and is not only associated with isolated systolic hypertension but also with diastolic dysfunction and heart failure, chronic kidney disease (CKD), and cognitive decline (Heredia et al., 2024).

Aging is associated with a physiological decline in kidney function. With normal aging, kidneys undergo various structural and functional changes, including renal arteriosclerosis, glomerulosclerosis, and impairment of tubular function. The overall number of functioning nephrons also steadily decreases with aging (Weinstein and Anderson, 2010). Impairments

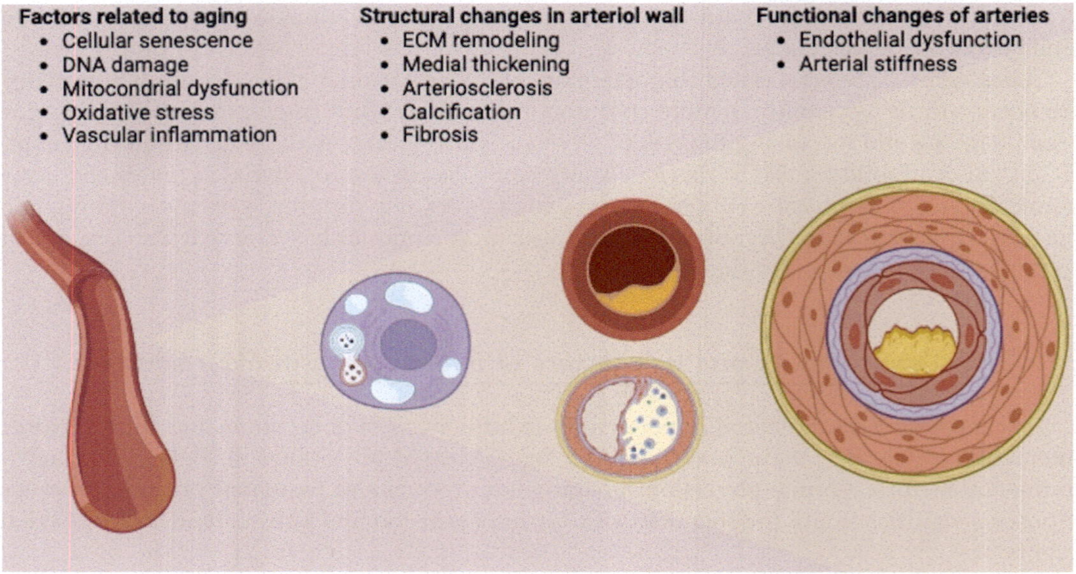

FIG. 16.1 Structural and functional changes in vascular aging. Factors related to aging, structural changes in the arterial wall, and functional changes in arteries with aging resemble vascular alterations associated with aging.

in renal sodium handling occur, causing salt sensitivity. All these changes can disrupt the delicate balance of fluids and hormones, contributing to the increased BP in older adults (Frame and Wainford, 2018).

Lifestyle factors and hypertension in the older adult

Epidemiological studies have shown a clear association between BP and lifestyle factors, suggesting that lifestyle modifications are essential for the prevention and management of hypertension, as evident in the guidelines (Whelton et al., 2017; Mancia et al., 2023). Hypertension is associated with unhealthy lifestyle factors, including nonadherence to recommended dietary guidelines, inadequate physical activity, excess body weight, tobacco use, and heavy alcohol consumption (Whelton et al., 2017; Mancia et al., 2023).

Comorbid conditions affecting hypertension in older adults

The presence of several comorbid conditions, including chronic lung disease, diabetes, sleep apnea, obesity, dyslipidemia, CKD, and arrhythmias, is frequent in older adults and contributes significantly to the risk of hypertension. In patients with hypertension, there is a common overlap in risk factors for obesity, type 2 diabetes, and CKD, conditions that often coexist. Both systolic and diastolic BP are significantly associated with body mass index, but the association is weaker in older adults compared to younger subjects (Li et al., 2018). Older adults are more vulnerable to adverse effects, and polypharmacy can lead to fluctuating BP and medication nonadherence (Mukete and Ferdinand, 2016). Cognitive decline also contributes to nonadherence to medications and lifestyle modifications in older adults (El-Saifi et al., 2018).

Symptoms and diagnosis of hypertension in older adults

Common symptoms

Hypertension itself rarely causes symptoms, and the majority of patients with arterial hypertension have no symptoms, even if BP readings reach dangerously high levels. The emergency symptoms depend on the organs affected and may include headaches, blurred vision, dizziness, chest pain, anxiety, nosebleeds, and confusion (Mancia et al., 2023). In older adults, these symptoms can be easily attributed to other conditions, making hypertension detection more challenging.

Diagnosis

Accurate BP measurement is crucial, and multiple readings are recommended. Because of the variability of BP, high BP should be confirmed over at least two to three visits (Mancia et al., 2023). Considering the high variability and increased predisposition to orthostatic hypotension (OH), both office and out-of-office BP measurements should be utilized to more accurately define the BP profile and guide therapeutic strategies. Therefore complementary to office BP, ambulatory BP monitoring (ABPM) and/or BP self-measurement should also be part of daily clinical practice in the elderly (Bahat et al., 2024).

Complications of hypertension in older adults

Epidemiological studies consistently demonstrate a strong association between hypertension and the development of various complications, substantially impacting morbidity and mortality in older adults (Table 16.2) (Zhou et al., 2018; Butler et al., 2011; Anderson et al., 2015; Kannel, 2000).

Cardiovascular disease

The association between hypertension and major cardiovascular events is well established. Hypertension results in considerable cardiovascular morbidity and mortality among older adults. Uncontrolled hypertension also increases the risk of all-cause and cardiovascular mortality (Zhou et al., 2018). High BP is an important risk factor for various heart diseases, such as coronary artery disease, heart failure, and atrial fibrillation (Mancia et al., 2023). Among older adults, there is a continuous increase in heart failure risk as systolic BP rises,

TABLE 16.2 Complications of hypertension in older adults.

Complication	Consequences	Key considerations
Cardiovascular disease	Left ventricular hypertrophy Atherosclerosis Heart failure Coronary artery disease Peripheral artery disease Aortic aneurysm	Older adults are at increased risk due to age-related changes in the cardiovascular system. Arterial stiffness and other age-related vascular changes exacerbate the effects of hypertension, increasing the risk of atrial fibrillation.
Kidney disease	Proteinuria Nephrosclerosis Chronic kidney disease Renovascular disease	Age-related decline in kidney function is compounded by hypertension. Hypertension can accelerate the progression of CKD. Kidney disease also causes hypertension, resulting in a vicious cycle.
Cerebrovascular disease	Stroke (hemorrhagic or ischemic) Transient Ischemic Attack Retinopathy Cognitive decline Dementia	Hypertension is a major risk factor for stroke in older adults. Hypertensive retinopathy can lead to gradual or sudden vision impairment. Hypertension can contribute to overall frailty and disability.

even at levels below 115 mmHg (Butler et al., 2011). However, the relationship between BP levels and cardiovascular risk is not linear and exhibits a U-shaped curve (Hong et al., 2021).

Kidney disease

Hypertension is common in patients with CKD, and high BP contributes to the progression of CKD. The kidney is one of the major organs damaged by high BP. Age-related changes in the kidneys and cardiovascular system lead to both a decline in kidney function and the development of hypertension. Reciprocally, high BP is strongly associated with the development and progression of CKD (Anderson et al., 2015). In fact, hypertensive nephropathy remains the second most common cause of CKD, leading to end-stage kidney disease.

Cerebrovascular disease

The dramatic increase in cerebrovascular disease observed with advancing age is largely attributed to age-related vascular changes and cardiovascular factors. Stroke is one of the leading causes of death. It is crucial to note that hypertension is the strongest modifiable risk factor for stroke. The Framingham Study showed that hypertension doubles the stroke risk in adults aged 65–94, with a higher risk for women (RR 2.3) than for men (RR 1.9) (Kannel, 2000). Atrial fibrillation is common in patients with hypertension, and both are associated with an increased risk of stroke. Clinical studies have demonstrated that treating hypertension significantly reduces the risk of both hemorrhagic and ischemic strokes (Perry et al., 2000).

Cognitive decline and dementia

Both cognitive decline and dementia are common in older adults. Cerebrovascular disease is a primary contributor to cognitive decline, driven by atherosclerosis and arterial stiffness. Epidemiological and observational studies suggest a connection between hypertension and an increased risk of cognitive decline and dementia. Particularly, hypertension in midlife (Bowling et al., 2021; Franklin et al., 1997; Carey et al., 2018; Giacona and Vongpatanasin, 2024; Noubiap et al., 2019; Wijkman et al., 2021; Daugherty et al., 2012; Hwang et al., 2017; Geng et al., 2023; Toh et al., 2023) is correlated with an increased risk for dementia in later life, including vascular dementia and Alzheimer's disease. The impact of hypertension on dementia risk in later life becomes more nuanced, with a stronger association with vascular dementia than Alzheimer's disease. The risk of dementia overall decreases with very advanced age (Lyon et al., 2024).

Management

Numerous randomized controlled trials and metaanalyses have demonstrated that lowering high BP significantly reduces the risk of cardiovascular events, cardiovascular death, all-cause mortality, and CKD in older adults (Williamson et al., 2016; Zhang et al., 2021; Beckett et al., 2008; Lv et al., 2013). As in younger patients, lifestyle interventions to prevent and treat hypertension play a crucial role in management.

Nonpharmacologic interventions

Optimal weight control, sodium restriction, increased potassium intake, physical activity, smoking cessation, and limited alcohol consumption are fundamental components of nonpharmacologic strategies (Mancia et al., 2023; Williamson et al., 2016). Reducing sodium intake has long been a cornerstone of hypertension management. The relationship between sodium-restricted diets and improved BP control is well established, with this effect being more pronounced in older adults (Appel et al., 2001). Lowering sodium intake is a highly effective nonpharmacologic therapy for hypertension in the elderly (Appel et al., 2001; Huang et al., 2020). However, older adults may have difficulty complying with dietary salt restrictions due to various factors, including taste changes and cognitive decline. Therefore dietary sodium intake should be moderately restricted to 100 to 120 mEq/day.

Adequate potassium, calcium, and magnesium intake contribute to reducing BP in older adults. Consistently, both the Mediterranean and the Dietary Approaches to Stop Hypertension (DASH) dietary patterns have been proven to lower BP and reduce the risk of cardiovascular disease (Bray et al., 2004). Along the same lines, the Mediterranean-style diet (rich in fruits, vegetables, legumes, nuts, and olive oil) is effective in reducing BP and arterial stiffness and improving cardiovascular health in older adults (Jennings et al., 2019).

Exercise in older adults plays an important role in controlling BP in the older adult population. Clinical trials have demonstrated that exercise results in reducing both systolic and diastolic BP in the elderly (Kazeminia et al., 2020; Henkin et al., 2023). As no specific exercise guidelines exist for elderly hypertensive patients, general adult population guidelines may be considered applicable.

Similarly, weight loss as a means to control BP in the older adult population was studied. In this population, weight loss should be approached with greater caution due to the risk of reductions in muscle mass, strength, and bone mineral density. The 2023 ESH/ESC guideline does not routinely recommend weight loss in patients over 80 years old unless obesity is severe (Mancia et al., 2023). Incorporating both aerobic and resistance exercise into weight loss can significantly reduce the potential adverse effects of weight loss. Therefore it is vital to monitor sarcopenia during weight control interventions.

In summary, lifestyle changes, including nutritional and exercise therapies, are essential nonpharmacological treatments for hypertension in the elderly. Nonpharmacological interventions not only improve BP control and enhance the effects of pharmacological therapies but may also improve quality of life, promoting overall health through balanced dietary habits. Overall, lifestyle changes are essential and beneficial for all individuals with hypertension, but pharmacological intervention is often necessary for those with higher BP levels or an insufficient response to lifestyle modifications.

Pharmacologic interventions

Drug therapy should be initiated in older adult hypertensive patients when lifestyle changes alone are not effective. Randomized trials have confirmed that older adults, including the very elderly over 80, derive clear benefits from antihypertensive therapy (Beckett et al., 2008; SHEP Cooperative Research Group, 1991). Prior to starting antihypertensive medication in older adults, a thorough evaluation of several key factors is essential. BP should be lowered to its ultimate goal gradually over a period of two to four months. Although older adults often require more medications than younger patients to reach target BP, lower initial doses should be used to minimize side effects (Mancia et al., 2023). In older adults with hypertension, especially those who are frail and exhibit significant OH, extra caution is imperative.

The Hypertension in the Very Old Trial (HYVET), focusing exclusively on patients aged 80 years or more, documented that antihypertensive therapy with indapamide, with or without perindopril, is beneficial (Beckett et al., 2008). With intensive treatment, a similar benefit was noted in the Systolic Blood Pressure Intervention Trial (SPRINT), studying the same group of patients (Zhang et al., 2021). The ESC/ESH guideline also advises initiating pharmacologic treatment for all patients under the age of 80 years with a systolic BP of 160 mmHg or higher and recommends a BP target for systolic BP < 140 mmHg (Mancia et al., 2023). As a result, antihypertensive drug treatment should be prescribed in most very old hypertensive patients.

Thiazide diuretics, angiotensin-converting enzyme (ACE) inhibitors, angiotensin II receptor blockers (ARBs), and calcium channel blockers (CCBs) have all been shown to improve cardiovascular outcomes in the elderly. Long-acting CCBs are effective and safe for older adults with hypertension, especially isolated systolic hypertension (Staessen et al., 1997; Hansson et al., 1999; Jamerson et al., 2008). Many older adult patients with hypertension have a specific indication for an ACE inhibitor or ARB. Olmesartan monotherapy effectively decreased BP and was well tolerated, with few adverse events in the elderly (Redon et al., 2018). The Avoiding Cardiovascular Events through Combination Therapy in Patients Living with Systolic Hypertension (ACCOMPLISH) trial demonstrated that benazepril and amlodipine significantly reduced cardiovascular events compared to benazepril and hydrochlorothiazide (9.6% vs. 11.8%, HR 0.80) (Jamerson et al., 2008).

In general, any of the three major drug classes (ACE inhibitor/ARB, CCB, or diuretic) can be used as initial therapy in the older population (Whelton et al., 2017; Mancia et al., 2023). Studies have shown that most patients will need combination therapy, which may include any two of these three drugs (Mancia et al., 2023). Despite this, some experts prefer initial therapy with a long-acting dihydropyridine CCB and add a long-acting ACE inhibitor/ARB as combination therapy based on the ACCOMPLISH trial (Jamerson et al., 2008). In general, once-daily prescriptions are often favored for better adherence, and guidelines recommend single-pill combination therapy to reduce pill burden and improve adherence.

The ESH guidelines included beta-blockers as an optional first-line therapy (Mancia et al., 2023). However, beta-blockers have a lesser antihypertensive effect and more side effects in the elderly population. Therefore beta-blockers should not be used as initial therapy in older adults in the absence of compelling indications such as heart failure and coronary artery disease (Whelton et al., 2017; Mancia et al., 2023). The recommended pharmacological therapy for heart failure with reduced ejection fraction consists of diuretics, ACE inhibitors (or ARBs), beta-blockers, and aldosterone receptor antagonists.

Certain classes of antihypertensives, like alpha and beta-blockers, are more strongly associated with OH. ACE inhibitors, ARBs, and CCBs are generally preferred, as they have less effect on the sympathetic compensatory response important in preventing OH. Diuretics, particularly loop diuretics, may also elevate the risk of OH.

In summary, before starting medications for hypertension in the older adult population, assessment should be done for OH, and the dose should be titrated gradually according to tolerance. Renal function should also be assessed to detect possible increases in serum creatinine and reductions in GFR. Electrolyte imbalances are also important side effects of drugs, which need to be monitored. Thiazide diuretics should be used with caution in the elderly because of the risk of hyponatremia.

Goals of treatment of hypertension in the older adult population and follow-up

While many studies designed to guide clinicians about the optimum goal for SBP in older adults were conducted, resulting in guidelines, the optimal target for diastolic BP in the elderly remains an unresolved issue.

Current clinical guidelines differ on the best BP target for older adults (Table 16.1). For most of the older adult population, a more aggressive systolic BP target of < 130 mmHg is recommended in the 2017 ACC/AHA guideline (Whelton et al., 2017). The SPRINT and the Strategy of Blood Pressure Intervention in the Elderly Hypertensive Patients (STEP) trials provided evidence supporting intensive BP control in older populations. In a prespecified subgroup analysis of participants aged 75 years or older in the SPRINT trial, intensive BP lowering (systolic BP target < 120 mmHg) was associated with a statistically significant reduction in both combined cardiovascular events (HR 0.66, 95% CI: 0.51–0.85) and all-cause mortality (HR 0.67, 95% CI: 0.49–0.91) compared to standard treatment (systolic BP target < 140 mmHg) (Williamson et al., 2016). On the other hand, the ESC/ESH guideline recommends a therapeutic target of systolic BP 130–139 mmHg and diastolic BP 70–79 mmHg for elderly patients aged 65 to 80 years (Mancia et al., 2023).

The HYVET trial showed that treating patients aged 80 years or older to a BP of 150/80 mmHg significantly lowered morbidity and mortality (Beckett et al., 2008). There is also evidence that lower BP targets (≤140/90 mmHg) decrease stroke risk and serious cardiovascular events when compared with higher BP targets (150–160/95–105 mmHg range) in hypertensive adults aged 65 years or older, although the effect on all-cause mortality is unclear (Falk et al., 2024). Furthermore, some studies suggest that lowering diastolic BP below 70 mmHg may increase cardiovascular risk (Somes et al., 1999; Fagard et al., 2007). Hypertension and frailty are strongly linked, and hypertension is more common in frail elderly patients. Plausibly, intensive BP control may influence the development of frailty, and frail older patients may not tolerate BP lowering.

In summary, current BP targets may be appropriate for the majority of older adults. A sensible clinical practice for managing hypertension in the older adult is cautiously targeting a systolic BP of 140 mmHg, while meticulously avoiding a diastolic BP below 70 mmHg to ensure adequate tissue perfusion. Hypertension treatment and control rates have improved in most countries since 1990 (NCDRF, 2021). Despite the easy diagnosis and available treatments, and the generally high awareness and treatment rates for hypertension among older adults, the control rates of hypertension remain low in this age group (Whelton et al., 2017). The percentage with controlled BP has generally been reported to be <50% (Bowling et al., 2021).

Special considerations

Isolated systolic hypertension

In the elderly, systolic BP increases more significantly compared to younger individuals, while diastolic BP decreases with age, resulting in a higher prevalence of isolated systolic hypertension (Franklin et al., 1997). The combination of high systolic BP and low diastolic BP, resulting in a high pulse pressure, indicates significant arterial stiffness, which is the most common manifestation of arterial aging.

Resistant hypertension

Resistant hypertension (RH) is defined by uncontrolled BP despite the use of at least three antihypertensive medications, commonly including RAS blockers, long-acting calcium channel blockers, and diuretics, or controlled BP that requires the use of ≥ 4 antihypertensive drugs (Carey et al., 2018).

The antihypertensive drugs should be used at maximally tolerated doses and at the appropriate dosing frequency. Accurate diagnosis of true RH necessitates careful evaluation of patient adherence to medications and recommended lifestyle changes, as well as accurate BP measurements. The initial step in evaluating possible RH is to exclude pseudo-resistance. White coat hypertension and nonadherence to medications are the main causes of pseudo-resistance. Ambulatory or home BP monitoring can be performed to identify the presence or absence of the white-coat effect. Similarly, various methods (e.g., pharmacy refill, questionnaires, and self-reports) may be used to assess medication adherence. Certain drugs or over-the-counter medications can increase BP and should be evaluated before establishing a diagnosis of RH (Giacona and Vongpatanasin, 2024).

The older adult population experiences a greater prevalence of true RH than the general population (Noubiap et al., 2019). The adoption of more stringent BP goals has contributed to a higher observed prevalence of RH (Wijkman et al., 2021). Observational studies have shown that patients with RH are at higher cardiovascular risk (Wijkman et al., 2021; Daugherty et al., 2012).

The etiology of RH is complex and multifactorial, encompassing contributions from obesity, an increase in the activity of the RAS and sympathetic system, and heightened renal sodium retention (Hwang et al., 2017). Higher body mass index, longer hypertension duration, and coronary artery disease are associated factors for RH in the elderly. High cardiac output and possible occult volume expansion are characteristics of RH in the elderly (Geng et al., 2023). Secondary causes of hypertension (primary aldosteronism, renal parenchymal disease, renovascular hypertension, and obstructive sleep apnea) are also more common in the elderly (Giacona and Vongpatanasin, 2024; Geng et al., 2023). Therefore proper screening and identification of secondary causes of hypertension are crucial for better management of RH in the elderly population.

Polypharmacy and drug interactions

A high comorbidity burden and polypharmacy (use of 5 or more medications) are common among the elderly population. As a fragile population that is more vulnerable to adverse effects, the elderly tend to have a higher risk of polypharmacy than the younger population. Drug-drug interactions can result in altered therapeutic effects or safety issues when two or more medications are taken together. Drug interactions and polypharmacy may be associated with worse outcomes, including falls, electrolyte abnormalities, hospitalization, and premature mortality (Mukete and Ferdinand, 2016; Toh et al., 2023). Both physiological changes due to aging and alterations in drug pharmacokinetics and pharmacodynamics make it more challenging in the elderly. Polypharmacy should be avoided as far as possible, and potential drug interactions must be considered in the elderly.

Conclusion

Both the incidence and prevalence of hypertension increase with aging. Aging-related changes in vessels, nerves, and kidneys contribute to rising BP. The diagnosis of hypertension requires repeated and careful measurement of BP. Home BP monitoring and ambulatory BP monitoring should be used prior to diagnosing hypertension, particularly to detect masked hypertension and white-coat hypertension. Therapy should be considered for all aging hypertensive patients, even in the very elderly. Most antihypertensive drugs can be used as initial therapy in the absence of compelling indications. More intensive antihypertensive treatment is recommended to achieve BP targets for these individuals.

References

Anderson, A.H., Yang, W., Townsend, R.R., Pan, Q., Chertow, G.M., Kusek, J.W., Charleston, J., He, J., Kallem, R.K., Lash, J.P., Miller, E.R., Rahman, M., Steigerwalt, S., Weir, M., Wright, J.T., Feldman, H.I., Appel, L.J., Go, A.S., 2015. Time-updated systolic blood pressure and the progression of chronic kidney disease: a cohort study. Ann. Intern. Med. 15393704. 162 (4), 258–265. Available from: http://annals.org/data/Journals/AIM/932765/0000605-201502170-00004.pdf. doi:10.7326/M14-0488.

Appel, L.J., Espeland, M.A., Easter, L., Wilson, A.C., Folmar, S., Lacy, C.R., 2001. Effects of reduced sodium intake on hypertension control in older individuals: results from the trial of nonpharmacologic interventions in the elderly (TONE). Arch. Intern. Med. 00039926. 161 (5), 685–693. Available from: http://archinte.jamanetwork.com/journal.aspx. doi:10.1001/archinte.161.5.685.

Bahat, G., Ribeiro, H., Sheppard, J.P., Bogaerts, J.M.K., Camafort, M., Dallmeier, D., De Backer, T., Desideri, G., Olszanecka, A., Persu, A., Protogerou, A., Rajzer, M., Virdis, A., Ungar, A., Weber, T., Benetos, A., 2024. Twelve hot questions in the management of hypertension in patients aged 80+ years and their answers with the help of the 2023 European Society of Hypertension Guidelines. J. Hypertens. 14735598. 42 (11), 1837–1847. Available from: http://journals.lww.com/jhypertension. doi:10.1097/HJH.0000000000003844.

Beckett, N.S., Peters, R., Fletcher, A.E., Staessen, J.A., Liu, L., Dumitrascu, D., Stoyanovsky, V., Antikainen, R.L., Nikitin, Y., Anderson, C., Belhani, A., Forette, F., Rajkumar, C., Thijs, L., Banya, W., Bulpitt, C.J., 2008. Treatment of hypertension in patients 80 years of age or older. N. Engl. J. Med. 15334406. 358 (18), 1887–1898. Available from: http://content.nejm.org/cgi/reprint/358/18/1887.pdf. doi:10.1056/NEJMoa0801369.

Bencivenga, L., Barreto, P.D.S., Rolland, Y., Hanon, O., Vidal, J.-S., Cestac, P., Vellas, B., Rouch, L., 2022. Blood pressure variability: a potential marker of aging. Ageing Res. Rev. 15681637. 80, 101677. doi:10.1016/j.arr.2022.101677.

Bowling, C.B., Lee, A., Williamson, J.D., 2021. Blood Pressure Control among Older Adults with Hypertension: narrative Review and Introduction of a Framework for Improving Care. J. Hypertens. 19417225. 34 (3), 258–266. Available from: https://academic.oup.com/ajh/issue. doi:10.1093/ajh/hpab002.

Bray, G.A., Vollmer, W.M., Sacks, F.M., Obarzanek, E., Svetkey, L.P., Appel, L.J., 2004. A further subgroup analysis of the effects of the DASH diet and three dietary sodium levels on blood pressure: results of the DASH-sodium trial. Am. J. Cardiol. 00029149. 94 (2), 222–227. Available from: www.elsevier.com/locate/amjcard. doi:10.1016/j.amjcard.2004.03.070.

Butler, J., Kalogeropoulos, A.P., Georgiopoulou, V.V., Bibbins-Domingo, K., Najjar, S.S., Sutton-Tyrrell, K.C., Harris, T.B., Kritchevsky, S.B., Lloyd-Jones, D.M., Newman, A.B., Psaty, B.M., 2011. Systolic blood pressure and incident heart failure in the elderly. The Cardiovascular Health Study and the Health, Ageing and Body Composition Study. Heart. 1468201X. 97 (16), 1304–1311. Available from: http://heart.bmj.com/content/97/16/1304.full.pdf. doi:10.1136/hrt.2011.225482

Carey, R.M., Calhoun, D.A., Bakris, G.L., Brook, R.D., Daugherty, S.L., Dennison-Himmelfarb, C.R., Egan, B.M., Flack, J.M., Gidding, S.S., Judd, E., Lackland, D.T., Laffer, C.L., Newton-Cheh, C., Smith, S.M., Taler, S.J., Textor, S.C., Turan, T.N., White, W.B., 2018. Resistant Hypertension: detection, Evaluation, and Management: a Scientific Statement From the American Heart Association. Hypertension. 0194-911X. 72 (5), e53–e90. doi:10.1161/hyp.0000000000000084.

Daugherty, S.L., Powers, J.D., Magid, D.J., Tavel, H.M., Masoudi, F.A., Margolis, K.L., O'Connor, P.J., Selby, J.V., Ho, P.M., 2012. Incidence and prognosis of resistant hypertension in hypertensive patients. Circulation. 15244539. 125 (13), 1635–1642. doi:10.1161/CIRCULATIONAHA.111.068064.

El-Saifi, N., Moyle, W., Jones, C., Tuffaha, H., 2018. Medication Adherence in Older Patients With Dementia: a Systematic Literature Review. J. Pharm. Pract. 0897-1900. 31 (3), 322–334. doi:10.1177/0897190017710524.

Fagard, R.H., Staessen, J.A., Thijs, L., Celis, H., Bulpitt, C.J., De Leeuw, P.W., Leonetti, G., Tuomilehto, J., Yodfat, Y., 2007. On-treatment diastolic blood pressure and prognosis in systolic hypertension. Arch. Intern. Med. 15383679. 167 (17), 1884–1891. Available from: http://archinte.ama-assn.org/cgi/reprint/167/17/1884. doi:10.1001/archinte.167.17.1884Belgium.

Falk, J.M., Froentjes, L., Kirkwood, J.E.M., Heran, B.S., Kolber, M.R., Allan, G.M., Korownyk, C.S., Garrison, S.R., 2024. Higher blood pressure targets for hypertension in older adults. Cochrane Database Syst. Rev. 14651858. 2024 (12). Available from: https://www.cochranelibrary.com/cdsr/table-of-contents. doi:10.1002/14651858.CD011575.pub3.

Frame, A.A., Wainford, R.D., 2018. Mechanisms of altered renal sodium handling in age-related hypertension. Am. J. Physiol. Renal Physiol. 15221466. 315 (1), F1. Available from: https://www.physiology.org/doi/pdf/10.1152/ajprenal.00594.2017. doi:10.1152/ajprenal.00594.2017.

Franklin, S.S., Gustin IV, W., Wong, N.D., Larson, M.G., Weber, M.A., Kannel, W.B., Levy, D., 1997. Hemodynamic patterns of age-related changes in blood pressure: the Framingham heart study. Circulation. 00097322. 96 (1), 308–315. Available from: http://circ.ahajournals.org. doi:10.1161/01.CIR.96.1.308.

Fuchs, F.D., Whelton, P.K., 2020. High Blood Pressure and Cardiovascular Disease. Hypertension. 15244563. 75 (2), 285–292. Available from: https://www.ahajournals.org/journal/hyp. doi:10.1161/HYPERTENSIONAHA.119.14240.

Geng, H., Chen, X., Liang, W., Liu, M., 2023. Associated factors and hemodynamic characteristics of resistant hypertension in the elderly. J. Clin. Hypertens. 1524-6175. 25 (3), 259–265. doi:10.1111/jch.14640.

Giacona, J.M., Vongpatanasin, W., 2024. Resistant Hypertension in Older Adults. Clin. Geriatr. Med. 18798853. 40 (4), 645–658. Available from: https://www.sciencedirect.com/science/journal/07490690. doi:10.1016/j.cger.2024.04.005.

Hansson, L., Lindholm, L.H., Ekbom, T., Dahlöf, B., Lanke, J., Scherstén, B., Wester, P.O., Hedner, T., De Faire, U., 1999. Randomised trial of old and new antihypertensive drugs in elderly patients: cardiovascular mortality and morbidity the Swedish trial in old patients with hypertension-2 study. Lancet. 01406736. 354 (9192), 1751–1756. Available from: http://www.journals.elsevier.com/the-lancet/. doi:10.1016/S0140-6736(99)10327-1.

Harvey, A., Montezano, A.C., Touyz, R.M., 2015. Vascular biology of ageing-Implications in hypertension. J. Mol. Cell. Cardiol. 10958584. 83, 112–121. Available from: http://www.elsevier.com/locate/yjmcc. doi:10.1016/j.yjmcc.2015.04.011.

Henkin, J.S., Pinto, R.S., Machado, C.L.F., Wilhelm, E.N., 2023. Chronic effect of resistance training on blood pressure in older adults with prehypertension and hypertension: a systematic review and meta-analysis. Exp. Gerontol. 18736815. 177. Available from: www.elsevier.com/locate/expgero. doi:10.1016/j.exger.2023.112193.

Heredia, C.P., Furman, D., Moreno, D.G., Tuday, E., 2024. Eric Tuday, The Role of Vascular Aging in the Development of Hypertension. Clin. Geriatr. Med. 07490690. 40 (4), 539–550. doi:10.1016/j.cger.2024.04.011.

Hong, S., Park, J.H., Han, K., Lee, C.B., Kim, D.S., Sung Hoon, Y., 2021. Blood Pressure and Cardiovascular Disease in Older Patients With Diabetes: retrospective Cohort Study. J. Am. Heart Assoc. 2047-9980. 10 (22). doi:10.1161/jaha.121.020999.

Huang, L., Trieu, K., Yoshimura, S., Neal, B., Woodward, M., Campbell, N.R.C., Li, Q., Lackland, D.T., Leung, A.A., Anderson, C.A.M., Macgregor, G.A., He, F.J., 2020. Effect of dose and duration of reduction in dietary sodium on blood pressure levels: systematic review and meta-analysis of randomised trials. BMJ. 17561833. 368. Available from: http://www.bmj.com/. doi:10.1136/bmj.m315.

Hwang, A.Y., Dietrich, E., Pepine, C.J., Smith, S.M., 2017. Resistant Hypertension: mechanisms and Treatment. Curr. Hypertens. Rep. 15343111. 19 (7). Available from: www.springer.com. doi:10.1007/s11906-017-0754-x.

Jamerson, K., Weber, M.A., Bakris, G.L., Dahlöf, B., Pitt, B., Shi, V., Hester, A., Gupte, J., Gatlin, M., Velazquez, E.J., 2008. Benazepril plus amlodipine or hydrochlorothiazide for hypertension in high-risk patients. N. Engl. J. Med. 15334406. 359 (23), 2417–2428. Available from: http://content.nejm.org/cgi/reprint/359/23/2417.pdf. doi:10.1056/NEJMoa0806182.

Jennings, A., Berendsen, A.M., de Groot, L.C.P.G.M., Feskens, E.J.M., Brzozowska, A., Sicinska, E., Pietruszka, B., Meunier, N., Caumon, E., Malpuech-Brugère, C., Santoro, A., Ostan, R., Franceschi, C., Gillings, R., O' Neill, C.M., Fairweather-Tait, S.J., Minihane, A.-M., Cassidy, A., 2019. Mediterranean-Style Diet Improves Systolic Blood Pressure and Arterial Stiffness in Older Adults. Hypertension. 0194-911X. 73 (3), 578–586. doi:10.1161/hypertensionaha.118.12259.

Kannel, W., 2000. Risk stratification in hypertension: new insights from the Framingham study. Am. J. Hypertens. 08957061. 13 (1), S3. doi:10.1016/S0895-7061(99)00252-6.

Kazeminia, M., Daneshkhah, A., Jalali, R., Vaisi-Raygani, A., Salari, N., Mohammadi, M., 2020. The Effect of Exercise on the Older Adult's Blood Pressure Suffering Hypertension: systematic Review and Meta-Analysis on Clinical Trial Studies. Int. J. Hypertens. 2090-0384. 2020, 1–19. doi:10.1155/2020/2786120.

Krug, A.W., Allenhöfer, L., Monticone, R., Spinetti, G., Gekle, M., Wang, M., Lakatta, E.G., 2010. Elevated mineralocorticoid receptor activity in aged rat vascular smooth muscle cells promotes a proinflammatory phenotype via extracellular signal-regulated kinase 1/2 mitogen-activated protein kinase and epidermal growth factor receptor-dependent pathways. Hypertension. 0194911X. 55 (6), 1476–1483. doi:10.1161/HYPERTENSIONAHA.109.148783.

Li, W., He, Y., Xia, L., Yang, X., Liu, F., Jingang, M., Hu, Z., Li, Y., Li, D., Jiang, J., Shan, G., Li, C., 2018. Association of Age-Related Trends in Blood Pressure and Body Composition Indices in Healthy Adults. Front. Physiol. 1664-042X. 9. doi:10.3389/fphys.2018.01574.

Lv, J., Ehteshami, P., Sarnak, M.J., Tighiouart, H., Jun, M., Ninomiya, T., Foote, C., Rodgers, A., Zhang, H., Wang, H., Strippoli, G.F.M., Perkovic, V., 2013. Effects of intensive blood pressure lowering on the progression of chronic kidney disease: a systematic review and meta-analysis. Can. Med. Assoc. J. 0820-3946. 185 (11), 949–957. doi:10.1503/cmaj.121468.

Lyon, M., Fullerton, J.L., Kennedy, S., Work, L.M., 2024. Hypertension & dementia: pathophysiology & potential utility of antihypertensives in reducing disease burden. Pharmacol. Ther. 01637258. 253, 108575. doi:10.1016/j.pharmthera.2023.108575.

Mancia, G., Kreutz, R., Brunström, M., Burnier, M., Grassi, G., Januszewicz, A., Muiesan, M.L., Tsioufis, K., Agabiti-Rosei, E., Algharably, E.A.E., Azizi, M., Benetos, A., Borghi, C., Hitij, J.B., Cifkova, R., Coca, A., Cornelissen, V., Cruickshank, J.K., Cunha, P.G., Danser, A.H.J., Pinho, R.M.D., Delles, C., Dominiczak, A.F., Dorobantu, M., Doumas, M., Fernández-Alfonso, M.S., Halimi, J.M., Járai, Z., Jelaković, B., Jordan, J., Kuznetsova, T., Laurent, S., Lovic, D., Lurbe, E., Mahfoud, F., Manolis, A., Miglinas, M., Narkiewicz, K., Niiranen, T., Palatini, P., Parati, G., Pathak, A., Persu, A., Polonia, J., Redon, J., Sarafidis, P., Schmieder, R., Spronck, B., Stabouli, S., Stergiou, G., Taddei, S., Thomopoulos, C., Tomaszewski, M., De Borne, P.V., Wanner, C., Weber, T., Williams, B., Zhang, Z.Y., Kjeldsen, S.E., 2023. 2023 ESH Guidelines for the management of arterial hypertension the Task Force for the management of arterial hypertension of the European Society of Hypertension: endorsed by the International Society of Hypertension (ISH) and the European Renal Association (ERA). J. Hypertens. 14735598. 41 (12), 1874–2071. Available from: http://journals.lww.com/jhypertension. doi:10.1097/HJH.0000000000003480.

Mukete, B.N., Ferdinand, K.C., 2016. Polypharmacy in Older Adults With Hypertension: a Comprehensive Review. J. Clin. Hypertens. 17517176. 18 (1), 10–18. Available from: http://onlinelibrary.wiley.com/journal/10.1111/(ISSN)1751-7176. doi:10.1111/jch.12624.

Muntner, P., Carey, R.M., Gidding, S., Jones, D.W., Taler, S.J., Wright, J.T. Jr., Whelton, P.K., 2018. Potential US Population Impact of the 2017 ACC/AHA High Blood Pressure Guideline. Circulation 137 (2), 109–118. doi:10.1161/CIRCULATIONAHA.117.032582.

NCD Risk Factor Collaboration (NCD-RisC), 2021. Worldwide trends in hypertension prevalence and progress in treatment and control from 1990 to 2019: a pooled analysis of 1201 population-representative studies with 104 million participants. Lancet 398, 957–980. doi:10.1016/S0140-6736(21)01330-1.

Noubiap, J.J., Nansseu, J.R., Nyaga, U.F., Sime, P.S., Francis, I., Bigna, J.J., 2019. Global prevalence of resistant hypertension: a meta-analysis of data from 3.2 million patients. Heart. 1468201X. 105 (2), 98–105. Available from: http://heart.bmj.com/. doi:10.1136/heartjnl-2018-313599.

Oliveros, E., Patel, H., Kyung, S., Fugar, S., Goldberg, A., Madan, N., Williams, K.A., 2020. Hypertension in older adults: assessment, management, and challenges. Clin. Cardiol. 19328737. 43 (2), 99–107. Available from: http://onlinelibrary.wiley.com/journal/10.1002/(ISSN)1932-8737. doi:10.1002/clc.23303.

Perry, H.M., Davis, B.R., Price, T.R., Applegate, W.B., Fields, W.S., Guralnik, J.M., Kuller, L., Pressel, S., Stamler, J., Probstfield, J.L., 2000. Effect of treating isolated systolic hypertension on the risk of developing of stroke: the systolic hypertension in the elderly program (SHEP). JAMA. 00987484. 284 (4), 465–471. Available from: http://jama.jamanetwork.com/journal.aspx. doi:10.1001/jama.284.4.465.

Pierdomenico, S.D., Pierdomenico, A.M., Coccina, F., Porreca, E., 2017. Prognosis of Masked and White Coat Uncontrolled Hypertension Detected by Ambulatory Blood Pressure Monitoring in Elderly Treated Hypertensive Patients. Am. J. Hypertens. 0895-7061. 30 (11), 1106–1111. doi:10.1093/ajh/hpx104.

SHEP Cooperative Research Group, 1991. Prevention of stroke by antihypertensive drug treatment in older persons with isolated systolic hypertension: final results of the Systolic Hypertension in the Elderly Program (SHEP). JAMA 265 (24), 3255–3264. doi:10.1001/jama.1991.03460240051028.

Redon, J., Weber, M.A., Reimitz, P.E., Wang, J.G., 2018. Comparative effectiveness of an angiotensin receptor blocker, olmesartan medoxomil, in older hypertensive patients. J. Clin. Hypertens. 17517176. 20 (2), 356–365. Available from: http://onlinelibrary.wiley.com/journal/10.1111/(ISSN)1751-7176. doi:10.1111/jch.13183.

Saren, J., Debain, A., Loosveldt, F., Petrovic, M., Bautmans, I., 2024. Elevated blood pressure variability is associated with an increased risk of negative health outcomes in adults aged 65 and above—a systematic review and meta-analysis. Age Ageing. 0002-0729. 53 (12). doi:10.1093/ageing/afae262.

Somes, G.W., Pahor, M., Shorr, R.I., Cushman, W.C., Applegate, W.B., 1999. The role of diastolic blood pressure when treating isolated systolic hypertension. Arch. Intern. Med. 00039926. 159 (17), 2004–2009. doi:10.1001/archinte.159.17.2004.

Staessen, J.A., Fagard, R., Thijs, L., Celis, H., Arabidze, G.G., Birkenhäger, W.H., Bulpitt, C.J., De Leeuw, P.W., Dollery, C.T., Fletcher, A.E., Forette, F., Leonetti, G., Nachev, C., O' Brien, E.T., Rosenfeld, J., Rodicio, J.L., Tuomilehto, J., Zanchetti, A., 1997. Randomised double-blind comparison of placebo and active treatment for older patients with isolated systolic hypertension. Lancet. 01406736. 350 (9080), 757–764. Available from: http://www.journals.elsevier.com/the-lancet/. doi:10.1016/S0140-6736(97)05381-6.

Toh, J.J.Y., Zhang, H., Soh, Y.Y., Zhang, Z., Wu, X.V., 2023. Prevalence and health outcomes of polypharmacy and hyperpolypharmacy in older adults with frailty: a systematic review and meta-analysis. Ageing Res. Rev. 18729649. 83. Available from: http://www.elsevier.com/locate/arr. doi:10.1016/j.arr.2022.101811.

Vasan, R.S., Larson, M.G., Leip, E.P., Kannel, W.B., Levy, D., 2001. Assessment of frequency of progression to hypertension in non-hypertensive participants in the Framingham Heart Study: a cohort study. Lancet. 01406736. 358 (9294), 1682–1686. Available from: http://www.journals.elsevier.com/the-lancet/. doi:10.1016/S0140-6736(01)06710-1.

Weinstein, J.R., Anderson, S., 2010. The Aging Kidney: physiological Changes. Adv. Chronic Kidney Dis. 15485595. 17 (4), 302–307. doi:10.1053/j.ackd.2010.05.002.

Whelton, P.K., Carey, R.M., Aronow, W.S., Casey Jr, D.E., Collins, K.J., Himmelfarb, D., et al., 2017. PCNA Guideline for the Prevention, Detection, Evaluation, and Management of High Blood Pressure in Adults: a Report of the American College of Cardiology/American Heart Association Task Force on Clinical Practice Guidelines. J. Am. Coll. Cardiol. 71 (19), 127.

Wijkman, M.O., Malachias, M.V.B., Claggett, B.L., Cheng, S., Matsushita, K., Shah, A.M., Jhund, P.S., Coresh, J., Solomon, S.D., Vardeny, O., 2021. Resistance to antihypertensive treatment and long-term risk: the Atherosclerosis Risk in Communities study. J. Clin. Hypertens. 17517176. 23 (10), 1887–1896. Available from: http://onlinelibrary.wiley.com/journal/10.1111/(ISSN)1751-7176. doi:10.1111/jch.14269.

Williamson, J.D., Supiano, M.A., Applegate, W.B., Berlowitz, D.R., Campbell, R.C., Chertow, G.M., Fine, L.J., Haley, W.E., Hawfield, A.T., Ix, J.H., Kitzman, D., Kostis, J.B., Marie, A.K.W., Launer, L.J., Oparil, S., Rodriguez, C.J., Roumie, C.L., Shorr, R.I., Sink, K.M., Gwadley, V., Whelton, P.K., Whittle, J., Wright, J.T., Pajewski, N.M., 2016. Intensive vs standard blood pressure control and cardiovascular disease outcomes in adults aged ≥75 years a randomized clinical trial. JAMA. 15383598. 315 (24), 2673–2682. Available from: http://jama.jamanetwork.com/article.aspx?articleid=2524266. doi:10.1001/jama.2016.7050.

Zhang, W., Zhang, S., Deng, Y., Shouling, W., Ren, J., Sun, G., Yang, J., Jiang, Y., Xinjuan, X., Wang, T.-D., Chen, Y., Yufeng, L., Yao, L., Dianfang, L., Wang, L., Shen, X., Yin, X., Liu, W., Zhou, X., Zhu, B., Guo, Z., Liu, H., Chen, X., Feng, Y., Tian, G., Gao, X., Kario, K., Cai, J., 2021. Trial of Intensive Blood-Pressure Control in Older Patients with Hypertension. N. Engl. J. Med. 0028-4793. 385 (14), 1268–1279. doi:10.1056/nejmoa2111437.

Zhou, D., Xi, B., Zhao, M., Wang, L., Veeranki, S.P., 2018. Uncontrolled hypertension increases risk of all-cause and cardiovascular disease mortality in US adults: the NHANES III Linked Mortality Study. Sci. Rep. 20452322. 8 (1). Available from: www.nature.com/srep/index.html. doi:10.1038/s41598-018-27377-2.

CHAPTER

17

Diabetes in kidney disease progression

Sheryl Cababat Caberto[a], *Lynn Schlanger*[a], *and Stephen Z. Fadem*[b]

[a]Division of Renal Medicine, Emory University School of Medicine, Atlanta, GA, United States

[b]Department of Medicine, Section of Nephrology, Baylor College of Medicine, Houston, TX, United States

Introduction

Age-related loss of kidney function has been observed for many years. The complex process of aging impacts the kidney at the molecular level, leading to gradual changes in the kidney's structure and function. Aging is ineluctable; thus the kidney naturally deteriorates due to the biological changes that occur with aging. During aging, there is a linear reduction in glomerular filtration rate, renal blood flow rate, and renal mass, and glomerulosclerosis becomes more evident (Anderson and Brenner, 1986). It is imperative to understand the aging process occurring in the kidney to prevent additional insults that may cause complications to an aging kidney (Table 17.1).

The kidney structurally changes with age. The structural changes include loss of renal mass, glomerulosclerosis, renal vasculature changes, and tubulointerstitial fibrosis. Reduction in renal mass results from the loss of the functional units of the kidney, called nephrons. The number of nephrons is related to the kidney's functional capacity. Nephron loss occurs as age advances, and this is reflected in the age-related decrease in glomerular filtration rate (GFR) (Denic et al., 2017, 2016). Age-related arterial wall thickening, intimal fibrosis, and decreased elasticity result in nephron loss and decreased renal blood flow, which further compromise kidney function (Weinstein and Anderson, 2010; Noronha et al., 2022). Nephrosclerosis (arteriosclerosis, glomerulosclerosis, and tubular atrophy with interstitial fibrosis) in the elderly increases because of the structural changes that occur in the kidney (Rule et al., 2010; Glassock and Rule, 2012). The glomerulus, the capillary network of the kidney that is significant for the filtration process, is vulnerable to scarring as the kidney ages. Glomerulosclerosis that results from aging may lead to further glomerular injury and subsequent reduction in the kidney's filtration capacity (Weinstein and Anderson, 2010).

Aging and the Kidney
https://doi.org/10.1016/B978-0-443-34069-7.00018-5

TABLE 17.1 A review of diabetic nephropathy.

Domain	Key findings or mechanisms	Clinical manifestations	Management or therapeutic strategies
Structural changes in the aging kidney	Loss of kidney tissue, loss of filtering units (nephrons), hardening of the glomeruli, stiffening of the blood vessels, and scarring of the kidney tissue	Decrease in kidney size and blood flow; higher risk of chronic kidney disease	Protect remaining kidney tissue, avoid kidney toxins, and maintain healthy blood pressure and blood sugar levels
Functional changes with aging	Decrease in kidney filtration, blood flow, the ability to concentrate urine, and the ability to maintain acid–base balance	Mild acid build-up, low or high sodium levels, and high potassium levels	Maintain adequate fluid intake, monitor electrolyte levels, and limit dietary acid load
Kidney injury accelerated by diabetes	Long-term high blood sugar leads to the buildup of advanced glycation products, inflammation, oxidative stress, and high blood pressure	Faster decline in kidney function, protein in the urine, and a higher risk of kidney failure	Maintain good control of blood sugar and blood pressure, and use kidney-protective medicines
Decline in filtration rate	Gradual decrease in kidney filtration occurs due to aging, with a faster decline observed in people with diabetes	Fatigue, swelling, and changes in body chemistry	Regular monitoring of kidney function and early treatment with protective medications
Protein in the urine	Damage to the filtering barrier of the kidney: an early sign of kidney disease progression	Presence of protein in the urine before major loss of function	Use kidney filtration rate and protein levels to classify and monitor disease, and control blood pressure
Multiple chronic conditions	Diabetes in older adults is often accompanied by high blood pressure, heart disease, high cholesterol, obesity, depression, and cognitive decline	Frailty, falls, and reduced quality of life	Coordinate care for all conditions, and set realistic treatment goals for each individual
Lifestyle changes	Balanced nutrition with limited protein and sodium, regular exercise, smoking cessation, and weight management	Improved blood sugar control, blood pressure, and cardiovascular health	Involve a dietitian, promote gentle aerobic and resistance exercises, and support smoking cessation
Blood sugar targets in older adults	The balance between preventing complications and avoiding low blood sugar	Individualized targets for long-term blood sugar control should be based on overall health and life expectancy	Avoid excessive lowering of blood sugar; select medications that have a lower risk of causing low blood sugar

Domain	Key findings or mechanisms	Clinical manifestations	Management or therapeutic strategies
Medication treatment	• Metformin: improves blood sugar control if kidney function is adequate • Sodium–glucose co-transporter inhibitors improve kidney and heart outcomes • Glucagon-like peptide-1 receptor medications: support weight and heart health • Mineralocorticoid receptor blockers: add kidney and heart protection • Angiotensin-converting enzyme inhibitors or angiotensin receptor blockers lower protein in urine and protect kidney function	Better kidney and heart outcomes, but an increased risk of high potassium or low blood sugar in some older adults	Use combinations based on tolerance and kidney function; monitor kidney function and electrolytes closely
Kidney replacement therapy	Decision to start dialysis or undergo a transplant depends on age, frailty, and personal goals	Decline in independence and physical function in many elderly people after starting dialysis	Shared decision-making among the healthcare team, patient, and family; consider conservative care or transplantation
Kidney transplant in older adults	Selected older adults can benefit from transplants despite their age	Longer survival and better quality of life compared to dialysis	Comprehensive evaluation, discussion of expected benefits and risks, and ongoing follow-up after transplant

The structural changes are correlated with the physiological changes in the kidney. These functional changes include a decline in GFR, impaired concentrating ability, decreased electrolyte handling, and altered acid–base balance. GFR is a measure of kidney function. Young, healthy individuals have a normal GFR of approximately 100–110 mL/min/1.73 m^2 which naturally declines with age; hence, older individuals without chronic kidney disease (CKD) are expected to have a lower GFR due to the aging kidney (Musso and Oreopoulos, 2011; Delanaye et al., 2016). After 30–40 years of age, a decline in GFR related to age is a normal physiological process. The age-related decrease in GFR is attributed to nephron loss because aging causes both functional and structural changes (Weinstein and Anderson, 2010; Hoang et al., 2003; Kielstein et al., 2003). The decline in GFR, as well as the increase in glomerulosclerosis and reduced renal plasma flow, may be associated with the impaired concentrating ability of the kidney (Schlanger et al., 2010). A reduction in urine concentrating ability has been reported in normal aging. In animal studies, transport proteins involved in urine concentration were found to be less abundant in the kidney medulla of aged rats, which may reflect similar mechanisms occurring in humans (Sands, 2012). In addition to the inability to excrete concentrated or dilute urine, electrolyte handling, particularly of ammonium, sodium, or potassium, is also affected. Regulation of electrolytes diminishes with aging, and the elderly are more likely to suffer from hyponatremia or hypernatremia, as well as hyperkalemia. Sodium is the most commonly affected electrolyte, with high mortality observed in old age (Musso and Oreopoulos, 2011; Schlanger et al., 2010). Aging kidneys also exhibit reduced excretion of acid and regeneration of bicarbonate, and mild metabolic acidosis may be seen in older healthy individuals. A low serum bicarbonate level is associated with higher mortality, irrespective of the cause, whether metabolic acidosis or respiratory alkalosis (Raphael et al., 2016).

Kidney damage in the elderly with diabetic kidney disease

The structural and functional changes caused by the normal process of aging in the kidney are further accelerated by diabetes, creating more damage to the kidneys. The accelerated kidney damage results from the multiple stresses that occur in diabetic kidney disease (DKD), such as AGEs accumulation, hypertension, oxidative stress, and inflammation (Guo et al., 2020). The consequences of these factors—decreased GFR and increased albuminuria—are risk factors for the progression of kidney failure (Delanaye and Pottel, 2016; Levey et al., 2015; Gansevoort et al., 2011).

Decline in estimated glomerular filtration rate

A decline in estimated glomerular filtration rate (eGFR) is evident in aging and DKD. There is a normal gradual decline of GFR in aging, and this is related to the decreased number of nephrons due to glomerulosclerosis, which is an important predictor of CKD progression. However, progressive CKD is not attributed to age-related glomerulosclerosis (Hommos et al., 2018). A study by Davies and Shock in 1950 on males aged between 20 and 90 years found an average decline in GFR of 0.96 mL/min/year, or about 10 mL/min/decade (Davies and Shock, 1950). The first systematic review of normal kidney function decline in aging determined that the normal decline rate may range between − 0.37 and − 1.07 mL/min/1.73 m^2/year in healthy individuals (Guppy et al., 2024). DKD is a clinical diagnosis characterized by decreased eGFR and albuminuria. Because of the complications of DKD, such as chronic hyperglycemia, hypertension, and proteinuria, a rapid decline in GFR may occur. The rate of decline of eGFR in DKD progression was reported to be 3.57 ± 1.45 mL/min/1.73 m^2/year (Altemtam et al., 2012). A reduction in eGFR is a significant sign of CKD progression, particularly when a declining trajectory is observed.

Albuminuria

The marker of kidney damage is albuminuria. Urine albumin-to-creatinine ratio is used to estimate albuminuria, and this eliminates the effect of urine volume on urine concentration (Elsayed et al., 2023). Albuminuria is an early sign of the progression of DKD, as it is directly related to a reduction in kidney function. It was reported that albuminuria increases more rapidly in the elderly, and increased albuminuria in elderly patients with diabetes was significantly higher than in those without diabetes (Mykkänen et al., 1994). Albuminuria is a complication of DKD and a significant indicator of CKD progression. Hence, guidelines recommend using albuminuria and eGFR in staging CKD ("KDIGO, 2024: Clinical Practice Guideline for the Evaluation and Management of Chronic Kidney Disease," 2024).

Complications and comorbidities in the elderly

Diabetes is a common disease in the elderly. The epidemiological prediction for diabetes in Americans indicates an increase of 165%, from 11 million in 2000 (prevalence of 4.0%) to 29 million in 2050 (prevalence of 7.2%). This projection is expected if the prevalence rates of diabetes continue to rise in a linear fashion (King et al., 1998). Diabetic nephropathy is the leading cause of chronic kidney disease (CKD). The significant risk factors for DKD are hyperglycemia and hypertension. Both factors worsen structural kidney damage and glomerular filtration rate if diabetes is poorly controlled, consequently leading to the progression of CKD to end-stage kidney disease (ESKD), which requires renal replacement therapy (Gregg et al., 2002). The morbidity and mortality rates of diabetes are predicted independently by aging and the duration of the disease (Huang et al., 2014). A nonconcurrent cohort study, which used claims data from the 1994–1996 Medicare 5% Standard Analytical Files, showed significantly higher all-cause mortality rates in elderly patients with diabetes mellitus (DM) compared to the general population (Bertoni et al., 2002). A longitudinal study, conducted from January 1, 1991 to December 31, 2004, analyzed the mortality and morbidity rates of elderly patients who were newly diagnosed with DM. During this 10-year follow-up, there was a higher rate of complications in elderly patients with DM compared to those without DM (Bethel et al., 2007). The microvascular complications of diabetes include retinopathy, nephropathy leading to ESKD, and neuropathy. The macrovascular complications include coronary heart disease, stroke, and peripheral arterial disease. Diabetic nephropathy is strongly associated with cardiovascular complications, although the mechanisms are not well established (Pálsson and Patel, 2014). According to cardiovascular (CVD) trials, diabetic patients with CKD have a higher risk for cardiovascular disease compared to those without CKD. Therefore CVD outcomes improve as the risk of CKD in diabetes decreases (Swamy et al., 2023). Diabetes has now become a very common disease in the elderly, but there are also less recognized complications that must not be overlooked because they can be debilitating. These complications include cognitive disorders, physical disability, falls and fractures, and other geriatric syndromes. The impact on quality of life presents a great challenge for clinicians due to the concurrence of aging-related complications and other chronic diseases (Gregg et al., 2002; Huang et al., 2014).

Multiple long-term conditions (MLTC) or multimorbidity refer to the presence of two or more chronic medical conditions. Long-term diabetes carries a higher risk of MLTC, including cardiovascular disease and ESKD (Seng et al., 2020). Diabetes and increasing age are associated with DKD, which has a strong association with many diseases such as hypertension, hyperlipidemia, and coronary artery disease (Roy et al., 2021). Elderly patients with diabetes commonly have comorbidities, and this significantly impacts their management and treatment. There is a high prevalence of hypertension, coronary heart disease, and CKD in patients with diabetes, as well as hyperlipidemia and obesity (Iglay et al., 2016). Mental health problems are also becoming common among patients with diabetes. Clinicians must not overlook examining patients for their mental health conditions because this certainly changes the management approach for these patients (Nowakowska et al., 2019).

Treatment and management of DKD in the elderly

Lifestyle changes

Lifestyle changes are necessary for a holistic approach to controlling diabetes, delaying CKD progression, and preventing complications. Nutrition is an essential part of these lifestyle changes becauseas kidney function declines, waste products accumulate; thus, the diet should be consistent with kidney function. Dietary modifications in DKD include a low-protein diet with a recommended range of 0.6–0.8 g/kg body weight per day, sodium intake ≤ 2.3 g/day for blood pressure control, a low-glycemic-index diet, and avoiding processed foods, as these are high in sodium and phosphorus (Ikizler et al., 2020). Exercise, such as aerobic and resistance training, improves cardiovascular well-being, including blood sugar and weight. Physical activity should be based on the overall health condition, particularly on what an individual can tolerate (Colberg et al., 2016). Blood pressure targets depend on the risks and benefits of cardiovascular or renal management and treatment. The American Diabetes Association (ADA) recommends that diabetic and hypertensive patients with high cardiovascular risk (10-year atherosclerotic cardiovascular disease [ASCVD] risk ≥ 15%) maintain a target BP of < 130/80 mm Hg, and those with low cardiovascular risk (10-year ASCVD risk < 15%) maintain a target BP of < 140/90 mm Hg. The results of the SPRINT trial showed that a target systolic BP of < 120 mm Hg is superior to < 140 mm Hg in high-risk nondiabetic patients with hypertension, including elderly patients (de Boer et al., 2022; Davies et al., 2022). Thus, KDIGO's (2024) Clinical Practice Guideline for the Management of Blood Pressure in Chronic Kidney Disease recommends a target systolic BP of < 120 mm Hg but with certain caveats concerning safety and limited evidence ("KDIGO, 2024: Clinical Practice Guideline for the Evaluation and Management of Chronic Kidney Disease," 2024). The International Diabetes Federation (IDF) published a guideline on HbA1c targets for the elderly in 2013. The guideline categorized elderly patients as functionally independent with an HbA1c goal of 7–7.5%, functionally dependent with HbA1c goal of 7–8%, and those in end-of-life care with no specific HbA1c goal, focusing on avoiding hyperglycemia symptoms (Cho et al., 2013; Leung et al., 2018). Smoking has been reported as an independent risk factor for the development of DKD. Smoking cessation decreases the incidence of CKD, cardiovascular and lung diseases, and cancers, and most importantly, reduces the risk of DKD progression (Yacoub et al., 2010; Abdel-Rahman and Reeves, 2012). Obesity is a risk factor for diabetes. Diabetes and obesity, combined with hypertension, are associated with the progression of kidney disease. Weight loss is important in managing diabetes, and it should be gradual, especially in the elderly, because rapid weight loss can lead to muscle loss. Sarcopenia starts to develop in middle age (~1%/year), becoming severe at ~ 50% in the eighth to ninth decade of life (Maric-Bilkan, 2013; Bertoni et al., 2002; Wilkinson et al., 2018). In addition to modifications in lifestyle factors, compliance with therapeutic management is also indispensable. Lifestyle changes improve health outcomes by reducing the risk of cardiovascular events and death for elderly patients with DKD (Onyenwenyi and Ricardo, 2015).

Glycemic control

Hemoglobin A1c target and risk of hypoglycemia

Glycemic control is essential in the management of elderly diabetic patients with CKD. Because of the serious consequences of glycemic control in the elderly, the benefits of tight glucose control and the risks of hypoglycemia must be carefully weighed to properly manage blood glucose levels. There are no age-specific recommendations for glycemic control due to the diversity of older patients with diabetes. Glycemic targets depend on patients' functionality, life expectancy, and risk of hypoglycemia (Casagrande et al., 2017). In general, HbA1c target of 7.0–8.0% is recommended for elderly patients. The HbA1c targets in the elderly are often set higher to reduce the risk of hypoglycemia (Leung et al., 2018; Cho et al., 2013), which is a common problem because elderly patients can be overtreated. Elderly patients over 70 years old on sulfonylureas or insulin had HbA1c of < 7% in a study conducted in the United Kingdom (Hambling et al., 2017; Clemens et al., 2019). The risk of hypoglycemia is more common in the elderly with lower kidney function, as demonstrated in a study of adults with a mean age of 75 years in Ontario, Canada, conducted from April 2002 through March 2013 (Hodge et al., 2017). Many diabetes drugs are renally excreted; therefore older patients with CKD are at increased risk for hypoglycemia due to the decline in kidney function (Moen et al., 2009) (Table 17.2).

Pharmacotherapy

In elderly patients with a long-term history of diabetes and other comorbidities, the HbA1c target is around 7.0–8.0% because the risk of hypoglycemia outweighs the benefit (Cho et al., 2013; Leung et al., 2018). HbA1c target is achieved through lifestyle changes and pharmacologic therapy. Low kidney function in CKD can impact the efficacy and safety of a drug. The current therapeutic drugs are not only effective for diabetes treatment; they have also been found to provide cardiovascular and renal protection in clinical trials.

The recommended first-line therapeutic treatment for DKD patients with eGFR above 30 mL/min/1.73 is metformin and sodium-glucose co-transporter 2 inhibitors (SGLT2i). In advanced CKD, glucagon-like peptide-1 receptor agonists (GLP-1 RAs) are considered because of their renal and cardiovascular benefits, as well as SGLT2i for patients with eGFR > 20. Thus, metformin, SGLT2i and GLP-1 RAs should be considered the first-line drugs for DKD patients (Tong and Adler, 2022). In addition, mineralocorticoid receptor antagonists (MRAs) are also drugs of choice for DKD, for the same reason of having protective cardiorenal effects (Pitt et al., 2021; Bakris et al., 2020).

Biguanides: Metformin

Metformin is the initial drug option to control glucose concentrations in diabetes patients. It is a cost-effective drug for the treatment of diabetes and the prevention of DKD. It may be safely used, with close monitoring, in patients with an eGFR of ≥ 30 mL/min/1.73 m^2. It is contraindicated in advanced CKD because of lactic acidosis, as metformin is renally excreted

TABLE 17.2 Medications used in the treatment of diabetes and its related conditions.

Drug class	Mechanism of action	Benefits for kidney and cardiovascular health	Special considerations in older adults
Biguanides (Metformin)	Reduces glucose production in the liver and improves the body's sensitivity to insulin	Improves blood sugar control and may help prevent the development of diabetic kidney disease	Use only when the kidney filtration rate is above 30 mL/min; monitor for lactic acid buildup; adjust the dose for reduced kidney function
Angiotensin-converting enzyme inhibitors	Block the formation of angiotensin, a hormone that narrows blood vessels	Lower blood pressure, reduce protein loss in urine, and slow the progression of kidney disease	May increase blood potassium levels or cause a rise in creatinine; careful monitoring is needed when starting treatment
Angiotensin receptor blockers	Prevent angiotensin from binding to its receptor on blood vessels	Similar kidney and cardiovascular protection as enzyme inhibitors; an alternative if a cough occurs	Monitor kidney function and potassium levels; avoid combining with enzyme inhibitors in most cases
Sodium–glucose co-transporter inhibitors	Reduce blood sugar by causing glucose to be excreted in the urine	Slow the decline in kidney function and reduce the risk of heart failure and cardiovascular death	May cause dehydration or low blood pressure; use caution in frail older adults or those with a low filtration rate
Glucagon-like peptide-1 receptor medications	Enhance insulin release, suppress appetite, and slow stomach emptying	Improve blood sugar control, reduce body weight, lower cardiovascular risk, and potentially provide kidney protection	May cause nausea or weight loss; adjust based on tolerance and monitor for dehydration
Mineralocorticoid receptor blockers (steroidal and non-steroidal).	Block mineralocorticoid activity, reducing fibrosis and inflammation in the kidneys and heart	Lower risk of kidney disease progression and heart events	Can increase blood potassium; use cautiously and monitor blood tests frequently
Insulin and sulfonylureas	Promote insulin availability or release to lower blood sugar	Strong glucose-lowering effect when oral agents are insufficient	High risk of low blood sugar, especially with reduced kidney function; simplify regimens and use with caution
Statins (cholesterol-lowering agents)	Reduce cholesterol production in the liver	Lower risk of heart attack and stroke in people with diabetes and kidney disease	Muscle pain or weakness may occur; monitor for interactions with other drugs
Diuretics	Increase urine output and help control fluid balance and blood pressure	Help manage swelling and high blood pressure in kidney disease	May cause dehydration or electrolyte imbalance; adjust the dose for kidney function and monitor weight and electrolytes
Aspirin and antiplatelet therapy	Reduce blood clot formation in arteries	Prevent heart attacks and strokes in high-risk diabetic patients	Use only if the clear cardiovascular benefit outweighs the risk of bleeding; assess gastrointestinal tolerance

(Inzucchi et al., 2014). Lactic acidosis rarely occurs; therefore, metformin may be used in older CKD patients, but it must be used with caution (Ralph Defronzo et al., 2016). The ADA recommends that metformin should be reduced in older adults because of the physiological decline in kidney function (Doyle-Delgado et al., 2020).

Angiotensin-converting enzyme inhibitor and angiotensin 2 receptor blocker

Renin–angiotensin system blockade with angiotensin-converting enzyme inhibitor (ACE-i) or angiotensin 2 receptor blocker (ARB) reduces the risk of DKD progression by lowering proteinuria. These drugs are most beneficial in patients with overt proteinuria (Brenner et al., 2001; Lewis et al., 1993). Combination therapy with these drugs results in a greater decrease in proteinuria but carries an increased risk of adverse events, including renal dysfunction and hyperkalemia (Fried et al., 2013; Yusuf et al., 2008). Monotherapy can also cause these complications, which limit its utilization in the elderly (Brenner et al., 2001; Lewis et al., 1993). Guidelines regarding the benefits of these drugs were published, and they are not different from those for younger individuals; however, the American Geriatrics Society (AGS) highlighted the risks of increased creatinine and hyperkalemia (Ahmed and Catic, 2019). Renal dysfunction can occur upon initiating these drugs, but it may not persist, and close monitoring is necessary (Ahmed and Catic, 2019; Pappoe and Winkelmayer, 2010). If there is an increase in creatinine of > 30% within the first two months, or if there is hyperkalemia with a serum potassium level of ≥ 5.6 mmol/L, the drug should be discontinued (Bakris and Weir, 2000).

SGLT2i—canagliflozin, dapagliflozin, and empagliflozin

SGLT2i are drugs for diabetes that have significant benefits apart from glycemic control (Krishnan et al., 2023). The landmark clinical trials of SGLT2i include the CREDENCE Trial (Canagliflozin and Renal Events in Diabetes with Established Nephropathy Clinical Evaluation), the DAPA-CKD Trial (Dapagliflozin and Prevention of Adverse Outcomes in Chronic Kidney Disease), and the EMPA-KIDNEY Trial (Study of Heart and Kidney Protection with Empagliflozin). All these trials demonstrated a lower risk of CKD progression or cardiovascular death. These benefits remain evident even in nondiabetic patients and advanced CKD patients with an eGFR of 20 ml/min per 1.73 m^2 (Perkovic et al., 2019; Heerspink et al., 2020; EMPA-KIDNEY Collaborative Group, 2023: "Empagliflozin in Patients with Chronic Kidney Disease," 2023). Thus, the mechanism of action of SGLT2i in the treatment of diabetes is independent of their renal and cardiovascular protective effects, and they are currently considered a mainstay therapy for CKD (Davies et al., 2022). However, SGLT2i are not consistent in their effects across all age groups. There is limited data concerning the potential adverse effects of these drugs in elderly patients due to their underrepresentation in clinical trials. For this reason, the benefits of SGLT2i in elderly patients remain uncertain (Amioka et al., 2023). The use of SGLT2i is not contraindicated in elderly patients with CKD; however, patients in the SGLT2i clinical trials were aged < 65 years (Perkovic et al., 2019; Heerspink et al., 2020; EMPA-KIDNEY Collaborative Group, 2023: "Empagliflozin in Patients with Chronic Kidney Disease," 2023). In DAPA-CKD trial, the prespecified data analysis showed significant benefit of dapagliflozin on eGFR of patients aged > 65 years and older versus placebo (Heerspink et al., 2020; Madero et al., 2024). Analyses of data from the CREDENCE and DAPA-CKD trials showed a reduced risk of kidney events in all age groups, with the lowest absolute risk of composite endpoints observed in patients aged ≥ 70 years in the CREDENCE trial and aged ≥ 80 years in the DAPA-CKD trial (Perkovic et al., 2019; Madero et al., 2024). It is necessary for clinicians to exercise caution when prescribing these drugs due to the age-related physiological changes that occur in elderly patients.

Glucagon-like peptide-1 receptor agonists (GLP-1 RAs)

Aging and obesity are risk factors for diabetes. In the United States, 12 million of the 30 million diabetic population are over the age of 65 (National Diabetes Statistics Report, 2017; Guidelines Abstracted from the American Geriatrics Society Guidelines for Improving the Care of Older Adults with Diabetes Mellitus: 2013 Update, 2013). A retrospective study, using an electronic medical record database, found that obesity is a common comorbidity in patients with diabetes, ranking next to hypertension as the most common (Iglay et al., 2016). Semaglutide, a drug that belongs to this class, was FDA-approved for obesity in 2021. Subcutaneous semaglutide among adults with overweight or obesity resulted in continued weight loss (Rubino et al., 2021). Furthermore, the FLOW clinical trial (Evaluate Renal Function with Semaglutide Once Weekly) investigated kidney outcomes in patients with type 2 diabetes and CKD. There was an early clinical trial cessation because of strong evidence of efficacy. The results of primary and secondary outcomes favored semaglutide, indicating a significant benefit in slowing CKD progression and reducing cardiovascular events. Serious adverse events were also lower in the semaglutide group (Perkovic et al., 2024). Data analyses of the SUSTAIN clinical trials revealed the efficacy and safety of semaglutide in elderly (≥65 years) patients (Warren et al., 2018).

Mineralocorticoid receptor antagonist

The MRAs are classified into steroidal—spironolactone and eplerenone—and nonsteroidal, finerenone (Agarwal et al., 2021). Steroidal MRAs have been reported to have an antiproteinuric effect, which indicates their impact on DKD, but the use of these drugs is limited due to hyperkalemia, as well as gynecomastia associated with spironolactone (Mehdi et al., 2009). The FIDELIO-DKD (Effect of Finerenone on Chronic Kidney Disease Outcomes in Type 2 Diabetes) study investigated the long-term effects of finerenone on the kidney and heart. The study demonstrated lower risks of CKD progression and cardiovascular events with finerenone in patients with CKD and type 2 diabetes (Bakris et al., 2020). Another clinical trial, the FIGARO-DKD (Cardiovascular Events with Finerenone in Kidney Disease and Type 2 Diabetes), showed that finerenone treatment improved cardiovascular outcomes in patients with type 2 diabetes and CKD stage 2 to 4 with moderately elevated albuminuria or CKD stages 1 to 2 with severely elevated albuminuria (Pitt et al., 2021). According to the FIDELITY analysis, which was a pooled analysis of the FIDELIO-DKD and FIGARO-DKD clinical trials, finerenone is effective across age groups, and no new safety concerns were identified in patients aged ≥ 65 years (Agarwal et al., 2022).

Renal replacement therapy: Dialysis and renal transplant

Diabetes and hypertension are the most common causes of CKD, and approximately 1 in 3 people with diabetes have kidney disease (Chronic Kidney Disease in the United States,

2023, 2023). According to the United States Renal Data System's 2023 Annual Data Report, more than 808,000 people in the United States have ESKD, with 68% on dialysis and 32% having a kidney transplant (2023 USRDS Annual Data Report: Epidemiology of Kidney Disease in the United States, 2023).

ESKD patients must understand the fact that the dialysis machine is their new kidney, which maintains fluid balance in the body and removes waste products. It is imperative that patients have a profound understanding of their condition, especially in the elderly, because dialysis is life-changing. Age is an important factor in determining when to start dialysis, considering the reduction in quality of life in the elderly. A study on nursing home elderly residents undergoing dialysis found that there is a substantial and sustained decline in functional status (Tamura et al., 2009). Older adults may experience a fair increase in life expectancy and less time at home when dialysis is initiated at eGFR $< 12\ mL/min/1.73\ m^2$ (Montez-Rath et al., 2024). Thus, multidisciplinary and family-engaged decision-making regarding dialysis in the elderly is necessary to reach a rational decision that aligns with the patient's and family's goals-of-care (Montez-Rath et al., 2024).

Kidney transplant has been growing as a treatment option for older adults with ESKD, and there has been significant improvement in outcomes over the years (McAdams-Demarco et al., 2014). Analysis of the data from the Scientific Registry of transplant recipients showed that patients older than 70 years of age experience a significant reduction in mortality with kidney transplant compared with dialysis. The elderly not only benefit from a reduction in mortality but also enjoy an improved quality of life (Rao et al., 2007). The SF-36 (36-item short form) health survey, with 8 scaled scores (vitality, physical functioning, bodily pain, general health perceptions, physical role functioning, emotional role functioning, social role functioning, and mental health), is widely used as an indicator of health-related quality of life (Huang et al., 2009). Older transplant patients have higher SF-36 scores compared with dialysis patients (Apostolou et al., 2007; Rebollo et al., 2000).

Conclusion

Diabetes is the most common cause of CKD and ESKD. The prevalence of diabetes is growing because life expectancy is improving; thus, the elderly are contributing to the diabetes population. DKD in the elderly is so complicated that it requires caution in managing these patients. Diabetes inflicts irreversible damage to the kidney and consequently causes DKD. The progression of DKD is multifactorial, including aging and comorbidities. The complications of diabetes, combined with the normal physiologic decline of aging and comorbidities in the elderly, make older adults vulnerable to rapid CKD progression. Early detection, lifestyle changes, glycemic control, and the use of reno-protective medications are crucially important in improving outcomes. Dialysis and kidney transplant are life-saving treatments for DKD patients. The goal of the multidisciplinary approach in the management and treatment of DKD is to improve patients' quality of life.

AI disclosure

During the preparation of this work, the author(s) used ChatGPT solely to check references. After using this tool/service, the author(s) reviewed and edited the content as needed and take full responsibility for the content of the publication.

References

2023 USRDS Annual Data Report: Epidemiology of Kidney Disease in the United States. (2023), Available from: https://usrds-adr.niddk.nih.gov/2023.

Abdel-Rahman, A., Reeves, A., 2012. Management of diabetic nephropathy in the elderly: special considerations. J. Nephrol. Ther. 2 (5), 124.

Agarwal, R., Filippatos, G., Pitt, B., Anker, S.D., Rossing, P., Joseph, A., Kolkhof, P., Nowack, C., Gebel, M., Ruilope, L.M., Bakris, G.L., 2022. Cardiovascular and kidney outcomes with finerenone in patients with type 2 diabetes and chronic kidney disease: the FIDELITY pooled analysis. Eur. Heart J. 15229645. 43 (6), 474–484. Available from: http://eurheartj.oxfordjournals.org/. doi:10.1093/eurheartj/ehab777.

Agarwal, R., Kolkhof, P., Bakris, G., Bauersachs, J., Haller, H., Wada, T., Zannad, F., 2021. Steroidal and non-steroidal mineralocorticoid receptor antagonists in cardiorenal medicine. Eur. Heart J. 15229645. 42 (2), 152–161. Available from: http://eurheartj.oxfordjournals.org/. doi:10.1093/eurheartj/ehaa736.

Ahmed, F.A., Catic, A.G., 2019. Decision-making in geriatric patients with end-stage renal disease: thinking beyond nephrology. J. Clin. Med. 20770383. 8 (1). Available from: https://www.mdpi.com/journal/jcm. doi:10.3390/jcm8010005.

Altemtam, N., Russell, J., Nahas, M.E., 2012. A study of the natural history of diabetic kidney disease (DKD). Nephrol. Dial. Transplant. 0931-0509. 27 (5), 1847–1854. doi:10.1093/ndt/gfr561.

Amioka, M., Sanada, R., Matsumura, H., Kinoshita, H., Sairaku, A., Morishima, N., Nakano, Y., 2023. Impact of SGLT2 inhibitors on old age patients with heart failure and chronic kidney disease. Int. J. Cardiol. 18741754. 370, 294–299. Available from: www.elsevier.com/locate/ijcard. doi:10.1016/j.ijcard.2022.09.059.

Anderson, S., Brenner, B.M., 1986. Effects of aging on the renal glomerulus. Am. J. Med. 00029343. 80 (3), 435–442. doi:10.1016/0002-9343(86)90718-7.

Apostolou, T., Hutchison, A.J., Boulton, A.J.M., Chak, W., Vileikyte, L., Uttley, L., Gokal, R., 2007. Quality of life in CAPD, transplant, and chronic renal failure patients with diabetes. Ren. Fail. 15256049. 29 (2), 189–197. doi:10.1080/08860220601098862.

Bakris, G.L., Agarwal, R., Anker, S.D., Pitt, B., Ruilope, L.M., Rossing, P., Kolkhof, P., Nowack, C., Schloemer, P., Joseph, A., Filippatos, G., 2020. Effect of finerenone on chronic kidney disease outcomes in type 2 diabetes. N. Engl. J. Med. 15334406. 383 (23), 2219–2229. Available from: http://www.nejm.org/medical-index. doi:10.1056/NEJMoa2025845.

Bakris, G.L., Weir, M.R., 2000. Angiotensin-converting enzyme inhibitor-associated elevations in serum creatinine: is this a cause for concern? Arch. Intern. Med. 00039926. 160 (5), 685–693.

Bertoni, A.G., Krop, J.S., Anderson, G.F., Brancati, F.L., 2002. Diabetes-related morbidity and mortality in a national sample of U.S. elders. Diabetes Care 25 (3), 471–475. doi:10.2337/diacare.25.3.471.

Bethel, M.A., Sloan, F.A., Belsky, D., Feinglos, M.N., 2007. Longitudinal incidence and prevalence of adverse outcomes of diabetes mellitus in elderly patients. Arch. Intern. Med. 15383679. 167 (9), 921–927. Available from: http://archinte.ama-assn.org/cgi/reprint/167/9/921. doi: 10.1001/archinte.167.9.921

Brenner, B.M., Cooper, M.E., De Zeeuw, D., Keane, W.F., Mitch, W.E., Parving, H.H., Remuzzi, G., Snapinn, S.M., Zhang, Z., Shahinfar, S., 2001. Effects of losartan on renal and cardiovascular outcomes in patients with type 2 diabetes and nephropathy. N. Engl. J. Med. 00284793. 345 (12), 861–869. doi:10.1056/NEJMoa011161.

Casagrande, S., Cowie, C.C., Fradkin, J.E., 2017. Intensive glycemic control in younger and older U.S. adults with type 2 diabetes. J. Diabetes Complications. 1873460X. 31 (8), 1299–1304. Available from: www.elsevier.com/locate/jdiacomp. doi:10.1016/j.jdiacomp.2017.05.006.

Cho, N.H., Colagiuri, S., Distiller, L, 2013. Managing older people with type 2 diabetes. Global Guideline, 30–31.

Chronic Kidney Disease in the United States, 2023, 2023. Available from: https://www.cdc.gov/kidney-disease/php/data-research/index.html.

Clemens, K.K., O'Regan, N., Rhee, J.J., 2019. Diabetes Management in Older Adults With Chronic Kidney Disease. Curr. Diabetes Rep. 15390829. 19 (3). Available from: www.springer.com. doi:10.1007/s11892-019-1128-3.

Colberg, S.R., Sigal, R.J., Yardley, J.E., Riddell, M.C., Dunstan, D.W., Dempsey, P.C., Horton, E.S., Castorino, K., Tate, D.F., 2016. Physical activity/exercise and diabetes: a position statement of the American Diabetes Association. Diabetes Care. 19355548. 39 (11), 2065–2079. Available from: http://care.diabetesjournals.org/content/39/11/2065.full-text.pdf. doi:10.2337/dc16-1728.

Davies, D.F., Shock, N.W., 1950. Age changes in glomerular filtration rate, effective renal plasma flow, and tubular excretory capacity in adult males. J. Clin. Invest. 0021-9738. 29 (5), 496–507. doi:10.1172/JCI102286.

Davies, M.J., Aroda, V.R., Collins, B.S., Gabbay, R.A., Green, J., Maruthur, N.M., Rosas, S.E., Prato, S.D., Mathieu, C., Mingrone, G., Rossing, P., Tankova, T., Tsapas, A., Buse, J.B., 2022. Management of Hyperglycemia in Type 2 Diabetes, 2022. A Consensus Report by the American Diabetes Association (ADA) and the European Association for the Study of Diabetes (EASD). Diabetes Care. 19355548. 45 (11), 2753–2786. Available from: http://care.diabetesjournals.org/content/by/year. doi:10.2337/dci22-0034.

de Boer, I.H., Khunti, K., Sadusky, T., Tuttle, K.R., Neumiller, J.J., Rhee, C.M., Rosas, S.E., Rossing, P., Bakris, G., 2022. Diabetes Management in Chronic Kidney Disease: a Consensus Report by the American Diabetes Association (ADA) and Kidney Disease: improving Global Outcomes (KDIGO). Diabetes Care. 19355548. 45 (12), 3075–3090. Available from: http://care.diabetesjournals.org/content/by/year. doi:10.2337/dci22-0027.

Delanaye, G., Pottel, R., 2016. An age-calibrated definition of chronic kidney disease: rationale and benefits. Clin. Biochem. Rev. 37 (1), 17–26.

Denic, A., Glassock, R.J., Rule, A.D., 2016. Structural and Functional Changes With the Aging Kidney. Adv. Chronic Kidney Dis. 15485609. 23 (1), 19–28. Available from: http://www.elsevier.com/wps/find/journaldescription.cws_home/703170/description#description. doi:10.1053/j.ackd.2015.08.004.

Denic, A., Lieske, J.C., Chakkera, H.A., Poggio, E.D., Alexander, M.P., Singh, P., Kremers, W.K., Lerman, L.O., Rule, A.D., 2017. The substantial loss of nephrons in healthy human kidneys with aging. J. Am. Soc. Nephrol. 15333450. 28 (1), 313–320. Available from: http://jasn.asnjournals.org/content/28/1/313.full.pdf+html. doi:10.1681/ASN.2016020154.

Doyle-Delgado, K., Chamberlain, J.J., Shubrook, J.H., Skolnik, N., Trujillo, J., 2020. Pharmacologic approaches to glycemic treatment of type 2 diabetes: synopsis of the 2020 American diabetes association's standards of medical care in diabetes clinical guideline. Ann. Intern. Med. 15393704. 173 (10), 813–821. Available from: https://www.acpjournals.org/doi/pdf/10.7326/M20-2470. doi:10.7326/M20-2470.

Elsayed, N.A., Aleppo, G., Aroda, V.R., Bannuru, R.R., Brown, F.M., Bruemmer, D., Collins, B.S., Hilliard, M.E., Isaacs, D., Johnson, E.L., Kahan, S., Khunti, K., Leon, J., Lyons, S.K., Perry, M.L., Prahalad, P., Pratley, R.E., Seley, J.J., Stanton, R.C., Gabbay, R.A., 2023. 11. Chronic Kidney Disease and Risk Management: standards of Care in Diabetes—2023. Diabetes Care. 19355548. 46, S191. Available from: http://care.diabetesjournals.org/content/by/year. doi:10.2337/dc23-S011.

EMPA-KIDNEY Collaborative Group, 2023. Empagliflozin in Patients with Chronic Kidney Disease. N. Engl. J. Med. 0028-4793. 388 (2), 117–127. doi:10.1056/nejmoa2204233.

Fried, L.F., Emanuele, N., Zhang, J.H., Brophy, M., Conner, T.A., Duckworth, W., Leehey, D.J., McCullough, P.A., O'Connor, T., Palevsky, P.M., Reilly, R.F., Seliger, S.L., Warren, S.R., Watnick, S., Peduzzi, P., Guarino, P., 2013. Combined angiotensin inhibition for the treatment of diabetic nephropathy. N. Engl. J. Med. 15334406. 369 (20), 1892–1903. Available from: http://www.nejm.org/doi/pdf/10.1056/NEJMoa1303154. doi:10.1056/NEJMoa1303154.

Gansevoort, R.T., Matsushita, K., Velde, M.V.D., Astor, B.C., Woodward, M., Levey, A.S., Jong, P.E.D., Coresh, J., 2011. Lower estimated GFR and higher albuminuria are associated with adverse kidney outcomes. A collaborative meta-analysis of general and high-risk population cohorts. Kidney Int. 15231755. 80 (1), 93–104. Available from: https://www.journals.elsevier.com/kidney-international. doi:10.1038/ki.2010.531.

Glassock, R.J., Rule, A.D., 2012. The implications of anatomical and functional changes of the aging kidney: with an emphasis on the glomeruli. Kidney Int. 15231755. 82 (3), 270–277. Available from: https://www.journals.elsevier.com/kidney-international. doi:10.1038/ki.2012.65.

Gregg, E.W., Engelgau, M.M., Narayan, V., 2002. Complications of diabetes in elderly people. BMJ. 09598146. 325 (7370), 916–917. Available from: http://www.bmj.com/. doi:10.1136/bmj.325.7370.916.

Guidelines Abstracted from the American Geriatrics Society Guidelines for Improving the Care of Older Adults with Diabetes Mellitus: 2013 Update, 2013. J. Am. Geriatr. Soc. 0002-8614. 61 (11), 2020–2026. doi:10.1111/jgs.12514.

Guo, J., Zheng, H.J., Zhang, W., Lou, W., Xia, C., Han, X.T., Huang, W.J., Zhang, F., Wang, Y., Liu, W.J., 2020. Accelerated Kidney Aging in Diabetes Mellitus. Oxid. Med. Cell. Longev. 19420994. 2020. Available from: http://www.hindawi.com/journals/oximed/. doi:10.1155/2020/1234059.

Guppy, M., Thomas, E.T., Glasziou, P., Clark, J., Jones, M., O'Hara, D.V., Doust, J., 2024. Rate of decline in kidney function with age: a systematic review. BMJ Open. 20446055. 14 (11). Available from: http://bmjopen.bmj.com/content/early/by/section. doi:10.1136/bmjopen-2024-089783.

Hambling, C.E., Seidu, S.I., Davies, M.J., Khunti, K., 2017. Older people with Type 2 diabetes, including those with chronic kidney disease or dementia, are commonly overtreated with sulfonylurea or insulin therapies. Diabet. Med. 0742-3071. 34 (9), 1219–1227. doi:10.1111/dme.13380.

Heerspink, H.J.L., Stefánsson, B.V., Correa-Rotter, R., Chertow, G.M., Greene, T., Hou, F.F., Mann, J.F.E., McMurray, J.J.V., Lindberg, M., Rossing, P., Sjöström, C.D., Toto, R.D., Langkilde, A.M., Wheeler, D.C., 2020. Dapagliflozin in patients with chronic kidney disease. N. Engl. J. Med. 15334406. 383 (15), 1436–1446. Available from: http://www.nejm.org/medical-index. doi:10.1056/NEJMoa2024816.

Hoang, K., Tan, J.C., Derby, G., Blouch, K.L., Masek, M., Ma, I., Lemley, K.V., Myers, B.D., 2003. Determinants of glomerular hypofiltration in aging humans. Kidney Int. 00852538. 64 (4), 1417–1424. Available from: https://www.journals.elsevier.com/kidney-international. doi:10.1046/j.1523-1755.2003.00207.x.

Hodge, M., McArthur, E., Garg, A.X., Tangri, N., Clemens, K.K., 2017. Hypoglycemia Incidence in Older Adults by Estimated GFR. Am. J. Kidney Dis. 15236838. 70 (1), 59–68. Available from: http://www.elsevier.com/inca/publications/store/6/2/3/2/7/6/index.htt. doi:10.1053/j.ajkd.2016.11.019.

Hommos, M.S., Zeng, C., Liu, Z., Troost, J.P., Rosenberg, A.Z., Palmer, M., Kremers, W.K., Cornell, L.D., Fervenza, F.C., Barisoni, L., Rule, A.D., 2018. Global glomerulosclerosis with nephrotic syndrome; the clinical importance of age adjustment. Kidney Int. 15231755. 93 (5), 1175–1182. Available from: https://www.journals.elsevier.com/kidney-international. doi:10.1016/j.kint.2017.09.028.

Huang, E.S., Laiteerapong, N., Liu, J.Y., John, P.M., Moffet, H.H., Karter, A.J., 2014. Rates of complications and mortality in older patients with diabetes mellitus: the diabetes and aging study. JAMA Intern. Med. 21686106. 174 (2), 251–258. Available from: http://archinte.jamanetwork.com/article.aspx?articleid=1785198. doi:10.1001/jamainternmed.2013.12956.

Huang, E., Segev, D.L., Rabb, H., 2009. Kidney Transplantation in the Elderly. Semin. Nephrol. 29 (6), 621–635. doi:10.1016/j.semnephrol.2009.07.011.

Iglay, K., Hannachi, H., Howie, P.J., Xu, J., Li, X., Engel, S.S., Moore, L.M., Rajpathak, S., 2016. Prevalence and co-prevalence of comorbidities among patients with type 2 diabetes mellitus. Curr. Med. Res. Opin. 14734877. 32 (7), 1243–1252. doi:10.1185/03007995.2016.1168291.

Ikizler, T.A., Burrowes, J.D., Byham-Gray, L.D., Campbell, K.L., Carrero, J.J., Chan, W., Fouque, D., Friedman, A.N., Ghaddar, S., Goldstein-Fuchs, D.J., Kaysen, G.A., Kopple, J.D., Teta, D., Wang, A.Y.-M., Cuppari, L., 2020. KDOQI Clinical Practice Guideline for Nutrition in CKD: 2020 Update. Am. J. Kidney Dis. 15236838. 76 (3), S1. Available from: http://www.elsevier.com/inca/publications/store/6/2/3/2/7/6/index.htt. doi:10.1053/j.ajkd.2020.05.006.

Inzucchi, S.E., Lipska, K.J., Mayo, H., Bailey, C.J., McGuire, D.K., 2014. Metformin in patientswith type 2 diabetes and kidney disease a systematic review. JAMA. 15383598. 312 (24), 2668–2675. Available from: http://jama.jamanetwork.com/article.aspx?articleid=2084896. doi:10.1001/jama.2014.15298.

KDIGO, 2024. 2024 Clinical Practice Guideline for the Evaluation and Management of Chronic Kidney Disease. Kidney Int. 105 (4S), S135.

Kielstein, J.T., Bode-Böger, S.M., Frölich, J.C., Ritz, E., Haller, H., Fliser, D., 2003. Asymmetric dimethylarginine, blood pressure, and renal perfusion in elderly subjects. Circulation 107 (14), 1891–1895. doi:10.1161/01.CIR.0000060496.23144.A7.

King, H., Aubert, R.E., Herman, W.H., 1998. Global burden of diabetes, 1995-2025: prevalence, numerical estimates, and projections. Diabetes Care. 01495992. 21 (9), 1414–1431. Available from: http://care.diabetesjournals.org/. doi:10.2337/diacare.21.9.1414.

Krishnan, A., Shankar, M., Lerma, E.V., Wiegley, N., 2023. Sodium Glucose Cotransporter 2 (SGLT2) Inhibitors and CKD: are You a #Flozinator? Kidney Med. 25900595. 5 (4), 100608. doi:10.1016/j.xkme.2023.100608.

Leung, E., Wongrakpanich, S., Munshi, M.N., 2018. Diabetes management in the elderly. Diabetes Spectr. 19447353. 31 (3), 245–253. Available from: http://spectrum.diabetesjournals.org/content/31/3/245.full-text.pdf. doi:10.2337/ds18-0033.

Levey, A.S., Becker, C., Inker, L.A., 2015. Glomerular filtration rate and albuminuria for detection and staging of acute and chronic kidney disease in adults: a systematic review. JAMA. 15383598. 313 (8), 837–846. Available from: http://jama.jamanetwork.com/article.aspx?articleid=2130322. doi:10.1001/jama.2015.0602.

Lewis, E.J., Hunsicker, L.G., Bain, R.P., Rohde, R.D., 1993. The Effect of Angiotensin-Converting-Enzyme Inhibition on Diabetic Nephropathy. N. Engl. J. Med. 15334406. 329 (20), 1456–1462. doi:10.1056/NEJM199311113292004.

Madero, M., Chertow, G.M., Mark, P.B., 2024. SGLT2 Inhibitor Use in Chronic Kidney Disease: supporting Cardiovascular. Kidney Med. 25900595. 6 (8), 100851. doi:10.1016/j.xkme.2024.100851.

Maric-Bilkan, C., 2013. Obesity and Diabetic Kidney Disease. Med. Clin. North Am. 00257125. 97 (1), 59–74. doi:10.1016/j.mcna.2012.10.010.

McAdams-Demarco, M.A., James, N., Salter, M.L., Walston, J., Segev, D.L., 2014. Trends in kidney transplant outcomes in older adults. J. Am. Geriatr. Soc. 15325415. 62 (12), 2235–2242. Available from: http://onlinelibrary.wiley.com/journal/10.1111/(ISSN)1532-5415. doi:10.1111/jgs.13130.

Mehdi, U.F., Adams-Huet, B., Raskin, P., Vega, G.L., Toto, R.D., 2009. Addition of angiotensin receptor blockade or mineralocorticoid antagonism to maximal angiotensin-converting enzyme inhibition in diabetic nephropathy. J. Am. Soc. Nephrol. 15333450. 20 (12), 2641–2650. Available from: http://jasn.asnjournals.org/cgi/reprint/20/12/2641. doi:10.1681/ASN.2009070737.

Moen, M.F., Zhan, M., Hsu, V.D., Walker, L.D., Einhorn, L.M., Seliger, S.L., Fink, J.C., 2009. Frequency of hypoglycemia and its significance in chronic kidney disease. Clin. J. Am. Soc. Nephrol. 1555905X. 4 (6), 1121–1127. Available from: http://cjasn.asnjournals.org/cgi/reprint/4/6/1121. doi:10.2215/CJN.00800209.

Montez-Rath, M.E., Thomas, I.C., Charu, V., Odden, M.C., Seib, C.D., Arya, S., Fung, E., O'Hare, A.M., Wong, S.P.Y., Tamura, M.K., 2024. Effect of Starting Dialysis Versus Continuing Medical Management on Survival and Home Time in Older Adults With Kidney Failure: a Target Trial Emulation Study. Ann. Intern. Med. 15393704. 177 (9), 1233–1243. Available from: https://www.acpjournals.org/doi/10.7326/M23-3028. doi:10.7326/M23-3028.

Musso, C.G., Oreopoulos, D.G., 2011. Aging and physiological changes of the kidneys including changes in glomerular filtration rate. Nephron Physiol. 16602137. 119 (1), 1. doi:10.1159/000328010.

Mykkänen, L., Haffner, S.M., Kuusisto, J., Pyorälä, K., Laakso, M., 1994. Microalbuminuria precedes the development of NIDDM. Diabetes. 00121797. 43 (4), 552–557. Available from: http://diabetes.diabetesjournals.org/. doi:10.2337/diab.43.4.552.

National Diabetes Statistics Report, 2017. Available from: https://www.cdc.gov/diabetes/php/data-research/index.html.

Noronha, I.L., Santa-Catharina, G.P., Andrade, L., Coelho, V.A., Jacob-Filho, W., Elias, R.M., 2022. Glomerular filtration in the aging population. Front. Med. 2296858X. 9. Available from: https://journal.frontiersin.org/journal/medicine. doi:10.3389/fmed.2022.769329.

Nowakowska, M., Zghebi, S.S., Ashcroft, D.M., Buchan, I., Chew-Graham, C., Holt, T., Mallen, C., Van Marwijk, H., Peek, N., Perera-Salazar, R., Reeves, D., Rutter, M.K., Weng, S.F., Qureshi, N., Mamas, M.A., Kontopantelis, E., 2019. The comorbidity burden of type 2 diabetes mellitus: patterns, clusters and predictions from a large English primary care cohort. BMC Med. 17417015. 17 (1). Available from: http://www.biomedcentral.com/bmcmed/. doi:10.1186/s12916-019-1373-y.

Onyenwenyi, C., Ricardo, A.C., 2015. Impact of Lifestyle Modification on Diabetic Kidney Disease. Curr. Diabetes Rep. 15390829. 15 (9). Available from: www.springer.com. doi:10.1007/s11892-015-0632-3.

Pálsson, R., Patel, U.D., 2014. Cardiovascular complications of diabetic kidney disease. Adv. Chronic Kidney Dis. 15485609. 21 (3), 273–280. Available from: http://www.elsevier.com/wps/find/journaldescription.cws_home/703170/description#description. doi:10.1053/j.ackd.2014.03.003.

Pappoe, L.S., Winkelmayer, W.C., 2010. ACE inhibitor and angiotensin II type 1 receptor antagonist therapies in elderly patients with diabetes mellitus: are they underutilized? Drugs Aging. 11791969. 27 (2), 87–94. doi:10.2165/11316430-000000000-00000.

Perkovic, V., Jardine, M.J., Neal, B., Bompoint, S., Heerspink, H.J.L., Charytan, D.M., Edwards, R., Agarwal, R., Bakris, G., Bull, S., Cannon, C.P., Capuano, G., Chu, P.L., De Zeeuw, D., Greene, T., Levin, A., Pollock, C., Wheeler, D.C., Yavin, Y., Zhang, H., Zinman, B., Meininger, G., Brenner, B.M., Mahaffey, K.W., 2019. Canagliflozin and renal outcomes in type 2 diabetes and nephropathy. N. Engl. J. Med. 15334406. 380 (24), 2295–2306. Available from: http://www.nejm.org/medical-index. doi:10.1056/NEJMoa1811744.

Perkovic, V., Tuttle, K.R., Rossing, P., Mahaffey, K.W., Mann, J.F.E., Bakris, G., Baeres, F.M.M., Idorn, T., Bosch-Traberg, H., Lausvig, N.L., Pratley, R., 2024. Effects of semaglutide on chronic kidney disease in patients with type 2 diabetes. N. Engl. J. Med. 15334406. 391 (2), 109–121. Available from: http://www.nejm.org/medical-index. doi:10.1056/NEJMoa2403347.

Pitt, B., Filippatos, G., Agarwal, R., Anker, S.D., Bakris, G.L., Rossing, P., Joseph, A., Kolkhof, P., Nowack, C., Schloemer, P., Ruilope, L.M., 2021. Cardiovascular events with finerenone in kidney disease and type 2 diabetes. N. Engl. J. Med. 15334406. 385 (24), 2252–2263. Available from: http://www.nejm.org/medical-index. doi:10.1056/NEJMoa2110956.

Ralph Defronzo, G.A.F., Chen, K., Bicsak, T.A., 2016. Metformin-associated lactic acidosis: current perspectives on causes and risk. Metabolism. 00260495. 65 (2), 20–29. doi:10.1016/j.metabol.2015.10.014.

Rao, P.S., Merion, R.M., Ashby, V.B., Port, F.K., Wolfe, R.A., Kayler, L.K., 2007. Renal transplantation in elderly patients older than 70 years of age: results from the scientific registry of transplant recipients. Transplantation. 00411337. 83 (8), 1069–1074. doi:10.1097/01.tp.0000259621.56861.31.

Raphael, K.L., Murphy, R.A., Shlipak, M.G., Satterfield, S., Huston, H.K., Sebastian, A., Sellmeyer, D.E., Patel, K.V., Newman, A.B., Sarnak, M.J., Ix, J.H., Fried, L.F., 2016. Bicarbonate concentration, acid-base status, and mortality in the health, aging, and body composition study. Clin. J. Am. Soc. Nephrol. 1555905X. 11 (2), 308–316. Available from: http://cjasn.asnjournals.org/content/11/2/308.full.pdf. doi:10.2215/CJN.06200615.

Rebollo, P., Ortega, F., Baltar, J.M., Badí, X., Alvarez-Ude, F., Díaz-Corte, C., Naves, M., Navascúes, R.A., Ureña, A., Alvarez-Grande, J., 2000. Health related quality of life (HRQOL) of kidney transplanted patients: variables that influence it. Clin. Transplant. 14 (3), 199–207. doi:10.1034/j.1399-0012.2000.140304.x.

Roy, S., Schweiker-Kahn, O., Jafry, B., Masel-Miller, R., Raju, R.S., O'Neill, L.M.O., Correia, C.R., Trivedi, A., Johnson, C., Pilot, C., Saddemi, J., Memon, A., Chen, A., McHugh, S.P., Patel, S., Daroshefski, N.M., Nguyen, T., Wissler, W., Sharma, E., Hunter, K., 2021. Risk Factors and Comorbidities Associated with Diabetic Kidney Disease. J. Prim. Care Community Health. 21501327. 12. Available from: http://www.sagepub.com/journalsProdDesc.nav?prodId=Journal201976. doi:10.1177/21501327211048556.

Rubino, D., Abrahamsson, N., Davies, M., Hesse, D., Greenway, F.L., Jensen, C., Lingvay, I., Mosenzon, O., Rosenstock, J., Rubio, M.A., Rudofsky, G., Tadayon, S., Wadden, T.A., Dicker, D., 2021. Effect of Continued Weekly Subcutaneous Semaglutide vs Placebo on Weight Loss Maintenance in Adults with Overweight or Obesity: the STEP 4 Randomized Clinical Trial. JAMA. 15383598. 325 (14), 1414–1425. Available from: http://jama.jamanetwork.com/journal.aspx. doi:10.1001/jama.2021.3224.

Rule, A.D., Amer, H., Cornell, L.D., Taler, S.J., Cosio, F.G., Kremers, W.K., Textor, S.C., Stegall, M.D., 2010. The association between age and nephrosclerosis on renal biopsy among healthy adults. Ann. Intern. Med. 15393704. 152 (9), 561–567. Available from: http://www.annals.org/contents-by-date.2008.shtml. doi:10.7326/0003-4819-152-9-201005040-00006.

Sands, J.M., 2012. Urine concentrating and diluting ability during aging. J. Gerontol. A Biol. Sci. Med. Sci. 1758535X. 67 (12), 1352–1357. doi:10.1093/gerona/gls128.

Schlanger, L.E., Bailey, J.L., Sands, J.M., 2010. Electrolytes in the Aging. Adv. Chronic Kidney Dis. 15485595. 17 (4), 308–319. doi:10.1053/j.ackd.2010.03.008.

Seng, J.J.B., Kwan, Y.H., Lee, V.S.Y., Tan, C.S., Zainudin, S.B., Thumboo, J., Low, L.L., 2020. Differential health care use, diabetes-related complications, and mortality among five unique classes of patients with type 2 diabetes in Singapore: a latent class analysis of 71,125 patients. Diabetes Care. 19355548. 43 (5), 1048–1056. Available from: https://care.diabetesjournals.org/content/43/5/1048. doi:10.2337/dc19-2519.

Swamy, S., Noor, S.M., Mathew, R.O., 2023. Cardiovascular Disease in Diabetes and Chronic Kidney Disease. J. Clin. Med. 20770383. 12 (22). Available from: https://www.mdpi.com/journal/jcm. doi:10.3390/jcm12226984.

Tamura, M.K., Covinsky, K.E., Chertow, G.M., Yaffe, K., Landefeld, C.S., McCulloch, C.E., 2009. Functional status of elderly adults before and after initiation of dialysis. N. Engl. J. Med. 15334406. 361 (16), 1539–1547. Available from: http://content.nejm.org/cgi/reprint/361/16/1539.pdf. doi:10.1056/NEJMoa0904655.

Tong, L.L., Adler, S.G., 2022. Diabetic kidney disease treatment: new perspectives. Kidney Res. Clin. Pract. 22119140. 41, S63. Available from: http://www.krcp-ksn.org/main.html#. doi:10.23876/j.krcp.21.288.

Warren, M., Chaykin, L., Trachtenbarg, D., Nayak, G., Wijayasinghe, N., Cariou, B., 2018. Semaglutide as a therapeutic option for elderly patients with type 2 diabetes: pooled analysis of the SUSTAIN 1-5 trials. Diabetes Obes. Metab. 1462-8902. 20 (9), 2291–2297. doi:10.1111/dom.13331.

Weinstein, J.R., Anderson, S., 2010. The Aging Kidney: physiological Changes. Adv. Chronic Kidney Dis. 15485595. 17 (4), 302–307. doi:10.1053/j.ackd.2010.05.002.

Wilkinson, D.J., Piasecki, M., Atherton, P.J., 2018. The age-related loss of skeletal muscle mass and function: measurement and physiology of muscle fibre atrophy and muscle fibre loss in humans. Ageing Res. Rev. 15681637. 47, 123–132. doi:10.1016/j.arr.2018.07.005.

Yacoub, R., Habib, H., Lahdo, A., Ali, R.A., Varjabedian, L., Atalla, G., Akl, N.K., Aldakheel, S., Alahdab, S., Albitar, S., 2010. Association between smoking and chronic kidney disease: a case control study. BMC Public Health. 14712458. 10. doi:10.1186/1471-2458-10-731.

Yusuf, S., Teo, K.K., Pogue, J., Dyal, L., Copland, I., Schumacher, H., Dagenais, G., Sleight, P., Anderson, C., Ramos, B., Richardson, L., Murphy, J., Haehl, M., Hilbrich, L., Svaerd, R., Martin, K., Murwin, D., Meinicke, T., Schlosser, A., Schmidt, G., Creek, R., Schumacher, H., Distel, M., Aubert, B., Pogue, J., Dyal, L., Schmieder, R., Unger, T., Asmar, R., Mancia, G., Diaz, R., Paolasso, E., Piegas, L., Avezum, A., Munoz, E.C., Probstfield, J., Weber, M., Young, J., Fagard, R., Jansky, P., Mallion, J., Mann, J., Böhm, M., Eber, B., 2008. Telmisartan, ramipril, or both in patients at high risk for vascular events. N. Engl. J. Med. 15334406. 358 (15), 1547–1559. Available from: http://content.nejm.org/cgi/reprint/358/15/1547.pdf. doi:10.1056/NEJMoa0801317.

CHAPTER

18

Glomerulonephritis

Akwe Nyabera and Gerald Appel

Nephrology, Columbia University Medical Center, New York, NY, United States

Introduction

Glomerular diseases often lead to chronic kidney disease (CKD) and end-stage kidney disease (ESKD) (Windpessl et al., 2022). Aging affects the glomerular response to injury, the frequency of glomerular diseases observed, and both the response to and side effects of therapy. Thus it is not surprising that the elderly require specialized evaluation, treatment, and clinical considerations. As the population increasingly ages, these will be challenges for most nephrologists, clinicians, and practitioners.

Distribution of glomerulopathies across different ages

As in other age groups, primary glomerular diseases in the elderly can present as asymptomatic urinary abnormalities, nephrotic syndrome, nephritic syndrome, chronic glomerulonephritis, or rapidly progressive glomerulonephritis (Sumnu et al., 2015). Presentation in the elderly can be more complex. For example, acute kidney injury (AKI) superimposed on nephrotic syndrome in conditions such as minimal change disease or IgA nephropathy is more common in older patients compared to younger patients (Windpessl et al., 2022; Sevillano et al., 2019). Moreover, many older individuals have concurrent diseases such as diabetes mellitus and hypertension, which can accelerate damage caused by other diseases involving the glomerulus, leading to worse outcomes (Windpessl et al., 2022; Denic et al., 2016; Hodgin et al., 2015).

IgA nephropathy, primary focal segmental glomerulosclerosis, and lupus nephritis appear most commonly in the younger population (Tarr et al., 2015; Wenderfer and Gaut, 2017), while other disorders such as minimal change glomerulonephritis and membranous glomerulonephritis are present across the age spectrum. Finally, conditions such as amyloidosis and ANCA-related crescentic glomerulonephritis are seen more commonly in older patients.

While a definitive diagnosis in most patients with glomerular diseases is achieved via kidney biopsy, this is not always necessary, especially in older patients with comorbidities that raise the risk-benefit ratio of a renal biopsy. Currently, positive values for certain

Aging and the Kidney
https://doi.org/10.1016/B978-0-443-34069-7.00019-7

diagnostic clinical tests, in association with classic clinical findings, may obviate the need for a biopsy. For example, a positive ANCA test for PR3 c-ANCA in the presence of signs of acute glomerulonephritis and pulmonary or ENT involvement may lead the clinician to avoid a biopsy. Likewise, in a very frail, elderly patient with nephrotic syndrome and a high-titer PLA2R antibody level, a clinical diagnosis of membranous nephropathy may suffice. Deciding whether to biopsy the patient or add immunosuppression to conservative therapy should be made after considering several factors, such as kidney function at the time of diagnosis, the likelihood of successful treatment, side effects of the drug, patient comorbidities, patient preference, and life-expectancy at the time of diagnosis (Sumnu et al., 2015).

Different forms of glomerular disease affect areas of the glomerulus in different ways

An increase in the number of glomerulosclerotic glomeruli in persons without kidney disease occurs with aging. Indeed, renal pathologists, when reviewing biopsies, often use a formula (Age/2 – 10) to account for percent of sclerotic glomeruli commonly present in all people as they age (Hodgin et al., 2015). Glomerulonephritis can be both primary and secondary, and the morphology and clinical course depend upon which cell types in the glomerulus are targeted. Cells within the glomerulus interact and communicate extensively. The different components of the glomerulus, including the podocyte, the glomerular basement membrane, endothelial cells, mesangial cells, and parietal epithelial cells, may react differently and have more limited reserve and flexibility in the elderly. Age-dependent glomerulosclerosis and a subsequent decline in eGFR are caused by changes in the number, structure, and function of the different glomerular cell types (Shankland et al., 2021). The nonspecific glomerular changes associated with the aging process itself, which include widening of the glomerular basement membrane, mesangial expansion, glomerular enlargement, and increased glomerulosclerosis, are all associated with a reduced eGFR, reduced ability to concentrate urine, and worse outcomes after glomerular injury (Shankland et al., 2021; Windpessl et al., 2022; Wiggins, 2012). There is evidence to suggest that the podocyte is a critical cell type when it comes to aging (Wiggins, 2012; Shankland et al., 2021; Floege et al., 1997; Hodgin et al., 2015). Different studies have described glomerulosclerosis associated with aging as a podocyte disorder. There is decreased podocyte density (owing to decreased podocyte number per glomerulus as well as increased glomerular volume) noted in older kidneys when compared to younger kidneys (Wiggins, 2012; Hodgin et al., 2015).

This decrease in podocyte density is associated with an accumulation of proteinaceous material in Bowman's space. Other observable changes include mass podocyte detachment, leading to wrinkling of glomerular capillaries, tuft collapse, and periglomerular fibrosis. Similar processes were observed in the kidneys of younger patients with focal segmental glomerulosclerosis. Studies have also shown a correlation between a decrease in podocyte density and worse outcomes in diabetic glomerulosclerosis, IgA nephropathy, hypertensive glomerulosclerosis, and transplant glomerulopathy. The effects of aging on the vasculature and tubulointerstitial compartment must also be considered, with interstitial fibrosis and tubular atrophy, as well as arterial and arteriolar sclerosis, presenting more frequently on kidney biopsies with increased aging (Hodgin et al., 2015; see Tables 18.1 and 18.2).

TABLE 18.1 Age-related glomerular changes and their clinical implications.

Structural or functional change	Features of aging	Clinical implications in older adults
Background glomerulosclerosis	Increased proportion of sclerotic (scarred) glomeruli, even in the absence of overt kidney disease	Reduces renal reserve and can complicate the interpretation of kidney biopsies or risk prediction models
Glomerular basement membrane (GBM) and mesangium	Thickening of the glomerular basement membrane, mesangial expansion, glomerular enlargement, and increased global sclerosis	Associated with a lower estimated glomerular filtration rate, a reduced ability to concentrate urine, and poorer outcomes after kidney injury
Podocytes	Decreased podocyte density (fewer podocytes with larger glomeruli); podocyte detachment, tuft collapse, periglomerular fibrosis, and accumulation of proteinaceous material in Bowman's space	Central to the development of age-related glomerulosclerosis; it correlates with worse outcomes across conditions such as diabetic glomerulosclerosis, immunoglobulin A nephropathy, hypertensive glomerulosclerosis, and transplant glomerulopathy
Interstitial and vascular changes	Interstitial fibrosis, tubular atrophy, and arterial or arteriolar sclerosis	Contributes to progressive functional decline and affects prognosis, as well as tolerance to therapies

TABLE 18.2 Clinical presentation, diagnostic features, treatment, and prognosis in specific glomerular disorders in the elderly.

Condition	Clinical presentation	Diagnostic features	Treatment considerations	Prognosis
Membranous nephropathy	Nephrotic syndrome in the elderly; acute kidney injury is more common; often accompanied by higher blood pressure, lower baseline kidney function, and a greater risk of infection and thrombosis	Antibodies to phospholipase A2 receptor (PLA2R); evaluate for cancer (approximately 10% in elderly), autoimmune disease—lupus nephropathy, infection—hepatitis B and C, hematopoietic stem cell transplant, or use of nonsteroidal antiinflammatory drugs; biopsy may be omitted in frail patients with strongly positive PLA2R antibodies	Avoid corticosteroids alone; consider calcineurin inhibitors (CNI) or rituximab; start immunosuppressive therapy if proteinuria > 4 g/day or if serum creatinine increases by at least 30% over 6–12 months despite conservative therapy	Older adults have more treatment complications; careful prevention of infection and thrombosis is essential

Continued

TABLE 18.2 Clinical presentation, diagnostic features, treatment, and prognosis in specific glomerular disorders in the elderly—cont'd

Condition	Clinical presentation	Diagnostic features	Treatment considerations	Prognosis
IgA nephropathy	Blood and protein in the urine (with or without acute kidney injury); more frequent hypertension, reduced kidney function, and increased tubulointerstitial scarring	Kidney biopsy is required for diagnosis; renin–angiotensin–aldosterone system blockade, endothelin antagonists, and SGLT2 inhibitors all offer protection; immunosuppression is often less effective in older adults	Emphasize blood pressure and proteinuria control; renin–angiotensin–aldosterone system (RAAS) blockade, endothelin antagonists, and SGLT2 inhibitors all offer protection; immunosuppression (corticosteroids, MMF, complement blockers, and drugs to reduce the formation of Galactose deficient IgA1 and IgA immune complexes) should be used cautiously in the elderly. Newer agents such as targeted release budesonide, iptacopan, and sibeprenlimab are FDA approved for treatment	Worse long-term outcomes, with about twice the risk of ESKD after age 50; progression can occur even with low levels of protein in the urine
Antineutrophil cytoplasmic antibody (ANCA)-associated vasculitis	Blood and protein in the urine, acute glomerulonephritis, systemic small-vessel inflammation	Classified histologically (focal, crescentic, mixed, sclerotic); renal risk scoring considers normal versus sclerotic glomeruli and kidney function; strong ANCA antibody positivity may allow biopsy deferral in selected cases	Cyclophosphamide or rituximab improves outcomes; advanced age alone should not preclude immunosuppression. Avacopan, a complement blocker, may be sterodi sparing	Focal pattern has the best outcome; sclerotic pattern, the worst; crescentic disease may be reversible with aggressive treatment; mortality rises with age but decreases with appropriate therapy
Minimal change disease	Sudden presentation of severe nephrotic syndrome, often with acute kidney injury and hypertension; older adults are more susceptible to acute tubular injury	Kidney biopsy typically required	Corticosteroids or CNIs are first line; alternatives include cyclophosphamide, MMF, or rituximab	Fewer relapses after age 40

Condition	Clinical presentation	Diagnostic features	Treatment considerations	Prognosis
Focal segmental glomerulo-sclerosis (FSGS)	Protein in urine, with or without nephrotic syndrome; secondary forms may arise from hyperfiltration, drugs (interferon, pamidro-nate, heroin), fibrils, or infections (COVID-19, HIV) or genetic mutations	Columbia classifica-tion variants (collapsing, tip, perihilar, cellular, not otherwise specified) are useful for prognosis and identifying second-ary causes	All forms: low-Na diet, BP control, RAAS blockade, SGLT2 inhibitors; primary forms: corticosteroids or CNI; consider MMF or rituximab if kidney function is severely reduced	Tip variant has the best prognosis; collapsing variant has the worst. Outcomes correlate with the amount of scarring, proteinuria, and baseline kidney function
Lupus nephritis (late-onset systemic lupus erythemato-sus)	Often milder systemic lupus activity but greater cumulative kidney damage; frequent acute kidney injury, lower creatinine clearance, and higher blood pressure; classes III, IV, V, or mixed are common; crescents are present in one-third of cases	Biopsy is required to determine the class; treatment is similar to that for younger patients but adjusted for frailty and infection risk	Use lower doses of corticosteroids and immunosuppressive therapy cautiously; prioritize infection prevention, as infections are a major cause of death. Newer FDA approved agents that can be self administered subcuta-neously at home (belimumab) or infrequently every 6 months 9 (obinutu-zumab) may have special advantages in the elderly.	Higher cumulative organ damage: A careful balance between efficacy and toxicity is needed
Amyloidosis with kidney involvement	Proteinuria, with or without nephrotic syndrome; neuropa-thy, gastrointestinal symptoms, CHF, or orthostatic hypotension	Congo red–positive biopsy and electron microscopy with diagnostic 10 nm fibrils of GBM; may involve sampling a fat pad or another organ; if AL amyloid is present, multiple myeloma may also be present; determine the amyloid type (e.g., AL light-chain, serum amyloid A, leukocyte chemotac-tic factor 2, etc.) to guide therapy	Management depends on the type of amyloid; incorrect classification can lead to harmful treatment	Organ-threatening amyloid type and regional prevalence vary (serum amyloid A is more common in developing regions, while leukocyte chemotactic factor 2 is prevalent among older Hispanic adults in North America)

Continued

TABLE 18.2 Clinical presentation, diagnostic features, treatment, and prognosis in specific glomerular disorders in the elderly—cont'd

Condition	Clinical presentation	Diagnostic features	Treatment considerations	Prognosis
Membrano-proliferative glomerulone-phritis (MPGN) pattern	Variable glomerulone-phritis features	Immunofluorescence differentiates immune complex, parapro-tein-mediated, and complement-mediated forms, as well as chronic thrombotic microangiopathy; in older adults, rule out monoclonal gammopa-thy, C3G and immune complex with IF and EM deposits; serum complement levels are low in these cases	Treat the underlying cause; provide support-ive care for kidney function. For C3 G and immune complex GN, complement blockers can be used	Prognosis depends on the underlying cause and the degree of chronic damage at diagnosis

Membranous nephropathy is the most frequent primary glomerular disease and a leading cause of nephrotic syndrome in individuals over the age of 65 worldwide. AKI is more common during the course of this disease compared to some other primary glomerular diseases, and advanced age has been recognized as a risk factor for AKI in patients with membranous nephropathy (Sumnu et al., 2015). Patients above the age of 60 are more likely to have hypertension and worse baseline kidney function at presentation. They also experience higher rates of infection with immunosuppression and increased rates of thrombosis compared to younger adults (O'Callaghan et al., 2002; Yamaguchi et al., 2014). Membranous nephropathy is a pattern of injury caused by autoantibodies binding to specific antigens, leading to the accumulation of immune complexes along the subepithelial region of the glomerular basement membrane. Over the last 20 years, 14 target antigens (and in some cases, their circulating antibodies) have been discovered, accounting for 80%–90% of membranous nephropathy cases. Currently, the two most common and therefore most frequently screened-for antibodies are the anti-phospholipase A2 receptor (anti-PLA2R) and the anti-neural epidermal growth factor-like 1 (anti-NELL 1) protein. Both are prevalent in adults and older patients, as opposed to other antigens such as semaphorin and exostosin, which are more commonly found in younger patients, children, or lupus patients. These antigens and their corresponding antibodies have enabled more precision medicine approaches and, in some cases, have negated the need for a kidney biopsy (Sethi et al., 2023). In addition to testing for these target antigens, screening for other causes of membranous nephropathy should also be performed. Membranous nephropathy is associated with malignancy in up to 10% of cases, and this association is more common in the elderly (Lefaucheur et al., 2006; Beck, 2010). Furthermore, screening for systemic diseases such as autoimmune conditions, infections, hematopoietic stem cell transplantation, and sarcoidosis, as well as obtaining a thorough history of medication use, including NSAIDs, should be conducted (Sumnu et al., 2015).

In older adults, treatment with steroids alone may lead to more complications, and immunosuppressive therapy with agents such as rituximab should be considered when appropriate, particularly in patients presenting with proteinuria exceeding 4 g/day or at least a 30% increase in serum creatinine levels over 6–12 months despite conservative therapy (Sumnu et al., 2015; Zent et al., 1997; Passerini et al., 1993).

IgA nephropathy (IgAN) across all ages is a very common cause of primary glomerulonephritis and one of the major causes of CKD and ESKD worldwide. Once diagnosed, most patients progress to ESKD during their lifetime. Even in patients with relatively low rates of proteinuria (< 0.88 g/g), there are high rates of progression to kidney failure over the course of 10 years (Pitcher et al., 2023). IgA nephropathy was traditionally thought to primarily affect children and young adults, with many patients diagnosed before the age of 40. However, over the last 30 years, there has been an increased incidence of IgA nephropathy being diagnosed in adults over the age of 50, with a common presentation being hematuria and AKI (Sevillano et al., 2019). Older patients diagnosed with IgA nephropathy tend to have higher rates of hypertension, worse kidney function, and greater tubulointerstitial fibrosis at the time of biopsy (Frimat et al., 1996). Long-term prognosis in older adults is poor, with about a 1.95 times higher incidence of progression to ESKD in those above the age of 50 (Duan et al., 2013). Renin-angiotensin-aldosterone system (RAAS) blockade appears to have a protective effect in this population; however, the use of immunosuppression may not be as beneficial (Frimat et al., 1996).

Anti-neutrophil cytoplasmic antibody (ANCA)-associated vasculitis (AAV) can be divided into granulomatosis with polyangiitis (GPA), microscopic polyangiitis (MPA), and eosinophilic granulomatosis with polyangiitis (EGPA). These conditions form a multisystemic group of vasculitides characterized by necrotizing involvement of small vessels. The incidence of AAV increases with age and represents the most common form of glomerulonephritis in the sixth decade of life and beyond (Aydın et al., 2023). Kidney involvement typically presents clinically as hematuria, proteinuria, and acute kidney failure. Histopathology often reveals a rapidly progressing form of pauci-immune necrotizing and crescentic glomerulonephritis (GN). Histopathologic classifications for ANCA-GN have been developed to assist in the prognosis of patients. The Berden classification system categorizes patients into focal, crescentic, mixed, and sclerotic patterns based on glomerular lesions. Different histological patterns correlate with kidney function and long-term outcomes. Focal lesions have the best prognosis, sclerotic lesions indicate the poorest outcomes, and crescentic patterns suggest a potentially reversible condition but require aggressive treatment. The renal risk score developed by Brix et al. stratifies AAV patients based on their risk of developing ESKD using histopathological and clinical parameters at diagnosis. It incorporates three key factors: the percentage of normal glomeruli (a higher percentage indicates a better prognosis), the percentage of sclerotic glomeruli (a higher percentage indicates a worse prognosis), and kidney function at presentation, measured as the estimated glomerular filtration rate (eGFR). Patients with a higher percentage of sclerotic glomeruli and lower eGFR at presentation are more likely to progress to ESKD. The renal risk score helps identify patients who may benefit from aggressive immunosuppressive therapy versus those who may require supportive care due to irreversible kidney damage. In older patients, age-related glomerulosclerosis complicates the interpretation of histopathology. Differentiating between disease- and age-related glomerular changes is essential for accurate prognostication and treatment decisions (Berden et al., 2010; Alves and Góis, 2022). Age-related glomerulosclerosis contributing to kidney dysfunction should be considered during prognostication, and not all globally sclerotic glomeruli should be presumed to be disease-related. This differentiation aids in determining appropriate therapy and avoids excessive immunosuppression in older populations (Aydın et al., 2023). While therapy with cyclophosphamide and rituximab has vastly improved the prognosis of this disease, some studies have found higher mortality and worse disease outcomes in older patients (Jones et al., 2010; Stone et al., 2010). However, older patients may still benefit from immunosuppressive treatment, with other studies showing significantly lower 2-year mortality risk and lower rates of ESKD in patients above the age of 75 who received immunosuppressive therapy. Therefore age alone should not be the sole limiting factor in determining eligibility for treatment (Morris et al., 2020; Bomback et al., 2011).

Systemic lupus erythematosus (SLE) and lupus nephritis typically present in younger populations, often in women of childbearing age. Those presenting above the age of 50 are known as late-onset SLE. The incidence of late-onset SLE is about 12%–18%, and the course of the disease is milder, with lower rates of relapse and systemic manifestations, including kidney involvement (Rovenský and Tuchynová, 2008; Sharma et al., 2023). Nevertheless, older patients with lupus nephritis develop more damage over time. They often present with kidney failure, lower creatinine clearance, and higher rates of hypertension (Mak et al., 2007). Acute kidney injury is a common presenting factor, with the potential to lead to ESKD and dialysis dependence. Histology showing classes IV, V, and IV + V is common in late-onset LN patients (Tang et al., 2011), but there are no significant differences in the histological class of disease across different age groups (Tang et al., 2011). Studies have observed crescents and lupus vasculopathy in about 33% and 7.5% of cases, respectively. Treatment is similar to that of the younger age group with LN, but with more judicious use of corticosteroids and other immunosuppressives. With the administration of immunosuppression, infectious complications should be emphasized, as infections are one of the major treatment complications leading to death in this cohort (Sharma et al., 2023).

Minimal change disease in the elderly is an important cause of nephrotic syndrome and frequently presents as AKI and hypertension. Older patients are also more susceptible to AKI and acute tubular necrosis. Relapses are less common in those above the age of 40 (Haas et al., 2000; Waldman et al., 2007). Corticosteroids are still the main initial form of therapy; however, for many elderly patients in whom glucocorticoids may be relatively contraindicated, initial therapy with a CNI, MMF, or rituximab can be considered (Rosenberg and Kopp, 2017).

FSGS is a histological pattern of injury caused by a wide spectrum of diseases. It can be classified as primary, secondary, genetic, or FSGS of undetermined cause and occurs due to podocyte injury (KDIGO, 2021; Rosenberg and Kopp, 2017). It occurs more commonly in Black individuals (with a fourfold increased risk) compared to White or Asian individuals (Kitiyakara et al., 2004). A study examining biopsy-proven kidney disease in a cohort of Chinese patients over the age of 65 found that FSGS accounted for less than 5% of cases (Jin et al., 2014). The APOL1 risk allele has been identified as one of the factors associated with FSGS in individuals of sub-Saharan African ancestry (Daneshpajouhnejad et al., 2022). Primary FSGS is attributed to a circulating plasma factor that targets the podocyte, whereas secondary FSGS is associated with an excessive workload on the nephron. This can be secondary to hemodynamic adaptations of the kidney due to a reduction in nephron capacity, increased body size, glomerular hyperfiltration, drugs (including interferon, pamidronate, and heroin), or infections (especially COVID-19 and HIV) (Rosenberg and Kopp, 2017; Rout et al., 2024). Initially, glomerulosclerosis is both focal, with only a minority of glomeruli involved, and segmental, affecting only a part of the glomerulus. Over time, global glomerulosclerosis develops (D'Agati et al., 2011; Rosenberg and Kopp, 2017). The Columbia classification system has traditionally been used for prognostication but cannot differentiate between primary and secondary forms of FSGS. It uses light microscopy to divide histological variants into collapsing, perihilar, cellular, tip, and not-otherwise-specified based on their location with respect to the vascular and tubular poles, as well as considering glomerular hypercellularity and capillary collapse (Rosenberg and Kopp, 2017). Collapsing FSGS has been noted more frequently in Black, younger patients, whereas tip lesions appear more frequently in patients over the age of 50 (Chun et al., 2004; Thomas et al., 2006). Tip lesions tend to have the best prognosis, whereas collapsing FSGS has the worst prognosis. Important predictors of outcomes in all patients, including the elderly, are the amount of tubulointerstitial injury at the time of diagnosis, level of proteinuria, and degree of kidney dysfunction (D'Agati et al., 2011; Sumnu et al., 2015). All cases of FSGS should be treated with basic supportive measures such as a low-sodium diet, blood pressure control, and reduction of proteinuria with RAAS and SGLT2 inhibitors as tolerated. Treatment of many individuals with presumed primary FSGS who present with nephrotic syndrome is achieved with glucocorticoids. However, in patients at high risk for glucocorticoid-induced toxicity (such as those over the age of 70), steroid-sparing therapy with a CNI should be pursued. CNI use is not recommended in individuals with an eGFR < 30, and in these cases, MMF or rituximab may be used (KDIGO, 2021).

Amyloidosis refers to a cluster of diseases that result in the tissue deposition of proteins in a beta-sheet configuration of fibrils. About 42 different proteins capable of amyloid formation have been identified, 16 of which affect the kidney (Leung and Nasr, 2024). Amyloidosis mainly affects older adults and is commonly diagnosed in those above the age of 50–60 (Said et al., 2013). Amyloid deposition may be localized—in the organ of formation—or systemic, with deposition in different tissues (Muchtar et al., 2021). The type of amyloidosis is named after the protein deposited and classified as either acquired (wild type) or mutant (due to a germline pathogenic variant) (Leung and Nasr, 2024). AL amyloidosis is largely due to the deposition of light chains, while AA amyloidosis is due to the deposition of AA protein. When deposited, these proteins cause organ failure, eventually leading to morbidity and mortality. Vital organs affected include the heart, liver, peripheral nerves, and kidney (Buxbaum et al., 2022). Patients with renal amyloidosis may present with proteinuria, with or without nephrotic syndrome. In patients presenting with proteinuria, a diagnosis of amyloidosis should be suspected in those with additional systemic symptoms such as neuropathy, gastrointestinal symptoms, heart failure, or orthostatic hypotension (Appel and Leung, 2025). The prevalence of different types of amyloid varies depending on the age of the population and the geographic population studied. AA amyloidosis has a higher prevalence in the developing world compared to AL amyloidosis due to higher rates of infection (Oliveira-Silva et al., 2023; Prakash et al., 2012). Most reported cases of ALECT2 amyloidosis in North America are in older adults of Hispanic descent (Said et al., 2014; Larsen et al., 2016). In the United States, 86% of amyloidosis identified on kidney biopsy is immunoglobulin-associated (usually associated with the deposition of a single abnormal light chain), followed by AA amyloidosis at 7% and leukocyte cell-derived chemotaxin 2 (ALECT2) amyloidosis at 3% (Said et al., 2013). Much like other plasma cell dyscrasias, the incidence of AL amyloidosis increases with each decade of life after the age of 40, with the median age of diagnosis being 64. Fewer than 5% of cases present under the age of 40 (Kyle et al., 1992; Shimazaki et al., 2018; Muchtar et al., 2019). Kidney biopsy is often required to make a diagnosis, with the classic finding of Congo red–positive material viewed in the glomerular mesangium and along the glomerular capillary loops on light microscopy. Biopsy may be deferred in cases of multiple myeloma where a fat pad biopsy or other organ involvement is confirmed. Typing should be performed once a kidney biopsy confirms amyloid deposits within the kidney to avoid misdiagnosis, improper management, or exposure to unnecessary cytotoxic agents (Appel and Leung, 2025).

Membranoproliferative glomerulonephritis (MPGN) is a pattern of glomerular injury. It is not a diagnosis and does not provide insight into an underlying etiology. It occurs secondary to four main entities: immune complex-mediated GNs, paraprotein-mediated GNs, complement-mediated GNs, or chronic TMA. Immunofluorescence is used to distinguish between the four groups (Sumnu et al., 2015), depending on the deposits seen. In the elderly, secondary causes of MPGN, such as monoclonal gammopathy, should always be ruled out.

Summary and conclusions (Table 18.3)

Aging profoundly influences the prevalence, progression, and management of glomerular diseases. It leads to structural and functional changes in the glomerulus, such as podocyte loss, glomerular sclerosis, and reduced glomerular filtration rate (eGFR). These changes predispose older adults to worse outcomes following glomerular injury. While younger populations are more affected by diseases like IgA nephropathy and lupus nephritis, conditions like minimal change disease and membranous nephropathy are more evenly

TABLE 18.3 Presentation and diagnostic approach to older adults with primary glomerular disease.

Topic	Summary
Common presentations	Asymptomatic urinary abnormalities; nephrotic syndrome; nephritic syndrome (hematuria, proteinuria, high blood pressure, oliguria, edema); chronic glomerulonephritis; rapidly progressive glomerulonephritis (RPGN)
Elder-specific nuances	Acute kidney injury (AKI) superimposed on nephrotic syndrome occurs more frequently in older adults; concurrent diabetes and hypertension accelerate glomerular damage and worsen outcomes
When biopsy may be deferred	Patients with strong antineutrophil cytoplasmic antibodies (c-ANCA or p-ANCA) and suggestive systemic findings, such as those involving the lungs or ear-nose-throat region, who present with acute glomerulonephritis. Patients who are frail and have nephrotic syndrome with high levels of phospholipase A2 receptor antibodies, suggesting membranous nephropathy
Factors guiding biopsy and treatment	Baseline kidney function; likelihood of response; drug toxicities; comorbidities; patient preferences; life expectancy at diagnosis

distributed, whereas amyloidosis and ANCA-associated glomerulonephritis are more prevalent in the elderly. Therefore diagnostic and treatment approaches need to be tailored to account for age-related changes, comorbidities, and patient preferences. Kidney biopsy remains the gold standard for diagnosis in most conditions. In a few conditions, such as ANCA vasculitis and membranous nephropathy, clinicians can instead rely on clinical findings and biomarkers for diagnosis when feasible. Immunosuppressive therapies are effective but associated with higher complication rates in the elderly. Precision medicine and steroid-sparing regimens should be employed, when possible, to reduce invasive procedures and optimize care.

References

Alves, P., Góis, M., 2022. The prognostic value of histopathological classifications in ANCA-associated vasculitis. Port. J. Nephrol. Hypertens. 08720169. doi:10.32932/pjnh.2022.10.203.

Appel, G., Leung, N., 2025. Renal amyloidosis. In: Glassock, R. (Ed.), UpToDate. Wolters Kluwer.

Aydın, M.F., Yıldız, A., Oruç, A., Aytaç Vuruşkan, B., Akgür, S., Ayar, Y., Güllülü, M., Dilek, K., Yavuz, M., Ortaç, H., Ersoy, A., 2023. Modified histopathological classification with age-related glomerulosclerosis for predicting kidney survival in ANCA-associated glomerulonephritis. Int. Urol. Nephrol. 55 (3), 741–748. doi:10.1007/s11255-022-03371-6.

Beck, L.H., 2010. Membranous nephropathy and malignancy. Semin. Nephrol. 30 (6), 635–644. doi:10.1016/j.semnephrol.2010.09.011.

Berden, A.E., Franco Ferrario, E.C.H., Jayne, D.R., Jennette, J.C., Joh, K., Neumann, I., Noël, L.-H., Pusey, C.D., Waldherr, R., Bruijn, J.A., Bajema, I.M., 2010. Histopathologic classification of ANCA-associated glomerulonephritis. J. Am. Soc. Nephrol. 21 (10), 1628–1636. doi:10.1681/ASN.2010050477.

Bomback, A.S., Appel, G.B., Radhakrishnan, J., Shirazian, S., Herlitz, L.C., Stokes, B., D'Agati, V.D., Markowitz, G.S., 2011. ANCA-associated glomerulonephritis in the very elderly. Kidney Int. 79 (7), 757–764. doi:10.1038/ki.2010.489.

Buxbaum, J.N., Dispenzieri, A., Eisenberg, D.S., Fändrich, M., Merlini, G., Saraiva, M.J.M., Sekijima, Y., Westermark, P., 2022. Amyloid nomenclature 2022: update, novel proteins, and recommendations by the International Society of Amyloidosis (ISA) Nomenclature Committee. Amyloid 29 (4), 213–219. doi:10.1080/13506129.2022.2147636.

Chun, M.J., Korbet, S.M., Schwartz, M.M., Lewis, E.J., 2004. Focal segmental glomerulosclerosis in nephrotic adults: presentation, prognosis, and response to therapy of the histologic variants. J. Am. Soc. Nephrol. 15 (8), 2169–2177.

D'Agati, V.D., Kaskel, F.J., Falk, R.J., 2011. Focal segmental glomerulosclerosis. N. Engl. J. Med. 365 (25), 2398–2411. doi:10.1056/NEJMra1106556.

Daneshpajouhnejad, P., Kopp, J.B., Winkler, C.A., Rosenberg, A.Z., 2022. The evolving story of apolipoprotein L1 nephropathy: the end of the beginning. Nat. Rev. Nephrol. 18 (5), 307–320. doi:10.1038/s41581-022-00538-3.

Denic, A., Glassock, R.J., Rule, A.D., 2016. Structural and functional changes with the aging kidney. Adv. Chronic Kidney Dis. 23 (1), 19–28.

Duan, Z.-Y., Cai, G.-Y., Chen, Y.-Z., Liang, S., Liu, S.-W., Jie, W., Qiu, Q., Lin, S.-P., Zhang, X.-G., Chen, X.-M., 2013. Aging promotes progression of IgA nephropathy: a systematic review and meta-analysis. Am. J. Nephrol. 38 (3), 241–252. doi:10.1159/000354646.

Floege, J., Hackmann, B., Kliem, V., Kriz, W., Alpers, C.E., Johnson, R.J., Kühn, K.W., Koch, K.M., Brunkhorst, R., 1997. Age-related glomerulosclerosis and interstitial fibrosis in Milan normotensive rats: a podocyte disease. Kidney Int. 51 (1), 230–243.

Frimat, L., Hestin, D., Aymard, B., Mayeux, D., Renoult, E., Kessler, M., 1996. IgA nephropathy in patients over 50 years of age: a multicentre, prospective study. Nephrol. Dial. Transplant. 11 (6), 1043–1047.

Haas, M., Spargo, B.H., Wit, E.J., Meehan, S.M., 2000. Etiologies and outcome of acute renal insufficiency in older adults: a renal biopsy study of 259 cases. Am. J. Kidney Dis. 35 (3), 433–447.

Hodgin, J.B., Bitzer, M., Wickman, L., Afshinnia, F., Wang, S.Q., O'Connor, C., Yang, Y., Meadowbrooke, C., Chowdhury, M., Kikuchi, M., Wiggins, J.E., Wiggins, R.C., 2015. Glomerular aging and focal global glomerulosclerosis: a podometric perspective. J. Am. Soc. Nephrol. 26 (12), 3162–3178. doi:10.1681/ASN.2014080752.

Jin, B., Zeng, C., Yongchun, G., Weibo, L., Xie, H., Chen, H., Liang, S., Feng, X., Jiang, S., Liu, Z., 2014. The spectrum of biopsy-proven kidney diseases in elderly Chinese patients. Nephrol. Dial. Transplant. 29 (12), 2251–2259. doi:10.1093/ndt/gfu239.

Jones, R.B., Tervaert, J.W.C., Hauser, T., Luqmani, R., Morgan, M.D., Peh, C.A., Savage, C.O., Segelmark, M., Tesar, V., Van Paassen, P., Walsh, D., Walsh, M., Westman, K., Jayne, D.R.W., 2010. Rituximab versus cyclophosphamide in ANCA-associated renal vasculitis. N. Engl. J. Med. 363 (3), 211–220. doi:10.1056/NEJMoa0909169.

KDIGO, 2021. Clinical practice guideline for the management of glomerular diseases. Kidney Int. 100 (4), S1–S276

Kitiyakara, C., Eggers, P., Kopp, J.B., 2004. Twenty-one-year trend in ESRD due to focal segmental glomerulosclerosis in the United States. Am. J. Kidney Dis. 44 (5), 815–825.

Kyle, R.A., Linos, A., Beard, C.M., Linke, R.P., Gertz, M.A., O'Fallon, W.M., Kurland, L.T., 1992. Incidence and natural history of primary systemic amyloidosis in Olmsted County, Minnesota, 1950 through 1989. Blood 79 (7), 1817–1822.

Larsen, C.P., Beggs, M.L., Wilson, J.D., Lathrop, S.L., 2016. Prevalence and organ distribution of leukocyte chemotactic factor 2 amyloidosis (ALECT2) among decedents in New Mexico. Amyloid 23 (2), 119–123. doi:10.3109/13506129.2016.1145110.

Lefaucheur, C., Stengel, B., Nochy, D., Martel, P., Hill, G.S., Jacquot, C., Rossert, J., 2006. Membranous nephropathy and cancer: epidemiologic evidence and determinants of high-risk cancer association. Kidney Int. 70 (8), 1510–1517.

Leung, N., Nasr, S.H., 2024. Update on classification, etiology, and typing of renal amyloidosis: a review. Am. J. Kidney Dis. 84 (3), 361–373.

Mak, A., Mok, C.C., Chu, W.P., To, C.H., Wong, S.N., Au, T.C., 2007. Renal damage in systemic lupus erythematosus: a comparative analysis of different age groups. Lupus 16 (1), 28–34.

Morris, A.D., Elsayed, M.E., Ponnusamy, A., Rowbottom, A., Martin, F., Geetha, D., Dhaygude, A.P., 2020. Treatment outcomes of anti-neutrophil cytoplasmic autoantibody-associated vasculitis in patients over age 75 years: a meta-analysis. Am. J. Nephrol. 51 (4), 327–335. doi:10.1159/000506532.

Muchtar, E., Dispenzieri, A., Magen, H., Grogan, M., Mauermann, M., McPhail, E.D., Kurtin, P.J., Leung, N., Buadi, F.K., Dingli, D., Kumar, S.K., Gertz, M.A., 2021. Systemic amyloidosis from A (AA) to T (ATTR): a review. J. Intern. Med. 289 (3), 268–292. doi:10.1111/joim.13169.

Muchtar, E., Gertz, M.A., Kyle, R.A., Lacy, M.Q., Dingli, D., Leung, N., Buadi, F.K., Hayman, S.R., Kapoor, P., Hwa, Y.L., Fonder, A., Hobbs, M., Gonsalves, W., Kourelis, T.V., Warsame, R., Russell, S., Lust, J.A., Lin, Y., Go, R.S., Steven Zeldenrust, S.V.R., Kumar, S.K., Dispenzieri, A., 2019. A modern primer on light chain amyloidosis in 592 patients with mass spectrometry-verified typing. Mayo Clin. Proc. 94 (3), 472–483.

O'Callaghan, C.A., Hicks, J., Doll, H., Sacks, S.H., Cameron, J.S., 2002. Characteristics and outcome of membranous nephropathy in older patients. Int. Urol. Nephrol. 33 (1), 157–165.

Oliveira-Silva, C., Marques, N., Pinho, A., Poínhos, R., Bergantim, R., Nunes, A.T., Sampaio, S., Rodrigues-Pereira, P., Silva, R., Praça, A., Frazão, J., Pestana, M., Tavares, I., 2023. Lessons from four decades of systemic amyloidosis with renal involvement. Nephron 147 (3-4), 158–169. doi:10.1159/000525675.

Passerini, P., Como, G., Viganò, E., Melis, P., Pozzi, C., Altieri, P., Ponticelli, C., 1993. Idiopathic membranous nephropathy in the elderly. Nephrol. Dial. Transplant. 8 (12), 1321–1325.

Pitcher, D., Braddon, F., Hendry, B., Mercer, A., Osmaston, K., Saleem, M.A., Steenkamp, R., Katie Wong, A.N.T., Wang, K., Gale, D.P., Barratt, J., 2023. Long-term outcomes in IgA nephropathy. Clin. J. Am. Soc. Nephrol. 18 (6), 727–738. doi:10.2215/CJN.0000000000000135.

Prakash, J., Brojen, T., Rathore, S.S., Choudhury, T.A., Gupta, T., 2012. The changing pattern of renal amyloidosis in Indian subcontinent: two decades of experience from a single center. Ren. Fail. 34 (10), 1212–1216. doi:10.3109/0886022X.2012.723514.

Rosenberg, A.Z., Kopp, J.B., 2017. Focal segmental glomerulosclerosis. Clin. J. Am. Soc. Nephrol. 12 (3), 502–517. doi:10.2215/CJN.05960616.

Rout, R., Hashmi, M.F., Baradhi, K.M., 2024. Focal Segmental Glomerulosclerosis Treasure Island. StatPearls Publishing, FL.

Rovenský, J., Tuchynová, A., 2008. Systemic lupus erythematosus in the elderly. Autoimmun. Rev. 7 (3), 235–239. doi:10.1016/j.autrev.2007.11.014.

Said, S.M., Sethi, S., Valeri, A.M., Chang, A., Nast, C.C., Krahl, L., Molloy, P., Barry, M., Fidler, M.E., Cornell, L.D., Leung, N., Vrana, J.A., Theis, J.D., Dogan, A., Nasr, S.H., 2014. Characterization and outcomes of renal leukocyte chemotactic factor 2-associated amyloidosis. Kidney Int. 86 (2), 370–377. doi:10.1038/ki.2013.558.

Said, S.M., Sethi, S., Valeri, A.M., Leung, N., Cornell, L.D., Fidler, M.E., Hernandez, L.H., Vrana, J.A., Theis, J.D., Quint, P.S., Dogan, A., Nasr, S.H., 2013. Renal amyloidosis: origin and clinicopathologic correlations of 474 recent cases. Clin. J. Am. Soc. Nephrol. 8 (9), 1515–1523. doi:10.2215/CJN.10491012.

Sethi, S., Beck, L.H., Glassock, R.J., Haas, M., De Vriese, A.S., Caza, T.N., Hoxha, E., Lambeau, G., Tomas, N.M., Madden, B., Debiec, H., D'Agati, V.D., Alexander, M.P., Amer, H., Appel, G.B., Barbour, S.J., Caravaca-Fontan, F., Cattran, D.C., Moura, M.C., D'Avila, D.O., Eick, R.G., Garovic, V.D., Greene, E.L., Hernandez, L.P.H., Jennette, J.C., Lieske, J.C., Markowitz, G.S., Nath, K.A., Nasr, S.H., Nast, C.C., Pani, A., Praga, M., Remuzzi, G., Rennke, H.G., Ruggenenti, P., Roccatello, D., Soler, M.J., Specks, U., Stahl, R.A.K., Singh, R.D., Theis, J.D., Velosa, J.A., Wetzels, J.F.M., Winearls, C.G., Yandian, F., Zand, L., Ronco, P., Fervenza, F.C., 2023. Mayo clinic consensus report on membranous nephropathy: proposal for a novel classification. Mayo Clin. Proc. 98 (11), 1671–1684. doi:10.1016/j.mayocp.2023.08.006.

Sevillano, A.M., Diaz, M., Caravaca-Fontán, F., Barrios, C., Bernis, C., Cabrera, J., Calviño, J., Castillo, L., Cobelo, C., Delgado-Mallén, P., Espinosa, M., Fernandez-Juarez, G., Fernandez-Reyes, M.J., Garcia-Osuna, R., Garcia, P., Goicoechea, M., Gonzalez-Cabrera, F., Guzmán, D.A., Heras, M., Martín-Reyes, G., Martinez, A., Olea, T., Peña, J.K., Quintana, L.F., Rabasco, C., López Revuelta, K., Rodas, L., Rodriguez-Mendiola, N., Rodriguez, E., Miguel, L.S., de la Nieta, M.D.S., Shabaka, A., Sierra, M., Valera, A., Velo, M., Verde, E., Ballarin, J., Noboa, O., Moreno, J.A., Gutiérrez, E., Praga, M., 2019. IgA nephropathy in elderly patients. Clin. J. Am. Soc. Nephrol. 14 (8), 1183–1192. doi:10.2215/CJN.13251118.

Shankland, S.J., Wang, Y., Shaw, A.S., Vaughan, J.C., Pippin, J.W., Wessely, O., 2021. Podocyte aging: why and how getting old matters. J. Am. Soc. Nephrol. 32 (11), 2697–2713. doi:10.1681/ASN.2021050614.

Sharma, H., Kaul, A., Mohakuda, S.S., Manas Ranjan Behera, D.S.B., Agrawal, V., Agarwal, V., Prasad, N., Singh, A., Patel, M.R., 2023. Clinicopathologic characteristics and outcomes of late onset lupus nephritis: a single centre experience. Rheumatol. Int. 43 (10), 1849–1858. doi:10.1007/s00296-023-05357-8.

Shimazaki, C., Hata, H., Iida, S., Ueda, M., Katoh, N., Sekijima, Y., Ikeda, S., Yazaki, M., Fukushima, W., Ando, Y., 2018. Nationwide survey of 741 patients with systemic amyloid light-chain amyloidosis in Japan. Intern. Med. 57 (2), 181–187. doi:10.2169/internalmedicine.9206-17.

Stone, J.H., Merkel, P.A., Spiera, R., Seo, P., Langford, C.A., Hoffman, G.S., Kallenberg, C.G.M., Clair, W.S., Turkiewicz, A., Tchao, N.K., Webber, L., Ding, L., Sejismundo, L.P., Mieras, K., Weitzenkamp, D., Ikle, D., Seyfert-Margolis, V., Mueller, M., Brunetta, P., Allen, N.B., Fervenza, F.C., Geetha, D., Keogh, K.A., Kissin, E.Y., Monach, P.A., Peikert, T., Stegeman, C., Ytterberg, S.R., Specks, U., 2010. Rituximab versus cyclophosphamide for ANCA-associated vasculitis. N. Engl. J. Med. 363 (3), 221–232. doi:10.1056/NEJMoa0909905.

Sumnu, A., Gursu, M., Ozturk, S., 2015. Primary glomerular diseases in the elderly. World J. Nephrol. 4 (2), 263–270. doi:10.5527/wjn.v4.i2.263.

Tang, Z., Chen, D., Yang, S., Zhang, H., Weixin, H., Liu, Z., Leishi, L., 2011. Late onset lupus nephritis: analysis of clinical manifestations and renal pathological features in Chinese patients. Rheumatol. Int. 31 (12), 1625–1629. doi:10.1007/s00296-010-1536-9.

Tarr, T., Dérfalvi, B., Győri, N., Szántó, A., Siminszky, Z., Malik, A., Szabó, A.J., Szegedi, G., Zeher, M., 2015. Similarities and differences between pediatric and adult patients with systemic lupus erythematosus. Lupus 24 (8), 796–803. doi:10.1177/0961203314563817.

Thomas, D.B., Franceschini, N., Hogan, S.L., Holder, S.T., Jennette, C.E., Falk, R.J., Jennette, J.C., 2006. Clinical and pathologic characteristics of focal segmental glomerulosclerosis pathologic variants. Kidney Int. 69 (5), 920–926.

Waldman, R.J.C.M., Valeri, A., Busch, J., Stokes, B., Markowitz, G., D'Agati, V., Appel, G., 2007. Adult minimal-change disease: clinical characteristics, treatment, and outcomes. Clin. J. Am. Soc. Nephrol. 2 (3), 445–453.

Wenderfer, S.E., Gaut, J.P., 2017. Glomerular diseases in children. Adv. Chronic Kidney Dis. 24 (6), 364–371.

Wiggins, J.E., 2012. Aging in the glomerulus. J. Gerontol. A Biol. Sci. Med. Sci. 67 (12), 1358–1364. doi:10.1093/gerona/gls157.

Windpessl, M., Odler, B., Bajema, I.M., Geetha, D., Säemann, M., Lee, J.M., Vaglio, A., Kronbichler, A., 2022. Glomerular diseases across lifespan: key differences in diagnostic and therapeutic approaches. Semin. Nephrol. 43 (4).

Yamaguchi, M., Ando, M., Yamamoto, R., Akiyama, S., Kato, S., Katsuno, T., Kosugi, T., Sato, W., Tsuboi, N., Yasuda, Y., Mizuno, M., Ito, Y., Matsuo, S., Maruyama, S., 2014. Patient age and the prognosis of idiopathic membranous nephropathy. PloS One 9 (10). doi:10.1371/journal.pone.0110376.

Zent, R., Nagai, R., Cattran, D.C., 1997. Idiopathic membranous nephropathy in the elderly: a comparative study. Am. J. Kidney Dis. 29 (2), 200–206.

CHAPTER

19

Peripheral vascular disease

Eric Peden[a], Omodele Durojaye[a,b], and Brianna Whithorn[a]

[a]Vascular Surgery, Houston Methodist Hospital, Houston, TX, United States

[b]Department of Cardiovascular Surgery, Houston Methodist Hospital, Houston, TX, United States

Introduction: Overview of atherosclerosis and peripheral artery disease in the elderly

Peripheral arterial disease (PAD) is characterized by an atherosclerotic stenosis or blockage of arteries in the lower extremities. Due to the increasing burden of chronic disease in older patient populations, PAD affects 8.5 million people in the United States and about 230 million worldwide, disproportionately affecting 20%–26% of patients over 80 years of age (Polonsky and McDermott, 2021; Aronow, 2004). It is especially important because it is linked to increased morbidity and mortality.

In patients with no previous history of lower-extremity revascularization, PAD is defined by an ankle-brachial index (ABI) of <0.90. Typically, it presents with exercise-induced calf pain (Treat-Jacobson et al., 2019). This can have a tangible effect on elderly patients, as PAD can be functionally impairing, leading to reduced quality of life and limiting their ability to perform their normal daily activities, such as meeting basic needs, walking longer distances, and maintaining gait speed (Kuo and Yu, 2008). Poor management of PAD can lead to serious complications, such as arterial insufficiency ulcers, chronic limb-threatening ischemia, and amputation (Aronow, 2004).

Furthermore, PAD is associated with an increased risk of cardiovascular events, including myocardial infarction and stroke, as well as all-cause and cardiovascular mortality (Polonsky and McDermott, 2021; Aronow, 2004). Therefore PAD in the elderly is a common yet serious condition that requires comprehensive management to reduce cardiovascular risks and improve functional outcomes.

In elderly patients, the prevalence of PAD increases with age and the severity of chronic kidney disease (CKD). The ACC/AHA Guidelines determined that up to 25% of patients with CKD have PAD, rising to 45% among those patients on dialysis due to end-stage kidney disease (ESKD) (Gornik et al., 2024). When stratified by age groups, PAD was found in 7% of individuals aged 60–69, 12.5% of those aged 70–79, and 23.2% of those aged 80 and older,

Aging and the Kidney
https://doi.org/10.1016/B978-0-443-34069-7.00023-9

with and without CKD. A similar trend is likely observed in elderly CKD patients, which may be attributed to the compounding risk factors associated with advanced age and CKD (Ostchega et al., 2007). The concentration of PAD in the elderly CKD population is seen in the NEFRONA study, which reported a PAD prevalence of 28% in CKD patients compared to 12.3% in non-CKD controls (Arroyo et al., 2017). In particularly susceptible patient populations, such as dialysis patients, research highlights PAD prevalence ranging from 17% to 48%, with hemodialysis patients exhibiting higher rates (21.8%) compared to those on peritoneal dialysis (4.8%) (Lee et al., 2012).

Epidemiology and impact

CKD in elderly populations exhibits significant variability across age, gender, ethnicity, and geographic factors. According to the Kidney Disease: Improving Global Outcomes (KDIGO) 2024 Clinical Practice Guideline, CKD prevalence increases with advancing age, particularly in those over 75 years old (Stevens et al., 2024). Gender differences are evident, as CKD is more common in women (12.6%) compared to men (9.7%). However, men face a greater risk of progression to ESKD, despite the higher lifetime risk of CKD stages 3–5 observed in women (Moyer, 2012).

Ethnic disparities documented in the literature show that African Americans are three to five times more likely to develop ESKD, even though they experience a similar CKD prevalence (11.2%) compared to Whites (11.6%) (Cheung et al., 2023). This may potentially be linked to genetic predispositions, particularly variants of the APOL1 gene, which contribute to the higher CKD risk observed in African Americans. In addition, elevated albuminuria has been linked to a greater risk of disease progression in Black individuals as compared to White individuals (Cheung et al., 2023). In non-Hispanic Black individuals, the lifetime risk of ESKD is higher compared to other ethnic groups, with rates of 8.0% for men and 6.8% for women (Albertus et al., 2016). Geographically, the "stroke belt" region of the southeastern United States has higher CKD prevalence, likely due to exacerbation of risk factors such as environmental, socioeconomic, and access-related disparities (Cheung et al., 2023).

PAD increases the burden of CKD in elderly patients, with a 2.5 times higher frequency of myocardial infarction and nearly three times higher in-hospital mortality compared to those without CKD (Go et al., 2005; Lüders et al., 2017). Lower limb amputations are 10–12 times more common in dialysis patients with PAD compared to those with normal kidney function (Gornik et al., 2024). The morbidity and mortality associated with CKD are considerable, as affected individuals face increased risks for cardiovascular disease, fractures, infections, and cognitive impairments. Mortality rates are particularly high among those with lower estimated glomerular filtration rate (eGFR) levels (Stengel et al., 2011).

Factors affecting diagnosis

Generally, the history and physical assessment are essential for diagnosing patients with PAD. ABI is a widely used measurement for evaluating PAD severity. Exercise ABI testing is recommended for patients exhibiting symptoms suggestive of PAD with normal or borderline ABI values (Conte et al., 2015). Tests such as segmental pressures, Doppler waveforms, and pulse volume recordings are alternative noninvasive physiological tests that may be used to further characterize symptoms when ABI is nondiagnostic (Sibley et al., 2017).

PAD diagnosis in elderly patients is less straightforward because ABI values may not accurately reflect the true severity of the disease. Factors such as vascular calcification, limitations of diagnostic tools, and atypical presentations can influence the accuracy of diagnostic criteria.

ABI values can be falsely elevated in elderly patients due to medial arterial calcifications. This calcification reduces the reliability of noninvasive diagnostic tools such as Doppler ultrasonography. Thus, when ABI values exceed 1.4, alternative assessments such as the toe-brachial index (TBI) and tibial waveform analysis are recommended. Other methods, such as CT angiography and magnetic resonance angiography (MRA), are useful for detailed evaluation. In patients with CKD, however, the risk of contrast-induced nephropathy should be assessed prior to imaging. Since these diagnostic tools may not be widely accessible or may be costly, they can lead to missed or delayed diagnoses.

High prevalence of comorbidities, such as diabetes mellitus and cardiovascular disease, can lead to the attribution of PAD symptoms to neuropathy and infections. Neuropathy can mask typical symptoms of claudication, and reduced mobility in the elderly can obscure exertion-related complaints (Aronow, 2004).

Unique challenges in performing research

Conducting research with a more vulnerable population, such as elderly patients, poses unique challenges ethically, experimentally, and logistically. Oftentimes, data involving elderly populations show worse outcomes, and applications of studies are limited in scope due to the need to maximize control over select variables. For these reasons, the elderly remain underrepresented in clinical studies, where researchers must pay close attention to addressing challenges and improving care and potential outcomes.

In clinical trials involving adults, researchers frequently limit the inclusion criteria by age and exclude those over 75. This practice is rationalized by concerns about increased comorbidities, frailty, logistical complexities, and the desire to increase the generalizability of their findings (Molitch et al., 2015; Jha et al., 2013). For example, prevalent conditions such as frailty and sarcopenia in elderly CKD patients can act as confounding variables and influence study outcomes by increasing the risk of morbidity and mortality (Go et al., 2005; Pizzarelli et al., 2023). Furthermore, the complex progression and categorization of CKD patients prevent the holistic development of standardized inclusion criteria (Kim and Caine, 2002; Butler et al., 2025).

Ethically, research among patient populations with a higher prevalence of cognitive impairments, such as dementia, raises concerns about their ability to provide informed consent and thus participate in trials (Rid et al., 2010). High-risk yet potentially treatable patients are usually excluded due to regulatory agencies' tendency to be more risk-averse.

Clinically, elderly patients are more likely to present with atypical symptoms, leading to misdiagnosis or exclusion/delay in studies. The dangers of polypharmacy to this population require careful drug dosing, further complicating trial protocols (Lattanzio et al., 2015). When examining outcomes of interventional studies in elderly CKD patients, this population experiences higher mortality rates due to an increased frequency of cardiovascular events and infections. As the need for individualized treatment regimens increases in older patients, recommended guidelines become less reliable due to smaller sample sizes, high dropout rates from health decline, and difficulty in establishing meaningful endpoints such as frailty, quality of life, and functional capacity.

Logistically, study enrollment and retention are limited by transportation burdens, additional caregiver requirements, and complex study protocols. Increasing reliance on digital devices and tools for data collection can lead to inaccurate or incomplete patient-provided data due to a lack of familiarity with and access to new technologies. Many elderly patients are also financially restricted to a fixed monthly income and are unable to support additional out-of-pocket travel costs, ultimately deterring participation.

To make the studies more applicable to a broader range of patients and reflect current populations, researchers should widen the inclusion age range and comorbidity criteria, consider a heterogeneous elderly CKD population, and focus on patient-based outcomes. Providing logistical and financial support can increase retention and recruitment. Analysis based on stratification criteria such as frailty and age can aid in clarifying the effects of treatment in a diverse group (Heller et al., 2014; Pizzarelli et al., 2023). By addressing these hurdles, researchers may produce results that are both robust and clinically meaningful, ultimately improving care in this growing demographic.

Progression of PAD and atherosclerosis

The pathophysiology of atherosclerosis is relatively well established and documented in the literature. This process can be outlined in a few general phases:

- Endothelial dysfunction triggers the first step of the atherosclerotic pathway. Damage to the endothelial surface allows the accumulation of apoB-containing lipoproteins (LDL, VLDL, and apoE remnants) in the subendothelial space. These retained lipoproteins are then oxidized by myeloperoxidase, lipoxygenase, and reactive oxygen species, along with other atherogenic factors that activate endothelial cells.
- In response to the higher levels of oxidized LDLs, monocytes transmigrate to the site using chemoattractants (MCP-1) produced by endothelial cells and anchor to the intimal space with adhesion molecules such as selectins and VCAM-1. Additional cells, including dendritic cells, mast cells, regulatory T cells, and Helper T1 cells, are also recruited by activated endothelial cells.
- The migrated monocytes transform into inflammatory M1 macrophages and utilize unique receptors to internalize VLDL, LDL, and apoE remnants, becoming foam cells. Simultaneously, these macrophages further amplify inflammatory signaling pathways to enhance cell recruitment and LDL modification.
- As the lesion grows and stabilizes into a well-established calcified plaque, dead cells accumulate within the lesion, forming a necrotic area due to poor clearance and increased apoptotic activity. This calcification plays a major role in determining rupture risk and plaque stability.

- To keep the plaque isolated from the circulating blood and protect against rupture, a fibrous cap forms over the plaque. This cap is composed of collagen and vascular smooth muscle cells (VSMCs) and may be degraded by MMPs, increased calcifications, and VSMC death. In the event of a rupture, the plaque may act as an embolus and lodge in the coronary arteries or cerebral vasculature (Linton et al., 2009).

Specific to this population, endothelial dysfunction is aggravated by uremic toxins, reduced nitric oxide availability, and oxidative stress (London et al., 2005). Higher levels of inflammation increase cytokine levels, such as tumor necrosis factor-alpha (TNF-α) and interleukin-6 (IL-6), expediting plaque formation (Himmelfarb et al., 2002). CKD further contributes to vascular calcification and plaque rigidity from prolonged mineral disturbances, such as hyperphosphatemia, increased ferritin, lower 25(OH) vitamin D levels, and secondary hyperparathyroidism (Gracia et al., 2016). CKD-associated anemia intensifies ischemic complications by compromising oxygen delivery and inhibiting angiogenesis (Norgren et al., 2007). Other traditional risk factors, such as hypertension, diabetes, and smoking, have additive effects that lead to rapid and unstable plaque formation, increasing the risk of rupture and subsequent thrombotic events (London et al., 2005; Gracia et al., 2016).

Altogether, the progression of atherosclerosis and PAD in elderly CKD patients is driven by both traditional and CKD-specific risk factors. The NEFRONA study and other research have highlighted the significant contributions of CKD-associated abnormalities in mineral metabolism, inflammation, and oxidative stress to these conditions (Gracia et al., 2016). The ACC/AHA identifies CKD as a significant risk amplifier for adverse cardiovascular and limb-related outcomes in PAD patients, emphasizing the need for aggressive management of cardiovascular risk factors to improve outcomes (Gornik et al., 2024).

Clinical progression with corresponding rates of intervention

Diagnostic tools, ranging from clinical assessment and ABI to CT angiography, help describe the clinical progression of chronic limb-threatening ischemia (CLTI). Classification systems, such as the Rutherford or Fontaine systems, categorize patients based on symptom severity and clinical presentation. This ultimately guides clinicians in management and options for interventions.

The Rutherford classification for CLTI is summarized below (Hardman et al., 2014):

- Stage 0 (asymptomatic): Management typically involves conservative approaches, such as medical therapy and risk factor control, with limited data suggesting that only a few patients require invasive intervention at this stage.
- Stage 1 (mild claudication): Minor exercise-induced leg pain that is relieved by rest.
- Stage 2 (moderate claudication): More severe pain limits walking distances. Atypically presenting symptoms, due to neuropathy or reduced physical activity, may occur in CKD patients. Management strategies include supervised exercise programs and medical therapies, with revascularization considered for refractory cases. Approximately 10%–15% of patients with intermittent claudication progress to requiring invasive interventions and revascularization due to worsening symptoms or functional impairment (Lüders et al., 2016).

- Stage 3 (severe claudication): Significant impact on mobility; pain occurs after very short distances or at rest.
- Stage 4 (ischemic rest pain): Limb-threatening ischemia presenting with pain at rest due to inadequate blood flow. Management of CLTI typically requires aggressive approaches, including wound care, infection control, and revascularization, with amputation considered for severe cases. Approximately 20%–40% of CLTI patients undergo revascularization, while major amputations occur in 26%–40% of cases (Lüders et al., 2016).
- Stage 5 (minor tissue loss): Nonhealing ulcers or focal gangrene.
- Stage 6 (major tissue loss): Extensive gangrene or nonhealing wounds, potentially leading to amputation.

Likewise, in the setting of acute limb ischemia (ALI), typically resulting from a sudden embolic or thrombotic event, the Rutherford Classification for ALI categorizes the patient's clinical presentation and helps to guide management. These patients experience a sudden onset of ischemic symptoms, such as severe pain, pallor, and pulselessness. Thirty to fifty percent of CKD patients with ALI face higher risks than the general population and typically require immediate revascularization, with in-hospital mortality rates reaching as high as 16.4% (Gornik et al., 2024; Lüders et al., 2016).

Overall, CKD significantly amplifies the consequences of PAD, causing 1.8 times higher amputation rates and doubling in-hospital mortality of patients (7.8% vs. 4.0%) compared to non-CKD patients, increasing in a stepwise fashion with increasingly advanced disease stages. Revascularization rates in CKD patients are lower than in non-CKD patients, likely due to higher procedural risks. The need for major amputation and hospitalizations increases with CKD severity, underscoring the critical interplay between these conditions and the necessity for specialized management strategies (Lüders et al., 2016).

Impact of CKD on PAD progression

Kidney disease has emerged as an independent risk factor for the development and progression of PAD. A metaanalysis comprising 817,084 individuals and 21 international cohorts demonstrated a strong association between PAD incidence with reduced eGFR and increased albuminuria (Matsushita et al., 2017). Individuals with PAD and an eGFR of 45 mL/min/1.73 m^2 increased their risk of PAD by 22% compared to those with an eGFR of 95 mL/min/1.73 m^2. For individuals with PAD and an eGFR of 15 mL/min/1.73 m^2, the risk rose by more than 100% (Matsushita et al., 2017). Similarly, the ARIC Study found a significant association between PAD and the progression of kidney disease, with PAD patients showing a higher risk of developing ESKD (Wattanakit et al., 2007). Taken together, these findings provide support for a bidirectional relationship between CKD and PAD, thereby emphasizing the need for early detection and management among high-risk populations.

Within the PAD patient population, those with CKD are associated with very poor clinical outcomes, including an increased risk of amputation, restenosis after revascularization, and further progression to CLTI. The metaanalysis showed that albuminuria is particularly predictive of poor outcomes, with a 50% increased risk for PAD at an albumin-to-creatinine ratio

(ACR) of 30 mg/g and a 2.3-times higher risk at an ACR of 300 mg/g (Matsushita et al., 2017). The association of albuminuria with amputation was particularly remarkable, with a 3.7-times increase in lower limb amputation in individuals with an ACR ≥ 300 mg/g (Matsushita et al., 2017). These outcomes suggest that albuminuria may be a strong indicator to identify PAD patients at the highest risk for severe complications.

Lastly, in CKD patients undergoing revascularization procedures such as angioplasty or bypass surgery, there is a higher incidence of restenosis and graft failure, diminishing the long-term benefits of such interventions (Kumada et al., 2008; Wattanakit et al., 2007). Furthermore, the transition from simple PAD to CLTI occurs at a much faster pace in CKD patients, likely due to the interactive effects of endothelial dysfunction, inherently poor healing, and microvascular disease (Matsushita et al., 2017).

Histologic differences

Distinct patterns of calcification in CKD patients

In PAD patients, distinct histological calcification may be observed between those with and without CKD. Vascular calcification in CKD patients is notably accelerated through disruptions in mineral metabolism, endothelial dysfunction patterns of the vasculature, and chronic inflammation. Two predominant forms of vascular calcification are medial arterial calcification (MAC) and intimal arterial calcification (IAC), with some patients exhibiting a combination of both. See Fig. 19.1.

Medial arterial calcification is particularly notable in dialysis patients with ESKD (Moe et al., 2002). Histologically, MAC is characterized by diffuse circumferential calcium deposits in the tunica media that increase artery stiffness while preserving lumen size. Immunohistochemical studies show the presence of bone matrix proteins such as bone sialoprotein, osteopontin, and alkaline phosphatase (Moe et al., 2002). This suggests that the calcification process in CKD mimics osteogenesis as opposed to passive mineral deposition. This process is facilitated by VSMC transdifferentiation into osteoblast-like cells, which actively contribute to the formation of calcified deposits (Fayed et al., 2019). This is further supported by studies analyzing intraoperative arterial biopsies in CKD patients, confirming that intimal fibrosis, rather than lipid-laden plaques, is the predominant histological feature of PAD in this population (Fayed et al., 2019). In contrast, isolated arterial calcification (IAC) is characterized by patchy calcification within atherosclerotic plaques and presents with similar pathophysiology to classic atherosclerosis, displaying lipid accumulation, inflammatory cell infiltration, and foam cell formation (O'Neill et al., 2015).

For patients exhibiting mixed arterial calcification within a single vascular segment, this pattern is associated with more severe vascular stiffness, poor response to revascularization procedures, and a higher risk of amputation (Fayed et al., 2019). Specifically, the iliac and femoral arteries demonstrate more intimal calcification, while the smaller/medium-sized arteries display more medial calcification. Due to the pattern of the vascular lesions, this suggests that traditional means of preventing atherosclerosis in this population may be less effective (O'Neill et al., 2015).

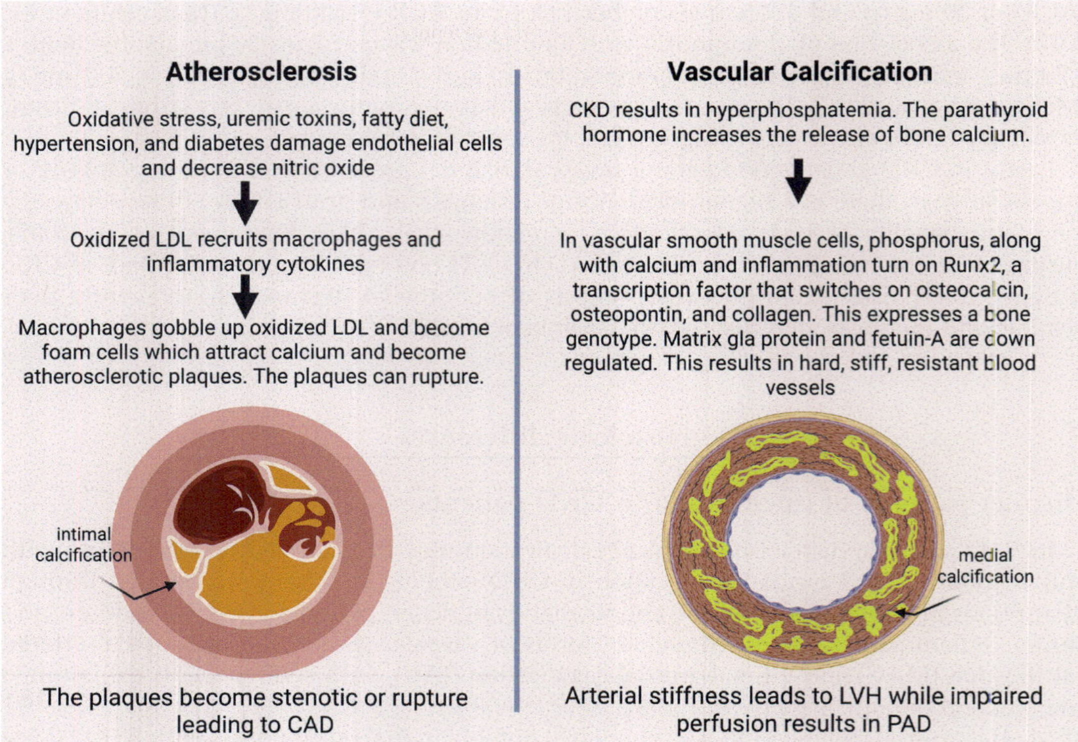

FIG. 19.1 Comparison of atherosclerosis and vascular calcification. This figure illustrates two pathological processes: atherosclerosis and vascular calcification. Atherosclerosis, characterized by the accumulation of oxidized LDL by macrophages, can lead to coronary artery disease (CAD) through plaque formation and potential rupture. In contrast, vascular calcification is linked to chronic kidney disease (CKD) and is driven by factors such as hyperphosphatemia, which induces bone-like deposition in vascular smooth muscle cells, resulting in arterial stiffness and heart failure. *Created in BioRender. Fadem, S. 2025.*

Amputation rates in elderly CKD patients with PAD

Statistics and risk factors

There are several risk factors associated with PAD, which include smoking/nicotine use, familial atherosclerosis, diabetes, hyperlipidemia, hypertension, and chronic kidney disease. The prevalence of PAD is notably higher in those with renal disease, reaching 24%–37% compared to the overall estimated US prevalence of PAD, which is around 7% (Garimella et al., 2012). In addition to the increased risk of PAD in CKD, the severity of PAD is directly correlated with higher stages of CKD and is particularly severe for patients requiring hemodialysis. In a crossover study, patients with end-stage kidney disease (ESKD) who also have PAD were significantly older (67 ± 10 years vs. 62 ± 11 years) and more likely to have other PAD risk factors, such as diabetes mellitus and anemia. They had significantly lower serum albumin levels, higher glucose values, C-reactive protein levels, and lower dialysis adequacy kinetics than the patients without PAD (Aščerić et al., 2019). Though these concurrent conditions do exist, the presence of renal disease alone is a poor prognostic factor for PAD-associated outcomes, such as failed limb revascularization.

One of the concerns in all patients with PAD is limb salvage, and when all revascularization options have been exhausted, major lower extremity amputation is often necessary and includes below-the-knee amputation, above-the-knee amputation, or, in extreme cases, hip disarticulation—depending on the level and severity of the disease. A higher amputation level required portends worse quality of life, immobility, and overall mortality. According to a large cohort study by Smilowitz et al., patients with concurrent CKD and PAD had an adjusted odds ratio of 1.33 when major lower extremity amputation was compared between CKD patients and those with normal renal function (Smilowitz et al., 2020). Beyond the two categories of CKD vs. no CKD, the risk of major lower extremity amputation increases as eGFR decreases and is highest in patients requiring renal replacement therapy.

Factors influencing amputation risk

Patients with CKD are at heightened risk of cardiovascular events and more severe PAD, with higher rates of intervention and amputation. While there is clearly an increased risk of amputation in patients with CKD, data and understanding of the procedures and treatments leading up to amputation are mixed. For example, a large cohort study by Lüders et al. noted significantly fewer revascularization procedures for patients with CKD compared to patients without CKD. In addition, there was an inverse correlation between CKD stage and the rate of revascularization, despite worse disease in the CKD patients. This study also noted a nearly doubled rate of lower extremity amputation in CKD patients compared to their counterparts with normal renal function during their index hospitalization (Lüders et al., 2016). Contrary to Lüders team's findings, a large retrospective cohort study by Subramanian et al. found that there was an increased likelihood of specialty care and similar rates of revascularization procedures in CKD patients in the 1 year leading up to amputation compared to their counterparts with normal GFR (Subramanian et al., 2021).

In addition to the diagnosis and the number of revascularization attempts, the pattern of disease must be considered. In general, intimal calcification is often seen in patients with atherosclerotic disease and is associated with risk factors such as diabetes, hyperlipidemia, hypertension, and tobacco use. Intimal calcification distribution often involves areas of change in diameter or turbulent flow, such as bifurcations, and does not appear to be caused by CKD, though impaired renal function may potentiate the process. In contrast to this "normal" PAD disease process, medial calcification is more prevalent in PAD patients with CKD, and the disease pattern is more widespread, affecting vessels often spared by atherosclerotic disease, such as small vessels. Development of medial calcification is secondary to dysregulated calcium-phosphate metabolism and deposition into the arterial wall. This process, accompanied by intimal narrowing due to concurrent atherosclerosis, inhibits compensatory mechanisms while at the same time increasing afterload on the heart, leading to left ventricular hypertrophy. Rather than just causing stenosis, medial calcification decreases vessel compliance, inhibiting its innate compensatory mechanisms and making it less elastic. These patients often have increased postprocedural complications and failed limb salvage (Lanzer et al., 2025).

Early diagnosis and treatment for preventing amputations

While there is a prevalence of PAD in the CKD population, classic symptoms such as claudication are often absent, and the development of wounds is therefore higher. Despite more severe and common PAD in CKD patients, the rate of revascularization procedures is not proportionally higher. This is not due to a lack of diagnostic criteria. In a large observational study, patients with CKD had higher rates of specialty care utilization and underwent diagnostic evaluations, with similar rates of revascularization attempts. As noted previously, there is an increased occurrence of adverse events and failed revascularization in those with CKD compared to those with normal renal function (Subramanian et al., 2021).

Since PAD in CKD patients often does not present with typical claudication, a low threshold for screening is advisable, along with controlling or eliminating concurrent risk factors such as hyperglycemia, smoking, or unattended wounds. The National Kidney Foundation's Kidney Disease Outcomes Initiative (KDOQI) guidelines recommend that patients undergo screening for PAD upon initiation of renal replacement therapy (Garimella and Hirsch, 2014; Garimella et al., 2012). Noninvasive studies are a mainstay for monitoring and screening for PAD. It is important to note that calcification in vessels often produces falsely elevated ABIs. However, as understanding of the disease process improves, so does the interpretation of these studies. As with any patient with PAD, management must be individualized (Table 19.1).

TABLE 19.1 Making the diagnosis of peripheral vascular disease.

Peripheral vascular disease diagnostic tools		
Diagnostic TOOL	**Use/finding**	**Limitations in CKD/elderly**
History & physical exam	Claudication, resting pain, ulcers, and decreased pulses	Atypical symptoms in CKD and the elderly (neuropathy, reduced mobility)
ABI (Ankle-Brachial Index)	ABI < 0.9 = PAD; ABI > 1.4 suggests noncompressible vessels	Medial calcification in CKD can lead to false elevation
Toe-brachial index (TBI) preferred in CKD and diabetics	Useful if ABI > 1.4	Toe vessels are less calcified in PAD
Doppler waveforms/ segmental pressures/pulse volume recordings	Characterize perfusion patterns	Reduced accuracy with severe calcification
Duplex ultrasound	Noninvasive arterial flow imaging	Operator dependent
Computed tomography angiography (CTA) and magnetic resonance angiography (MRA)	Detailed arterial anatomy, revascularization planning	Require either iodinated contrast, which can cause acute kidney injury, or gadolinium (Gd); early Gd compounds caused nephrogenic systemic fibrosis, though this is rare now; MRA is preferred in CKD
Plain X-ray/CT (noncontrast)	Detects vascular calcification	Does not quantify functional perfusion
Histology (biopsy, rare)	Differentiates intimal vs medial calcification	Rarely performed in clinical practice

Medical management of PAD in elderly CKD patients

Pharmacological interventions

The mainstay of medical management of PAD revolves around decreasing the effects of risk factors and improving functional capacity. This includes the management of modifiable risk factors such as dyslipidemia (with a goal of LDL < 70 and HDL > 40), glycemic control (oral regimen vs. insulin), control of hypertension (first-line treatment is ACE inhibitors), smoking cessation, and participation in a PAD walking program. A PAD walking program is a monitored regimen that tracks the distance a patient can walk without claudication and incrementally increases this distance over time (Conte et al., 2015). The addition of an antiplatelet agent has been found to be beneficial in this population. In addition, cilostazol, a phosphodiesterase-3 inhibitor, is often used in conjunction with the above and has both antiplatelet and vasodilatory effects, which may increase a patient's functional capacity. Due to the mechanism of action of cilostazol, however, heart failure is a contraindication for its use. Therefore its use may be limited in higher stages of CKD and in ESKD, as heart failure may be a coexisting condition. The data and understanding of these treatments and their effects on the disease process of PAD in those with concurrent CKD are limited. For patients with varying stages of renal disease, the deposition of calcium phosphate into the media as a result of dysregulated metabolism prompts investigations into managing this process. There is no clear evidence supporting the slowing or regression of this process. However, agents of potential interest include calcimimetics, phosphate binders, magnesium supplementation, and vitamin K. These adjuncts require further investigation and are not part of the treatment regimen for managing PAD (Nelson et al., 2020).

Management recommendations

Differences in lipid management and other medications

Dyslipidemia is exceedingly common in patients with CKD and ESKD and is a contributing factor to CV-related events. According to the American Heart Association Guidelines, the goal for LDL is < 70 mg/dL. The initial medical management is generally a high-intensity statin as long as it is tolerated. If LDL remains > 70 mg/dL. Additional therapies may be added, such as PCSK9 inhibitors or ezetimibe (Grundy et al., 2019). In contrast, the European Society of Cardiology includes CKD as a risk modifier, classifying patients with moderate CKD (GFR 30–59 mL/min) as "high risk," who, like in the AHA guidelines, have an LDL goal of < 70 mg/dL. Patients with severe CKD (GFR < 30 mL/min) are also recommended to receive statin therapy, with adjunct therapy (e.g., ezetimibe or PCSK9 inhibitors) as needed (Gornik et al., 2024). Statin therapy has not been shown to be effective in ESKD (Wanner et al., 2005).

Surgical outcomes in elderly CKD patients versus nonrenal patients

When medical management fails or there is advanced PAD involving rest pain or tissue loss, intervention is often necessary. There are many options for revascularization, ranging from open surgery, including bypass creation and endarterectomy, to endovascular approaches. Oftentimes, the calcification of arteries in CKD patients makes open surgery quite difficult, and even in cases where this is accomplished, both short- and long-term outcomes in severe CKD patients differ from those with mild CKD. In a retrospective analysis of the American College of Surgeons National Surgical Quality Improvement Program (NSQIP) database involving patients with CKD and chronic limb-threatening ischemia (CLTI), 6978 patients had undergone infrainguinal lower extremity arterial bypass during their study period. Their outcomes were compared based on CKD stage—Stage 3 or less, Stage 4–5, and ESKD (Ambur et al., 2019). Unfavorable outcomes were observed more frequently in the severe CKD and HD group, including graft failure (OR 1.67) in the severe CKD group (Ambur et al., 2019).

Endovascular outcomes in elderly CKD patients versus nonrenal patients

Comparative outcomes

Per the TASC II classifications of femoropopliteal disease, endovascular management is recommended for patients with Type A or B lesions and for high surgical risk patients with Type C lesions (Norgren et al., 2007). This primarily incorporates stenting, balloon angioplasty, and/or, less commonly, atherectomy. The success of the intervention, as determined by the subjective resolution of symptoms and the objective timeframe of patency, depends on many factors, including the patient's overall health and activity level. Studies that analyzed the trend between endovascular interventions over time, major amputation rates, and lower extremity bypass surgeries demonstrated a three-fold increase in endovascular management with a simultaneous decrease in major amputations (Goodney et al., 2009; Clair et al., 2021). However, these studies, like many other studies on endovascular management of PAD, tend to exclude patients with ESKD or do not provide multivariate analysis of patients with CKD.

Balloon angioplasty is another option for endovascular management, typically performed with either a paclitaxel drug-coated balloon or a plain balloon. Studies reviewing femoropopliteal patency rates after angioplasty demonstrated that ESKD patients on dialysis had statistically significantly lower five-year primary patency rates at 51.7%, compared to nondialysis patients at 68%. Yet, most patients were in their late 60 s and early 70 s (Heideman et al., 2016). Freedom rates from clinically indicated reintervention at 12 months postintervention in this population were estimated to be around 70%, compared to nondialysis patients, who were estimated to be around 90% (Heideman et al., 2016). Although the rare study examining treatment with angioplasty or stent in the CKD population reported that age was not associated with an increased risk for restenosis, most studies that provide multivariate analysis with age as a variable tend to conclude that age greater than 80 is a primary indicator of mortality (Heideman et al., 2016; Nakano et al., 2015).

Compared to endovascular management, open surgical management within the CKD population shows no statistically significant difference in the amputation-free survival rate (AFS), according to a study by Meyer et al. (2018). Considering most patients in this study were above 70 years old, this data is helpful in deciding between endovascular versus open management. Elderly patients with CKD who require intervention for infrapopliteal peripheral artery disease may be offered either option, depending on baseline fitness and clearance to undergo surgical management.

Deep venous arterialization (DVA) for elderly CKD patients

Brief introduction to DVA

Deep venous arterialization (DVA) is a relatively new approach to lower extremity revascularization in patients with PAD. It involves connecting an arterial inflow segment to a venous outflow segment, using veins to restore flow. DVA is typically reserved for patients considered "no-option" patients, meaning they are not candidates for open or endovascular options due to inadequate arterial outflow targets or advanced occlusive disease of their pedal arteries (Ilyas and Powell, 2022). For these patients, DVA is sometimes attempted as a last resort prior to eventual amputation. The concept is to drive more blood flow into the capillary bed through arterialization of the venous system, since these patients are thought to have arterial disease that is beyond repair (Zaman and Rundback, 2023). This is, intuitively, an attractive concept in the advanced CKD patient with severe PAD because of advanced small vessel disease and severe calcification of the distal vessels.

DVA can be performed via an open, endovascular, or hybrid approach. The open approach involves a surgical arteriovenous bypass and mechanical disruption of distal venous valves. Its success, in part, relies on selecting an appropriate inflow artery through preoperative planning with angiography. Choices for inflow include proximal options such as the common femoral or superficial femoral arteries, as well as distal options such as the proximal tibial artery. The preferred conduit is the native great saphenous vein. However, other options described in the literature for conduits include the cephalic vein and polytetrafluoroethylene (PTFE) graft—a vascular prosthesis made from synthetic material. Choices for outflow include the posterior tibial vein or a target on the dorsal venous arch (Ho et al., 2020).

The endovascular approach, also termed percutaneous DVA, is similar to open DVA, although it may be suitable for patients who are unable to tolerate open procedures. The concept is to create a connection between the arteries and veins of the proximal calf and use covered stents to drive flow down into the venous system of the foot, increasing perfusion of the capillary bed (Zaman and Rundback, 2023). One example is the LimFlow (LimFlow Inc.) system, which has been approved by the Food and Drug Administration (FDA) for exactly this purpose.

Currently published outcomes, including patients with CKD

Although most elderly patients with PAD and concomitant CKD fall into the "no-option" category and would theoretically benefit from DVA, clinical evidence supporting its use in this population is lacking. PROMISE I was a clinical trial investigating the management of "no-option" CLTI with DVA using LimFlow (LimFlow Inc.). Of the 32 patients enrolled in the trial, the average age was 71 years, and although 11 had CKD, none of the patients were ESKD or dialysis-dependent. The results from this trial demonstrated a 74% and 70% AFS rate at 6 months and 12 months, respectively (Clair et al., 2021). As interest in this topic grew, PROMISE II was conducted with similar endpoints, although it had a larger population sample, more closely representative of the real world. The average patient age was 70 years, 41 (39%) had CKD, and 19 (18%) were ESKD on dialysis. The overall amputation-free survival in the group was 66% at one year. A sobering finding, however, was that the amputation-free survival was much worse in the dialysis-dependent group at 37% compared to 73% in the non-ESKD group, despite initial technical success in nearly all patients (Shishehbor et al., 2023). Although no control group existed, all of these patients had advanced limb-threatening ischemia with no other revascularization options.

Conclusion

The elderly patient with CKD and PAD poses a significant clinical challenge. Mortality rates are very high in this group, and the disease has often progressed to end-stage. A patient's clinical status, including ambulation, independent living, and the presence or absence of wounds or rest pain, helps guide clinical decision-making. For many patients, palliative wound care with Betadine paint to prevent secondary infections will suffice. Pharmacological management to slow disease progression plays less of a role in this group than in younger patients. Revascularization procedures are performed less commonly in this group than in others due to higher rates of morbidity and mortality with worse outcomes. Early experience with newer revascularization methods, such as deep venous arterialization, has shown very poor outcomes as well. Prevention of advancement to severe PAD with large wounds should be practiced through foot checks at dialysis units, utilization of foot specialists, and medical optimization. Carefully planned and performed revascularization can be undertaken, but with diminished expectations compared to other patient groups that are younger and do not have CKD.

AI disclosure

During the preparation of this work, the author(s) used ChatGPT to identify the highlights of the research articles for use within the textbook chapter. After using this tool/service, the author(s) reviewed and edited the content as needed and take full responsibility for the content of the publication.

References

Albertus, P., Morgenstern, H., Robinson, B., Saran, R., 2016. Risk of ESRD in the United States. Am. J. Kidney Dis. 02726386. 68 (6), 862–872. doi:10.1053/j.ajkd.2016.05.030.

Ambur, V., Park, P., Gaughan, J.P., Golarz, S., Schmieder, F., Van Bemmelen, P., Choi, E., Dhanisetty, R., 2019. The impact of chronic kidney disease on lower extremity bypass outcomes in patients with critical limb ischemia. J. Vasc. Surg. 07415214. 69 (2), 491–496. doi:10.1016/j.jvs.2018.05.229.

Aronow, W.S., 2004. Management of peripheral arterial disease of the lower extremities in elderly patients. J. Gerontol. A Biol. Sci. Med. Sci. 1079-5006. 59 (2), M172. doi:10.1093/gerona/59.2.M172.

Arroyo, D., Betriu, A., Valls, J., Gorriz, J.L., Pallares, V., Abajo, M., Gracia, M., Valdivielso, J.M., Fernandez, E., Investigators from the NEFRONA study, 2017. Factors influencing pathological ankle-brachial index values along the chronic kidney disease spectrum: the NEFRONA study. Nephrol. Dial. Transplant. 32 (3), 513-520. doi: 10.1093/ndt/gfw039.

Ašćerić, R.R., Dimković, N.B., Trajković, G.Ž., Ristić, B.S., Janković, A.N., Durić, P.S., Ilijevski, N.S., 2019. Prevalence, clinical characteristics, and predictors of peripheral arterial disease in hemodialysis patients: a cross-sectional study. BMC Nephrol. 1471-2369. 20 (1). doi:10.1186/s12882-019-1468-x.

Butler, C.R., Nalatwad, A., Cheung, K.L., Hannan, M.F., Hladek, M.D., Johnston, E.A., Kimberly, L., Liu, C.K., Nair, D., Ozdemir, S., Saeed, F., Scherer, J.S., Segev, D.L., Sheshadri, A., Tennankore, K.K., Washington, T.R., Wolfgram, D., Ghildayal, N., Hall, R., McAdams-DeMarco, M., 2025. Establishing research priorities in geriatric nephrology: a delphi study of clinicians and researchers. Am. J. Kidney Dis. 15236838. 85 (3), 293–302. Available from: https://www.sciencedirect.com/science/journal/02726386. doi:10.1053/j.ajkd.2024.09.012.

Cheung, K.L., Crews, D.C., Cushman, M., Yuan, Y., Wilkinson, K., Long, D.L., Judd, S.E., Shlipak, M.G., Ix, J.H., Bullen, A.L., Warnock, D.G., Gutiérrez, O.M., 2023. Risk factors for incident CKD in black and white Americans: the REGARDS study. Am. J. Kidney Dis. 15236838. 82 (1), 11. Available from: http://www.elsevier.com/inca/publications/store/6/2/3/2/7/6/index.htt. doi:10.1053/j.ajkd.2022.11.015.

Clair, D.G., Mustapha, J.A., Shishehbor, M.H., Schneider, P.A., Henao, S., Bernardo, N.N., Deaton, D.H., PROMISE, I., 2021. Early feasibility study of the LimFlow System for percutaneous deep vein arterialization in no-option chronic limb-threatening ischemia: 12-month results. J. Vasc. Surg. 10976809. 74 (5), 1626–1635. Available from: https://www.sciencedirect.com/journal/journal-of-vascular-surgery. doi:10.1016/j.jvs.2021.04.057.

Conte, M.S., Pomposelli, F.B., Clair, D.G., Geraghty, P.J., McKinsey, J.F., Mills, J.L., Moneta, G.L., Murad, M.H., Powell, R.J., Reed, A.B., Schanzer, A., Sidawy, A.N., 2015. Society for Vascular Surgery practice guidelines for atherosclerotic occlusive disease of the lower extremities: management of asymptomatic disease and claudication. J. Vasc. Surg. 10976809. 61 (3), 2. Available from: http://www.elsevier.com/inca/publications/store/6/2/3/1/5/2/index.htt. doi:10.1016/j.jvs.2014.12.009.

Fayed, A., Soliman, A., Mahdy, H.E., Hamza, W., Abdulazim, D.O., Salem, M.M., Din, U.A.S.E., 2019. Intraoperative arterial biopsy in incident hemodialysis patients: differences observed. Nephron. 1660-8151. 143 (1), 54–61. doi:10.1159/000500486.

Garimella, P.S., Hart, P.D., O'Hare, A., Deloach, S., Herzog, C.A., Hirsch, A.T., 2012. Peripheral artery disease and CKD: a focus on peripheral artery disease as a critical component of CKD care. Am. J. Kidney Dis. 15236838. 60 (4), 641–654. doi:10.1053/j.ajkd.2012.02.340.

Garimella, P.S., Hirsch, A.T., 2014. Peripheral artery disease and chronic kidney disease: clinical synergy to improve outcomes. Adv. Chronic Kidney Dis. 15485609. 21 (6), 460–471. Available from: http://www.elsevier.com/wps/find/journaldescription.cws_home/703170/description#description. doi:10.1053/j.ackd.2014.07.005.

Go, A.S., Chertow, G.M., Fan, D., 2005. Chronic kidney disease and the risks of death, cardiovascular events, and hospitalization. J. Vasc. Surg. 07415214. 41 (1), 177. doi:10.1016/j.jvs.2004.10.020.

Goodney, P.P., Beck, A.W., Nagle, J., Welch, H.G., Zwolak, R.M., 2009. National trends in lower extremity bypass surgery, endovascular interventions, and major amputations. J. Vasc. Surg. 07415214. 50 (1), 54–60. doi:10.1016/j.jvs.2009.01.035.

Gornik, H.L., Aronow, H.D., Goodney, P.P., Arya, S., Brewster, L.P., Byrd, L., Chandra, V., Drachman, D.E., Eaves, J.M., Ehrman, J.K., Evans, J.N., Getchius, T.S.D., Gutiérrez, J.A., Hawkins, B.M., Hess, C.N., Ho, K.J., Jones, W.S., Kim, E.S.H., Kinlay, S., Kirksey, L., Kohlman-Trigoboff, D., Long, C.A., Pollak, A.W., Sabri, S.S., Sadwin, L.B., Secemsky, E.A., Serhal, M., Shishehbor, M.H., Treat-Jacobson, D., Wilkins, L.R., 2024. Correction to: 2024 ACC/AHA/AACVPR/APMA/ABC/SCAI/SVM/SVN/SVS/SIR/VESS guideline for the management of lower extremity peripheral artery disease: a report of the American College of Cardiology/American Heart Association Joint Committee on Clinical Practice Guidelines. Circulation. 0009-7322. 151 (14). doi:10.1161/cir.0000000000001329.

Gracia, M., Betriu, À., Martínez-Alonso, M., Arroyo, D., Abajo, M., Fernández, E., Valdivielso, J.M., 2016. Predictors of subclinical atheromatosis progression over 2 years in patients with different stages of CKD. Clin. J. Am. Soc. Nephrol. 1555-9041. 11 (2), 287–296. doi:10.2215/cjn.01240215.

Grundy, S.M., Stone, N.J., Bailey, A.L., Beam, C., Birtcher, K.K., Blumenthal, R.S., Braun, L.T., de Ferranti, S., Faiella-Tommasino, J., Forman, D.E., Goldberg, R., Heidenreich, P.A., Hlatky, M.A., Jones, D.W., Lloyd-Jones, D., Lopez-Pajares, N., Ndumele, C.E., Orringer, C.E., Peralta, C.A., Saseen, J.J., Smith, S.C., Sperling, L., Virani, S.S., Yeboah, J., 2019. AHA/ACC/AACVPR/AAPA/ABC/ACPM/ADA/AGS/APhA/ASPC/NLA/PCNA guideline on the management of blood cholesterol: executive summary: a report of the American College of Cardiology/American Heart Association task force on clinical practice guidelines. Circulation. 0009-7322. 139 (25). doi:10.1161/cir.0000000000000624.

Hardman, R., Omid Jazaeri, J.Y., Smith, M., Gupta, R., 2014. Overview of classification systems in peripheral artery disease. Semin. Interv. Radiol. 0739-9529. 31 (04), 378–388. doi:10.1055/s-0034-1393976.

Heideman, P.P., Rajebi, M.R., McKusick, M.A., Bjarnason, H., Oderich, G.S., Friese, J.L., Fleming, M.D., Stockland, A.H., Harmsen, W.S., Mandrekar, J., Misra, S., 2016. Impact of chronic kidney disease on clinical outcomes of endovascular treatment for femoropopliteal arterial disease. J. Vasc. Interv. Radiol. 15357732. 27 (8), 1204–1214. Available from: http://www.elsevier.com. doi:10.1016/j.jvir.2016.04.036.

Heller, C., Balls-Berry, J.E., Nery, J.D., Erwin, P.J., Littleton, D., Kim, M., Kuo, W.P., 2014. Strategies addressing barriers to clinical trial enrollment of underrepresented populations: a systematic review. Contemp. Clin. Trials. 15517144. 39 (2), 169–182. doi:10.1016/j.cct.2014.08.004.

Himmelfarb, J., Stenvinkel, P., Ikizler, T.A., Hakim, R.M., 2002. The elephant in uremia: oxidant stress as a unifying concept of cardiovascular disease in uremia. Kidney Int. 00852538. 62 (5), 1524–1538. doi:10.1046/j.1523-1755.2002.00600.x.

Ho, V.T., Gologorsky, R., Kibrik, P., Chandra, V., Prent, A., Lee, J., Dua, A., 2020. Open, percutaneous, and hybrid deep venous arterialization technique for no-option foot salvage. J. Vasc. Surg. 10976809. 71 (6), 2152–2160. Available from: https://www.sciencedirect.com/journal/journal-of-vascular-surgery. doi:10.1016/j.jvs.2019.10.085.

Ilyas, S., Powell, R.J., 2022. Management of the no-option foot: deep vein arterialization. Semin. Vasc. Surg. 15584518. 35 (2), 210–218. Available from: http://www.elsevier.com/inca/publications/store/6/2/3/1/9/3/index.htt. doi:10.1053/j.semvascsurg.2022.05.002.

Jha, V., Garcia-Garcia, G., Iseki, K., Zuo, L., Naicker, S., Plattner, B., Saran, R., Wang, A.Y.-M., Yang, C.-W., 2013. Chronic kidney disease: global dimension and perspectives. Lancet. 01406736. 382 (9888), 260–272. doi:10.1016/s0140-6736(13)60687-x.

Kim, S.Y.H., Caine, E.D., 2002. Utility and limits of the mini mental state examination in evaluating consent capacity in Alzheimer's disease. Psychiatr. Serv. 53 (10), 1322–1324. doi:10.1176/appi.ps.53.10.1322.

Kumada, Y., Aoyama, T., Ishii, H., Tanaka, M., Kawamura, Y., Takahashi, H., Toriyama, T., Aoyama, T., Yuzawa, Y., Maruyama, S., Matsuo, S., Murohara, T., 2008. Long-term outcome of percutaneous transluminal angioplasty in chronic haemodialysis patients with peripheral arterial disease. Nephrol. Dial. Transplant. 0931-0509. 23 (12), 3996–4001. doi:10.1093/ndt/gfn378.

Kuo, H.-K., Yu, Y.-H., 2008. The relation of peripheral arterial disease to leg force, gait speed, and functional dependence among older adults. J. Gerontol. A Biol. Sci. Med. Sci. 1079-5006. 63 (4), 384–390. doi:10.1093/gerona/63.4.384.

Lanzer, P., Schurgers, L., Twarda-Clapa, A., Ferraresi, R., Hui, H., Kamenskiy, A., Chen, Y., Hamana, T., Fok, P.-W., Millán, Á., Virmani, R., St. Hilaire, C., 2025. Medial arterial calcification in ageing and disease: current evidence and knowledge gaps. Eur. Heart J. 0195–668X. doi:10.1093/eurheartj/ehaf341.

Lattanzio, F., Corsonello, A., Montesanto, A., Abbatecola, A.M., Lofaro, D., Passarino, G., Fusco, S., Corica, F., Pedone, C., Maggio, M., Volpato, S., Incalzi, R.A., 2015. Disentangling the impact of chronic kidney disease, anemia, and mobility limitation on mortality in older patients discharged from hospital. J. Gerontol. A Biol. Sci. Med. Sci. 1079-5006. 70 (9), 1120–1127. doi:10.1093/gerona/glv068.

Lee, C.C., Wu, C.J., Chou, L.H., Shen, S.M., Chiang, S.F., Jen, P.C., Yeh, M.C., Pan, C.F., 2012. Peripheral artery disease in peritoneal dialysis and hemodialysis patients: single-center retrospective study in Taiwan. BMC Nephrol. 14712369. 13 (1). doi:10.1186/1471-2369-13-100.

Linton, M.F., Yancey, P.G., Davies, S.S., Jerome, W.G., Linton, E.F., Song, W.L., Doran, A.C., Vickers, K.C., 2009. The Role of Lipids and Lipoproteins in Atherosclerosis. In: Feingold K.R, et al. (eds.), Endotext. MDText.com, Inc., South Dartmouth, MA.

London, G.M., Marchais, S.J., Guérin, A.P., Métivier, F., 2005. Arteriosclerosis, vascular calcifications and cardiovascular disease in uremia. Curr. Opin. Nephrol. Hypertens. 10624821. 14 (6), 525–531. Available from: http://journals.lww.com/co-nephrolhypertens/pages/default.aspx. doi:10.1097/01.mnh.0000168336.67499.c0.

Lüders, F., Bunzemeier, H., Engelbertz, C., Malyar, N.M., Meyborg, M., Roeder, N., Berger, K., Reinecke, H., 2016. CKD and acute and long-term outcome of patients with peripheral artery disease and critical limb ischemia. Clin. J. Am. Soc. Nephrol. 1555-9041. 11 (2), 216–222. doi:10.2215/cjn.05600515.

Lüders, F., Fürstenberg, T., Engelbertz, C., Gebauer, K., Meyborg, M., Malyar, N.M., Reinecke, H., 2017. The impact of chronic kidney disease on hospitalized patients with peripheral arterial disease and critical limb ischemia. Angiology. 0003-3197. 68 (2), 145–150. doi:10.1177/0003319716638797.

Matsushita, K., Ballew, S.H., Coresh, J., Arima, H., Ärnlöv, J., Cirillo, M., Ebert, N., Hiramoto, J.S., Kimm, H., Shlipak, M.G., Visseren, F.L.J., Gansevoort, R.T., Kovesdy, C.P., Shalev, V., Woodward, M., Kronenberg, F., Chalmers, J., Arima, H., Perkovic, V., Grams, M.E., Sang, Y., Schaeffner, E., Martus, P., Levin, A., Djurdjev, O., Tang, M., Heine, G., Seiler, S., Zawada, A., Emrich, I., Sarnak, M., Katz, R., Brenner, H., Schöttker, B., Rothenbacher, D., Saum, K.-U., Köttgen, A., Schneider, M., Eckardt, K.-U., Jamie Green, H.L.K., Chang, A.R., Black, C., Marks, A., Prescott, G., Clark, L., Fluck, N., Jee, S.H., Mok, Y., Chodick, G., Shalev, V., Wetzels, J.F.M., Blankestijn, P.J., van Zuilen,

A.D., Bots, M., Peralta, C., Hiromoto, J., Katz, R., Sarnak, M., Bottinger, E., Nadkarni, G.N., Ellis, S.B., Nadukuru, R., Timothy Kenealy, C.R.E., Collins, J.F., Drury, P.L., Bakker, S.J.L., Heerspink, H.J.L., Jassal, S.K., Bergstrom, J., Ix, J.H., Barrett-Connor, E., Kalantar-Zadeh, K., Carrero, J.J., Gasparini, A., Qureshi, A.R., Barany, P., Algra, A., van der Graaf, Y., Evans, M., Segelmark, M., Stendahl, M., Schön, S., Tangri, N., Sud, M., Naimark, D., Lannfelt, L., Larsson, A., Hallan, S., Levey, A.S., Chen, J., Kwak, L., Grams, M.E., Sang, Y., 2017. Measures of chronic kidney disease and risk of incident peripheral artery disease: a collaborative meta-analysis of individual participant data. Lancet Diabetes Endocrinol. 22138587. 5 (9), 718–728. doi:10.1016/s2213-8587(17)30183-3.

Meyer, A., Schilling, A., Kott, M., Rother, U., Lang, W., Regus, S., 2018. Open Versus Endovascular Revascularization of Below-Knee Arteries in Patients with End-Stage Renal Disease and Critical Limb Ischemia. Vasc. Endovasc. Surg. 1538-5744. 52 (8), 613–620. doi:10.1177/1538574418789036.

Moe, S.M., O'Neill, K.D., Duan, D., Ahmed, S., Chen, N.X., Leapman, S.B., Fineberg, N., Kopecky, K., 2002. Medial artery calcification in ESRD patients is associated with deposition of bone matrix proteins. Kidney Int. 00852538. 61 (2), 638–647. Available from: https://www.journals.elsevier.com/kidney-international. doi:10.1046/j.1523-1755.2002.00170.x.

Molitch, M.E., Adler, A.I., Flyvbjerg, A., Nelson, R.G., So, W.Y., Wanner, C., Kasiske, B.L., Wheeler, D.C., De Zeeuw, D., Mogensen, C.E., 2015. Diabetic kidney disease: a clinical update from kidney disease: improving global outcomes. Kidney Int. 15231755. 1 (87), 20–30. https://www.journals.elsevier.com/kidney-international. doi:10.1038/ki.2014.128.

Moyer, V.A., 2012. Screening for chronic kidney disease: U.S. Preventive Services Task Force recommendation statement. Ann. Intern. Med. 15393704. 157 (8), 567–570. Available from: http://annals.org/data/Journals/AIM/25337/0000605-201210160-00008.pdf. doi:10.7326/0003-4819-157-8-201210160-00533.

Nakano, M., Hirano, K., Iida, O., Yamauchi, Y., Soga, Y., Kawasaki, D., Tazaki, J., Suzuki, K., Fujiwara, M., Yamaoka, T., 2015. Clinical efficacy of infrapopliteal endovascular procedures for hemodialysis patients with critical limb ischemia. Ann. Vasc. Surg. 08905096. 29 (6), 1225–1234. doi:10.1016/j.avsg.2015.03.034.

Nelson, A.J., Raggi, P., Wolf, M., Gold, A.M., Chertow, G.M., Roe, M.T., 2020. Targeting vascular calcification in chronic kidney disease. JACC Basic Transl. Sci. 2452302X. 5 (4), 398–412. Available from: http://www.journals.elsevier.com/jacc-basic-to-translational-science. doi:10.1016/j.jacbts.2020.02.002.

Norgren, L., Hiatt, W.R., Dormandy, J.A., Nehler, M.R., Harris, K.A., Fowkes, F.G.R., 2007. Inter-society consensus for the management of peripheral arterial disease (TASC II). J. Vasc. Surg. 07415214. 45 (1), S5. doi:10.1016/j.jvs.2006.12.037.

O'Neill, W.C., Han, K.H., Schneider, T.M., Hennigar, R.A., 2015. Prevalence of nonatheromatous lesions in peripheral arterial disease. Arterioscler. Thromb. Vasc. Biol. 15244636. 35 (2), 439–447. Available from: https://www.ahajournals.org/journal/atvb. doi:10.1161/ATVBAHA.114.304764.

Ostchega, Y., Paulose-Ram, R., Dillon, C.F., Qiuping, G., Hughes, J.P., 2007. Prevalence of peripheral arterial disease and risk factors in persons aged 60 and older: data from the National Health and Nutrition Examination Survey 1999–2004. J. Am. Geriatr. Soc. 0002-8614. 55 (4), 583–589. doi:10.1111/j.1532-5415.2007.01123.x.

Pizzarelli, F., Basile, C., Aucella, F., Dattolo, P.C., 2023. Chronic kidney disease in the elderly and frail patient: perspectives with opinions and comments. J. Nephrol. 1724-6059. 36 (6), 1565–1570. doi:10.1007/s40620-023-01676-y.

Polonsky, T.S., McDermott, M.M., 2021. Lower extremity peripheral artery disease without chronic limb-threatening ischemia: a review. JAMA 15383598. 325 (21), 2188–2198. Available from: http://jama.jamanetwork.com/journal.aspx. doi:10.1001/jama.2021.2126.

Rid, A., Emanuel, E.J., Wendler, D., 2010. Evaluating the risks of clinical research. JAMA. 0098-7484. 304 (13), 1472. doi:10.1001/jama.2010.1414.

Shishehbor, M.H., Powell, R.J., Montero-Baker, M.F., Dua, A., Martínez-Trabal, J.L., Bunte, M.C., Lee, A.C., Mugglin, A.S., Mills, J.L., Farber, A., Clair, D.G., 2023. Transcatheter arterialization of deep veins in chronic limb-threatening ischemia. N. Engl. J. Med. 15334406. 388 (13), 1171–1180. Available from: http://www.nejm.org/medical-index. doi:10.1056/NEJMoa2212754.

Sibley, R.C., Reis, S.P., MacFarlane, J.J., Reddick, M.A., Kalva, S.P., Sutphin, P.D., 2017. Noninvasive physiologic vascular studies: a guide to diagnosing peripheral arterial disease. Radiographics. 15271323. 37 (1), 346–357. Available from: http://pubs.rsna.org/doi/pdf/10.1148/rg.2017160044. doi:10.1148/rg.2017160044.

Smilowitz, N.R., Bhandari, N., Berger, J.S., 2020. Chronic kidney disease and outcomes of lower extremity revascularization for peripheral artery disease. Atherosclerosis. 18791484. 297, 149–156. Available from: https://www.elsevier.com/locate/atherosclerosis. doi:10.1016/j.atherosclerosis.2019.12.016.

Stengel, B., Metzger, M., Froissart, M., Rainfray, M., Berr, C., Tzourio, C., Helmer, C., 2011. Epidemiology and prognostic significance of chronic kidney disease in the elderly—the Three-City prospective cohort study. Nephrol. Dial. Transplant. 1460-2385. 26 (10), 3286–3295. doi:10.1093/ndt/gfr323.

Stevens, P.E., Ahmed, S.B., Carrero, J.J., Foster, B., Francis, A., Hall, R.K., Herrington, W.G., Hill, G., Inker, L.A., Kazancıoğlu, R., Lamb, E., Lin, P., Madero, M., McIntyre, N., Morrow, K., Roberts, G., Sabanayagam, D., Schaeffner, E., Shlipak, M., Shroff, R., Tangri, N., Thanachayanont, T., Ulasi, I., Wong, G., Yang, C.W., Zhang, L., Levin, A., 2024. KDIGO 2024 clinical practice guideline for the evaluation and management of chronic kidney disease. Kidney Int. 15231755. 105 (4), S117. Available from: https://www.sciencedirect.com/science/journal/00852538. doi:10.1016/j.kint.2023.10.018.

Subramanian, N., Han, J., Leeper, N.J., Ross, E.G., Montez-Rath, M.E., Chang, T.I., 2021. Comparison of pre-amputation evaluation in patients with and without chronic kidney disease. Am. J. Nephrol. 0250-8095. 52 (5), 388–395. doi:10.1159/000516017.

Treat-Jacobson, D., McDermott, M.M., Bronas, U.G., Campia, U., Collins, T.C., Criqui, M.H., Gardner, A.W., Hiatt, W.R., Regensteiner, J.G., Rich, K., 2019. Optimal exercise programs for patients with peripheral artery disease: a scientific statement from the american heart association. Circulation. 0009-7322. 139 (4). doi:10.1161/cir.0000000000000623.

Wanner, C., Krane, V., März, W., Olschewski, M., Mann, J.F.E., Ruf, G., Ritz, E., 2005. Atorvastatin in patients with type 2 diabetes mellitus undergoing hemodialysis. N. Engl. J. Med. 353 (3), 238–248. Available from: http://content.nejm.org/cgi/reprint/353/3/238.pdf. doi:10.1056/NEJMoa043545.

Wattanakit, K., Folsom, A.R., Selvin, E., Coresh, J., Hirsch, A.T., Weatherley, B.D., 2007. Kidney function and risk of peripheral arterial disease. J. Am. Soc. Nephrol. 1046-6673. 18 (2), 629–636. doi:10.1681/asn.2005111204.

Zaman, N., Rundback, J., 2023. Deep venous arterialization: background, patient selection, technique, outcomes and follow-up, and future implementation. Semin. Interv. Radiol. 0739-9529. 40 (02), 183–192. doi:10.1055/s-0043-57264.

PART 4

Management and prevention

CHAPTER

20

Diagnosis of CKD in an elderly individual, due to a decline in GFR with normal healthy aging

Bryce M. Churilla[a], *Jae Hun Son*[a], *Khan Shabtab*[b,c], *Sheryl Cababat Caberto*[c], *and Stephen Z. Fadem*[d]

[a]Division of Renal Medicine, Emory University, Atlanta, GA, United States
[b]Renal Medicine, Atlanta VA Medical Center, Atlanta, GA, United States
[c]Division of Renal Medicine, Emory University School of Medicine, Atlanta, GA, United States
[d]Department of Medicine, Section of Nephrology, Baylor College of Medicine, Houston, TX, United States

Introduction

Chronic kidney disease (CKD) affects one in seven adults in the United States, while less than 10% are aware of its presence (Farrell and Vassalotti, 2024). The effect of kidney disease is wide-ranging. A sustained, reduced glomerular filtration rate has been associated with increased mortality, bone dysregulation, anemia, and more (Vassalotti et al., 2016).

As advancements in science and medicine have extended human lifespans, the aging population in the world faces a growing burden of health issues, including higher rates of cardiovascular disease, cancer, diabetes, and, in particular, CKD (Tang et al., 2024). The prevalence of CKD rises significantly with age, affecting nearly 30% of individuals over 65 (Tang et al., 2024) as does the risk of developing it with increasing life expectancy (Grams et al., 2013). CKD is typically diagnosed across all age groups using serum creatinine levels, estimated glomerular filtration rate, or creatinine clearance. However, it is crucial to account for normal age-related physiological changes and to evaluate whether these diagnostic methods are precise and reliable in distinguishing between age-associated variations and true pathological CKD. This distinction is critical for reducing the disease burden, optimizing treatment strategies, and improving patient outcomes. By refining current testing methods, clinicians

https://doi.org/10.1016/B978-0-443-34069-7.00022-7

can make more accurate diagnoses, tailor interventions more effectively, and minimize the risk of overdiagnosis or underdiagnosis in this vulnerable population.

Evolution of renal function measurement

The history of urinary diagnostic testing and, by extension, the understanding of kidney disease, can be traced back to ancient Greece, when early physicians recognized urine as a vital window into human health. Hippocrates of Kos, often regarded as the father of medicine, observed that the presence of bubbles in urine could be associated with kidney disease, hinting at early clinical correlations between urine characteristics and renal pathology (Diamantis et al., 2008). In the Middle Ages, the technique of uroscopy, which is the precursor to modern-day urinalysis, was utilized to understand a patient's overall health and detect renal or systemic illnesses by analyzing the color, clarity, and other visible characteristics of urine (Armstrong, 2007). Ancient practitioners also discovered that warming the urine could cause substances to precipitate, including proteins—a rudimentary method of proteinuria detection. In the late 17th century, Dutch chemist Frederik Dekkers built upon this principle by systematically describing the coagulation of urinary proteins upon heating, a technique that laid the groundwork for modern urinalysis (Diamantis et al., 2008). The evolution of kidney diagnostics further advanced in the 19th century with Richard Bright, who is known as the father of nephrology. Bright linked specific clinical symptoms to pathological changes in the kidneys, describing what came to be known as Bright's disease, which has been inferred as various forms of nephritis (Diamantis et al., 2008). These early insights marked the beginning of nephrology as a medical discipline, highlighting the enduring significance of urine in diagnosing kidney ailments.

Creatinine is a nitrogenous waste product formed by the breakdown of creatinine phosphate, a molecule involved in energy production in muscle tissue. It is produced at a relatively constant rate, depending on muscle mass, and excreted almost entirely by the kidneys, making it a valuable marker of renal function (Shahbaz and Gupta, 2025).

The discovery of creatinine dates back to the 19th century. By the early 1900s, researchers observed that creatinine levels in the blood rose when renal function declined, as impaired kidneys were unable to efficiently excrete it. This realization led to the use of serum creatinine concentration as an indirect indicator of glomerular filtration. The development of the creatinine clearance test in the mid-20th century, measuring both serum and urine creatinine, marked a major advancement and offered a more accurate estimation of renal function (Shahbaz and Gupta, 2025; Losito, 2023). Over time, creatinine became a cornerstone of nephrology. Today, it remains one of the most widely used and accessible indicators for assessing kidney health. It plays a central role in calculating the estimated glomerular filtration rate (eGFR), which guides the diagnosis and staging of CKD.

Urea is a nitrogen-containing compound that serves as the primary endproduct of protein metabolism in humans. It is synthesized in the liver through the urea cycle, where excess nitrogen, primarily derived from the breakdown of amino acids, is converted into urea, a less toxic compound than ammonia (Gounden et al., 2026). Once urea is formed, it is transported via the bloodstream to the kidneys, where it is filtered and excreted in urine. Because of this pathway, urea levels in the blood and urine serve as important indicators of both metabolic and renal function.

The discovery of urea dates back to the 18th century; however, the connection between urea and kidney disease began to emerge in the 19th century as physicians observed that patients with severe renal dysfunction exhibited elevated levels of urea in the blood. The condition was later termed uremia (History of Urine Testing, 2016). This accumulation occurred because damaged kidneys were unable to effectively excrete urea, leading to a toxic buildup. The measurement of blood urea nitrogen (BUN) eventually became a standard diagnostic tool for assessing renal function, particularly in the setting of acute and chronic kidney failure. Urea, once just a chemical curiosity, became a critical biomarker in the clinical evaluation of kidney health.

In the 1960s, a new molecule, Cystatin C, was described. It was found to be produced by all nucleated cells. In the 1980s and 1990s, researchers began to study Cystatin C more closely as a potential marker and a better alternative for assessing renal function, particularly when muscle mass was variable or when creatinine-based estimation equations became unreliable. Since its discovery and increasing utilization, Cystatin C has been incorporated into the most recent eGFR equations that are used, such as the CKD-EPI (Chronic Kidney Disease Epidemiology Collaboration) Cystatin C equation and the CKD-EPI Creatinine-Cystatin C equations (Levey et al., 2009; Inker et al., 2011).

The measurement of renal function has evolved significantly over time, beginning with early observations that waste products like urea and creatinine accumulate in the blood when renal function declines. As the understanding of creatinine's origin in muscle metabolism and its renal excretion became clearer in the early 20th century, scientists recognized its potential as a marker for renal function. This led to the development of the creatinine clearance test (Gounden et al., 2026), which estimates the eGFR by comparing the measured amount of creatinine in a timed urine collection and the level of serum creatinine. In spite of the fact that this was a cumbersome method, it provided a more direct assessment of kidney filtration capacity.

Creatinine clearance (CrCl) equation

$$CrCl\,(mL\,/\,min) = \frac{Urine\ Creatinine\,(mg\,/\,dL) \times Urine\ Volume\,(mL)}{Serum\ Creatinine\,(mg\,/\,dL) \times Time\,(min)} \tag{1}$$

Creatinine clearance (Eq. 1) estimates the volume of plasma cleared of creatinine by the kidneys per minute and is calculated using both serum and urine creatinine measurements (Gounden et al., 2026). We still utilize creatinine clearance in cases when someone has unstable serum creatinine, abnormal muscle mass, or when precise GFR is needed for drug dosing or in cases of kidney donation (Shahbaz and Gupta, 2025). However, inaccuracy is inevitable because of incomplete 24-h urine collection and slight overestimation of true GFR. Creatinine is not only filtered in the glomerulus but also secreted by renal tubules.

In 1976, the Cockcroft-Gault equation (Eq. 2) was introduced to estimate creatinine clearance using serum creatinine, age, weight, and sex, providing a practical alternative to urine collection (Cockcroft and Gault, 1976).

Cockcroft-Gault equation (Cockcroft and Gault, 1976)

$$CrCl\,(mL/min) = \frac{(140 - Age) \times Weight\,(kg) \times [0.85\ if\ female]}{72 \times Serum\ Creatinine\,(mg/dL)} \tag{2}$$

This formula was adjusted for sex, age, and weight. It accounted for sex, recognizing that women generally have lower muscle mass than men. Age was included due to the natural decline in renal function over time. Weight was considered as a muscle mass surrogate for creatinine production in estimating creatinine clearance. The Cockcroft-Gault equation became valuable for drug dosing, and it is still used for renal dosing of medications, as many drug studies still reference this equation (Gounden et al., 2026). However, there were some limitations because it overestimated eGFR for obese patients (Winter et al., 2012).

In the 1990s, the Modification of Diet in Renal Disease (MDRD) equation (Eq. 3) shifted the focus toward estimating GFR directly from serum creatinine, adjusting for age, sex, and race (Levey et al., 2006; Levey et al., 2007). It aimed to improve the early detection of CKD, where estimating GFR would be more useful than estimating creatinine clearance. The idea was that creatinine clearance tended to overestimate renal function in patients with higher GFR, and this could be problematic when dealing with patients who have normal or mildly impaired renal function (Coresh and Stevens, 2006). The formula was further refined by the CKD-EPI equation in 2009 (Eq. 4), which improved accuracy, especially at higher levels of renal function.

MDRD equation

$$\begin{aligned} GFR &= 175x\,[Scr\,(mg/dL)/88.4]^{-1.154}\,x\,Age^{-0.203} \\ &\quad x(1.212\ [if\ black]\ x0.742\ [if\ female]) \end{aligned} \tag{3}$$

2009 CKD-EPI creatinine equation (race-based)

$$\begin{aligned} GFR2_{009CKD-EPI} &= 141 \times [min(Scr/\kappa, 1)]^{\alpha} \times [max(Scr/\kappa, 1)]^{-1.209} \times \\ &\quad (0.993)^{Age} \times (1.018\ if\ female)\ or \times (1.159\ if\ Black) \end{aligned} \tag{4}$$

where Scr is serum creatinine, κ is 0.7 for females and 0.9 for males, α is −0.329 for females and −0.411 for males, min indicates the minimum of Scr/κ or 1, and max indicates the maximum of Scr/κ or 1.

The CKD-EPI equation is an improved method for estimating GFR based on serum creatinine, along with age and sex, compared to the MDRD equation, particularly for individuals with normal or mildly reduced renal function. This allowed for a broader range of the population to be included in its development.

In 2021, in response to increasing concerns about the use of race in clinical algorithms, a revised CKD-EPI equation (Eq. 5) was introduced. It eliminated the race coefficient. This updated version was developed using a diverse population and incorporated refitted coefficients to maintain accuracy across racial groups without requiring race-based adjustments (Inker et al., 2021).

2021 CKD-EPI equation

$$eGFR = 142 \times min\ (standardized\ Scr\ /\ K,1)^{\alpha} \times max(standardized\ Scr\ /\ K,1)^{-1.200} \times 0.9938\ age\ in\ years \times 1.012[if\ female] \quad (5)$$

where Scr is serum creatinine in mg/dL, K is 0.7 (females) or 0.9 (males), α is −0.241 (females) or − 0.302 (males), min(standardized Scr/K, 1) is the minimum of Scr/K or 1, and max(standardized Scr/K, 1) is the maximum of Scr/K or 1.

The increasing utilization of cystatin C values has led to incorporating cystatin C into the CKD-EPI equation along with creatinine for a more precise estimation of GFR without relying on a race-based algorithm (Eq. 6). Looking ahead, we can expect the future of renal function assessment to focus on more personalized, race-free, and biomarker-integrated models, potentially incorporating genomics and real-time biomonitoring to improve early detection and precision care in nephrology.

2021 CKD-EPI creatinine-cystatin C equation

$$eGFR_{cr-cys} = 135x min\ (Scr\ /\ \kappa,1)^{\alpha} \times max\ (Scr\ /\ \kappa,1)^{-0.544} \times min\ (Scys\ /\ 0.8,1)^{-0.323} \times max\ (Scys\ /\ 0.8,1)^{-0.778} \times 0.9961^{Age} \times 0.963[if\ female] \quad (6)$$

where S_{cr} is standardized serum creatinine in mg/dL, κ is 0.7 (females) or 0.9 (males), α is −0.219 (females) or −0.144 (males), min(S_{cr}/κ, 1) is the minimum of S_{cr}/κ or 1.0, max(S_{cr}/κ, 1) is the maximum of S_{cr}/κ or 1.0, and S_{cys} is standardized serum cystatin C in mg/L, Age (years). The eGFR equations can be found online at http://mdrd.com.

How is CKD diagnosed?

CKD is diagnosed after three or more months of kidney damage and subsequent decreased filtration (Farrell and Vassalotti, 2024). Reduced filtration is assessed using a surrogate calculation called the estimated glomerular filtration rate (eGFR). This estimation can be made using validated equations that utilize serum markers of filtration, such as creatinine (Inker et al., 2021). These equations were created by the Chronic Kidney Disease Epidemiology Collaboration (CKD-EPI) research group, which analyzes large datasets from multiple studies (Ebert et al., 2022).

CKD is divided into five stages based on GFR: G1 (greater than or equal to 90 mL/min), G2 (60–89 mL/min), G3a (45–59 mL/min), G3b (30–44 mL/min), G4 (15–29 mL/min), and G5 (<15 mL/min), which is kidney failure. The measurement of urine microalbumin can also help identify those at risk for progression to end-stage kidney disease (ESKD), in conjunction with GFR. The degree of albuminuria (A) and GFR, using heatmaps provided by KDIGO, can provide this insight (KDIGO, 2021).

Albumin in the urine is a sign of renal damage, and its presence is a risk factor for ESKD. Large amounts of albumin in the urine can be indicative of dysfunction in both the glomerular basement membrane and the proximal tubule, the early portion of the nephron that reabsorbs filtered albumin (Farrell and Vassalotti, 2024). Like GFR, albuminuria is categorized into stages: A1 (<30 mg), A2 (30–300 mg), A3 (><30 mg), A2 (30–300 mg), A3 Nephrotic

TABLE 20.1 Stages of albuminuria (KDIGO classification). This table outlines the stages of albuminuria, their corresponding cutoff values, and brief descriptions. KDIGO does not have an A4 category but keeps nephrotic-range as a subset of A3.

Category	Degree of severity	Alb/cr ratio	Stage (description)
A1	Mild	<30 mg/g	Normal to mildly increased
A2	Moderate	30-300 mg/g	Moderately increased
A3	Severe	>300 mg/g	Severely increased
	Nephrotic	>2000	Nephrotic range

Adapted from KDIGO, 2021. Clinical Practice Guideline for the Management of Blood Pressure in CKD.

(>2000 mg), with nephrotic-range albuminuria defined as >2000 mg (KDIGO, 2021) (Table 20.1). Albuminuria can be measured by 24-hour urine collection or a spot level test. The spot albumin evaluation correlates with 24-hour collection (Farrell and Vassalotti, 2024), which is a less tedious task for patients. Albumin is not the only protein that can be detected in the urine. As such, total protein can also be measured. However, total protein assays are not recommended for staging CKD, as urine albumin assays are better at quantifying even small amounts of albuminuria (Chen et al., 2019).

Renal disease is evaluated not only with blood markers and urine studies but also through imaging of the kidneys themselves. There are multiple modalities for imaging in such assessments: Ultrasound, CT, and MRI. Imaging can be helpful not only in identifying the cause of renal dysfunction, such as stones, hydronephrosis, new cysts, or masses, but also in determining its chronicity. A reduction in kidney size and/or cortical thickness can be a sign of chronic kidney damage (KDIGO, 2021). Macroscopic changes occur with the aging kidney, for which imaging can be particularly useful (Hommos et al., 2017).

Estimating renal function: Age-related eGFR decline or CKD

As our kidneys age, they become more sensitive to substances that cause blood vessels to constrict and less responsive to those that cause them to dilate. Nitric oxide (NO), which helps dilate blood vessels and control cell growth, decreases. There is also a decrease in levels of renin and aldosterone with aging. The overall effect of these changes is an elevation in blood pressure and subsequent kidney damage. Sex-specific changes also occur: estrogen slows CKD progression, while testosterone accelerates it. Additionally, physiological changes in other organs contribute to kidney damage. For example, age-related changes in heart function and increased oxidative stress play a key role in renal dysfunction (Weinstein and Anderson, 2010).

At birth, the glomerular filtration rate (GFR) is low, but it reaches adult levels by age two. The GFR remains around 140 mL/min/1.73 m^2 until about age 40. After this age, it declines by about 1 mL/min/1.73 m^2 per year (Lindeman et al., 1985). Factors such as high blood pressure, lead exposure, smoking, high cholesterol, atherosclerosis, inflammation, advanced glycation end products, obesity, and male gender can accelerate this decline. Prior episodes of acute kidney injury also increase the risk of CKD (Weinstein and Anderson, 2010).

Pathogenesis of age-related CKD

As we age, our kidneys undergo structural changes. The number of nephrons, which are the kidney's filtering units, decreases. In people under 40, less than 5% of glomeruli are sclerosed. This increases to about 30% by the age of 80, leading to a loss of 20%–25% of kidney mass, which is mostly in the outer part of the kidney. When glomeruli become damaged, the remaining nephrons increase in size to compensate. This adaptive change helps maintain overall kidney function; however, glomerular pressure subsequently increases, causing high blood pressure and further damage. The enlargement of glomeruli can also harm podocytes, which are cells essential for filtration. These changes, along with aging, lead to more podocyte loss, reduced podocyte density, and eventually, wrinkling of capillaries, collapse of the glomerular tuft, and fibrosis around the glomeruli (Noronha et al., 2022).

There are multiple determinants that affect how the kidney handles filtrate. These include hemodynamics, renal blood flow, hormones, and peptides (Epstein, 1996). In older adults, the renin-angiotensin system (RAS) is less active. To compensate for the decline in renin and aldosterone levels, the body becomes more sensitive to these hormones. Aging reduces the kidney's ability to concentrate or dilute urine, and the glomerular filtration rate declines. Older adults are unable to conserve water and solutes with the same effectiveness as younger people, which makes them more prone to hypovolemia and dehydration. This is particularly important, as studies have shown that older adults are more prone to orthostatic hypotension in this setting (Epstein, 1996).

The kidney's ability to manage various electrolytes also declines with age. Older adults are unable to effectively adapt to daily dietary salt intake via reabsorption and excretion, leading to sodium retention and fluid buildup. Not only is potassium excretion less efficient in older individuals, but a decreased response to aldosterone may also attenuate hyperkalemia in these patients (Epstein, 1996). The decrease in GFR with age also reduces the kidney's ability to handle metabolic changes and excrete excess hydrogen ions, making these patients prone to acidosis. Calcium balance is altered as older adults produce less vitamin D, which impairs calcium absorption, leading to higher levels of parathyroid hormone and fibroblast growth factor 23, which can lead to bone disease (Noronha et al., 2022).

Clinical risk factors and historical features of CKD in older adults

Clinical history

In any clinical setting, a careful and detailed history can be a key feature in understanding the underlying pathology behind a patient's clinical presentation. A renal-focused history is broad and necessitates an understanding of the many risk factors that make people prone to kidney disease. The REGARDS study (The Risk Factors for Incident CKD in Black and White Americans) was one of the most recent meta-analyses to investigate these risk factors, which include age, sex, sociodemographic factors, blood pressure, body mass index, diabetes, hyperlipidemia, heart disease, angiotensin-converting enzyme (ACE) inhibitor and angiotensin II receptor blocker (ARB) use, and nonsteroidal antiinflammatory drug (NSAID) use (Cheung, 2023). Other aspects of history-taking in these patients include screening for hematuria, foamy urine, urinary frequency or infrequency, edema, flank pain, rashes, and more (Chen et al., 2019). It is similarly important to understand a patient's baseline when considering what changes occurred prior to their presentation.

Further examination of common risk factors for CKD

Diabetic nephropathy is a major microvascular complication of diabetes mellitus (DM), and it is responsible for up to 50% of all cases of ESKD in Western populations. The earliest detectable clinical manifestation of CKD is microalbuminuria, and in the absence of early intervention, approximately 50% of patients with established microalbuminuria will progress to macroalbuminuria. This is associated with a 10-fold higher risk of progression to ESKD than that of patients without albuminuria altogether. The incidence of microalbuminuria in patients with type 1 diabetes is around 30%, which largely depends on medication compliance and tight blood glucose control. The incidence of microalbuminuria in patients with type 2 diabetes is also around 30%, but it is usually associated with hypertension (HTN). In both cases, albuminuria does not occur in the absence of hyperglycemia, and glucose control is the main determinant of progression to overt diabetic kidney disease (DKD). Other risk factors for DKD include morbid obesity, low birthweight, and genetic susceptibility factors, which may explain why some, but not all, patients with DM develop DKD (Natesan and Kim, 2021).

Hypertension is the second most common cause of CKD in elderly populations. It results from systemic vascular resistance and cardiac output. Pressure natriuresis involves increased renal sodium excretion in response to elevated blood pressure, but it is impaired in advanced age or CKD, which leads to extracellular volume expansion, increased systemic vascular resistance, and hypertension (Ivy and Bailey, 2014). Activation of the renin-angiotensin-aldosterone system (RAAS), particularly through the angiotensin II type 1 receptor, results in vasoconstriction, sodium retention, aldosterone synthesis, fibrosis, and vascular injury (Ma et al., 2010). Arterial stiffness, often considered a consequence of hypertension, may precede its onset (Mitchell, 2014). The pulsatile load from ventricular contraction fractures arteriolar elastin fibers, which are replaced by less distensible collagen, reducing vascular compliance (Laurent and Boutouyrie, 2020).

The SPRINT (Systolic Blood Pressure Intervention Trial) study compared the effects of antihypertensive treatment targeting a systolic blood pressure of < 120 mm Hg versus < 140 mm Hg in adults aged 50 and older with hypertension and cardiovascular disease (CVD) risk. The < 120 mm Hg group was found to have a 25% reduction in primary composite outcomes (myocardial infarction, nonMI acute coronary syndrome, stroke, acute heart failure, and CVD death) and a 27% reduction in all-cause mortality (Cushman et al., 2010). The ACCORD BP trial (Effects of Intensive Blood-Pressure Control in Type 2 Diabetes Mellitus), which targeted the same blood pressure levels in patients with diabetes, found a 12% reduction in the < 120 mm Hg group, though this was not statistically significant (Cushman et al., 2010).

Despite these findings, blood pressure targets remain a topic of debate. The ACC/AHA (American College of Cardiology and the American Heart Association) 2017 guidelines recommend a target of < 130/80 mm Hg for CKD patients (Whelton, 2018), while the European Society of Hypertension 2023 guidelines suggest < 140/90 mm Hg (Mancia et al., 2023). KDIGO (Kidney Disease Improving Global Outcomes) recommends a target of < 120 mm Hg (KDIGO, 2021). These differing recommendations contribute to inconsistent blood pressure management. Additionally, there is a need for more standardized and reliable blood pressure measurement technology, especially for out-of-office settings.

The interaction between hypertension and CKD is complex, increasing the risk of adverse cardiovascular and cerebrovascular outcomes. The pathophysiology of CKD-associated hypertension involves multiple mechanisms, including sodium dysregulation, increased sympathetic nervous system activity, and alterations in RAAS activity.

History of acute kidney injury

Older age is associated with an increased likelihood that renal function will not return to baseline after a kidney injury. Several studies have demonstrated that, even after adjustment for several important covariates, acute kidney injury (AKI) is independently associated with an increased risk for both CKD and ESRD. In elderly patients, the risk for ESRD after a single episode of AKI is elevated twofold in those with mild AKI, and it is elevated by 3- to 13-fold in those with more severe AKI (Coca et al., 2011).

Polypharmacy and its impact

Patients are prone to developing more comorbidities and acquiring chronic illnesses over the years as they age. As a result, polypharmacy is a growing problem for older adults. This is particularly true for those with CKD, as medications that are renally excreted need to be dose-adjusted. Approximately 50% of medications approved by the FDA (Food and Drug Administration) are renally excreted (Farrell and Vassalotti, 2024). One can imagine the problems that arise with polypharmacy, as many people may be unaware that they have kidney disease; thus they are at increased risk of medication toxicity. Many medications that require such dose reductions can have harmful effects when poorly cleared. These include opioids, blood thinners, antibiotics, and chemotherapy agents (Chen et al., 2019). The CKD-EPI equations can be useful in assessing clearance for medication dosing (Chen et al., 2019).

Screening the urinary system

The urinary system is composed not only of the kidneys but also the ureters, bladder, and urethra, which makes it an important focus of the history and physical exam. Obstructive uropathy refers to renal disease caused by impairment of urine flow. Congenital urinary tract obstruction (UTO), which is usually a result of posterior urethral valves, occurs early during fetal development and may lead to kidney failure. In adults, acquired UTO can result from many causes, including stones, masses, or benign prostatic hyperplasia (BPH). Urinary retention from strictures, spinal cord injury, infections, medications, trauma, or post-surgical procedures can also cause obstructive uropathy. Chronic obstructive uropathy can lead to structural and functional changes in the kidney, resulting in a reduction in GFR and altered handling of electrolytes and water excretion. Altered renal hemodynamics due to UTO can lead to acute kidney injury and, eventually, to irreversible renal injury, scarring, and CKD. Therefore, it is crucial, during history gathering, to inquire about congenital obstructive pathologies, history of stones, voiding dysfunction, or BPH. Screening for urinary retention in acutely ill geriatric patients should have a low threshold because of the high prevalence of urinary retention in this age group. Urinary retention is also very frequent in the postoperative phase in elderly patients, especially after abdominal and orthopedic surgeries, due to multiple precipitating factors, including limited mobility, pain, drugs (anesthesia, analgesia), advanced age, and male gender (Martin et al., 2019).

Physical examination

The assessment of renal disease is multifaceted and includes a comprehensive physical exam. There are multiple physical manifestations of renal disease, and patients can present with different signs and symptoms indicative of the underlying cause of CKD or its complications. Clinical manifestations generally occur with CKD stages 4–5, with eGFR < 30 mL/min/1.73 m^2. Important physical clues include new-onset edema, such as in the lower extremities or other areas prone to dependent swelling. Visually, one might observe new rashes, palpable purpura, or areas of skin excoriation (Chen et al., 2019). On auscultation, cardiac friction rubs or pulmonary crackles may be present. Neurologic exams may reveal worsening confusion or decreased sensation to touch due to peripheral neuropathy, such as in the case of diabetic kidney disease or cryoglobulinemic glomerulonephritis (Sethi et al., 2022). CKD is clinically silent and may present without physical findings; thus routine screening in asymptomatic patients is crucial (Table 20.2).

TABLE 20.2 A comparison of serum creatinine (cr) and serum cystatin C (cys).

Characteristic	Serum creatinine	Serum cystatin C
Source of production	Creatinine is produced by muscle metabolism and varies with muscle mass and diet.	Cystatin C is produced by all nucleated cells at a constant rate and is independent of muscle mass.
Are you affected by muscle mass?	Yes, creatinine is affected by low muscle mass. Frailty, sarcopenia, malnutrition, and amputations can falsely lower creatinine levels despite a low glomerular filtration rate (GFR).	No, cystatin C is mainly independent of muscle mass, making it a more reliable indicator of glomerular filtration in patients with sarcopenia or advanced age.
Affected by diet or other factors?	A high protein intake and creatinine supplements can raise serum creatinine levels. Hydration status can dilute creatinine.	Inflammation, thyroid dysfunction, and high adiposity can independently increase serum cystatin C levels, regardless of GFR.

Characteristic	Serum creatinine	Serum cystatin C
Excretion route	The glomerulus freely filters creatinine, but the proximal tubules also secrete it. At high serum creatinine levels, secretion contributes more significantly.	The glomerulus filters cystatin C. Filtered cystatin C is metabolized by the tubules and is not returned to the blood, so it is not present in urine in significant amounts.
Assay considerations	The creatinine assay is widely available, inexpensive, and standardized worldwide.	The cystatin C assay is more expensive, but standardization and availability are improving, making it increasingly accessible in major labs.
Prognostic value	The creatinine-based eGFR is a validated predictor of CKD outcomes. However, it is less sensitive to mild changes in kidney function in the elderly due to low muscle mass.	The serum cystatin C may detect changes in GFR earlier in some cases. It has a stronger association with cardiovascular outcomes and mortality in CKD patients, especially when the serum creatinine is falsely reassuring.
Use in eGFR equations	The serum creatinine is used in traditional equations such as Cockcroft-Gault, MDRD, and CKD-EPI 2009.	The serum cystatin C has been incorporated into newer equations, such as CKD-EPI 2012 and 2021, either alone or as a dual-marker. This has improved accuracy. This test is useful in older adults or individuals with abnormal body composition.

Laboratory tests and imaging

Assessment of altered renal function includes a comprehensive diagnostic workup. A suggested initial evaluation includes complete urinalysis, urine albumin-to-creatinine ratio, creatinine with estimated GFR, BUN, electrolytes, glucose, calcium, phosphorus, albumin, and complete blood count (Identify & Manage Patients with Chronic Kidney Disease, 2025). The clinical history and physical exam findings can greatly aid in diagnosis. For example, if a patient with diabetes has retinopathy, albuminuria, and negative screening tests, it is reasonable to assume the diagnosis is diabetic kidney disease. However, if further evaluation is needed due to concern for acute glomerular pathology, additional work-up must be completed. Tests such as hepatitis B and hepatitis C serologies, ANA (antinuclear antibody), rheumatoid factor, complement levels, serum electrophoresis (SPEP), and urine electrophoresis (UPEP) can be ordered (Sethi et al., 2022).

Creatinine versus cystatin C

Estimated glomerular filtration rate (eGFR) is one of the first screening methods for the evaluation of CKD (KDIGO, 2021). Over several decades, there have been advances in estimating glomerular filtration rate in an attempt to circumvent the complexities of direct GFR measurement, including the development of prediction equations (Miller and Jones, 2018). Multiple validated equations for surrogate GFR measurement are utilized, as noted in the KDIGO CKD Guidelines, which use various markers of filtration (KDIGO, 2021). Creatinine is the most utilized marker, given its cost-effectiveness, availability, and ease of measurement

(Miller and Jones, 2018). However, despite its accessibility, creatinine also has its limitations. Creatinine, which is derived from muscle, can be influenced by multiple factors, notably dietary intake and muscle mass (Table 20.2).

There has been ongoing research into other markers of filtration in recent years. Cystatin C is a small, freely filtered protein that is reabsorbed by proximal tubule cells and catabolized, making it an attractive surrogate for filtration. It is also produced by all nucleated cells rather than solely muscle cells (McMurray et al., 2009). There have been multiple barriers to the universal utilization of Cystatin C—a lack of standardization, testing costs, and availability among them (KDIGO, 2021; Miller and Jones, 2018). Cystatin C is also not without external factors that influence its testing, including thyroid disease, inflammation, and high adiposity (KDIGO, 2021).

Creatinine and cystatin C are two prevalent filtration markers that are used in the eGFR equations. These can be used alone; however, growing evidence has shown improved accuracy in eGFR assessment when they are both used in the same calculation (KDIGO, 2021). This may be related to the adjustment for each marker's limitations. For older adults, the interpretation of eGFR can be complex when using the aforementioned filtration markers. Sarcopenia, defined by low muscle mass and its impact on strength and performance (Cruz-Jentoft et al., 2010), is a common condition among older adults. Interpretation of serum creatinine can be impacted by low muscle mass in these patients, which may make the utilization of both cystatin C and serum creatinine more useful in CKD evaluation in this population.

Urinary test and creatinine clearance

Serum creatinine in a younger adult can correspond to a higher eGFR than that in an older adult. This phenomenon is the result of a change in urinary creatinine clearance with age. The decrease in urinary creatinine clearance may be due to decreased muscle mass associated with aging. A normalized serum creatinine with a reduced eGFR has important ramifications, as relying on serum creatinine alone may lead to inappropriate drug dosing and clinical decision-making (Epstein, 1996).

Renal ultrasound and imaging findings

Anatomical changes occur with aging not only microscopically but can also be visible on imaging. This includes the presence of renal cysts, which increase in size and number with age (Hommos et al., 2017). The increase in renal cyst size may be associated with hypertension (HTN). The kidneys lose mass with aging (Epstein, 1996; Fang et al., 2020), which has been noted to be more pronounced in the cortex than in the medulla. We lose cortex with age, but our renal mass is sustained in the early decades of life due to initial compensation with hypertrophy from the medulla (Hommos et al., 2017).

Complications of CKD in elderly

Progression of CKD leads to various problems. Bone mineral disease (BMD) is a common complication that is particularly important in frail older adults. BMD in CKD is characterized by dysregulation of phosphate, and its accumulation leads to decreased 1,25-dihydroxyvitamin D3 synthesis and a fall in serum calcium levels, which can result in increased serum parathyroid hormone (PTH) levels. Elevated PTH can lead to abnormal bone turnover and remodeling, which is a risk factor for the development of bone disorders (Hsu et al., 2020). Fractures are a major concern in bone disease, especially for older adults. Mortality is increased when a fracture has occurred. In patients with hip fractures, there is a 12%–20% increase in mortality compared to those without hip fractures, despite a similar demographic profile (Kelsey and Hoffman, 1987). Any new fracture in older adults signifies a high risk of additional fractures, especially within the following year. The risk of fracture is a consideration, as fall prevention is essential to avoid the increased mortality in older adults. During the patient encounter, measures should be taken to screen for gait abnormalities, unsafe home environments, and polypharmacy (LeBoff et al., 2022). Anemia is another common complication of CKD due to decreased erythropoietin production. Patients should be screened for additional causes of anemia, such as nutritional insufficiency of folate and B12, and iron deficiency. Erythropoietin-stimulating agents may be needed for iron-repleted patients with persistently low hemoglobin of < 10 g/dL (Chen et al., 2019).

Management and treatment

The management of CKD is centered not just on treating renal disease but also on addressing the various comorbidities that either worsen it or stem from it. Hypertension and kidney disease often go hand in hand. Hypertensive disease can be a significant factor toward the development of CKD, but it can also occur in the setting of renal damage. Pharmacologic therapy is largely based on the overall clinical picture. Patients with proteinuria or diabetic kidney disease are treated with ACE inhibitors or ARB therapy to prevent disease progression (Farrell and Vassalotti, 2024). These medications are also useful in patients with concurrent cardiac disease to prevent cardiac remodeling by modulating the RAAS, thereby managing hypertension with a blood pressure goal of < 130/80 (Farrell and Vassalotti, 2024). Management of diabetes is also important, as uncontrolled blood sugar can lead to disease progression (Chen et al., 2019). The A1C goal is typically < 7 (Chen et al., 2019). The use of antiglycemic pharmacologic therapy should be carefully monitored in patients with concurrent diabetes and renal disease, as many of these agents are renally excreted, which can lead to toxicity (Chen et al., 2019). Patients with CKD should be screened for cardiovascular disease due to the increased risk associated with renal dysfunction. Primary prevention with statin therapy should be considered in patients with CKD to reduce cardiovascular mortality (Farrell and Vassalotti, 2024). A cornerstone of CKD management is nutrition. Studies have shown the possible benefit of low-protein diets in patients with advanced CKD (stages 4 and 5) in preventing disease progression (Farrell and Vassalotti, 2024; KDIGO, 2021). Diets with lower acid intake may also help achieve this goal (Chen et al., 2019). Monitoring and limiting dietary intake is essential in patients with elevated blood pressure or issues of volume overload (Chen et al., 2019). Dietary modifications should be cautiously implemented, particularly in patients at risk of malnutrition, sarcopenia, or cachexia (KDIGO, 2021). As with any disease, CKD management and prevention of progression and complications should be tailored to the patient. It is crucial for clinicians to have an understanding of the medications

TABLE 20.3 Clinical pearls in CKD.

Risk factor/history item	Details/clinical notes	References
Age and sex	Increasing age is an independent risk factor. The incidence of CKD is more common in women.	(Cheung, 2023; Vosters et al., 2024)
Sociodemographic factors	Lower socioeconomic status is associated with a higher risk of CKD.	(Cheung, 2023)
Hypertension	Hypertension is closely associated with CKD, abnormal pressure natriuresis, RAAS activation, and arterial stiffness.	(Ivy and Bailey, 2014; Ma et al., 2010; Laurent and Boutouyrie, 2020)
Diabetes mellitus (DM)	Diabetic nephropathy accounts for around 50% of cases of ESKD in the West. Thirty percent develop proteinuria. The risk of advanced kidney disease rises with poor glycemic control and hypertension.	(Natesan and Kim, 2021)
Obesity & low birthweight	These may increase the risk of diabetic kidney disease (DKD).	(Natesan and Kim, 2021)
Heart disease & hyperlipidemia	Heart disease is common in CKD, and if untreated, it leads to poor outcomes.	(Cheung, 2023)
Medication exposure	NSAID use increases the risk of CKD.	(Cheung, 2023)
History of AKI	AKI increases the risk of progression to CKD/ESKD. Severe AKI can increase the risk by up to 13-fold.	(Coca et al., 2011)
Polypharmacy	Fifty percent of FDA-approved drugs are renally excreted; dose adjustment is critical; ↑ risk of toxicity in unrecognized CKD.	(Chen et al., 2019; Farrell and Vassalotti, 2024)
Obstructive uropathy (UTO)	Congenital (posterior urethral valves) or acquired (stones, BPH, strictures, tumors, trauma, medications). Causes scarring and CKD.	(Martin et al., 2019)
Other historical features	Concerning signs include hematuria, foamy urine, changes in urinary frequency, edema, flank pain, and rashes.	(Chen et al., 2019)

and how CKD affects drug excretion due to the risks of polypharmacy in older adults (Table 20.3).

Conservative management

It is essential to provide patients with clear and accurate information about dialysis prognosis and ESKD treatment options, including palliative and supportive care. While estimating prognosis in ESKD can be challenging, the surprise question, "Would you be surprised if the patient died in the next 6 or 12 months?", has been shown to improve prognostic predictions. Although this question is subjective and has its limitations, it is commonly used by healthcare providers to identify patients who are at the highest risk for morbidity and mortality. Physicians should initiate advanced care planning discussions as part of renal replacement therapy planning and continue these conversations regularly during the evaluation of patients on dialysis, particularly when there is a change in their health status.

In a study of elderly patients, less than 50% of those aged 75 years and older survive more than one year on dialysis. For individuals aged 70 to 74 on dialysis, the average remaining lifespan is approximately 3.9 years, compared to about 12.1 years for their peers in the general US population not on dialysis. Similarly, dialysis patients aged 75 to 79 have an expected remaining lifespan of about 3.3 years, compared to 9.1 years for nondialysis individuals of the same age group (Bello et al., 2022). Research, primarily from single-center studies, indicates that elderly patients who start dialysis generally live longer than those who do not, except in cases of ischemic heart disease, where dialysis does not improve survival rates (Chou et al., 2022).

Conservative, nondialytic management is a viable option for frail, elderly patients with CKD when dialysis is unlikely to improve quality or length of life. Effective decision-making involves advance care planning, focusing on patient values, goals, and treatment preferences (Raghavan and Holley, 2016). Hospice care should be considered for patients with a life expectancy of six months or less, focusing on comfort and symptom relief (Romero et al., 2023). The decision must involve a multidisciplinary approach, including nephrologists, primary care physicians, palliative care specialists, and other healthcare providers.

Elderly patients with CKD often experience a high symptom burden. Effective symptom management is crucial, addressing issues such as pain, fatigue, insomnia, pruritus, anorexia, and nausea. Pain management involves the use of acetaminophen, NSAIDs, weak opioids like tramadol, and strong opioids such as fentanyl, with adjuvants like gabapentin for neuropathic pain (Roy et al., 2020). Fatigue can be addressed by evaluating and treating sleep disorders, anemia, and depression, with erythropoietin and physical therapy as potential interventions (Ju et al., 2018). Sleep disturbances may be managed through lifestyle changes, sleep hygiene techniques, and medications such as trazodone. Pruritus treatment includes dietary phosphate restriction, phosphate binders, and emollient therapy, with additional options like antihistamines and UVB (ultraviolet B) light therapy (Lipman et al., 2021). Anorexia management involves antiemetics, promotility agents, and appetite stimulants. Nausea can be treated with haloperidol, while dyspnea management may include morphine and nonmedical interventions such as fans and relaxation techniques. Hospice care is recommended for patients expected to die within six months, focusing on symptom management and psychosocial support. A multidisciplinary approach is necessary to ensure comprehensive and compassionate care for elderly CKD patients (Raghavan and Holley, 2016).

Discussion of outcomes, ESKD planning, and the importance of individualized therapy

As CKD progresses, it is imperative to prepare for the possibility of dialysis. The IDEAL (The Initiating Dialysis Early and Late) study showed that there was no specific GFR threshold to begin dialysis, suggesting no overt benefit of early versus late dialysis initiation in patients with stage 5 CKD (Cooper et al., 2010). There are multiple forms of maintenance dialysis—hemodialysis, peritoneal dialysis, and home hemodialysis therapies. The availability of multiple treatment options underscores the importance of individualized care, focusing not only on the patient's goals of care but also on the patient's quality of life. Initiating early discussions about dialysis planning is important, including whether the patient desires dialysis, as inadequate preparation can lead to serious consequences. Urgent-start dialysis, performed within 48 h, has a high impact on morbidity and survival. Dialysis preparation should also address nonclinical aspects of patient care—social support, physical home space, caretakers, transportation, out-of-pocket costs, and more. In older adults, survival is decreased after starting dialysis, which makes shared decision-making very important (Chan et al., 2019).

Patients are living longer and reaching end-stage disease at later ages due to advances in multiple areas of renal disease management. One important option to consider for older adults is kidney transplantation. Kidney transplantation has become an increasingly popular choice among older adults, demonstrating improved 1-, 3-, and 5-year survival rates compared to previous years; however, it remains a complex discussion involving candidacy, available support, and patient safety (McAdams-Demarco et al., 2014).

Conclusion

The incidence of kidney disease is rapidly growing around the world. This is a result of not only the many risk factors for kidney disease but also the growing commitment to its screening, treatment, and prevention. In parallel, older adults are one of the fastest-growing demographic groups. The incidence of renal disease in those aged 65 or older is now rapidly rising. It becomes imperative to understand not only the complex effects that aging has on our kidneys and their physiology but also how to tailor individualized care for our older patients. This includes the assessment of individual goals of care, social support, nutrition, effects of medications, and more. As CKD becomes more prevalent, clinicians must possess the tools to treat patients into the later stages of life to limit the many effects of an aging kidney.

References

Identify & Manage Patients with Chronic Kidney Disease. National Institute of Diabetes and Digestive and Kidney Diseases, Bethesda, MD, 2025. Available from: https://www.niddk.nih.gov/health-information/professionals/clinical-tools-patient-management/kidney-disease/identify-manage-patients.

Armstrong, J.A., 2007. Urinalysis in Western culture: a brief history. Kidney Int. 00852538. 71 (5), 384–387. doi:10.1038/sj.ki.5002057.

Bello, A.K., Okpechi, I.G., Osman, M.A., Cho, Y., Htay, H., Jha, V., Wainstein, M., Johnson, D.W., 2022. Epidemiology of haemodialysis outcomes. Nat. Rev. Nephrol. 1759507X. 18 (6), 378–395. Available from: http://www.nature.com/nrneph/archive/index.html. doi:10.1038/s41581-022-00542-7.

Chan, C.T., Blankestijn, P.J., Dember, L.M., Gallieni, M., Harris, D.C.H., Lok, C.E., Mehrotra, R., Stevens, P.E., Wang, A.Y.M., Cheung, M., Wheeler, D.C., Winkelmayer, W.C., Pollock, C.A., Abu-Alfa, A.K., Bargman, J.M., Bleyer, A.J., Brown, E.A., Davenport, A., Davies, S.J., Finkelstein, F.O., Flythe, J.E., Goffin, E., Golper, T.A., Gómez, R., Hamano, T., Hecking, M., Heimbürger, O., Hole, B., Hothi, D.K., Ikizler, T.A., Isaka, Y., Iseki, K., Jha, V., Kawanishi, H., Kerr, P.G., Komenda, P., Kovesdy, C.P., Lacson, E., Laville, M., Lee, J.P., Lerma, E.V., Levin, N.W., Lichodziejewska-Niemierko, M., Liew, A., Lindley, E., Lockridge, R.S., Madero, M., Massy, Z.A., McCann, L., Meyer, K.B., Morton, R.L., Nadeau-Fredette, A.C., Okada, H., Perez, J., Perl, J., Polkinghorne, K.R., Riella, M.C., Robinson, B.M., Rocco, M.V., Rosansky, S.J., Rotmans, J.I., Roblero, M.F.S., Tangri, N., Tonelli, M., Tong, A.,

Tsukamoto, Y., Tungsanga, K., Vachharajani, T.J., van Loon, I., Watnick, S., Weiner, D.E., Wilkie, M., Zakharova, E., 2019. Dialysis initiation, modality choice, access, and prescription: conclusions from a Kidney Disease: improving Global Outcomes (KDIGO) Controversies Conference. Kidney Int. 15231755. 96 (1), 37–47. Available from: https://www.journals.elsevier.com/kidney-international. doi:10.1016/j.kint.2019.01.017.

Chen, T.K., Knicely, D.H., Grams, M.E., 2019. Chronic kidney disease diagnosis and management: a review. JAMA. 15383598. 322 (13), 1294–1304. Available from: http://jama.jamanetwork.com/journal.aspx. doi:10.1001/jama.2019.14745.

Cheung, K., 2023. Risk factors for incident CKD in black and white Americans: the REGARDS study. Am. J. Kidney Dis. 82 (1), 11–21. doi:10.1053/j.ajkd.2022.11.015.

Chou, A., Li, K.C., Brown, M.A., 2022. Survival of older patients with advanced CKD managed without dialysis: a narrative review. Kidney Med. 25900595. 4 (5). Available from: https://www.journals.elsevier.com/kidney-medicine. doi:10.1016/j.xkme.2022.100447.

Coca, S.G., Cho, K.C., Hsu, C.Y., 2011. Acute kidney injury in the elderly: predisposition to chronic kidney disease and vice versa. Nephron Clin. Pract. 16602110. 119 (1), c19. doi:10.1159/000328023.

Cockcroft, D.W., Gault, M.H., 1976. Prediction of creatinine clearance from serum creatinine. Nephron. 00282766. 16 (1), 31–41. doi:10.1159/000180580.

Cooper, B.A., Branley, P., Bulfone, L., Collins, J.F., Craig, J.C., Fraenkel, M.B., Harris, A., Johnson, D.W., Kesselhut, J., Jing Jing, L., Luxton, G., Pilmore, A., Tiller, D.J., Harris, D.C., Pollock, C.A., Randomized, A., 2010. Controlled trial of early versus late initiation of dialysis. N. Engl. J. Med. 0028-4793. 363 (7), 609–619. doi:10.1056/nejmoa1000552.

Coresh, J., Stevens, L.A., 2006. Kidney function estimating equations: where do we stand? Curr. Opin. Nephrol. Hypertens. 10624821. 15 (3), 276–284. doi:10.1097/01.mnh.0000222695.84464.61.

Cruz-Jentoft, A.J., Baeyens, J.P., Bauer, J.M., Boirie, Y., Cederholm, T., Landi, F., Martin, F.C., Michel, J.P., Rolland, Y., Schneider, S.M., Topinková, E., Vandewoude, M., Zamboni, M., 2010. Sarcopenia: european consensus on definition and diagnosis. Age Ageing. 14682834. 39 (4), 412–423. doi:10.1093/ageing/afq034.

Cushman, W.C., Evans, G.W., Byington, R.P., Goff, D.C., Grimm, R.H., Cutler, J.A., Simons-Morton, D.G., Basile, J.N., Corson, M.A., Probstfield, J.L., Katz, L., Peterson, K.A., Friedewald, W.T., Buse, J.B., Bigger, J.T., Gerstein, H.C., Ismail-Beigi, F., 2010. Effects of intensive blood-pressure control in type 2 diabetes mellitus. N. Engl. J. Med. 15334406. 362 (17), 1575–1585. Available from: http://content.nejm.org/cgi/reprint/362/17/1575.pdf. doi:10.1056/NEJMoa1001286.

Diamantis, A., Magiorkinis, E., Androutsos, G., 2008. Proteinuria: from ancient observation to 19th century scientific study. J. Urol. 0022-5347. 180 (6), 2330–2332. doi:10.1016/j.juro.2008.08.043.

Ebert, N., Pottel, H., van der Giet, M., Kuhlmann, M.K., Delanaye, P., Schaeffner, E., 2022. The impact of the new CKD-EPI equation on GFR estimation in the elderly. Dtsch. Arztebl. Int. 1866-0452. 119 (41). doi:10.3238/arztebl.m2022.0258.

Epstein, M., 1996. Aging and the kidney. J. Am. Soc. Nephrol. 1046-6673. 7 (8), 1106–1122. doi:10.1681/asn.v781106.

Fang, Y., Gong, A.Y., Haller, S.T., Dworkin, L.D., Liu, Z., Gong, R., 2020. The ageing kidney: molecular mechanisms and clinical implications. Ageing Res. Rev. 18729649. 63. Available from: http://www.elsevier.com/locate/arr. doi:10.1016/j.arr.2020.101151.

Farrell, D.R., Vassalotti, J.A., 2024. Screening, identifying, and treating chronic kidney disease: why, who, when, how, and what? BMC Nephrol. 14712369. 25 (1). Available from: https://bmcnephrol.biomedcentral.com/. doi:10.1186/s12882-024-03466-5.

Gounden, V., Bhatt, H., Jialal, I., Jan. 2026. Renal Function Tests. StatPearls, Treasure Island, FL. Available from: https://www.ncbi.nlm.nih.gov/books/NBK507821/.

Grams, M.E., Chow, E.K.H., Segev, D.L., Coresh, J., 2013. Lifetime incidence of CKD stages 3-5 in the United States. Am. J. Kidney Dis. 15236838. 62 (2), 245–252. doi:10.1053/j.ajkd.2013.03.009.

Hommos, M.S., Glassock, R.J., Rule, A.D., 2017. Structural and functional changes in human kidneys with healthy aging. J. Am. Soc. Nephrol. 15333450. 28 (10), 2838–2844. Available from: http://jasn.asnjournals.org/content/28/10/2838.full.pdf+html. doi:10.1681/ASN.2017040421.

Hsu, C.Y., Chen, L.R., Chen, K.H., 2020. Osteoporosis in patients with chronic kidney diseases: a systemic review. Int. J. Mol. Sci. 14220067. 21 (18), 1–24. Available from: https://www.mdpi.com/1422-0067/21/18/6846/pdf. doi:10.3390/ijms21186846.

Inker, L.A., Eckfeldt, J., Levey, A.S., Leiendecker-Foster, C., Rynders, G., Manzi, J., Waheed, S., Coresh, J., 2011. Expressing the CKD-EPI (Chronic Kidney Disease Epidemiology Collaboration) cystatin C equations for estimating GFR with standardized serum cystatin C Values. Am. J. Kidney Dis. 15236838. 58 (4), 682–684. doi:10.1053/j.ajkd.2011.05.019.

Inker, L.A., Eneanya, N.D., Coresh, J., Tighiouart, H., Wang, D., Sang, Y., Crews, D.C., Doria, A., Estrella, M.M., Froissart, M., Grams, M.E., Greene, T., Grubb, A., Gudnason, V., Gutiérrez, O.M., Kalil, R., Karger, A.B., Mauer, M., Navis, G., Nelson, R.G., Poggio, E.D., Rodby, R., Rossing, P., Rule, A.D., Selvin, E., Seegmiller, J.C., Shlipak, M.G., Torres, V.E., Yang, W., Ballew, S.H., Couture, S.J., Powe, N.R., Levey, A.S., 2021. New creatinine- And cystatin C-based equations to estimate GFR without race. N. Engl. J. Med. 15334406. 385 (19), 1737–1749. Available from: http://www.nejm.org/medical-index. doi:10.1056/NEJMoa2102953.

Ivy, J.R., Bailey, M.A., 2014. Pressure natriuresis and the renal control of arterial blood pressure. J. Physiol. 14697793. 592 (18), 3955–3967. Available from: http://www.wiley.com/bw/editors.asp?ref=0022-3751&site=1. doi:10.1113/jphysiol.2014.271676.

Ju, A., Strippoli, G.F.M., Craig, J.C., Tong, A., Saglimbene, V.M., Unruh, M.L., 2018. Interventions for fatigue in people with chronic kidney disease requiring dialysis. Cochrane Database Syst. Rev. 1469493X. 2018 (8). Available from: http://as.wiley.com/WileyCDA/Brand/id-6.html. doi:10.1002/14651858.CD013074.

KDIGO, 2021. Clinical practice guideline for the management of blood pressure in chronic kidney disease. Kidney Int. 99 (3S), S1–S87.

Kelsey, J.L., Hoffman, S., 1987. Risk factors for hip fracture. N. Engl. J. Med. 15334406. 316 (7), 404–406. doi:10.1056/NEJM198702123160709.

Laurent, S., Boutouyrie, P., 2020. Arterial stiffness and hypertension in the elderly. Front. Cardiovasc. Med. 2297-055X. 7. doi:10.3389/fcvm.2020.544302.

LeBoff, M.S., Greenspan, S.L., Insogna, K.L., Lewiecki, E.M., Saag, K.G., Singer, A.J., Siris, E.S., 2022. The clinician's guide to prevention and treatment of osteoporosis. Osteoporos. Int. 0937-941X. 33 (10), 2049–2102. doi:10.1007/s00198-021-05900-y.

Levey, A.S., Coresh, J., Greene, T., Marsh, J., Stevens, L.A., Kusek, J.W., Van Lente, F., 2007. Expressing the modification of diet in renal disease study equation for estimating glomerular filtration rate with standardized serum creatinine values. Clin. Chem. 0009-9147. 53 (4), 766–772. doi:10.1373/clinchem.2006.077180.

Levey, A.S., Coresh, J., Greene, T., Stevens, L.A., Zhang, Y., Hendriksen, S., Kusek, J.W., Van Lente, F., 2006. Using standardized serum creatinine values in the modification of diet in renal disease study equation for estimating glomerular filtration rate. Ann. Intern. Med. 00034819. 145 (4), 247–254. Available from: http://annals.org/issues.aspx. doi:10.7326/0003-4819-145-4-200608150-00004.

Levey, A.S., Stevens, L.A., Schmid, C.H., Zhang, Y., Castro, A.F., Feldman, H.I., Kusek, J.W., Eggers, P., Lente, F.V., Greene, T., Coresh, J., 2009. A new equation to estimate glomerular filtration rate. Ann. Intern. Med. 15393704. 150 (9), 604–612. Available from: http://www.annals.org/cgi/reprint/150/9/604.pdf. doi:10.7326/0003-4819-150-9-200905050-00006.

Lindeman, R.D., Tobin, J., Shock, N.W., 1985. Longitudinal studies on the rate of decline in renal function with age. J. Am. Geriatr. Soc. 15325415. 33 (4), 278–285. doi:10.1111/j.1532-5415.1985.tb07117.x.

Lipman, Z.M., Paramasivam, V., Yosipovitch, G., Germain, M.J., 2021. Clinical management of chronic kidney disease-associated pruritus: current treatment options and future approaches. Clin. Kidney J. 20488513. 14, I16. Available from: http://ckj.oxfordjournals.org/. doi:10.1093/ckj/sfab167.

Losito, A., 2023. History of creatinine clearance: tribute to a forerunner. Clin. Kidney J. 16 (6), 891–895. doi:10.1093/ckj/sfad024.

Ma, T.K.W., Kam, K.K.H., Yan, B.P., Lam, Y.Y., 2010. Renin-angiotensin-aldosterone system blockade for cardiovascular diseases: current status. Br. J. Pharmacol. 14765381. 160 (6), 1273–1292. Available from: http://onlinelibrary.wiley.com/journal/10.1111/%28ISSN%291476-5381. doi:10.1111/j.1476-5381.2010.00750.x.

Mancia, G., Kreutz, R., Brunström, M., Burnier, M., Grassi, G., Januszewicz, A., Muiesan, M.L., Tsioufis, K., Agabiti-Rosei, E., Algharably, E.A.E., Azizi, M., Benetos, A., Borghi, C., Hitij, J.B., Cifkova, R., Coca, A., Veronique Cornelissen, J.K.C., Cunha, P.G., Danser, A.H.J., de Pinho, R.M., Delles, C., Dominiczak, A.F., Dorobantu, M., Doumas, M., Fernández-Alfonso, M.S., Halimi, J.-M., Járai, Z., Jelaković, B., Jordan, J., Kuznetsova, T., Laurent, S., Lovic, D., Lurbe, E., Mahfoud, F., Manolis, A., Miglinas, M., Narkiewicz, K., Niiranen, T., Palatini, P., Parati, G., Pathak, A., Persu, A., Polonia, J., Redon, J., Sarafidis, P., Schmieder, R., Spronck, B., Stabouli, S., Stergiou, G., Taddei, S., Thomopoulos, C., Tomaszewski, M., Van de Borne, P., Wanner, C., Weber, T., Williams, B., Zhang, Z.-Y., Kjeldsen, S.E., 2023. ESH Guidelines for the management of arterial hypertension. The Task Force for the management of arterial hypertension of the European Society of Hypertension. J. Hypertens. 0263-6352. 41 (12), 1874–2071. doi:10.1097/hjh.0000000000003480.

Martin, J., Chandler, W., Speakman, M., 2019. Investigating chronic urinary retention. BMJ. 0959-8138. 366, l4590. doi:10.1136/bmj.l4590.

McAdams-Demarco, M.A., James, N., Salter, M.L., Walston, J., Segev, D.L., 2014. Trends in kidney transplant outcomes in older adults. J. Am. Geriatr. Soc. 15325415. 62 (12), 2235–2242. Available from: http://onlinelibrary.wiley.com/journal/10.1111/(ISSN)1532-5415. doi:10.1111/jgs.13130United.

McMurray, M.D., Trivax, J.E., McCullough, P.A., 2009. Serum cystatin C, renal filtration function, and left ventricular remodeling. Circ. Heart Fail. 1941-3289. 2 (2), 86–89. doi:10.1161/circheartfailure.109.856393.

Miller, W.G., Jones, G.R.D., 2018. Estimated glomerular filtration rate; laboratory implementation and current global status. Adv. Chronic Kidney Dis. 15485609. 25 (1), 7–13. Available from: http://www.elsevier.com/wps/find/journaldescription.cws_home/703170/description#description. doi:10.1053/j.ackd.2017.09.013.

Mitchell, G., 2014. Recent advances in hypertension: arterial stiffness and hypertension. Hypertension 64 (1), 13–18.

Natesan, V., Kim, S.-J., 2021. Diabetic nephropathy - a review of risk factors, progression, mechanism, and dietary management. Biomol. Ther. 1976-9148. 29 (4), 365–372. doi:10.4062/biomolther.2020.204.

Noronha, I.L., Santa-Catharina, G.P., Andrade, L., Coelho, V.A., Jacob-Filho, W., Elias, R.M., 2022. Glomerular filtration in the aging population. Front. Med. 2296858X. 9. Available from: https://journal.frontiersin.org/journal/medicine. doi:10.3389/fmed.2022.769329.

Raghavan, D., Holley, J.L., 2016. Conservative care of the elderly CKD patient: a practical guide. Adv. Chronic Kidney Dis. 15485609. 23 (1), 51–56. Available from: http://www.elsevier.com/wps/find/journaldescription.cws_home/703170/description#description. doi:10.1053/j.ackd.2015.08.003.

Romero, K., Widera, E., Wachterman, M.W., 2023. Breaking the link between enrollment in hospice and discontinuation of dialysis. JAMA Intern. Med. 21686114. 183 (3), 177–178. Available from: http://archinte.jamanetwork.com/issues.aspx. doi:10.1001/jamainternmed.2022.6390.

Roy, P.J., Weltman, M., Dember, L.M., Liebschutz, J., Jhamb, M., 2020. Pain management in patients with chronic kidney disease and end-stage kidney disease. Curr. Opin. Nephrol. Hypertens. 14736543. 29 (6), 671–680. Available from: http://journals.lww.com/co-nephrolhypertens/pages/default.aspx. doi:10.1097/MNH.0000000000000646.

Sethi, S., De Vriese, A.S., Fervenza, F.C., 2022. Acute glomerulonephritis. Lancet. 1474547X. 399 (10335), 1646–1663. Available from: http://www.journals.elsevier.com/the-lancet/. doi:10.1016/S0140-6736(22)00461-5.

Shahbaz, R., Gupta, M., 2025. Creatinine Clearance. StatPearls [Internet]. Available from: https://www.ncbi.nlm.nih.gov/books/NBK544228/.

Tang, Y., Jiang, J., Zhao, Y., Dunfeng, D., 2024. Aging and chronic kidney disease: epidemiology, therapy, management and the role of immunity. Clin. Kidney J. 2048-8505. 17 (9). doi:10.1093/ckj/sfae235.

Vassalotti, J.A., Centor, R., Turner, B.J., Greer, R.C., Choi, M., Sequist, T.D., 2016. Practical approach to detection and management of chronic kidney disease for the primary care clinician. Am. J. Med. 15557162. 129 (2), 153. Available from: https://www.elsevier.com/locate/amjmed. doi:10.1016/j.amjmed.2015.08.025.

Vosters, T.G., Kingma, F.M., Stel, V.S., van den Born, B.-J.H., Huisman, B.J.M.V., van Ittersum, F.J., Jager, K.J., Vogt, L., van Valkengoed, I.G.M., 2024. Sex differences in CKD risk factors across ethnic groups. Nephrol. Dial. Transplant. 0931-0509. 39 (7), 1194–1197. doi:10.1093/ndt/gfae038.

Weinstein, J.R., Anderson, S., 2010. The aging kidney: physiological changes. Adv. Chronic Kidney Dis. 15485595. 17 (4), 302–307. doi:10.1053/j.ackd.2010.05.002.

Whelton, P.K., 2018. ACC/AHA/AAPA/ABC/ACPM/AGS/APhA/ASH/ASPC/NMA/PCNA guideline for the prevention, detection, evaluation, and management of high blood pressure in adults. Hypertension 71 (6), e13.

Winter, M.A., Guhr, K.N., Berg, G.M., 2012. Impact of various body weights and serum creatinine concentrations on the bias and accuracy of the cockcroft-gault equation. Pharmacotherapy. 02770008. 32 (7), 604–612. doi:10.1002/j.1875-9114.2012.01098.x.

CHAPTER

21

Myths about chronic kidney disease in the elderly

Ahmed Awan and Sarwar Khan

Department of Internal Medicine, Baylor College of Medicine, Houston, TX, United States

Introduction

The diagnosis of chronic kidney disease (CKD) and the subsequent illness perception can affect quality of life (Knowles et al., 2023). The importance of this finding lies in preventing unnecessary stress on patients, especially when the label of disease does not actually change the overall prognosis of the patient in a meaningful way. Properly defining kidney disease in the elderly is of great importance. Subsequently, when there is a diagnosis of kidney disease, the next challenge is determining what to do about it. There are many things that are purported to work "to help the kidneys." These can include medicines, supplements, or food products. Patients are vulnerable and often seek solutions wherever they can find them. With the proliferation of the internet, it can be very easy for incorrect information to disseminate to patients, even in the most well-intentioned cases. Even for medical practitioners, there are gaps in knowledge and commonly held beliefs that may not be backed by evidence, or the evidence may have changed. The dizzying amount of scientific evidence being generated every day also contributes to this difficulty in proper knowledge acquisition. Here, we will attempt to demystify some of the common myths and misunderstandings about kidney disease in the elderly, which also apply to the larger group of the adult population in general in terms of kidney disease (Fig. 21.1).

Aging and the Kidney
https://doi.org/10.1016/B978-0-443-34069-7.00027-6

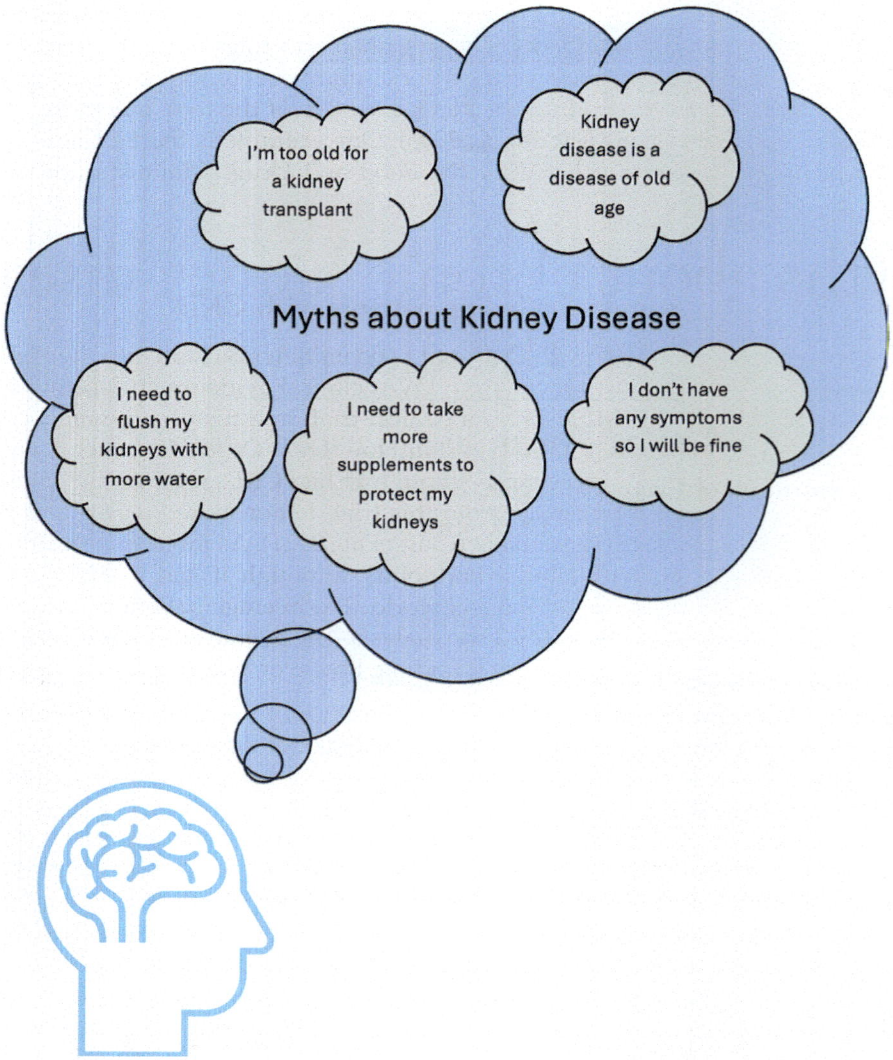

FIG. 21.1 Myths about kidney disease. There are many false conceptions about kidney disease and its management.

Myth: Aging is always associated with a decline in kidney function

All of the organs in our body undergo senescence, which is the normal deterioration of function with age. The kidneys are not immune to this fate. While the kidneys do experience age-related decline in function, this deterioration usually progresses slowly. In most people, the kidneys continue to perform adequately throughout life. In fact, many individuals die from other age-related conditions such as cardiovascular disease, stroke, or cancer before kidney function declines enough to cause serious health problems. Our kidneys will often outlive us. Even with normal healthy aging, there will be a loss of nephrons, the functional units of the kidney. This is similar to wrinkles on the skin, which inevitably form, although there are methods to reduce their number and extent. The aging process of the kidneys has been studied in biopsies from living kidney donors, where the donor has to meet many stringent criteria that deem them healthy. This ensures the kidney being donated will be of good quality and provides insights into what healthy aging may look like in the kidney. As expected, with increasing age, there is a trend toward more scarring in the kidney, otherwise called nephrosclerosis (Rule et al., 2010; Emmons et al., 2023). Nephrosclerosis can simply be thought of as the breakdown of the nephrons that give the kidneys their ability to filter the blood. These studies are conducted on healthy people without the typical chronic diseases such as hypertension and diabetes, both of which are associated with poorer kidney function. The only common variable that may correlate to the damage is aging. Interestingly, the estimated glomerular filtration rate (eGFR), our common tool for assessing total filtration ability, does not seem to adequately predict the nephrosclerosis observed in the biopsy data from living donors.

The eGFR does decline with normal aging in the majority of persons. Different studies exploring this finding in multiple ways have confirmed this but do not exactly agree on the rate of decline. One important study following healthy men over 20 years showed a decline of about 7 mL/min per decade (Lindeman et al., 1985). Other studies in different populations are in line with this glomerular filtration rate (GFR) decline. This decline usually starts around 30–40 years of age (Glassock and Winearls, 2009).

It is not clear what the exact implication of this reduced eGFR is for a patient, other than that it is a normal part of aging. KDIGO defines a GFR of <60 mL/min/1.73 m^2 as the threshold for defining a person as having CKD. One large prospective study examined patients over 70 years of age, and between 38% to 62% of people had an eGFR of <60 mL/min/1.73 m^2 (Ebert et al., 2017). This cohort was a reflection of the general population, with an accurate representation of all the associated comorbidities found in this age group. In the same study, a urine albumin-to-creatinine ratio of greater than 30 mg/g was associated with higher cardiovascular risk factors, emphasizing the important role of proteinuria, more than GFR alone, in predicting adverse outcomes.

When eGFR in older adults falls below 60 mL/min/1.73 m^2, some studies show there is an increase in mortality risk compared to age-matched controls with preserved eGFR (Warnock et al., 2017; Malmgren et al., 2015; Hallan et al., 2012). However, not all studies support this finding. What appears more consistent is that small eGFR declines seen in patients younger than 60 years old are associated with a mortality risk that is significantly higher (Jonsson et al., 2020). This suggests that the decrease in eGFR, which is part of normal kidney senescence as one ages, may be relatively benign and does not convey a major risk for death as it does in younger patients with similar declines. In one large metaanalysis of over 2 million people, an eGFR above 105 mL/min/1.73 m^2 in the elderly was associated with the unexpected finding of having worse mortality compared to the normal range of 90 mL/min/1.73 m^2. While this observation remains unclear, it underscores the incomplete understanding of kidney function in the elderly and its implications for overall health. What is consistent across studies, however, is that worsening albuminuria—rather than a modest decline in eGFR—predicts poorer outcomes in the elderly.

Considering the above discussion, one can think about a hypothetical case of an otherwise healthy elderly patient who has an eGFR listed just below 60 mL/min/1.73 m^2 and normal-range albuminuria, who would have the label of CKD placed on them by the KDIGO standards. It is unclear whether being labeled this way is the appropriate approach for a patient like this. There is no clear consensus on whether mildly reduced GFR leads to appreciable adverse outcomes, and even if it does, whether those outcomes can be mitigated. Undue stress and anxiety may be placed on a patient by assigning this label. Reassurance can be provided to elderly patients who find themselves with this diagnosis, as long as there are no other signs of more serious kidney disease. Risk calculators, such as the Kidney Failure Risk Equation (KFRE)—a version of which can be found online at https://ckd-epi.com (last accessed July 23, 2025)—are simple, validated tools that can provide clear percentages regarding a patient's risk for progressive kidney disease and the need for kidney replacement therapy at two and five years. This tool helps both patients and providers alike gain a sense of where things stand. In addition, as circumstances change over time, proper follow-up and monitoring of kidney function are essential, though not at the same frequency as for a younger individual who has a higher risk for adverse outcomes.

Myth: A decline in kidney function is always associated with symptoms

In our experience, many patients, when first told they have kidney disease, indicate that they have no pain in their kidneys or say they now understand where the pain in their back was coming from. This highlights a simple misunderstanding the general public has regarding their kidneys. The assumption is that only if there is a symptom, there is a problem. This is unfortunate, as in most types of kidney disease, it is a silent disease until significant damage has been done. Except in cases of kidney stones, urinary tract infections, cyst ruptures, or physical trauma, there are no physical symptoms of early CKD. The symptoms of CKD, when they do manifest, are subtle, such as fatigue, decreased appetite, and changed sleep patterns. These usually don't appear until stage 4 or 5 CKD. In addition, these symptoms are not specific to kidney disease and can be associated with many other illnesses. Some of these symptoms may also be falsely attributed to "normal aging," which can prevent early recognition and treatment. Furthermore, urine output can remain normal even in end-stage kidney disease requiring dialysis, at least when the patient has first started.

Given the silent nature of most kidney diseases, screening should be conducted in at-risk individuals. Some of these risks include individuals with diabetes, hypertension, heart disease, those over the age of 60, and those with a positive family history of kidney disease. Interaction with the health care system in general usually results in some test that will detect kidney disease, whether through blood or urine analysis. An important point is to have routine follow-ups with a provider who can reassess patient risks over time and repeat screening as their health changes. In the management of established CKD, the recommendation by KDIGO is to monitor patients with CKD at Stage 1 and 2 disease every year, Stage 3 every 6 months, Stage 4 every 3 months, and Stage 5 every 6 weeks. This strategy encompasses the idea that kidney disease progresses silently, and a systematized way of monitoring is necessary. Of course, if there is a concern for faster progression or a specific symptom, then more timely evaluation can be done. Thus some physicians prefer to follow Stage 4 patients every 6 weeks. This approach also allows patients to ease into their new diagnosis. It often is a shock for patients to hear they have kidney disease, given the lack of symptoms, and they need time to process their diagnosis. In addition, repeated encounters with a provider will allow them to understand their disease further and plan ahead. As the disease progresses, they will eventually need to plan for kidney replacement therapy. Approximately 80% of patients in the United States start with a central line dialysis catheter. This is far from the ideal of either kidney transplant, arteriovenous fistula, or PD catheter, which eventually result in better outcomes and reduced morbidity. The KFRE discussed above can help predict which patients need planning for kidney replacement sooner rather than later.

Myth: Dialysis is not an option since I'm elderly; it's too harsh

Frailty is an important concept in the elderly and can loosely be defined as a syndrome of decreased functional and physical capacity in domains such as energy level, strength, cognitive ability, and body weight. All of these factors can lead to worse overall health outcomes. Dialysis, whether through hemodialysis or peritoneal dialysis, is an intensive procedure and takes a toll on the body both mentally and physically. The elderly often have higher rates of frailty and may be less suited for the rigors of dialysis. There is no absolute cut off at which dialysis should not be offered, but with increasing age, there are diminishing survival advantages. For example, at 70 years old, there is a survival advantage over conservative care, but beyond 80 years old, that advantage disappears (Verberne et al., 2016). Patients can be counseled on what they may expect to benefit by starting dialysis at later stages in their life. This does not tell the whole story, though, and requires an experienced clinician to navigate the complexities of a choice like this. Later in this book, an approach to conservative kidney care will be explored that avoids interventions such as dialysis or transplant. With that said, patients who have fewer comorbidities and less frailty may benefit from starting dialysis regardless of their age. There are patients above 90 years old who still derive benefit from dialysis, and for them, the burdens of the procedure are acceptable. Dialysis also does not have to be an all-or-nothing intervention. Incremental dialysis is an approach to dialysis where the amount and duration of dialysis are based on the patient's residual kidney function and symptoms (Mathew et al., 2016). For example, instead of three sessions of hemodialysis a week, a patient may only need two. Or with peritoneal dialysis, fewer exchanges on the cycler could be attempted. This would reduce the burden of multiple trips to a dialysis unit, which comes with many hazards, particularly for a frail elderly population.

Dialysis vascular access is another important consideration in the elderly. It refers to the way blood is mobilized for dialysis, either through an arteriovenous fistula (AVF), graft (AVG), or catheter. In older patients, comorbidities such as diabetes, hypertension, and peripheral vascular disease result in suboptimal blood vessels, making it more difficult to create an appropriate arteriovenous access. For example, maturation failure of the AVF, which is the inability to use a newly created AVF, is higher in the elderly than in younger individuals (Moist et al., 2012). Repeat procedures and maturation time could take even a few months for the fistula to be ready. In general, there is a "fistula first" approach to dialysis access, meaning attempts are made to create an AVF before other methods, such as an AVG or catheter, are used. This is done because catheters and AVGs have higher rates of infections and thrombosis than AVFs. However, this same logic may not apply to the elderly, as it may be difficult to even create the AVF in the first place and put the patient through excessive procedures for limited benefit. This takes into account life expectancy in elderly patients on dialysis. The benefits derived from an AVF take time to materialize, which an elderly patient might not have. An AVG or catheter may be more suited to an elderly individual, as they may be used immediately or within a few days and do not require maturation.

Home modalities of dialysis are also important to consider in the elderly. Peritoneal dialysis (PD) may be a more suitable option. It works by using a catheter embedded into the peritoneum that allows dialysis fluid to be exchanged in and out, ultimately clearing the blood of toxins and excess fluid. This method avoids the vascular access issues discussed above, which are common in the elderly. PD is generally described as a "gentler" form of dialysis. In particular, it is more hemodynamically tolerable as it is done daily over many hours compared to the short, thrice-weekly sessions of hemodialysis. In PD, there are no rapid fluid shifts as seen with hemodialysis, which can cause a variety of symptoms that are less tolerable in the elderly. Some of these symptoms may include hypotension, muscle cramps, nausea, and headaches that may last for hours after a hemodialysis session and cause a significant decrease in quality of life. PD also has the added benefit of being done from home with minimal interactions with the health care system compared to the frequent visits required for in-center hemodialysis. Usually, only one visit per month to a dialysis center is needed. PD allows for more customization in prescription and can fit around a patient's lifestyle more easily. There are some limitations to PD in the elderly. PD requires some hand-eye coordination to make the connections from the catheter to the PD machine or dialyzate bags, along with specific hygiene precautions. In general, if a patient can drive, they likely can do PD on their own, as the skills are somewhat similar. If the elderly patient can not do it themselves, they would require a care-giver to assist, which may or may not be feasible. In addition, there are some reported higher rates of peritoneal infections in the elderly compared to a younger population (Peng et al., 2023). None of these are absolute barriers but rather considerations.

Home hemodialysis is another modality that may be well suited for the elderly. It allows the patient to perform dialysis in their own home, but the technical barriers might be higher than those of peritoneal dialysis. It does not avoid the various problems associated with vascular access, as discussed above.

Myth: Kidney transplants should be avoided in the elderly

A kidney transplant often brings anxieties to patients and their families. Some attitudes include, "I'm too old and shouldn't take a kidney from someone else" or "I won't be able to handle a surgery like that." Patient's family members also want to see if they can donate and what they need to do. There are no absolute age cut offs for receiving a kidney transplant; however, some individual transplant centers have age limits. The decision whether or not to proceed with a kidney transplant is often made through a holistic process that includes the patient's comorbidities, frailty, cognitive function, and social support system. Frailty, as discussed above in the previous section, is a multifactorial assessment of physical and functional capacity. Frailty is often magnified in the kidney disease population due to complications associated with kidney disease, including anemia, volume overload, higher risk for fractures, muscle loss, uremic toxins contributing to mental slowing, and a sense of unwellness, among other factors. With all these potential contributors, frailty should be scrutinized closely. The Fried Frailty Phenotype (FFP) and the Short Performance Physical Battery (SPPB) are two potential tests that can gauge a potential patient's eligibility for transplant. The FFP looks at five domains, including unintentional weight loss, exhaustion, weakness in grip strength, slow ambulation speed, and low perceived physical activity. All these categories are assessed through a questionnaire completed by patients. The SPPB is an actual physical test that the patient completes to provide a sense of how functional they are in daily tasks. Another test that many centers use is the timed up and go test (TUG), also referred to as the "get up and go test." It times a patient from a seated position to get up, walk three meters, turn around, and sit back down. A time of less than 10 s is somewhat associated with better outcomes after a transplant. It is a useful and quick in-clinic test that captures many of the components of frailty seen in the more comprehensive tests. Regardless of all these tests, it ultimately is a multifactorial discussion between all members of a transplant team, along with the patient and their family, about whether they are physically strong enough for a transplant.

Living donor transplant is better for the elderly for a number of reasons. One logistical reason is that the deceased donor waiting list can be longer than 5 years in many cases, which, for an elderly patient, might be prohibitively long as the mortality rate on dialysis at 5 years can be very high. A living donor evaluation and subsequent transplant can happen much more quickly compared to the longer wait times on the deceased donor list. In addition, although not unique to the elderly, living donor donation usually results in a healthier kidney being transplanted.

Another consideration is the immunosuppression regimen in elderly individuals. The elderly are more susceptible to infections than younger individuals, as they have a less robust immune system. In contrast to this, and to their benefit, this means their immune system will be less able to reject their transplanted kidney. A less powerful initial immunosuppression regimen should be used in the elderly because of these two reasons. Cancer rates are also higher in the elderly as a normal fact of aging. Normal cancer screening should be done as for any patient, but posttransplant extra vigilance in the form of skin exams and other age-appropriate cancer screenings should be undertaken. This is because one of the effects of immunosuppression is an increased risk of cancer through the dampening effects on cancer-killing cells of the immune system.

Overall, elderly patients should be considered for kidney transplants, as it can have an overall beneficial effect on their lives.

Myth: Drinking water helps prevent and treat kidney disease

An intuitive question that patients often ask providers when first learning about their kidney disease is, "Am I drinking enough water?" This is because people tend to associate kidney health with the amount of fluid they consume. Some individuals may even take it upon themselves to drink excessive amounts of water, to the extent that they need to urinate multiple times per hour. Staying "hydrated" is a common piece of advice in the general public, and the recommendation to drink eight cups of water a day is widely circulated.

However, even among health care providers, there isn't a clear consensus on what should be recommended regarding water intake, despite it being a substance that constitutes approximately 50% of a person's body. Normal thirst signals are typically sufficient to keep a person adequately hydrated, as the hypothalamus regulates the body's osmolality—another term for hydration. This raises the question: is more hydration necessarily better? There are only a few specific conditions, such as kidney stones and autosomal dominant polycystic kidney disease, where drinking more water than dictated by normal thirst signals has a clear, evidence-based benefit (Wang et al., 2013). This issue is particularly significant in the elderly population, given their mobility challenges. An intervention that leads to frequent trips to the bathroom could increase the risk of falls and should only be recommended if it provides a clear and substantial benefit as a treatment strategy. The hypothesis that dehydration plays a role in the progression of CKD is based on preclinical data showing the harmful effects of antidiuretic hormone (ADH), also known as vasopressin. Excess levels of ADH can lead to several detrimental outcomes, including increased systemic blood pressure, elevated glomerular pressure, heightened proteinuria, and direct effects on kidney mesangial cell proliferation. All of these mechanisms contribute directly to the development and progression of kidney disease.

The clinical data on the impact of high water consumption on the development and progression of kidney disease is more complex, beyond the known areas of benefit in polycystic kidney disease (PKD) and kidney stones. In the case of preventing CKD in the general population, it does appear that there is reasonable evidence suggesting that increasing fluid intake is beneficial. Four large studies—two prospective and two cross-sectional—have examined this question. The first study separated patients into groups based on urine volumes, in liters (L), ranging from low (<1 L), normal (1–2 L) moderate (2–3 L), and high urine volumes (>3 L) to assess the impact on kidney function changes over a 7 year period. The groups were compared to the "normal" urine output group as a reference, and those producing over 3 L of urine per day demonstrated a significant difference in GFR decline compared not only to the normal group but also to the moderate group. This translated to a 0.6 mL/min/1.73 m^2 per year slower decline in kidney function. Taken over a lifetime, this could represent a significant change in GFR and a meaningful low-burden intervention for patient care (Clark et al., 2011).

A later study did not support these same conclusions (Palmer et al., 2014). This study similarly examined prospective cohorts split between varying levels of fluid intake. It went a step further than examining the development of worsening kidney function and also looked at all-cause and cardiovascular mortality. No signal of benefit was found in any of the fluid consumption levels: low, medium, or high.

The other large cross-sectional studies showed decreased rates of CKD associated with increased fluid intake. One of these studies demonstrated this effect in patients with an average age of 66 (Strippoli et al., 2011). The other study included adults of all ages as part of the National Health and Nutrition Examination Survey (NHANES) (Sontrop et al., 2013). This study specifically showed that plain water intake was associated with less CKD compared to other forms of fluid intake.

The only randomized controlled trial (RCT) that has addressed kidney function decline in a healthy population without CKD was conducted in elderly men defined as 55–75 years of age (Spigt et al., 2006). The intervention group received advice to increase their water intake by 1.5 L a day, and the control group was given a small aliquot of placebo syrup to take daily. The goal of increasing fluid intake was not reached in the intervention group. No effect was observed in improving GFR or quality of life in the higher water intake group. Importantly, no harm was observed in the intervention group that increased fluid intake, including the incidence of hyponatremia.

As a whole, these studies show that increased fluid intake, and in particular water, may have a beneficial effect on reducing the development of kidney disease. The studies all have methodological limitations, with varying populations studied and different criteria for fluid intake, which does make their interpretation more difficult. Importantly, though, even with all the varied studies, it does not seem that an obvious trend toward harm was noted, even in the one study with an average age of 66. Without an indication of harm, it may be appropriate to recommend this simple intervention to motivated patients. So it still remains: what is the right amount of fluid intake to prevent the development of CKD? About 3 L of fluid intake seems to provide some benefit, and greater than 4.5 L does not appear to have more benefit. Also, drinking less than 2 L of water might be associated with the development of CKD. This supports the popularly held belief that drinking at least 8 cups of water a day, which is approximately 2 L, is generally a healthy practice. It would be very beneficial to have a low-cost, easily implementable solution that could prevent a serious disease such as CKD. It is important to note that the patients in these studies were generally healthier than the sicker patients for whom fluid limitations are often prescribed by providers, such as in advanced CKD or heart failure.

So far, what has been discussed relates fluid intake to the development of CKD. However, what is equally important is determining the optimal fluid intake when CKD is already present. Up until recently, there were no RCTs examining this question, despite how fundamental fluid intake is (Clark et al., 2016). Observational and animal data suggested that increased fluid intake might slow the progression of CKD, but the evidence was very minimal. A re-analysis of the Modification of Diet in Renal Disease study, a large RCT investigating the effects of protein restriction and blood pressure control in CKD patients, indicated that higher urine volumes did not slow the progression of CKD and may have even accelerated the decline in kidney function (Hebert et al., 2003). The CKD-REIN study was another large cohort-based study designed to assess a multitude of factors related to the progression of CKD. One group analyzed a subset of the data in relation to water intake and CKD progression (Wagner et al., 2022). The authors found a U-shaped distribution related to water intake and CKD risk. The extremes of water intake—less than 0.5 L and more than 2 L—were associated with faster progression of the disease. They concluded that CKD patients should consume between 1 and 2 L of water per day as a general recommendation, tailored as needed to the individual patient. The Chronic Kidney Disease Water Intake Trial (CKD-WIT) was the first large RCT to specifically explore this (Clark et al., 2018). In this 1-year trial, participants with CKD stage 3 were randomized to either continue their current water intake or be coached to drink 1 to 1.5 L more water. At the end of the trial, there was no significant difference in the primary outcome of GFR decline between the two groups, although there was a statistically significant decrease in vasopressin levels in the extra-hydration group. Decreased vasopressin levels have been associated with slowing kidney disease progression through reduced glomerular hyperfiltration and a reduction in proteinuria, pointing to a possible benefit that might not have been evident in a one-year trial.

There are harms associated with drinking excessive fluid in CKD. One potential issue is the development of hyponatremia, especially in elderly individuals. Another concern is the potential for the development or worsening of edema, particularly when there is a concomitant increase in salt intake. Both of these issues can be life-threatening if not monitored closely. In addition, more frequent trips to the bathroom would be expected, which can be problematic for individuals with mobility issues and may predispose them to a greater risk of falls. Urinary incontinence could also worsen with a higher urine volume. These problems could arise if the recommendation to increase fluid intake is given as a blanket statement without proper guidance and monitoring from a medical professional. Therefore caution should be exercised when making sweeping statements such as "drink more fluid."

Another important point for the elderly is achieving adequate hydration in the first place, let alone the more ambitious goal of increased hydration as discussed above. Dehydration is the most frequent fluid and electrolyte problem in the elderly, and this issue is even more prevalent among those who live in long-term care facilities such as nursing homes. Dehydration is broadly defined as a deficiency in total body water content, failing to meet the baseline value required to achieve homeostasis. Dehydration can lead to a number of problems, including poor quality of life, confusion, falls, and constipation, all of which can exacerbate other medical issues. There are some strategies for increasing fluid intake that can be applied to those prone to dehydration and to those advised to increase their fluid intake for other reasons (Bruno et al., 2021). Strategies that have proven effective include verbal prompting and increasing the availability and variety of beverages. Verbal prompting, such as a simple daily reminder to stay hydrated, was found to be effective in one study. Making water and other beverages easily accessible also helps. For example, setting aside the daily water requirement in a large container allows for easy portioning throughout the day. In addition, offering more appealing options—such as water infused with flavors like lemon, mint, or cucumber—can make hydration more enjoyable. Some interesting strategies that were studied but did not prove effective included providing a straw, implementing a nonalcoholic cocktail hour, and introducing a more colorful beverage cart.

Myth: Supplements can prevent or slow the progression of kidney disease

There are many supplements on the market, and patients are often bombarded with information through the internet about how to support their kidney health. Ideally, an individualized plan tailored to each patient and their specific goals is necessary. Here, we discuss the most commonly sought-after nutrients and supplements that have been suggested to promote kidney health, with a quick summary provided in Table 21.1.

Vitamin D supplementation shows some potential benefits in the prevention and progression of CKD. Vitamin D can be obtained from foods or supplements in its precursor forms, vitamin D2 and D3, which then need to be converted by the body into the active form. These supplements can be purchased over-the-counter and are readily available. It can also be taken in its active form as either calcitriol or a vitamin D analog which works in a similar manner but requires a prescription. The end result of both these medications is the stimulation of the vitamin D receptor (VDR), which is present in many different organs. Notably, vitamin D is able to suppress renin production, which is the first effector molecule

TABLE 21.1 Nutrients and supplements in preventing and slowing CKD.

Nutrient	Myth	Reality
Water	Excess water will help the kidneys by "flushing them"	2–3 L of plain water is a safe target for healthy individuals and CKD patients. Excess water can be harmful, and low water intake can also cause the progression of kidney disease.
Vitamin D	High doses of vitamin D will protect me from a variety of diseases	Supplementation should target 30 ng/mL in all patients.
Vitamin A, B, C, E	Taking high doses of these vitamins will help "boost" my kidneys	There is no specific role in the prevention of kidney disease.
PUFAs	Taking fish oil will help my kidneys	Should be encouraged if other heart disease risk factors are present, but it has no specific role in preventing kidney disease.
Protein	Protein is bad for my kidneys.	In those with CKD, 0.8 g/kg/day should be taken to prevent progression.
Prebiotics/ Probiotics	"Good" bacteria will help my kidneys	No specific role in kidney disease, but suitable for other indications, such as gastrointestinal (GI) health. While many over-the-counter (OTC) probiotics are not specifically formulated for kidney health, Renadyl has been explicitly formulated for chronic kidney disease (CKD). Further studies are necessary to demonstrate its efficacy.
Diet	I can't eat fruits and vegetables because they contain potassium	The Mediterranean and DASH diets, which are rich in fruits and vegetables, are beneficial for kidney health. Foods with high potassium can be limited as needed. Ultra-processed foods should be avoided.
Traditional Chinese Medicine/ Ayurvedic Medicine	I want a natural approach to protect my kidneys	Although there are potentially promising herbs, harm can be caused due to a lack of regulation and the avoidance of known beneficial medications.

in the renin-angiotensin-aldosterone-system (RAAS). In pathological states such as kidney disease, overactivation of the local kidney RAAS leads to excess angiotensin II, which causes increased intra-glomerular pressures, elevated inflammatory cytokines and immune pathway activation, podocyte damage, and other deleterious effects, all resulting in worsening kidney disease. Vitamin D in its active form essentially downregulates the expression of genes that produce renin. Studies have shown that over or underexpressing the VDR has the expected effect of decreasing and increasing renin expression, respectively. The NF-κB pathway is also influenced by vitamin D. NF-κB is a key regulator in the inflammatory cascade, particularly in the kidney. It has been shown to increase macrophages in the kidney, which in turn promote inflammation. Angiotensin II also promotes NF-κB expression. Vitamin D is able to block the binding of NF-κB to the genome and prevent downstream transcription of inflammatory proteins. These data on vitamin D so far are at the preclinical level and have been tested in animals or in vitro, showing promise. In some human studies, the results are promising as well. Vitamin D deficiency has been associated with higher levels of albuminuria. In other studies, vitamin D analogs have shown beneficial effects in reducing proteinuria, particularly in diabetic nephropathy, where kidney-level RAAS activation is very high. There may be more benefit from vitamin D-mediated downregulation of the RAAS in this population (Li, 2010). To date, however, despite all the promising data, no RCTs are available that show relevant improved outcomes in treatment with vitamin D, whether through achieving normal levels or above-target levels. In general, it is a low-risk intervention with proper monitoring, so it is reasonable to aim for the target goal to potentially avoid worsening kidney disease. The KDIGO guidelines recommend 30 ng/mL as the target level of serum 25(OH)D. The data on general supplementation in a non-CKD population is lacking with regard to the development of kidney disease. However, more attention should be paid to vitamin D supplementation in those with risk factors for developing CKD, as some protective effects might be present in this population as well. Various societies list anywhere from 20–30 ng/mL as the target goal for 25(OH)D levels. Vitamin D3 at 600–2000 IU should be taken daily to maintain these levels. Other essential vitamins, such as A, B-complex, C, and E, have no specific role in preventing or treating CKD. Recommendations suggest supplementing only those who have a deficiency or are at risk of developing one.

Polyunsaturated fatty acids (PUFAs) are another potential supplement that may help prevent or slow down kidney disease. PUFAs are categorized into omega-3 and omega-6 fatty acids, with many different molecules in each category. Fish oil is a common supplement that contains high levels of omega-3, and patients often take it for cardiovascular reasons or to prevent various diseases. These fatty acids have varied effects on inflammation in the body and can act as antioxidants. Higher blood PUFA levels have been linked to reduced development of incident CKD, and higher DHA levels have been associated with slower progression of CKD to kidney failure (Koh et al., 2024). In addition, there is some evidence suggesting decreased proteinuria with omega-3 supplementation. Even with some promising results, no RCTs have demonstrated a benefit to supplementing PUFAs in any form, such as fish oil. At this point, the KDOQI guidelines do not support the routine use of these supplements (Lin et al., 2021). However, there is no clear evidence of harm in kidney disease. If PUFAs are being taken for other indications, such as cardiovascular disease or hyperlipidemia, their use should be encouraged.

Protein intake is a heavily studied intervention in preventing the progression of CKD. Excess protein consumption causes glomerular hyperfiltration, which can accelerate glomerular damage. The recommended consumption of protein is 0.8 g/kg/day of bodyweight. For example, a 70 kg person should eat 56 g of protein in a day from a variety of sources. KDIGO also recommends avoiding excess protein intake above 1.3 g/kg/day. To take it a step further, a motivated person could also further reduce their protein intake to 0.3–0.4 g/kg of body weight along with supplemented amino acids, which is also endorsed by the KDIGO guidelines. A robust metaanalysis on this question found a 13% lower progression to ESRD compared to those following the 0.8 g/kg protein-restricted diet (Rhee et al., 2018). The 1 year GFR benefit from the more restrictive diet was approximately 4 mL/min/1.73 m^2. Averaged over a few years, this is a substantial benefit. The potential harms are clear in regard to malnourishment with protein wasting, although none of the trials noted harms when done properly. Therefore this intervention should not be undertaken without close supervision to avoid the harms of malnourishment. In particular, with the elderly, caution should be taken as this group suffers from sarcopenia due to a variety of other factors, and a recommendation toward extremes of low protein intake may be detrimental. These recommendations apply to patients with CKD, and the same recommendations do not apply to those without kidney disease who are trying to prevent its onset. Higher intake of protein may be reasonable for those individuals with varying levels of physical activity.

The old adage told to kids, "eat your vegetables," applies to kidney disease as well. Increased fruit and vegetable intake can help both in the prevention of kidney disease and in slowing its progression. One large prospective cohort study of over 9000 patients followed over eight years showed that those with the highest rates of fruit and vegetable consumption had significantly lower rates of CKD development and proteinuria (Jhee et al., 2019). In addition, higher vegetable and fruit intake has been associated with lower blood pressure through a variety of mechanisms. Lower blood pressure can also protect against the development of CKD. The importance of fruits and vegetables has been better studied in patients already diagnosed with CKD. The KDIGO guidelines recommend greater reliance on a plant-based diet for persons with CKD. Less importance should be placed on animal products and ultraprocessed foods. However, animal products can still be part of a healthy diet when eaten in moderation. A focus on plant-based food sources can decrease the daily acid load, which may aid in slowing the progression of CKD. Increased fiber intake may decrease uremic toxin production in the gut. There is also lower absorption of phosphorus from plant sources compared to processed or animal foods. In addition, an increase in fruits and vegetables likely guards against the development of cardiovascular disease, which CKD patients are at an increased risk for (Carrero et al., 2020). All of this should be weighed against the risks of elevated potassium levels in patients, as certain fruits and vegetables can sometimes contribute to this. However, patients should not avoid fruits and vegetables solely because of the potential to develop elevated potassium. If elevated potassium does develop, there are many strategies to combat it that will still allow for a plant-based diet.

Some diets that meet these goals in kidney disease are the Dietary Approaches to Stop Hypertension (DASH) Diet and the Mediterranean Diet. These diets focus on whole foods, meaning unprocessed ingredients such as fruits, vegetables, grains, and lean protein. The DASH diet, in particular, emphasizes low sodium intake at approximately 2 g per day, and if dairy products are consumed, they should be low-fat or nonfat. The Mediterranean Diet places additional focus on olive oil as the primary fat source, along with other high omega-3 fat sources. Both diets allow for moderate intake of red meats but caution against processed foods. They are both very versatile and can serve as the foundation of a sustainable diet. If possible, a kidney-focused dietitian can be utilized as well. It can sometimes be difficult for patients to change their dietary habits alone without the help of a professional, and many medical providers may not be familiar with the practical aspects of diet. Kidney dietitians can provide a more nuanced approach tailored to a patient's specific needs at different stages of kidney disease and personal preferences. They are also experts at targeting the right amounts of sodium, phosphorus, potassium, protein, and fluid for a patient after discussion with the medical provider.

Probiotics and prebiotics have been studied in CKD and its relation to cardiac disease. One large meta-analysis showed they can reduce some inflammatory markers and improve lipid profiles, but data has not suggested clear benefits in the progression of CKD (Zheng et al., 2021). There is a diversity of different types of prebiotics and probiotics, and it is unclear what dose, strain, and combination may have a beneficial effect. At this time, no specific guidance can be given, but it is likely not harmful to patients, and if it helps with other medical issues, it can be continued. Renadyl has been specifically formulated and studied in CKD. While early RCTs show promise, further studies are necessary (Natarajan et al., 2014).

A special note will be made regarding alternative medications such as traditional Chinese medicine (TCM) and Ayurvedic medicine, which are often sought after by patients for a variety of ailments, including kidney disease. This is to highlight what providers may encounter in their practice and to ensure they are at least equipped to answer questions from patients or potentially look out for complications. TCM is a long-practiced medical system with its roots in China and is now practiced in many parts of the world. It uses herbs, among other therapies, for treatments. One herb, called *Tripterygium wilfordii Hook F,* commonly known as the thunder god vine, is routinely used in TCM for the treatment of various nephropathies. Its active ingredient, triptolide, may have beneficial effects on kidney fibrosis, at least in non-human models, which is the final pathway of CKD (Zhong et al., 2015). A number of other herbs have been studied that have varying effects on kidney disease. One combination of these herbs is called the "Shenqi particle." It is a combination of thirteen different herbs, with some having known active compounds and others having unclear active compounds. A large RCT published in the American Journal of Kidney Disease compared the Shenqi particle to a typical regimen of cyclophosphamide plus prednisone for the treatment of idiopathic membranous nephropathy (Chen et al., 2013). The Shenqi particle showed similar remission rates to the standard regimen and fewer adverse events. It is thought that the herb *Astragalus* in the compound might be a key active ingredient, given its previously reported effects on kidney disease. There were many limitations with this study, but it showed some interesting results and new therapeutic options to a Western audience that could be explored further. It should be noted that this treatment is not recognized by any large kidney disease organization across the globe. With the active ingredient not known, it is hard to use it in an allopathic medical setting due to multiple important regulatory barriers. In addition, the preparation of these herbs must be done with care, as mishandling may lead to overtly toxic compounds. In China, the long history of these herbs has led to an understanding of their proper preparation and the avoidance of overt harm. One harmful compound contained in some herbal products is called aristolochic acid. This compound is responsible for "Balkan endemic nephropathy" and "Chinese Herb Nephropathy," which are now more properly termed "Aristolochic acid nephropathy" (AAN) since the culprit toxin has been identified. It leads to a sometimes rapidly progressive tubulointerstitial nephritis, resulting in ESKD within as early as two years. The incidence of AAN is unclear but may represent a significant proportion of those who ingest it, with resulting variable presentations and degrees of harm, as there is likely no safe dose (Gökmen et al., 2013). This has led to many countries banning the sale of herbs that contain it. However, this does not stop the import of these harmful herbs, which can be mixed with other herbs. The regulation of these herbs in TCM, at least in the United States, is not at the same standard as other medications regulated by the FDA. It is difficult to recommend a particular approach because of the nonstandardized formulation of the herbal preparations. Proper guidance should be sought, and a thorough risk-benefit analysis should be conducted with patients if they wish to try these therapies.

Ayurvedic medicine has its origins in India and, like TCM, claims herbal remedies to prevent or treat kidney disease. A quick search online will yield various treatment options, as there is a large market for these alternative therapies. One specific formulation of herbs, called NEERI-KFT, is purported to work on some of the common final pathways of CKD progression (Gautam et al., 2021). It faces similar problems to those of herbal preparations in TCM, including the absence of identified active ingredients, the absence of published safety analyses, and a lack of proper RCTs. This is not to say that individual components of these herbs may not have therapeutic value in certain patients, but there is a risk of unforeseen harms and diversion away from treatments with proven benefits.

Conclusion

The chapter highlights how the diagnosis and labeling of CKD, particularly in older adults, significantly influence quality of life and clinical decision-making. It underscores that age-related declines in eGFR are common and not necessarily predictive of poor outcomes. Albuminuria serves as a more reliable indicator of kidney risk. Given that CKD often remains asymptomatic until its later stages, we recommend targeted screening and scaled follow-up, emphasizing tools like the Kidney Failure Risk Equation to personalize care without polypharmacy.

It is a myth that CKD invariably causes symptoms or that older age rules out renal replacement therapy. A nuanced, individualized approach includes incremental dialysis, careful selection of vascular access based on vessel integrity and life expectancy, and strong consideration of home-based therapies like peritoneal dialysis to reduce cardiovascular strain. Kidney transplantation for well-selected older patients can be successful when guided by assessments of frailty, functional status, and tailored immunosuppression strategies.

High water intake is often promoted as "flushing the kidneys"; however, it has limited and mixed support outside of kidney stones and autosomal dominant polycystic kidney disease (ADPKD). In established CKD, excessive hydration has not been shown to slow disease progression. Nutritional recommendations favor plant-dominant diets such as Mediterranean or DASH, reduced sodium intake, moderate protein consumption (around 0.8 g/kg/day for CKD patients), and avoidance of ultraprocessed foods. While omega-3 fatty acids and vitamin D show potential renal benefits, the evidence remains inconclusive. Probiotics, including kidney-specific formulations like Renadyl, are promising but not yet proven. Finally, unregulated herbal supplements, particularly those containing aristolochic acid, can be nephrotoxic. Clinicians are urged to guide patients toward safe, evidence-based treatments and away from misleading online health claims.

References

Bruno, C., Collier, A., Holyday, M., Lambert, K., 2021. Interventions to improve hydration in older adults: a systematic review and meta-analysis. Nutrients 13 (10). doi:10.3390/nu13103640.

Carrero, J.J., González-Ortiz, A., Avesani, C.M., Bakker, S.J.L., Bellizzi, V., Chauveau, P., Clase, C.M., Cupisti, A., Espinosa-Cuevas, A., Molina, P., Moreau, K., Piccoli, G.B., Post, A., Sezer, S., Fouque, D., 2020. Plant-based diets to manage the risks and complications of chronic kidney disease. Nat. Rev. Nephrol. 16 (9), 525–542. doi:10.1038/s41581-020-0297-2.

Chen, Y., Deng, Y., Ni, Z., Chen, N., Chen, X., Shi, W., Zhan, Y., Yuan, F., Deng, W., Zhong, Y., 2013. Efficacy and safety of traditional Chinese medicine (Shenqi particle) for patients with idiopathic membranous nephropathy:

a multicenter randomized controlled clinical trial. Am. J. Kidney Dis. 62 (6), 1068–1076. doi:10.1053/j.ajkd.2013.05.005.

Clark, W.F., Sontrop, J.M., Huang, S.-H., Gallo, K., Moist, L., House, A.A., Cuerden, M.S., Weir, M.A., Bagga, A., Brimble, S., Burke, A., Muirhead, N., Pandeya, S., Garg, A.X., 2018. Effect of coaching to increasewater intake on kidney function decline in adults with chronic kidney disease the CKD WIT randomized clinical trial. JAMA 319 (18), 1870–1879. doi:10.1001/jama.2018.4930.

Clark, W.F., Sontrop, J.M., Huang, S.-H., Moist, L., Bouby, N., Bankir, L., 2016. Hydration and chronic kidney disease progression: a critical review of the evidence. Am. J. Nephrol. 43 (4), 281–292. doi:10.1159/000445959.

Clark, W.F., Sontrop, J.M., Macnab, J.J., Suri, R.S., Moist, L., Salvadori, M., Garg, A.X., 2011. Urine volume and change in estimated GFR in a community-based cohort study. Clin. J. Am. Soc. Nephrol. 6 (11), 2634–2641. doi:10.2215/CJN.01990211.

Ebert, N., Jakob, O., Gaedeke, J., van der Giet, M., Kuhlmann, M.K., Martus, P., Mielke, N., Schuchardt, M., Tölle, M., Wenning, V., Schaeffner, E.S., 2017. Prevalence of reduced kidney function and albuminuria in older adults: the Berlin Initiative Study. Nephrol. Dial. Transplant. 32 (6), 997–1005. doi:10.1093/ndt/gfw079.

Emmons, B.R., Batal, I., Radhakrishnan, J., Husain, S.A., 2023. Age-related changes in nephrosclerosis in a multiethnic living kidney donor cohort. Kidney Int. 104 (2), 394–397. doi:10.1016/j.kint.2023.04.012.

Gautam, G., Parveen, B., Umar Khan, M., Sharma, I., Kumar Sharma, A., Parveen, R., Ahmad, S., 2021. A systematic review on nephron protective AYUSH drugs as constituents of NEERI-KFT (a traditional Indian polyherbal formulation) for the management of chronic kidney disease. Saudi J. Biol. Sci. 28 (11), 6441–6453. doi:10.1016/j.sjbs.2021.07.008.

Glassock, R.J., Winearls, C., 2009. Ageing and the glomerular filtration rate: truths and consequences. Trans. Am. Clin. Climatol. Assoc. 120, 419–428.

Gökmen, M.R., Cosyns, J.-P., Arlt, V.M., Stiborová, M., Phillips, D.H., Schmeiser, H.H., Simmonds, M.S.J., Cook, H.T., Vanherweghem, J.-L., Nortier, J.L., Lord, G.M., 2013. The epidemiology, diagnosis, and management of aristolochic acid nephropathy: a narrative review. Ann. Intern. Med. 158 (6), 469–477. doi:10.7326/0003-4819-158-6-201303190-00006.

Hallan, S.I., Matsushita, K., Sang, Y., Mahmoodi, B.K., Black, C., Ishani, A., Kleefstra, N., Naimark, D., Roderick, P., Tonelli, M., Wetzels, J.F.M., Astor, B.C., Gansevoort, R.T., Levin, A., Wen, C.-P., Coresh, J., 2012. Age and association of kidney measures with mortality and end-stage renal disease. JAMA 308 (22), 2349–2360. doi:10.1001/jama.2012.16817.

Hebert, L.A., Greene, T., Levey, A., Falkenhain, M.E., Klahr, S., 2003. High urine volume and low urine osmolality are risk factors for faster progression of renal disease. Am. J. Kidney Dis. 41 (5), 962–971.

Jhee, J.H., Kee, Y.K., Park, J.T., Chang, T.-I., Kang, E.W., Yoo, T.-H., Kang, S.-W., Han, S.H., 2019. A diet rich in vegetables and fruit and incident CKD: a community-based prospective cohort study. Am. J. Kidney Dis. 74 (4), 491–500. doi:10.1053/j.ajkd.2019.02.023.

Jonsson, A.J., Lund, S.H., Eriksen, B.O., Palsson, R., Indridason, O.S., 2020. The prevalence of chronic kidney disease in Iceland according to KDIGO criteria and age-adapted estimated glomerular filtration rate thresholds. Kidney Int. 98 (5), 1286–1295. doi:10.1016/j.kint.2020.07.028.

Knowles, S.R., Apputhurai, P., Jenkins, Z., O'flaherty, E., Ierino, F., Langham, R., Ski, C.F., Thompson, D.R., Castle, D.J., 2023. Impact of chronic kidney disease on illness perceptions, coping, self-efficacy, psychological distress and quality of life. Psychol. Health Med. 28 (7), 1963–1976. doi:10.1080/13548506.2023.2179644.

Koh, H.B., Kim, H.W., Joo, Y.S., Jung, C.-Y., Kim, H.J., Chang, T.I., Park, J.T., Yoo, T.-H., Kang, S.-W., Han, S.H., 2024. Plasma levels of polyunsaturated fatty acids and adverse kidney outcomes. Am. J. Kidney Dis. 84 (2), 179–184.

Li, Y.C., 2010. Renoprotective effects of vitamin D analogs. Kidney Int. 78 (2), 134–139. doi:10.1038/ki.2009.175.

Lin, P.-C., Chou, C.-L., Ou, S.-H., Fang, T.-C., Chen, J.-S., 2021. Systematic review of nutrition supplements in chronic kidney diseases: a grade approach. Nutrients 13 (2), 1–21. doi:10.3390/nu13020469.

Lindeman, R.D., Tobin, J., Shock, N.W., 1985. Longitudinal studies on the rate of decline in renal function with age. J. Am. Geriatr. Soc. 15325415. 33 (4), 278–285. doi:10.1111/j.1532-5415.1985.tb07117.x.

Malmgren, L., McGuigan, F.E., Berglundh, S., Westman, K., Christensson, A., Åkesson, K., 2015. Declining estimated glomerular filtration rate and its association with mortality and comorbidity over 10 years in elderly women. Nephron. 130 (4), 245–255. doi:10.1159/000435790.

Mathew, A., Obi, Y., Rhee, C.M., Chen, J.L.T., Shah, G., Lau, W.-L., Kovesdy, C.P., Mehrotra, R., Kalantar-Zadeh, K., 2016. Treatment frequency and mortality among incident hemodialysis patients in the United States comparing incremental with standard and more frequent dialysis. Kidney Int. 90 (5), 1071–1079.

Moist, L.M., Lok, C.E., Vachharajani, T.J., Xi, W., AlJaishi, A., Polkinghorne, K.R., Vazquez, M., Lee, T.C., 2012. Optimal hemodialysis vascular access in the elderly patient. Semin. Dial. 25 (6), 640–648. doi:10.1111/sdi.12037.

Natarajan, R., Pechenyak, B., Vyas, U., Ranganathan, P., Weinberg, A., Liang, P., Mallappallil, M.C., Norin, A.J., Friedman, E.A., Saggi, S.J., 2014. Randomized controlled trial of strain-specific probiotic formulation (renadyl) in dialysis patients. Biomed Res. Int. 2314-6141. 2014. Available from: http://www.hindawi.com/journals/biomed/. doi:10.1155/2014/568571.

Palmer, S.C., Wong, G., Iff, S., Yang, J., Jayaswal, V., Craig, J.C., Rochtchina, E., Mitchell, P., Wang, J.J., Strippoli, G.F.M., 2014. Fluid intake and all-cause mortality, cardiovascular mortality and kidney function: a population-based longitudinal cohort study. Nephrol. Dial. Transplant. 29 (7), 1377–1384. doi:10.1093/ndt/gft507.

Peng, Y.-K., Tai, T.-S., Wu, C.-Y., Tsai, C.-Y., Lee, C.-C., Chen, J.-J., Hsiao, C.-C., Chen, Y.-C., Yang, H.-Y., Yen, C.-L., 2023. Clinical outcomes between elderly ESKD patients under peritoneal dialysis and hemodialysis: a national cohort study. Sci. Rep. 13 (1). doi:10.1038/s41598-023-43476-1.

Rhee, C.M., Ahmadi, S.-F., Kovesdy, C.P., Kalantar-Zadeh, K., 2018. Low-protein diet for conservative management of chronic kidney disease: a systematic review and meta-analysis of controlled trials. J. Cachexia Sarcopenia Muscle 9 (2), 235–245. doi:10.1002/jcsm.12264.

Rule, A.D., Amer, H., Cornell, L.D., Taler, S.J., Cosio, F.G., Kremers, W.K., Textor, S.C., Stegall, M.D., 2010. The association between age and nephrosclerosis on renal biopsy among healthy adults. Ann. Intern. Med. 152 (9), 561–567. doi:10.7326/0003-4819-152-9-201005040-00006.

Sontrop, J.M., Dixon, S.N., Garg, A.X., Buendia-Jimenez, I., Dohein, O., Huang, S.-H.S., Clark, W.F., 2013. Association between water intake, chronic kidney disease, and cardiovascular disease: a cross-sectional analysis of NHANES data. Am. J. Nephrol. 37 (5), 434–442. doi:10.1159/000350377.

Spigt, M.G., Knottnerus, J.A., Westerterp, K.R., Olde Rikkert, M.G.M., Schayck, C.P., 2006. The effects of 6 months of increased water intake on blood sodium, glomerular filtration rate, blood pressure, and quality of life in elderly (aged 55–75) men. J. Am. Geriatr. Soc. 54 (3), 438–443.

Strippoli, G.F.M., Craig, J.C., Rochtchina, E., Flood, V.M., Wang, J.J., Mitchell, P., 2011. Fluid and nutrient intake and risk of chronic kidney disease. Nephrology 16 (3), 326–334. doi:10.1111/j.1440-1797.2010.01415.x.

Verberne, W.R., Geers, A.B.M.T., Jellema, W.T., Vincent, H.H., van Delden, J.J.M., Bos, W.J.W., 2016. Comparative survival among older adults with advanced kidney disease managed conservatively versus with dialysis. Clin. J. Am. Soc. Nephrol. 11 (4), 633–640. doi:10.2215/CJN.07510715.

Wagner, S., Merkling, T., Metzger, M., Bankir, L., Laville, M., Frimat, L., Combe, C., Jacquelinet, C., Fouque, D., Massy, Z.A., Stengel, B., 2022. Water intake and progression of chronic kidney disease: the CKD-REIN cohort study. Nephrol. Dial. Transplant. 37 (4), 730–739. doi:10.1093/ndt/gfab036.

Wang, C.J., Grantham, J.J., Wetmore, J.B., 2013. The medicinal use of water in renal disease. Kidney Int. 84 (1), 45–53. doi:10.1038/ki.2013.23.

Warnock, D.G., Delanaye, P., Glassock, R.J., 2017. Risks for all-cause mortality: stratified by age, estimated glomerular filtration rate and albuminuria. Nephron. 136 (4), 292–297. doi:10.1159/000455197.

Zheng, H.J., Guo, J., Wang, Q., Wang, L., Wang, Y., Zhang, F., Huang, W.-J., Zhang, W., Liu, W.J., Wang, Y., 2021. Probiotics, prebiotics, and synbiotics for the improvement of metabolic profiles in patients with chronic kidney disease: a systematic review and meta-analysis of randomized controlled trials. Crit. Rev. Food Sci. Nutr. 61 (4), 577–598. doi:10.1080/10408398.2020.1740645.

Zhong, Y., Menon, M.C., Deng, Y., Chen, Y., He, J.C., 2015. Recent advances in traditional Chinese medicine for kidney disease. Am. J. Kidney Dis. 66 (3), 513–522. doi:10.1053/j.ajkd.2015.04.013.

CHAPTER

22

The living donor and aging

Catherine Cecelia Vatsis[a] *and Sean Hebert*[b]

[a]Southwest Kidney Institute, Phoenix, AZ, United States

[b]MaineHealth Transplant Program, Maine Medical Center, Portland, ME, United States

Introduction

As of March 2025, there are 90,432 patients on the waiting list for kidney transplants in the United States (Current U.S. Waiting list, 2025). Although the number of kidney transplants performed each year has grown over the past two decades, the demand for organs continues to exceed supply, resulting in a persistent shortage. In 2024, a total of 27,759 kidney transplants were performed, up from 16,007 in 2004; however, this only allows for the removal of about one-third of patients from the waitlist. This rise is primarily attributed to an increase in kidney transplants from deceased donors, which grew from 9359 in 2004 to 21,341 in 2024 (U.S. Transplants performed : January 1, 1988—February 28, 2025, 2025). Meanwhile, the number of live donor kidney transplants has remained relatively constant, increasing only slightly from 6648 in 2004 (42% of the donor pool) to a peak of 6856 in 2019. In 2024, the number of live transplants was 6418 in 2024, representing 23% of the donor pool (Fig. 22.1A–D).

The majority of kidney donors are non-Hispanic White, female, and between 40 and 54 years old. To expand live kidney donation, legislative efforts have focused on reducing financial disincentives as well as addressing incompatible donor-recipient pairs. In 2006, the National Living Donor Assistance Center (NLDAC) was established to remove travel costs and cover lost wages (Warren et al., 2014). In addition, in 2007, federal legislation legalized kidney-paired donation, enabling incompatible donor-recipient pairs to exchange kidneys with other pairs to secure a compatible match (Legality of alternative organ donation practices under 42 U.S.C. § 274e, 2007). While these efforts have led to an increase in the percentage of donors participating in paired donation, they have had little impact on the overall number of live kidney donors.

A recent national survey of US adults aged 25 to 66 found that 87% of respondents would consider donating a kidney while still alive (Kaplow et al., 2024). The most commonly cited concern was the potential negative impact on their health. In addition, 75% of participants indicated that receiving more information about the health risks associated with live kidney

Aging and the Kidney
https://doi.org/10.1016/B978-0-443-34069-7.00025-2

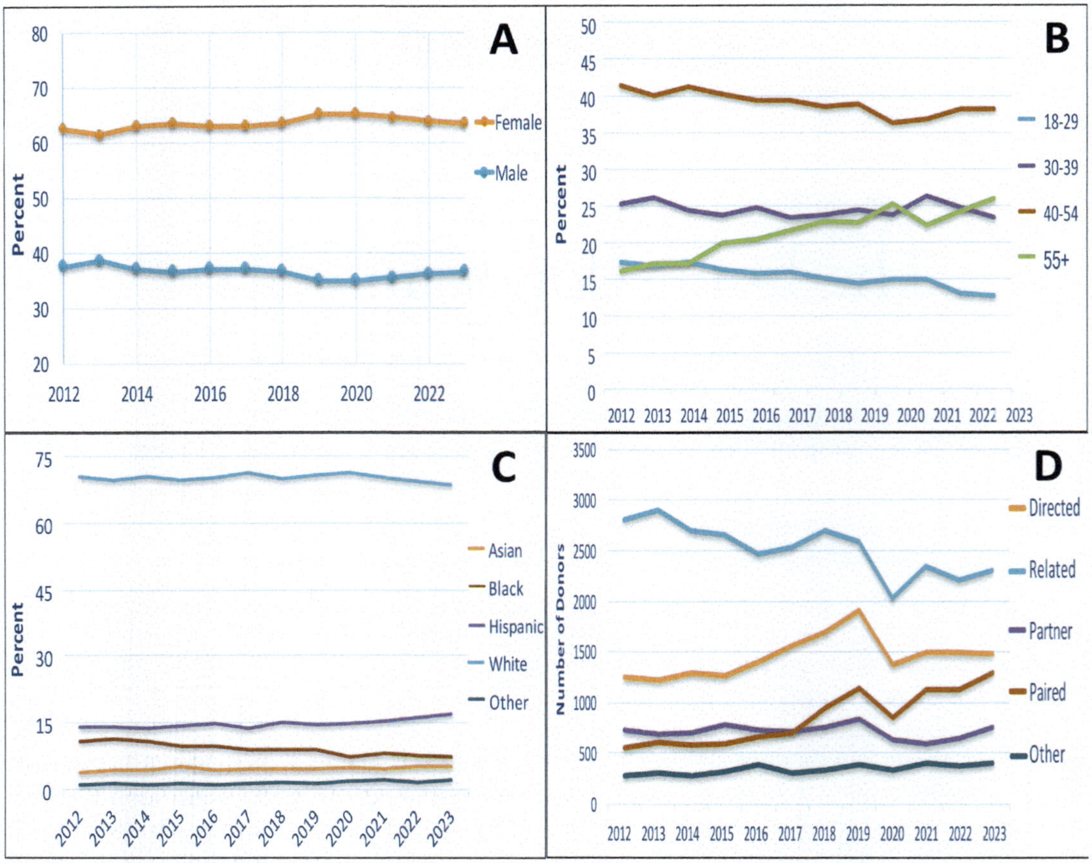

FIG. 22.1 (A–D) Live kidney donor demographics from 2012 to 2023, categorized by sex (A), age (B), race/ethnicity (C), and donor relation (D). *Modified from Lentine, K.L., Smith, J.M., Lyden, G.R., Miller, J.M., Booker, S.E., Dolan, T.G., Temple, K.R., Weiss, S., Handarova, D., Israni, A.K., Snyder, J.J., 2025. OPTN/SRTR 2023 annual data report: kidney. Am. J. Transplant. 25 (2). doi:10.1016/j.ajt.2025.01.020.*

donation would increase their willingness to donate. Notably, these findings suggest that many potential live kidney donors have not yet engaged with transplant centers, indicating room for further growth in live kidney donation. In line with these results, we believe that targeted public education efforts—highlighting overall health outcomes and expected kidney function post-donation—are essential next steps to help address the ongoing organ shortage.

Improved graft and patient survival

The 1 year and 5 year post-kidney transplant patient survival rates are 97.4% and 86.2%, respectively, greatly exceeding the 5 year survival rate of 40%–50% in those on maintenance dialysis (Poggio et al., 2021). Importantly, this longer life expectancy occurs in recipients of both deceased and live kidney donations. However, this improved survival is influenced by two factors: donor type and time on dialysis. Live kidney donation is associated with significantly longer graft and patient survival than deceased donor transplants, as demonstrated in the 2023 annual data report. The 1-year and 5 year patient survival rates are 99% and 91.9% in live donor kidney recipients compared with 96.9% and 84.8% in deceased donor recipients. The 1-year and 5 year graft survival rates are 98.1% and 87.8% in those receiving live donor kidneys versus 94.5% and 77.2% in those receiving kidneys from deceased donors. Moreover, Poggio et al. showed that the median graft survival for live donor kidney transplants was 19.2 years compared with 11.7 years for deceased donor kidney transplants (Poggio et al., 2021).

The reasons for this improved graft and patient survival are multiple. First, the organ quality from a live donor kidney is typically better, as potential donors go through a litany of tests to exclude the presence of clinical kidney disease prior to organ donation. Second, the cold ischemia time is significantly reduced with live kidney donation because there is minimal delay from the time of organ procurement to placement in the recipient. Third, the transplant surgery can be scheduled at an optimal time, even preemptively (prior to the initiation of maintenance dialysis). A retrospective study of 8481 US patients undergoing live donor kidney transplantation found that preemptive living donor kidney transplants (PKT) were associated with a reduction in allograft failure during the first year (rate ratio 0.48; $p = 0.002$), an 82% reduction in the second year (rate ratio 0.18; $p = 0.001$), followed by an 86% reduction in subsequent years (rate ratio 0.14; $p = 0.001$) (Mange et al., 2001). Fourth, there is the potential for improved immunologic compatibility, as live donation allows for better matching between donors and recipients via participation in a paired exchange program (Hariharan et al., 2021).

These results are consistent in the pediatric population as well. Vats et al. showed that long-term cumulative graft survival in pediatric kidney transplant recipients was 88% and 75% for live kidney donors at 5 and 10 years, respectively, compared with 72% and 46% for deceased donors (Vats et al., 2002). As pediatric recipients have increased longevity, many will outlive their first transplant and will require a second transplant. In those with a potential live donor candidate, the optimal timing strategy for utilizing this live donor kidney—whether as the first donor or as a second option if a first deceased donor transplant fails—remains uncertain. Using the Scientific Registry of Transplant Recipients (SRTR), Van Arendonk et al. analyzed first and second allograft survival among 14,799 pediatric kidney recipients between 1987 and 2010 (Van Arendonk et al., 2013). They found that pediatric recipients who received a live donor kidney had longer graft survival compared to a deceased donor kidney, whether performed first (adjusted hazard ratio [aHR] = 0.78, 95% CI: 0.73–0.84; $p < 0.001$) or second (aHR = 0.74, 95% CI: 0.64–0.84; $p < 0.001$). When a live donor kidney transplant was performed second, the better graft survival was maintained over a deceased donor transplant, regardless of whether the first transplant was from a living donor (aHR = 0.68, 95% CI: 0.56–0.83; $p < 0.001$) or a deceased donor (aHR = 0.77, 95% CI: 0.63–0.95; $p = 0.02$). Thus the graft survival of the live kidney transplant was not negatively influenced by a prior deceased donor transplant.

Donor nephrectomy

Evolution of surgical techniques

The first live donor nephrectomy was performed via open surgical technique by Dr. Joseph Murray in 1954. Introduced in 1991, laparoscopic nephrectomy (LN) provided a minimally invasive surgical alternative, and by 1995, Drs. Lloyd Ratner and Louis Kavoussi performed the first laparoscopic live-donor nephrectomy in the United States. This newer technique was well received as it decreased the size of incisions, significantly reduced blood loss, postoperative analgesia requirements, and shortened hospital stays by 2.7 days (Kavoussi, 2000). Moreover, a Cochrane review of five randomized controlled trials of primary outcomes after donor nephrectomy demonstrated that analgesia requirements were lower after laparoscopic nephrectomy compared to open nephrectomy (ON) (standardized mean difference 0.45 higher in the ON group) (Kourounis et al., 2024). In 2002, Dr. Horgan et al. published the first series of robotic-assisted live-donor nephrectomies performed in Chicago (Vella et al., 2024). While minimally invasive surgeries provide a more efficient alternative to the open surgical technique, the advancement of robotic-assisted surgery over conventional laparoscopy remains under debate.

Laparoscopic nephrectomy remains the most common surgical technique among US transplant centers performing live-donor nephrectomies. Lentine et al. surveyed 97 centers between 2008 and 2012 and found that 93.8% used the laparoscopic technique, while 2.4% utilized robotic-assisted methods, and 3.7% had planned open nephrectomies (Lentine et al., 2016). Laparoscopic hand-assisted nephrectomy was more frequently performed (57.4%) than pure laparoscopy (40.8%), as reported in the OPTN Living Donor Registration Form (OPTN/SRTR 2023 Annual data report: kidney, 2023).

Perioperative and postoperative period

Complication incidence

Regardless of the surgical technique employed, potential peri-operative complications may include pain, organ injury, hemorrhage, blood clots, hernias, infections, wound complications, and death. These complications are typically classified as major (renal failure, multi-organ failure, and death) or minor, as specified by the Clavien classification, with reported rates of 3%–6% for major and 22% for minor complications. Most studies demonstrate similar complication rates. One study documented complication rates as follows: gastrointestinal (4.4%), bleeding (3.0%), respiratory (2.5%), surgical/anesthesia-related (2.4%), and "other" (6.6%). Notably, higher-volume centers (>50 cases/year) had a 44% lower risk of perioperative complications compared to mid-sized centers (11–50 cases/year) (Lentine et al., 2016).

One less well-recognized complication is postoperative testicular pain. Between 3% and 55% of male donors experience this, likely due to intraoperative gonadal vein ligation (Schoephoerster et al., 2022). Another study by Gandhi et al. evaluated male donors from the Renal and Lung Donor Evaluation (RELIVE) Study to determine the incidence of testicular pain in the 2551 male donors for whom data on testicular status was available (Gandhi et al., 2022). Fifty-four patients, or 2.12%, developed testicular pain. They found that non-Hispanic White patients and older donors (4 years older, 42 vs. 38 years old) were more likely to develop this symptom. Furthermore, laparoscopic nephrectomy, but not the laterality of nephrectomy, was also associated with the increased incidence.

Mortality

Historically, studies have shown that the risk of mortality with donor nephrectomy is about 3.1 per 10,000. However, more recent trends show a significantly lower risk. Compared to the time intervals of 1993–2002 and 2003–2012, the most recent time frame of 2013–2022 has shown a mortality rate of 0.9 per 10,000 (Massie et al., 2024). They found that males, individuals with hypertension, and Black individuals had a higher mortality risk.

Physiological changes in the post-donation period

Hemodynamic changes

Hyperfiltration and eGFR trajectory post-donation

Following donor nephrectomy, there is an immediate 50% reduction in renal mass and glomerular filtration rate (GFR). The remaining kidney undergoes physiological adaptive hyperfiltration with glomerular hypertrophy and an increase in the single nephron glomerular filtration rate (SNGFR), which subsequently reaches approximately 60%–70% of the pre-donation value.

The adaptive changes that occur in the remaining kidney can begin as early as one week post-donation (Akoh and Mathuram Thiyagarajan, 2013). However, the long-term effects of reduced GFR, and whether the trajectory of kidney function loss in donors mirrors that of individuals with two kidneys, have been central questions driving the following studies. Lam et al. compared the change in estimated glomerular filtration rate (eGFR) among 566 live kidney donors (LKD) with 2259 nondonor controls (Lam et al., 2020). The time intervals measured were 6 weeks to < 2 years, 2 years to < 5 years, and ≥ 5 years. Those in the LKD group had an eGFR increase of + 1.06, + 0.64, and − 0.06 versus a decline of − 0.89, − 0.64, and − 0.97 in the nondonor controls, respectively. The overall change was + 0.35 in the donor group and − 0.85 in the control group. These findings show that, unlike nondonors who experience a gradual decline in kidney function over time, kidney donors actually exhibit an increase in eGFR during the first few years following donation. These findings were consistent among patients of different ages, pre-donation eGFRs, socioeconomic statuses, presence of pre-donation hypertension, and distance to the transplant center.

Similarly, Kasiske et al. conducted a study to determine the eGFR changes at a longer post-donation follow-up period. At the 9 year follow-up visit, there was no evidence of eGFR decline in the donor group, as the eGFR change was + 0.02 mL/min/1.73 m^2 in the donor group compared with an eGFR decline of 1.26 mL/min/1.73 m^2 in the control group. Since previous studies primarily relied on estimating equations for GFR follow-up, which are subject to variability, using measured GFR (mGFR) based on plasma clearance of iohexol offers a more precise assessment with the lowest coefficient of variability (Kasiske et al., 2020). Berglund et al. conducted such a study involving 214 randomly selected live kidney donors, with follow-up extending to 16.9 ± 9.1 years post-donation. They found that 84.6% had an mGFR ≥ 60 mL/min/1.73 m^2, 14% had an mGFR of 45–60 mL/min/1.73 m^2 and only

1.4% had an mGFR < 45 mL/min/1.73 m². No donors had an mGFR < 30 mL/min/1.73 m². By 20 years post-donation, 56.5% of donors had experienced an mGFR decline, while 36% continued to have an mGFR increase, and 7.5% had no change. On average, mGFR declined by 0.42 mL/min/1.73 m² per year of age, similar to the reported GFR decline of 0.4–2.5 mL/min per year of age in the general population. Importantly, there was no evidence of long-term hyperfiltration injury as a result of live donor nephrectomy (Berglund et al., 2018).

Cardiovascular changes post-donation

Left ventricular mass and cardiovascular mortality

Compared to healthy controls, kidney donors exhibit adverse changes in left ventricular (LV) mass, systolic function, aortic stiffness, and cardiovascular disease biomarkers at 12 months post-donation. However, it remains uncertain whether these changes persist in the long-term. In the CRIB (Chronic Renal Impairment in Birmingham)-DONOR Study in 2021, Moody et al. found increased LV mass, mass-to-volume ratio, and greater aortic stiffness, along with decreased global circumferential strain on cardiac MRI at 12 months following nephrectomy. Donors also had a higher risk of elevated troponin T levels, a biomarker indicative of cardiac injury (Moody et al., 2016).

Similarly, Altmann et al. performed cardiac and renal magnetic imaging studies in kidney donors prior to and at 4 and 12 months post-donation. Among 23 donors (mean age 54 ± 10 years, 52% male), there was a statistically significant increase in LV mass (from 112 ± 22 to 115 ± 23 g, $p < 0.001$), though no changes in ejection fraction or in end-diastolic and end-systolic pressures at either follow-up time point (Altmann et al., 2017).

The long-term cardiovascular impact of kidney donation remains unclear, as some studies suggest these early changes may not be sustained. For instance, Price et al. demonstrated that while LV mass was increased at 12 months post-donation, there was no difference at a longer follow-up period of 5 years (Price et al., 2021) Similarly, a Canadian study comparing 2028 donors and 20,280 matched nondonors demonstrated no difference in major cardiovascular event risks (Garg et al., 2012a). In line with these findings, Munch et al. observed no differences in the incidence of major adverse cardiovascular events (MACE) or atrial fibrillation between donors and nondonor controls at 8 years post-donation (Munch et al., 2021).

Recent evidence suggests that short-term cardiovascular changes following kidney donation tend to resolve over time and may not have a lasting impact on donors' long-term cardiovascular health. The underlying mechanisms driving these early changes remain unclear, though several hypotheses have been proposed. One possibility is the presence of transient, unmeasured hemodynamic or circulatory alterations within the first 12 months post-donation. In addition, the initial decline in GFR observed after donation often stabilizes and may even surpass baseline levels over time. It is plausible that the observed cardiovascular changes parallel these adaptive renal hemodynamic responses.

Metabolic changes post-donation

Mineral and bone disease

Immediately post-nephrectomy, parathyroid hormone (PTH) and fibroblast growth factor 23 (FGF23) increase by 40%, accompanied by a 10%–15% decrease in calcium and phosphorus levels. By two weeks, Duque et al. showed that calcium, phosphorus, and PTH levels had returned to baseline values. FGF23, on the other hand, remained higher than baseline over the first year (Duque et al., 2024). After normalizing at 14 days, serum phosphorus levels declined and were significantly lower 1 year post-donation. Their study demonstrated that this decrease in phosphorus levels correlated with increased FGF23 resulting in increased phosphaturia. At 10 years, FGF23 and phosphorus levels returned to normal. While this study is limited by a lack of data between the first and 10th year post-donation, Young et al. found that significantly elevated FGF23 levels persisted at follow-up of 5.3 years (Young et al., 2012).

In the Assessing Long-Term Outcomes in Living Kidney Donors (ALTOLD) study, Kasiske et al. confirmed that this low phosphorus level persisted within the first five years post-donation (Kasiske et al., 2016). Their study did not collect data on FGF23, but they were able to chronicle the PTH trends up to three years after nephrectomy and showed that donors had significantly increased PTH levels (52.5 ± 24.1 vs. 43.2 ± 17.5; $p < 0.001$) compared to nondonor controls.

Whether this secondary hyperparathyroidism led to bone fragility prompted survey studies on post-donation fracture risk. Among more than 2,000 Canadian kidney donors, Garg et al. showed that the overall fracture risk was not significantly higher in donors (16.4) than in nondonor cohorts (18.7 events/10,000 person-years) (Garg et al., 2012b). However, this study was limited by a younger cohort (mean age: 43 years) with a mean follow-up time of 6 years. A more recent survey study, with a mean donor age of 67 years and 58% women, assessed overall fracture risk in kidney donors after a mean follow-up of 25 years (Maradit Kremers et al., 2024). Their results showed a lower rate of overall fractures (SIR: 0.89; 95% CI: 0.81–0.97) in donors compared to nondonor controls. Yet, they did find significantly more vertebral fractures (SIR: 1.42; 95% CI: 1.05–1.83) among donors.

To better delineate bone health changes, Grossardt et al. compared 139 donors from the survey study with 139 age and sex-matched controls (Grossardt et al., 2024). They measured bone formation and resorption markers, bone mineral density, as well as bone microstructure and strength via high-resolution peripheral quantitative computed tomography and micro-finite element analysis (HRpQCT) at a mean of 22 years post-donation. They found that donors had decreased 1,25-dihydroxyvitamin D concentrations (33.89 pg/mL vs. 38.79 pg/mL, percent difference = – 12.6%; $p < 0.001$), increased PTH (52.98 pg/mL vs. 46.89 pg/mL, percent difference = 13%; $p = 0.03$), increased serum calcium, as well as differences in bone resorption and formation markers (procollagen type I N-terminal propeptide [P1NP], osteocalcin, N-terminal telopeptide [NTx], and C-terminal telopeptide [CTx]). There was no significant difference in overall bone mineral density after adjusting for age, sex, and BMI. Microstructural findings were also not significantly different, but there was a trend toward a thinner cortical shell in donors, which has also been observed in people with primary hyperparathyroidism.

In summary, kidney donors experience long-term alterations in mineral metabolism, including persistently elevated PTH and calcium, reduced 1,25-vitamin D, and initially elevated FGF23. While overall bone density remains largely unaffected, subtle microstructural changes and increased vertebral fracture risk have been observed more than 20 years post-donation. Further long-term studies are needed to determine if these changes become clinically significant and whether vitamin D analog therapy may improve outcomes.

Other changes post-donation

Pregnancy after donation—Maternal and fetal outcomes

A cohort study by Ibrahim et al. compared various maternal and fetal outcomes in the pre-donation and post-donation periods (Ibrahim et al., 2009b). They found that post-donation, there were higher rates of pre-term deliveries and perinatal death. Maternal outcomes, including higher rates of preeclampsia, gestational hypertension, gestational diabetes, and proteinuria, were higher post-donation than pre-donation in women who had both pre- and post-donation pregnancies. Interestingly, these rates were no different when compared to the general population.

Reisæter et al. compared maternal and fetal risks of donors both before and after donation and reported no differences in preterm deliveries, perinatal deaths, or birth weight (Reisæter et al., 2009). With regard to maternal outcomes, there was an increased risk of preeclampsia but not gestational hypertension.

A third study by Garg et al., comparing donors and nondonors reported no difference in pre-term deliveries, perinatal death, or birth weight (Garg et al., 2015). However, there was an increased risk of gestational hypertension and preeclampsia.

The data suggest that potential donors who are women of childbearing age should be informed of their higher risks of preeclampsia and should be counseled about the possibility of worse fetal and/or maternal outcomes post-donation.

Clinical implications of a solitary kidney

Is reduced GFR post-donation considered CKD?

Chronic kidney disease, per the KDIGO guidelines, is defined by at least one marker of kidney damage or an eGFR < 60 for at least three months, regardless of the cause (KDIGO 2024 clinical practice guideline for the evaluation and management of chronic kidney disease, 2024). Based on the expected decline in kidney function after donation, a donor with an initial GFR of 80 mL/min/1.73 m^2 would have a post-donation GFR between 50 and 60 mL/min/1.73 m^2. By the conventional definition of CKD, a donor such as this one would be labeled as having CKD Stage 3. Whether these patients should be labeled as having CKD has been a topic of debate, as such a diagnosis has various diagnostic and treatment implications. Subsequent follow-up visits, unnecessary referrals, laboratory and/or imaging tests, along with the added stress of having the diagnosis of "kidney disease," pose unnecessary problems in the kidney donor population. Furthermore, some individuals have difficulty obtaining life and health insurance because the aforementioned CKD diagnosis is considered a "pre-existing condition." In fact, 2%–11% of kidney donors have faced issues with obtaining insurance (Matas and Ibrahim, 2013).

Comparison to those with tumor nephrectomy (TN)

Timsit et al. compared 248 patients, half of whom had a nephrectomy for localized renal cell carcinoma (RCC) and the other half of whom had living donor nephrectomies (Timsit et al., 2012). Results did not demonstrate a statistically significant difference in the postoperative

MDRD-eGFR (30.4% vs. 32.4% in the RCC vs. LD group). At the 4 year postoperative mark, there was a 16.2% and 5.3% risk of CKD with MDRD-eGFR < 45 mL/min/m^2 in the RCC and LD groups, respectively. However, the indication for nephrectomy was not a predictor for postoperative decline in kidney function.

Another study by Laksanabunsong et al. comparing 552 patients who had TN and 496 patients who had living donor nephrectomy demonstrated similar results (Laksanabunsong et al., 2024). The rates of CKD Stage ≥ 3 at approximately 5–6 year follow-up times were 26.4% and 24.5% in the TN and LD groups (p = 0.308). 10 year post-follow-up results were also statistically insignificant.

In contrast to these two aforementioned studies demonstrating no difference in the risk of developing post-nephrectomy CKD, a study from 2022 by Wang et al. demonstrated a dramatic difference in CKD risk when comparing those with TN and living donor nephrectomy. They found that the 5 year cumulative incidence of CKD in patients undergoing TN was 43.4% (189 of 500 patients). The mean interval at which CKD developed was three months postoperatively, with most developing CKD by the 1 year mark. Moreover, older patients, those with lower preoperative GFR in the contralateral kidney, and lower immediate postoperative GFR were predictors of CKD risk (Wang et al., 2022).

Using data from over 1000 patients in Manitoba, Canada, who underwent either partial or full nephrectomy for nonmetastatic renal cell carcinoma, Harasemiw et al. assessed the risk of developing CKD at the 5 year postoperative mark (10.3%) and developed a predictive model, the Kidney Cancer Risk Equation (KCRE), to estimate the risk of postoperative kidney failure, defined as the need for dialysis, transplantation, or an eGFR < 15 mL/min/1.73 m^2. Six variables—age, sex, eGFR, nephrectomy type, diabetes, and UACR—were included in their development model, which they successfully externally validated by comparing the patient cohort to an external validation cohort of over 12,000 patients from Ontario, Canada, who had the same preoperative diagnosis and underwent either partial or radical nephrectomy (Harasemiw et al., 2023). The KCRE is a clinically useful tool for guiding discussions about treatment options for patients with nonmetastatic renal cell carcinoma.

Does kidney donation increase the risk of proteinuria?

As previously mentioned, immediately following donor nephrectomy, there is a 50% reduction in kidney mass and GFR. The remaining kidney compensates within a few weeks as the GFR returns to around 70% of the pre-nephrectomy function. This adaptive hyperfiltration occurs due to an increase in single nephron GFR in the remaining kidney.

Concerns over this hyperfiltration leading to proteinuria stem from micropuncture studies conducted on nephrectomized mice. Following nephrectomy, Hostetter et al. performed segmental infarction on five-sixths of the remaining kidney in mice (Hostetter et al., 1981). Nephron loss and the subsequent sustained increase in single-nephron GFR resulted in glomerular hypertension, leading to glomerulosclerosis and proteinuria.

Epidemiologic studies have shown small increases in urinary protein post-donation. Many attribute this proteinuria to single-nephron hyperfiltration due to reduced nephron mass. However, whether this proteinuria leads to a progressive decline in kidney function remains uncertain. A systematic review of 48 studies, including 5048 donors across 27 countries, explored this issue (Garg et al., 2006). They found a pooled incidence of approximately 10% of kidney donors developing proteinuria, defined as 24 h urine protein > 300 mg. To determine whether these increases were due to aging, they compared donors to age-matched controls. Donors exhibited more proteinuria, with a weighted mean difference of 66 mg/day (147 mg/day vs. 83 mg/day in controls) at an average of 11 years post-donation, and levels increased over time. Notably, there was no evidence of accelerated GFR decline beyond that expected with normal aging, leaving the clinical significance of this low-grade proteinuria in donors unclear.

Ibrahim et al. showed that approximately 6% of 3534 White kidney donors had proteinuria after a median of 18 years following donation (Ibrahim et al., 2016). Proteinuria was more common among those with a higher body mass index (BMI) (HR 1.10; 95% CI, 1.06 to 1.13, $p < 0.001$) and males (HR, 1.56; 95% CI, 1.18 to 2.05; $p < 0.001$). In addition, 16.7% of those with an estimated GFR < 45 mL/min/1.73 m^2 had proteinuria, compared to 4.9% of those with eGFR > 45 mL/min/1.73 m^2. While the overall prevalence of proteinuria was low, the study highlighted associations between proteinuria, reduced eGFR, and the development of de novo diabetes and hypertension. These findings underscore the importance of early detection and proactive management to mitigate long-term risks.

Similarly, Dhalla et al. reported that 8% of 590 Canadian kidney donors developed either low eGFR or moderate to severe albuminuria (Dhalla et al., 2024). During a median follow-up of 8.6 years (maximum 16.9 years), 21 donors had eGFR < 45 mL/min/1.73 m^2, 23 developed moderate to severe albuminuria, and 3 donors received dialysis. These outcomes likely arose in donors without preexisting albuminuria, though a study limitation was the lack of pre-donation albuminuria data for 24.4% of participants. Key risk factors for either kidney outcome included lower pre-donation eGFR, pre-donation hypertension, and post-donation diabetes.

In contrast, Janki et al. demonstrated no difference in albuminuria post-donation compared with Dutch nondonors. Their study utilized a propensity score-matched comparison of 761 live kidney donors with 1522 general population nondonor cohorts (Janki et al., 2020). In addition, there was no difference in BMI, diabetes incidence, cardiovascular events, and mortality between the two groups. A lower risk of hypertension (OR 0.45, 95% CI 0.33–0.62) was found among the donor group, potentially reflective of the selection bias associated with live kidney donors. Another potential reason for no difference in albuminuria is the shorter median follow-up of 8 years. Given the prior findings that proteinuria increases with longer time since donation, it is possible that the follow-up period was too short to detect a difference.

Overall, 6%–10% of kidney donors develop clinically significant proteinuria, with the prevalence increasing over time post-donation. The underlying cause remains uncertain. While single-nephron hyperfiltration due to reduced nephron mass may contribute, it does not appear to drive the rapid kidney function decline observed in animal models.

Lenihan et al. tracked glomerular dynamics in 21 live kidney donors from pre-donation to a median follow-up of 6.3 years (Lenihan et al., 2016). Their findings showed an immediate 40% rise in renal plasma flow and up to a 33% increase in renocortical volume in the late post-donation period. Unlike animal models, post-donation hyperfiltration in humans occurred through increased renal plasma flow and a higher ultrafiltration coefficient. Notably, this increase resulted from compensatory glomerular hypertrophy rather than the glomerular hypertension seen in mouse studies. In addition, a sensitivity analysis of donors with well-controlled pre-donation hypertension confirmed similar glomerular hypertrophy without elevated glomerular pressure.

Moreover, individuals who develop proteinuria from hyperfiltration injury would be expected to show a secondary focal segmental glomerulosclerosis (FSGS) pattern. However, Mjøen et al. analyzed the pathology findings in nine kidney donors who progressed to end-stage kidney disease (ESKD), and all cases were linked to the recipient's condition rather than donor-related hyperfiltration injury (Mjøen et al., 2014).

The primary causes of ESKD among these donors were immunologic diseases, including glomerulonephritis (3 cases), systemic lupus erythematosus (1 case), ANCA-associated vasculitis (2 cases), sarcoidosis (1 case), and diabetes (2 cases). Notably, none of the donors exhibited a secondary FSGS pattern, indicating that proteinuria leading to ESKD was not typically a result of maladaptive hyperfiltration injury (Grupper et al., 2019).

Long-term outcomes

Survival

Ibrahim et al. reported that, of 3698 kidney donors who donated kidneys between 1963 and 2007, 3404 donors were documented as being alive. After excluding the 26 foreign nationals whose vital status was unknown, they found that the survival rate among kidney donors was similar to the survival rate of the general population, as estimated by the National Center for Health Statistics (Ibrahim et al., 2009a). Similar reassuring results have been observed in various international studies. Another study examined survival rates in Swedish living kidney donors who donated between 1964 and 1994. It found that, at the 20 year follow-up mark, the survival rate was actually higher (85%) compared to the expected survival rate (66%) (Fehrman-Ekholm et al., 1997). Yet another study of living kidney donors in New Zealand who donated a kidney between 1988 and 2018 reported that 99% (98.2%–99.5%) were alive at 10 years post-nephrectomy (Chan et al., 2025). Lastly, a retrospective observational study of 188 Japanese living kidney donors who donated between April 2009 and July 2022 demonstrated a 96.8% (182 of 188 LKDs) survival rate at a median follow-up of 5.7 years (Ogata et al., 2024). Such reassuring results provide great promise for the future of living donor transplantation.

CKD and ESKD onset

While the remaining kidney is able to compensate, at least in the initial 5 + years post-donation, the new baseline GFR in donors is lower than in their nondonor counterparts. It is important to consider that the natural decline in GFR that occurs with aging, along with the potential to develop kidney disease in the future, can lead to the development of ESKD sooner (Matas and Rule, 2022).

Ibrahim et al. reviewed the outcomes of 3698 living donor nephrectomies (LDN) performed at the University of Minnesota between 1963 and 2007 (Ibrahim et al., 2009a). Of the 255 patients who completed formal measurement of iohexol GFR at 12.2 ± 9.2 years post-transplant, 85.5% had a GFR of at least 60 mL/min/1.73m^2 m^2, and none had a GFR <30 mL/min/1.73 m^2. Age, BMI, and female sex were risk factors associated with having a GFR <60 mL/min/1.73 m^2.

At a later time mark of 22.5 ± 10.4 years, they found that only 11 donors had developed ESKD. This rate of 180 cases per million persons per year was lower than the rate of 268 per million persons per year in the White population of the United States. All 11 donors were related to their recipients, which raises the question of whether the higher incidence in this population is due to hereditary factors and not solely due to nephrectomy.

In contrast, two other studies showed a higher risk of ESKD among living donors compared with healthy nondonors.

Muzale et al. reported a higher incidence of ESKD at 15 years (3.9 versus 30.8 per 10,000, $p < 0.001$) (Muzaale et al., 2014). This higher incidence was present in Black, Hispanic, and Caucasian individuals at rates of 75, 33, and 23 per 10,000 in the three groups, respectively. They did note that the lifetime risk for ESKD was lower than that of the general population. The estimated lifetime risk of ESKD was 90 per 10,000 donors, 14 per 10,000 healthy nondonors, compared to 326 per 10,000 in the general US population.

Mjøen et al. similarly showed a rate of 302 versus 100 per million per year (adjusted hazard ratio 11.38, $p < 0.001$) in a living donor group of 190 donors versus a matched nondonor group in Norway (Mjøen et al., 2014). All nine donors who developed ESKD were related to the recipients, similar to what was reported in the aforementioned cohort study by Ibrahim et al. It is plausible that the increased incidence seen in the donor population is related to hereditary factors, not just due to nephrectomy (Ibrahim et al., 2009a).

Risk calculators

Massie et al. used data from the National Donor Registry to predict the 20 year donor risk of kidney failure (Massie et al., 2017). Some limitations of this calculator include the exclusion of blood pressure and urine albumin-to-creatinine ratio, as hypertension and albuminuria are known risk factors for the development of kidney disease. Furthermore, this model is limited in its assessment of long-term outcomes, as the data only include 20 years of follow-up.

Using seven nondonor cohorts, Grams et al. estimated the 15 year and lifetime risk of kidney failure without donation (Grams et al., 2016). While this model does incorporate lifetime risk for ESKD, it is based on cohort data with a short follow-up time and, therefore, may have some inaccuracies. Further, this model may underestimate the risk of kidney failure, particularly in young, obese donor candidates.

Palzer et al. developed an online calculator to estimate the 40 year donor risk of hypertension, diabetes mellitus (DM), proteinuria, and eGFRs of < 60 mL/min/1.73 m^2, < 45 mL/min/1.73 m^2, and < 30 mL/min/1.73 m^2 at a median follow-up of 22.8 years (Palzer et al., 2020). A significant limitation of this model is that it may not be generalizable, particularly to non-White donors, as the cohort group was composed of 94.2% White donors.

Despite limitations, these calculators help potential kidney donors make more informed decisions by predicting clinical outcomes.

Subclinical histological changes at donation

A potential live kidney donor evaluation that reveals normal kidney function, no diabetes or hypertension, no proteinuria, and no active urine sediment is typically reassuring that kidney histology is normal. Thus pre-donation kidney biopsies are usually not performed, as they are invasive and potentially harmful. Yet, the implications of incidental findings on implantation biopsies in an otherwise healthy individual are unclear.

Emmons et al. described such implantation biopsy findings among 1104 live kidney donors. Their study found histological "chronic changes" of glomerulosclerosis > 25%, interstitial fibrosis and tubular atrophy > 25%, or at least moderate arteriosclerosis in 14% of their donors. Age, Hispanic ethnicity, and hypertension were associated with higher odds of chronic changes, but the "abnormal" implantation biopsies were not predictive of eGFR six months post-donation (Emmons et al., 2024).

Although pre-donation screening showed no signs of proteinuria or hematuria, 1% of donors were found to have possible glomerular disease. Importantly, all 12 of these donors had first-degree relatives with ESKD. Eight had possible IgA nephropathy, two had possible immune complex-mediated GN, one had possible membranous nephropathy, and one had possible fibrillary GN. Four donors with possible IgA nephropathy had a family member with ESKD from IgA, and the one donor with possible fibrillary GN donated to a family member with the same diagnosis, suggesting that some of these biopsies identified true subclinical pathology. While rare, this finding illustrates the need for a low threshold for possible additional evaluation in donor candidates with a positive family history, especially if there is transient hematuria or proteinuria.

As noted earlier, donors who are first-degree relatives of their recipients face a higher risk of developing ESKD. Matas et al. proposed that if this increased risk were due to shared familial factors, the donor and recipient would likely have the same underlying cause of ESKD (Matas et al., 2017). However, analysis of kidney donors listed for transplant in the Organ Procurement and Transplantation Network (OPTN) revealed that while 88% were biologically related to their recipients, only 23% shared the same ESKD etiology. This discrepancy underscores the lack of key data needed to fully understand ESKD risk post-donation. A more plausible explanation for this increased ESKD risk is reduced nephron endowment. Denic et al. showed that among 1638 live kidney donors with implantation biopsies, each kidney had an estimated 873,696 nephrons. Those with a family history of ESKD had 56,175 fewer nephrons (Denic et al., 2017).

Findings from the Aging Kidney Anatomy study have revealed links between microstructural kidney features and adverse outcomes such as reduced GFR, albuminuria, and hypertension. Issa et al. reported that donors with glomerular volume and interstitial fibrosis/tubular atrophy (IFTA) above the 95th percentile for age were modestly predictive of a measured GFR below 60 mL/min/1.73 m^2 at a median of 4.4 months post-donation (Issa et al., 2019). In addition, larger cortical volume combined with a low nephron number was associated with albuminuria exceeding 5 mg/24 h, while severe arterial luminal stenosis predicted post-donation hypertension.

In a study with longer follow-up, Merzkani et al. analyzed nephron number, size, and nephrosclerosis in 807 living kidney donors over a mean follow-up of 10.5 years (Merzkani et al., 2021). They found that 6.4% developed an eGFR below 45 mL/min/1.73 m^2 and 5.1% reported proteinuria. Larger glomerular volume at the time of donation was linked to both outcomes, and donors with nephron numbers in the lowest 5% for their age had an increased risk of this low eGFR. However, no association was found between these microstructural features and the development of hypertension, indicating the need for further research to confirm these findings.

Overall, given the low incidence of reduced GFR and proteinuria after donation, these studies do not support the routine use of pre-donation kidney biopsies in live donor evaluations. However, they highlight microstructural features that may signal subclinical kidney disease. While these biopsy techniques are quite labor-intensive for routine clinical use, newer research is leveraging these findings to develop machine learning tools that improve imaging-based assessments. In one such study, Gregory et al. used a validated algorithm on contrast-enhanced CT scans from donor evaluations to differentiate the renal cortex from the medulla. They discovered that both cortical volume and the number of medullary pyramids were surrogates of nephron endowment, and fewer pyramids were linked to an eGFR < 60 mL/min/1.73 m^2 at 10 year follow-up (Gregory et al., 2023). Given the promising potential of these approaches, further validation of advanced imaging techniques could significantly improve donor counseling, informed consent, and long-term follow-up strategies.

CKD risk factors

Diabetes mellitus

Diabetes mellitus (DM) is the leading cause of end-stage kidney disease (Annual data report, 2024). Understanding the risk of developing ESKD in living kidney donors is thus of paramount importance. Grupper et al. found similar rates of DM in kidney donors compared to a matched control group; however, donors who were pre-diabetic (hemoglobin A1C 5.7%–6.4%) or who had a family history of diabetes mellitus had a higher risk of developing DM (Grupper et al., 2019). Ibrahim et al. found that 7.7% (309 of 4014) of kidney donors developed diabetes mellitus post-donation, with incidence increasing over longer periods following donation (2.4% at year 10, 7.0% at year 20, and 14.5% at year 30) (Ibrahim et al., 2017).

In comparing 761 living kidney donors to 1,522 matched nondonors, Janki et al. found no difference in the incidence of diabetes mellitus at a median of 8 years of follow-up (Janki et al., 2020). Moreover, Lin et al. compared 1081 kidney donors and 1082 age and sex-matched nondonors and demonstrated no difference in the incidence of diabetes mellitus (Lin et al., 2019).

Ibrahim et al. reported that donors who developed diabetes mellitus were more likely to have hypertension and proteinuria, but there was no difference in the annual change in eGFR between this group and those without diabetes (Ibrahim et al., 2010). However, in donors developing diabetes and proteinuria, the slope of eGFR decline was steeper (Ibrahim et al., 2017).

Hypertension

While older studies report an increased risk of hypertension post-donation, more recent evidence has demonstrated no increased hypertension risk. A retrospective cohort study from 2008 demonstrated a 40% higher risk of developing hypertension (prevalence of 16.3% vs. 11.9% in the group of 1278 LKDs compared to 6359 healthy nondonors, respectively), with no effect modification by age or sex. It is worth noting, though, that the donor group was seen more frequently by their physician, so it is possible that the more frequent monitoring explains these findings (Garg et al., 2008).

Others have reported that the prevalence of hypertension post-donation is affected by race. For example, Doshi et al. compared African American donors with healthy matched nondonors and found that the donor group had a higher risk of developing hypertension (40.8% versus 17.9%) (Doshi et al., 2013). This study, however, was limited by a small sample size.

The most promising evidence comes from a recently published 2024 prospective cohort study comparing 924 standard-criteria LKDs and 397 nondonors. There was no statistically significant increase in hypertension found at the median follow-up period of 7.3 years (Garg et al., 2024).

Despite conflicting reports regarding the risk of hypertension, more recent evidence demonstrating no increased risk of hypertension in the first 6–7 years post-donation is reassuring and can certainly be used to counsel potential donors during the preoperative evaluation process.

Weight gain and obesity

Obesity can be associated with an increased risk of hypertension and diabetes mellitus and is also an independent risk factor for the development of end-stage kidney disease (Hsu et al., 2006).

The risk of developing obesity after donation is no different from the risk in the nondonor population. Janki et al. compared 761 living kidney donors with 1522 nondonors, whose average baseline BMI was 25.9 and 25.5 kg/m^2, respectively (Janki et al., 2020). At the 8 year follow-up, they found no significant difference (+0.02 kg/m^2, 95% CI − 0.04–0.07) between BMI in the two groups.

In contrast to the aforementioned study, Grupper et al. found different outcomes regarding post-donation BMI. They compared 211 living kidney donors with both pair-matched controls and healthy controls and followed them over a mean of 5.5 years (Grupper et al., 2019). At baseline, the healthy controls had a lower BMI (25 kg/m^2) compared to donors (25.64 kg/m^2) and matched controls (25.3 kg/m^2). They found that the healthy controls had less weight gain (BMI change − 0.3 kg/m^2) at follow-up compared to both the donors (BMI change + 0.65 kg/m^2) and matched controls (BMI change + 0.41 kg/m^2). Of note, patients with a BMI greater than or equal to 32 kg/m^2 were excluded from this study, so assessing obesity risk from this data is not possible.

Issa et al. assessed weight gain trends in 940 donors over a median follow-up time of 22.3 years (IQR range, 15.4–35.8 years). They found that the risk of gaining weight was no different than in the general population; however, those who did gain weight post-donation had an increased relative risk of developing both hypertension (RR 1.93, 95% CI, 1.51–2.46, $p < 0.001$) and diabetes mellitus (RR 4.18, 95% CI 2.05–8.5, $p < 0.001$). It is worth noting that this study consisted predominantly of non-Hispanic White donors so the risk may be underscored because the prevalence of hypertension and diabetes is higher in Blacks and Hispanics. Furthermore, the relative risks increased as donors gained more weight. Predictive factors for post-donation weight gain included female sex, older age and higher BMI at the time of donation. This study also investigated the risk of post-donation weight gain in individuals who lost weight to meet the inclusion criteria of BMI ≤ 30 kg/m^2. According to OPTN guidelines, having a BMI > 35 kg/m^2 is a relative contraindication to being a living donor, and most transplant centers have an accepted cutoff between BMI 30–35 kg/m^2. In the particular transplant center used for the study, the BMI cutoff was 30 kg/m^2. The researchers found that those who initially lost weight to become eligible for kidney donation ultimately gained the most weight (mean 3.8 kg/m^2, 15.5% increase in BMI) post-donation (Issa et al., 2018). These findings highlight the importance of counseling prospective donors on the risks of weight gain after donation and encouraging healthy lifestyle choices.

Live kidney donation in older adults

Kidney waitlist demographics

In the United States, most kidney transplant candidates are over 50 years old. In 2023, individuals aged 50 to 64 made up 42.3% of the waitlist. In addition, the proportion of candidates aged 65 and older increased from 15% in 2012 to 26.7% in 2023. Despite this growing demographic, live kidney donation remains uncommon. In 2024, only 18% of kidney transplants in recipients over 65 came from live donors. The reasons for the reluctance to use older live kidney donors are unclear. To assess whether kidneys from older live donors could help address the organ shortage, we will examine donor risks and transplant outcomes.

Donor risks

Although the Organ Procurement and Transplantation Network (OPTN) does not set an upper age limit for live donors, acceptance criteria vary across transplant centers. In Europe, 43% of centers impose an upper age limit (Lafranca et al., 2017). In the United States, a study by Berger et al. found that only 29% (80/279) of transplant centers reported using live donors aged ≥ 70, with half of those centers reporting just a single such donor. Notably, survival rates for these older donors were high—99.5% at 1 year and 90% at ten years—exceeding those of matched nondonors (99.1% and 73%, respectively).

Dols et al. studied the impact of age on post-donation outcomes among 539 live kidney donors, comparing those < 60 years ($n = 422$) with those ≥ 60 years ($n = 117$) (Dols et al., 2011). With a median of 5.5 years of follow-up, they found the older group had a lower baseline eGFR pre-donation (80 vs. 96 mL/min, respectively; $p < 0.001$). The post-donation eGFR trajectory was followed up to 13 years post-donation, and, importantly, there was no statistical difference in percent eGFR change between the two groups, showing there was no accelerated decline in kidney function among older donors. Significantly more older donors did have an eGFR ≤ 60 mL/min/1.73 m^2 (80% versus 31% in those ≥ 60 mL/min/1.73 m^2 vs. < 60 mL/min/1.73 m^2, respectively), but no donors developed an eGFR ≤ 30 mL/min/1.73 m^2 nor was there a difference in proteinuria between the two groups. The authors concluded the lower post-donation eGFR in the older group was merely a reflection of their lower eGFR pre-donation.

Concerns about higher perioperative risks in older donors stem from their increased likelihood of comorbidities. In the previously mentioned study, Dols et al. included 25 donors over 70 years of age (Dols et al., 2011). There were no significant differences in operative time or perioperative complications in comparison to donors younger than 70 years. Hospital stay was significantly longer by one day (5 vs. 4 days, $p < 0.001$), which was attributed to additional time needed to arrange for adequate care at home. Moreover, O'Brien et al. found no significant differences in operative time, hospital stay, blood loss, or early postoperative complications between donors over 60 and those aged 42.3 ± 10.4 years (O'Brien et al., 2012). Similarly, Hiramitsu et al. analyzed 1226 live kidney donors aged 30–49, 50–69, and 70–89 and found that nephrectomies were performed safely across all age groups (Hiramitsu et al., 2021). While donors aged 70–89 had longer arterial lengths and heavier kidneys, major surgical outcomes—including graft quality, warm ischemia time, operative time, and blood loss—were similar across groups. Collectively, these studies confirm that older donor age does not negatively impact perioperative safety, and survival rates are comparable to the general population.

Transplant outcomes

Recipients of live donor kidneys generally have better survival outcomes than those receiving organs from deceased donors. However, studies have explored whether these benefits extend to kidneys from older living donors.

Berger et al. found that recipients of kidneys from live donors aged ≥ 70 had a higher risk of graft loss (subhazard ratio [SHR] 1.62, 95% CI 1.16–2.28, $p = 0.005$) compared to recipients of kidneys from 50–59 year-old live donors (Berger et al., 2011). However, their outcomes were similar to those of recipients of 50–59 year-old deceased donor kidneys (SHR 1.19, 95% CI 0.87–1.63, $p = 0.3$). One-year, five-year, and ten-year survival rates for recipients of kidneys from donors aged ≥ 70 were 93.1%, 74.5%, and 56.2%, respectively, with no significant difference from recipients of younger donor kidneys.

In contrast, Patel et al. found no significant difference in graft survival between recipients of older live donor (OLD) kidneys (≥60) and those receiving kidneys from younger live donors. Their study supported the use of OLD kidneys, showing significantly lower graft loss and all-cause mortality compared to standard-criteria deceased donor kidneys. Receiving an OLD kidney also provided a significant reduction in all-cause mortality (HR 0.163, 95% CI 0.141–0.189, $p < 0.001$) compared to remaining on the waitlist. However, a subgroup analysis revealed that recipients of kidneys from donors ≥ 70 had higher mortality than those receiving standard-criteria deceased donor kidneys, though survival was comparable to recipients of extended-criteria donor kidneys. Importantly, all age groups of OLD kidney recipients had a survival advantage over remaining on the waitlist (Patel et al., 2024).

While these studies support the use of kidneys from older live donors, the optimal recipient age remains uncertain. Hiramitsu et al. found that recipients aged ≥ 70 had the highest graft loss and mortality rates. Similarly, Berger et al. and Patel et al. reported higher risks for recipients of kidneys from donors aged ≥ 70.

Considerations for older recipients

Before concluding that older recipients should not receive kidneys from donors aged 70 or older, several factors should be considered:

Sampling bias due to era effect: Berger et al.'s study included recipients from 1990 to 2010, a period when outcomes for older recipients were worse. McAdams et al. reported a 59% improvement in death-censored graft survival among older recipients in the modern transplant era. This may explain the difference in graft loss observed in Patel et al.'s study, which analyzed patients from 2000 to 2019 (McAdams-DeMarco et al., 2014).

Recipient age at transplant: In both Berger et al.'s and Patel et al.'s studies, recipients of older donor kidneys were, on average, 8–11 years older than those receiving younger donor kidneys. Naturally, older recipients have higher mortality rates, which could influence survival outcomes.

Informative censoring: Vanhove et al. demonstrated that standard outcome metrics, such as death-censored graft failure and death with a functioning graft, overestimate failure rates in recipients aged ≥ 65 by up to 9.9% (±3.4%). The Scientific Registry of Transplant Recipients (SRTR) now routinely uses competing risk models to account for this bias (Vanhove et al., 2022).

Given these factors, we urge caution in interpreting study conclusions about older live kidney donors and their recipients. Despite potential risks, using kidneys from older live donors offers key advantages, including shorter wait times and an overall survival benefit compared to remaining on the waitlist. In addition, older patients may feel more comfortable accepting a kidney from a donor of a similar age rather than from a younger relative.

Quality of life

Jacobs et al. obtained questionnaires from 524 kidney donors to assess the effect of donation on their well-being (Jacobs et al., 1998). They found that the overall quality of life was better in donors than in the general population, and 96% stated they would donate again. Over half of the participants reported higher self-worth and a sense of purpose. In contrast, only 12% of donors reported stress related to the donation process, with more females than males being likely to report this. Postoperative complications in the recipient were also associated with higher stress levels in the donor.

While the RELIVE (Renal and Lung Living Donors Evaluation) trial demonstrated that the percentage of donors who developed depressive symptoms was similar to that of the general population (as assessed by the National Health and Nutrition Examination Survey participants), others have reported higher rates of anxiety and depression.

A small observational, cross-sectional study by Bhurtyal et al. in Nepal evaluated 147 kidney donors using the Hospital Anxiety and Depression Scale (HADS) (Bhurtyal et al., 2012). Twenty-eight percent reported anxiety, and 6% reported depression. Nearly 70% of the donor pool was female. In another larger study by Levea et al., 2479 living donors were evaluated to assess their mental health post-donation (Levea et al., 2024). Both depression and anxiety were reported in 18% of participants. Seventy-three percent of donors were female. Given prior data by Jacobs et al. showing that females were more likely to report stress in the post-donation period, it is plausible that if the donor pool were more evenly distributed between men and women, the percentage of donors reporting these symptoms would be lower.

Furthermore, the RELIVE trial evaluated factors that affected donors' mental health. They found that older donation age, higher education, and donation to a first-degree relative were protective factors, whereas a history of a psychiatric condition was a risk factor for poorer mental health after donation (Gross et al., 2013). A history of psychiatric illness, obesity, and non-White race were risk factors for decreased physical health. Younger age at the time of donation, greater financial burden, longer recovery time after donation, and a moral obligation to donate were risk factors for developing depressive symptoms (Jowsey et al., 2014).

Conclusion

As demonstrated in this chapter, consideration and implementation of live kidney donation is an effective and safe way to address organ shortages in the United States and worldwide. The evolution of surgical techniques, coupled with the use of living kidney donation, has resulted in improved graft and patient survival in recipients and improved surgical outcomes for donors. Newer studies documenting the long-term effects of kidney donation and overall donor health provide valuable information that can not only improve patient education and informed consent but also enhance the medical care physicians provide.

References

Legality of alternative organ donation practices under 42 U.S.C. § 274e, 2007. Available from: https://www.justice.gov/sites/default/files/olc/opinions/2007/03/31/organtransplant.pdf.

OPTN/SRTR 2023 Annual data report: kidney, 2023. Available from: https://srtr.transplant.hrsa.gov/ADR/Chapter?name=Kidney&year=2023.

Annual data report, 2024. Available from: https://www.niddk.nih.gov/about-niddk/strategic-plans-reports/usrds/data-query-tools/esrd-incident-count.

KDIGO 2024 clinical practice guideline for the evaluation and management of chronic kidney disease, 2024. https://www.kidney-international.org/action/showPdf?pii=S0085-2538%2823%2900766-4

Current U.S. Waiting list. 2025. Available from: https://optn.transplant.hrsa.gov/data/view-data-reports/national-data.

U.S. Transplants performed: January 1, 1988—February 28, 2025, 2025. Available from: https://optn.transplant.hrsa.gov/data/view-data-reports/national-data.

Akoh, J.A., Mathuram Thiyagarajan, U., 2013. Renal transplantation from elderly living donors. J. Transplant. 2013. doi:10.1155/2013/475964

Altmann, U., Böger, C.A., Farkas, S., Mack, M., Luchner, A., Hamer, O.W., Zeman, F., Debl, K., Fellner, C., Jungbauer, C., Banas, B., Buchner, S., 2017. Effects of reduced kidney function because of living kidney donation on left ventricular mass. Hypertension 69 (2), 297–303. doi:10.1161/HYPERTENSIONAHA.116.08175.

Berger, J.C., Muzaale, A.D., James, N., Hoque, M., Garonzik, J.M.W., Montgomery, R.A., Massie, A.B., Hall, E.C., Segev, D.L., 2011. Living kidney donors ages 70 and older: recipient and donor outcomes. Clin. J. Am. Soc. Nephrol. 6 (12), 2887–2893. doi:10.2215/CJN.04160511.

Berglund, D.M., Zhang, L., Matas, A.J., Ibrahim, H.N., 2018. Measured glomerular filtration rate after kidney donation: no evidence of accelerated decay. Transplantation 102 (10), 1756–1761. doi:10.1097/TP.0000000000002215.

Bhurtyal, N., Paudel, K., Shah, S., Paudel, S., Kafle, M.P., Shah, D.S., 2012. Anxiety and depression among living kidney donors in tertiary care hospital of low resource country setting Nepal. Ann. Med. Surg. 80. doi:10.1016/j.amsu.2022.104119

Chan, L.W., Irish, G.L., Goh, T.L., Alnasrallah, B., Davies, C.E., Sypek, M.P., Clayton, P.A., Collins, M.G., 2025. Outcomes of living kidney donors following donor nephrectomy in aotearoa New Zealand. Kidney Int. Rep. 10 (3), 762–771. doi:10.1016/j.ekir.2024.11.1362.

Denic, A., Lieske, J.C., Chakkera, H.A., Poggio, E.D., Alexander, M.P., Singh, P., Kremers, W.K., Lerman, L.O., Rule, A.D., 2017. The substantial loss of nephrons in healthy human kidneys with aging. J. Am. Soc. Nephrol. 28 (1), 313–320. doi:10.1681/ASN.2016020154.

Dhalla, A., Ravani, P., Quinn, R.R., Garg, A.X., Clarke, A., Al-Wahsh, H., Lentine, K.L., Klarenbach, S., Hemmelgarn, B.R., Wang, C., Lam, N.N., 2024. Risk factors for developing low estimated glomerular filtration rate and albuminuria in living kidney donors. Kidney Med. 6 (2). doi:10.1016/j.xkme.2023.100767.

Dols, L.F.C., Kok, N.F.M., Roodnat, J.I., Tran, T.C.K., Terkivatan, T., Zuidema, W.C., Weimar, W., Ijzermans, J.N.M., 2011. Living kidney donors: impact of age on long-term safety. Am. J. Transplant. 11 (4), 737–742. doi:10.1111/j.1600-6143.2011.03465.x.

Doshi, M.D., Garg, A.X., Li, L., Kim, S.J., Gibney, E.M., Parikh, C.R., Segev, D.L., 2013. Medical outcomes in African American live kidney donors: a matched cohort study. Am. J. Transplant. 13 (1), 111–118. doi:10.1111/j.1600-6143.2012.04303.x.

Duque, E.J., Ferreira, G.F., Oliveira, I.B., Dominguez, W., Agena, F., Jorgetti, V., Lemos, F., Wolf, M., David-Neto, E., Moysés, R.M.A., 2024. Short and long-term effects of kidney donation on mineral and bone metabolism. BMC Nephrol. 25 (1). doi:10.1186/s12882-024-03827-0.

Emmons, B.R., Batal, I., King, K.L., Yu, M., Canetta, P.A., Sandoval, P.R., Mohan, S., Tsapepas, D., Adler, J.T., Ratner, L.E., Husain, S.A., 2024. Association of implantation biopsy findings in living donor kidneys with donor and recipient outcomes. Am. J. Kidney Dis. 83 (3), 306–317. doi:10.1053/j.ajkd.2023.09.010.

Fehrman-Ekholm, I., Elinder, C.G., Stenbeck, M., Tydén, G., Groth, C.G., 1997. Kidney donors live longer. Transplantation 64 (7), 976–978. doi:10.1097/00007890-199704150-00007.

Gandhi, N.V., Murad, D.N., Hebert, S.A., Morgan, M., Nguyen, D.T., Graviss, E.A., Ibrahim, H.N., 2022. Incidence and correlates of testicular pain after kidney donation. Front. Urol. 2. doi:10.3389/fruro.2022.986255

Garg, A.X., Arnold, J.B., Cuerden, M.S., Dipchand, C., Feldman, L.S., Gill, J.S., Karpinski, M., Klarenbach, S., Knoll, G., Lok, C.E., Miller, M., Monroy-Cuadros, M., Nguan, C., Prasad, G.V.R., Sontrop, J.M., Storsley, L., Boudville, N., 2024. Hypertension and kidney function after living kidney donation. JAMA. 332 (4), 287–299. doi:10.1001/jama.2024.8523.

Garg, A.X., Meirambayeva, A., Huang, A., Kim, J., Prasad, G.V.R., Knoll, G., Boudville, N., Lok, C., McFarlane, P., Karpinski, M., Storsley, L., Klarenbach, S., Lam, N., Thomas, S.M., Dipchand, C., Reese, P., Doshi, M., Gibney, E., Taub, K., Young, A., 2012a. Cardiovascular disease in kidney donors: matched cohort study. BMJ 344 (7850). doi:10.1136/bmj.e1203.

Garg, A.X., Muirhead, N., Knoll, G., Yang, R.C., Prasad, G.V.R., Thiessen-Philbrook, H., Rosas-Arellano, M.P., Housawi, A., Boudville, N., 2006. Proteinuria and reduced kidney function in living kidney donors: a systematic review, meta-analysis, and meta-regression. Kidney Int. 70 (10), 1801–1810.

Garg, A.X., Nevis, I.F., McArthur, E., Sontrop, J.M., Koval, J.J., Lam, N.N., Hildebrand, A.M., Reese, P.P., Storsley, L., Gill, J.S., Segev, D.L., Habbous, S., Bugeja, A., Knoll, G.A., Dipchand, C., Monroy-Cuadros, M., Lentine, K.L., 2015. Gestational hypertension and preeclampsia in living kidney donors. N. Engl. J. Med. 372 (2), 124–133. doi:10.1056/NEJMoa1408932.

Garg, A.X., Pouget, J., Young, A., Huang, A., Boudville, N., Hodsman, A., Adachi, J.D., Leslie, W.D., Cadarette, S.M., Lok, C.E., Monroy-Cuadros, M., Prasad, G.V.R., Thomas, S.M., Naylor, K., Treleavan, D., 2012b. Fracture risk in living kidney donors: a matched cohort study. Am. J. Kidney Dis. 59 (6), 770–776. doi:10.1053/j.ajkd.2012.01.013.

Garg, A.X., Prasad, G.V.R., Thiessen-Philbrook, H.R., Ping, L., Melo, M., Gibney, E.M., Knoll, G., Karpinski, M., Parikh, C.R., Gill, J., Storsley, L., Vlasschaert, M., Mamdani, M., 2008. Cardiovascular disease and hypertension risk in living kidney donors: an analysis of health administrative data in Ontario, Canada. Transplantation. 86 (3), 399–406. doi:10.1097/TP.0b013e31817ba9e3.

Grams, M.E., Sang, Y., Levey, A.S., Matsushita, K., Ballew, S., Chang, A.R., Chow, E.K.H., Kasiske, B.L., Kovesdy, C.P., Nadkarni, G.N., Shalev, V., Segev, D.L., Coresh, J., Lentine, K.L., Garg, A.X., 2016. Kidney-failure risk projection for the living kidney-donor candidate. N. Engl. J. Med. 374 (5), 411–421. Available from: http://transplantmodels.com/. doi:10.1056/NEJMoa1510491.

Gregory, A.V., Denic, A., Moustafa, A., Dasaraju, P.G., Poudyal, B., Augustine, J.J., Mullan, A.F., Korfiatis, P., Rule, A.D., Kline, T.L., 2023. The number and size of individual kidney medullary pyramids is associated with clinical characteristics, kidney biopsy findings, and CKD outcomes among kidney donors. J. Am. Soc. Nephrol. 34 (10), 1752–1763. doi:10.1681/ASN.0000000000000203.

Gross, C.R., Messersmith, E.E., Hong, B.A., Jowsey, S.G., Jacobs, C., Gillespie, B.W., Taler, S.J., Matas, A.J., Leichtman, A., Merion, R.M., Ibrahim, H.N., 2013. Health-related quality of life in kidney donors from the last five decades: results from the RELIVE study. Am. J. Transplant. 13 (11), 2924–2934. doi:10.1111/ajt.12434.

Grossardt, B.R., Kremers, H.M., Miller, A.R., Kasiske, B.L., Matas, A.J., Khosla, S., Kremers, W.K., Amer, H., Kumar, R., 2024. Persistent changes in calcium-regulating hormones and bone turnover markers in living kidney donors more than 20 years after donation. JBMR Plus 8 (7). doi:10.1093/jbmrpl/ziae067.

Grupper, A., Angel, Y., Baruch, A., Schwartz, I.F., Schwartz, D., Nakache, R., Goykhman, Y., Katz, P., Nachmany, I., Lubezky, N., Weinstein, T., Shashar, M., Ben-Bassat, O.K., Berliner, S., Rogowski, O., Zeltser, D., Shapira,

I., Shenhar-Tsarfaty, S., 2019. Long term metabolic and renal outcomes of kidney donors compared to controls with excellent kidney function. BMC Nephrol. 20 (1). doi:10.1186/s12882-019-1214-4.

Harasemiw, O., Nayak, J.G., Grubic, N., Ferguson, T.W., Sood, M.M., Tangri, N., 2023. A predictive model for kidney failure after nephrectomy for localized kidney cancer: the kidney cancer risk equation. Am. J. Kidney Dis. 82 (6), 656–665. doi:10.1053/j.ajkd.2023.05.016.

Hariharan, S., Israni, A.K., Danovitch, G., 2021. Long-term survival after kidney transplantation. N. Engl. J. Med. 385 (8), 729–743. doi:10.1056/NEJMra2014530.

Hiramitsu, T., Tomosugi, T., Futamura, K., Okada, M., Matsuoka, Y., Goto, N., Ichimori, T., Narumi, S., Takeda, A., Kobayashi, T., Uchida, K., Watarai, Y., 2021. Adult living-donor kidney transplantation, donor age, and donor-recipient age. Kidney Int. Rep. 6 (12), 3026–3034. doi:10.1016/j.ekir.2021.10.002.

Hostetter, T.H., Olson, J.L., Rennke, H.G., 1981. Hyperfiltration in remnant nephrons: a potentially adverse response to renal ablation. Am. J. Physiol. Renal Physiol. 241 (1), F85–F93. doi:10.1152/ajprenal.1981.241.1.F85.

Hsu, C.-Y., McCulloch, C.E., Iribarren, C., Darbinian, J., Go, A.S., 2006. Body mass index and risk for end-stage renal disease. Ann. Intern. Med. 144 (1), 21–28. doi:10.7326/0003-4819-144-1-200601030-00006.

Ibrahim, H.N., Akkina, S.K., Leister, E., Gillingham, K., Cordner, G., Guo, H., Bailey, R., Rogers, T., Matas, A.J., 2009b. Pregnancy outcomes after kidney donation. Am. J. Transplant. 9 (4), 825–834. doi:10.1111/j.1600-6143.2008.02530.x.

Ibrahim, H.N., Berglund, D.M., Jackson, S., Vock, D.M., Foley, R.N., Matas, A.J., 2017. Renal consequences of diabetes after kidney donation. Am. J. Transplant. 17 (12), 3141–3148. doi:10.1111/ajt.14416.

Ibrahim, H.N., Foley, R.N., Reule, S.A., Spong, R., Kukla, A., Issa, N., Berglund, D.M., Sieger, G.K., Matas, A.J., 2016. Renal function profile in white kidney donors: the first 4 decades. J. Am. Soc. Nephrol. 27 (9), 2885–2893. doi:10.1681/ASN.2015091018.

Ibrahim, H.N., Foley, R., Tan, L., Rogers, T., Bailey, R.F., Guo, H., Gross, C.R., Matas, A.J., 2009a. Long-term consequences of kidney donation. N. Engl. J. Med. 360 (5), 459–469. doi:10.1056/NEJMoa0804883.

Ibrahim, H.N., Kukla, A., Cordner, G., Bailey, R., Gillingham, K., Matas, A.J., 2010. Diabetes after kidney donation. Am. J. Transplant. 10 (2), 331–337. doi:10.1111/j.1600-6143.2009.02944.x.

Issa, N., Sánchez, O.A., Kukla, A., Riad, S.M., Berglund, D.M., Ibrahim, H.N., Matas, A.J., 2018. Weight gain after kidney donation: association with increased risks of type 2 diabetes and hypertension. Clin. Transplant. 32 (9). doi:10.1111/ctr.13360.

Issa, N., Vaughan, L.E., Denic, A., Kremers, W.K., Chakkera, H.A., Park, W.D., Matas, A.J., Taler, S.J., Stegall, M.D., Augustine, J.J., Rule, A.D., 2019. Larger nephron size, low nephron number, and nephrosclerosis on biopsy as predictors of kidney function after donating a kidney. Am. J. Transplant. 19 (7), 1989–1998. doi:10.1111/ajt.15259.

Jacobs, C., Johnson, E., Anderson, K., Gillingham, K., Matas, A., 1998. Kidney transplants from living donors: how donation affects family dynamics. Adv. Ren. Replace. Ther. 5 (2), 89–97. doi:10.1016/s1073-4449(98)70002-0.

Janki, S., Dehghan, A., van de Wetering, J., Steyerberg, E.W., Klop, K.W.J., Kimenai, H.J.A.N., Rizopoulos, D., Hoorn, E.J., Stracke, S., Weimar, W., Völzke, H., Hofman, A., Ijzermans, J.N.M., 2020. Long-term prognosis after kidney donation: a propensity score matched comparison of living donors and non-donors from two population cohorts. Eur. J. Epidemiol. 35 (7), 699–707. doi:10.1007/s10654-020-00647-y.

Jowsey, S.G., Jacobs, C., Gross, C.R., Hong, B.A., Messersmith, E.E., Gillespie, B.W., Beebe, T.J., Kew, C., Matas, A., Yusen, R.D., Hill-Callahan, M., Odim, J., Taler, S.J., 2014. Emotional well-being of living kidney donors: findings from the RELIVE study. Am. J. Transplant. 14 (11), 2535–2544. doi:10.1111/ajt.12906.

Kaplow, K., Ruck, J.M., Levan, M.L., Thomas, A.G., Stewart, D., Massie, A.B., Sung, H.C., Pisano, S.F., Sidoti, C., Segev, D.L., Sinacore, J., Waterman, A.D., 2024. National attitudes toward living kidney donation in the United States: results of a public opinion survey. Kidney Med. 6 (3). doi:10.1016/j.xkme.2023.100788.

Kasiske, B.L., Anderson-Haag, T.L., Duprez, D.A., Kalil, R.S., Kimmel, P.L., Pesavento, T.E., Snyder, J.J., Weir, M.R., 2020. A prospective controlled study of metabolic and physiologic effects of kidney donation suggests that donors retain stable kidney function over the first nine years. Kidney Int. 98 (1), 168–175. doi:10.1016/j.kint.2020.02.026.

Kasiske, B.L., Kumar, R., Kimmel, P.L., Pesavento, T.E., Kalil, R.S., Kraus, E.S., Rabb, H., Posselt, A.M., Anderson-Haag, T.L., Steffes, M.W., Israni, A.K., Snyder, J.J., Singh, R.J., Weir, M.R., 2016. Abnormalities in biomarkers of mineral and bone metabolism in kidney donors. Kidney Int. 90 (4), 861–868. doi:10.1016/j.kint.2016.05.012.

Kavoussi, L.R., 2000. Laparoscopic donor nephrectomy. Kidney Int. 57 (5), 2175–2186. doi:10.1046/j.1523-1755.2000.00069.x.

Kourounis, G., Tingle, S.J., Hoather, T.J., Thompson, E.R., Rogers, A., Page, T., Sanni, A., Rix, D.A., Soomro, N.A., Wilson, C., 2024. Robotic versus laparoscopic versus open nephrectomy for live kidney donors. Cochrane Database Syst. Rev. 5 (5). doi:10.1002/14651858.CD006124.pub3.

Lafranca, J.A., Spoon, E.Q.W., van de Wetering, J., IJzermans, J.N.M., Dor, F.J.M.F., 2017. Attitudes among transplant professionals regarding shifting paradigms in eligibility criteria for live kidney donation. PloS One 12 (7). doi:10.1371/journal.pone.0181846.

Laksanabunsong, P., Hansomwong, T., Suk-ouichai, C., Woranisarakul, V., Jitpraphai, S., Chotikawanich, E., Taweemonkongsap, T., 2024. Comparison of renal function of patients after tumor nephrectomy versus donor nephrectomy: long term outcome using a propensity score matching analysis. Heliyon 10 (17). doi:10.1016/j.heliyon.2024.e36625.

Lam, N.N., Lloyd, A., Lentine, K.L., Quinn, R.R., Ravani, P., Hemmelgarn, B.R., Klarenbach, S., Garg, A.X., 2020. Changes in kidney function follow living donor nephrectomy. Kidney Int. 98 (1), 176–186. doi:10.1016/j.kint.2020.02.027.

Lenihan, C.R., Myers, B.D., Tan, J.C., 2016. Glomerular function and structure in living donors: lessons from single nephron studies. Curr. Transplant. Rep. 3, 24–32.

Lentine, K.L., Lam, N.N., Axelrod, D., Schnitzler, M.A., Garg, A.X., Xiao, H., Dzebisashvili, N., Schold, J.D., Brennan, D.C., Randall, H., King, E.A., Segev, D.L., 2016. Perioperative complications after living kidney donation: a national study. Am. J. Transplant. 16 (6), 1848–1857. doi:10.1111/ajt.13687.

Lentine, K.L., Smith, J.M., Lyden, G.R., Miller, J.M., Booker, S.E., Dolan, T.G., Temple, K.R., Weiss, S., Handarova, D., Israni, A.K., Snyder, J.J., 2025. OPTN/SRTR 2023 annual data report: kidney. Am. J. Transplant. 25 (2). doi:10.1016/j.ajt.2025.01.020.

Levea, S.-L., Prasadh, J.G., Wang, B.K., Salcedo-Betancourt, J.D., Matevish, L., Vivaldi, J.S., Lieber, S.R., Shah, J.A., Hwang, C.S., Wojciechowski, D., Vagefi, P.A., Patel, M.S., 2024. A contemporary analysis of mental well-being among living donor kidney applicants. Transplant. Direct 10 (6). doi:10.1097/TXD.0000000000001631.

Lin, S.-Y., Lin, C.-L., Sung, F.-C., Chang, C.-H., Wu, H.-C., Chen, W.-C., Wang, I.-K., Chen, C.-J., Chou, A.-K., Kao, C.-H., 2019. Risk of subsequent health disorders among living kidney donors. Medicine 98 (7). doi:10.1097/MD.0000000000014494.

Mange, K.C., Joffe, M.M., Feldman, H.I., 2001. Effect of the use or nonuse of long-term dialysis on the subsequent survival of renal transplants from living donors. N. Engl. J. Med. 344 (10), 726–731. doi:10.1056/NEJM200103083441004.

Maradit Kremers, H.M., Grossardt, B.R., Miller, A.R., Kasiske, B.L., Matas, A.J., Khosla, S., Kremers, W.K., Amer, H., Kumar, R., 2024. Fracture risk among living kidney donors 25 years after donation. JAMA Netw. Open 7 (1). doi:10.1001/jamanetworkopen.2023.53005.

Massie, A.B., Motter, J.D., Snyder, J.J., Levan, M.L., Segev, D.L., 2024. Thirty-year trends in perioperative mortality risk for living kidney donors. JAMA 332 (12), 1015–1017. doi:10.1001/jama.2024.14527.

Massie, A.B., Muzaale, A.D., Luo, X., Chow, E.K.H., Locke, J.E., Nguyen, A.Q., Henderson, M.L., Snyder, J.J., Segev, D.L., 2017. Quantifying postdonation risk of ESRD in living kidney donors. J. Am. Soc. Nephrol. 28 (9), 2749–2755. doi:10.1681/ASN.2016101084.

Matas, A.J., Hays, R.E., Ibrahim, H.N., 2017. A case-based analysis of whether living related donors listed for transplant share ESRD causes with their recipients. Clin. J. Am. Soc. Nephrol. 12 (4), 663–668. doi:10.2215/CJN.11421116.

Matas, A.J., Ibrahim, H.N., 2013. The unjustified classification of kidney donors as patients with CKD: critique and recommendations. Clin. J. Am. Soc. Nephrol. 8 (8), 1406–1413. doi:10.2215/CJN.02110213.

Matas, A.J., Rule, A.D., 2022. Long-term medical outcomes of living kidney donors. Mayo Clin. Proc. 97 (11), 2107–2122. doi:10.1016/j.mayocp.2022.07.010.

McAdams-DeMarco, M.A., James, N., Salter, M.L., Walston, J., Segev, D.L., 2014. Trends in kidney transplant outcomes in older adults. J. Am. Geriatr. Soc. 62 (12), 2235–2242. doi:10.1111/jgs.13130.

Merzkani, M.A., Denic, A., Narasimhan, R., Lopez, C.L., Larson, J.J., Kremers, W.K., Chakkera, H.A., Park, W.D., Taler, S.J., Stegall, M.D., Alexander, M.P., Issa, N., Rule, A.D., 2021. Kidney microstructural features at the time of donation predict long-term risk of chronic kidney disease in living kidney donors. Mayo Clin. Proc. 96 (1), 40–51. doi:10.1016/j.mayocp.2020.08.041.

Mjøen, G., Hallan, S., Hartmann, A., Foss, A., Midtvedt, K., Øyen, O., Reisæter, A., Pfeffer, P., Jenssen, T., Leivestad, T., Line, P.-D., Øvrehus, M., Dale, D.O., Pihlstrøm, H., Holme, I., Dekker, F.W., Holdaas, H., 2014. Long-term risks for kidney donors. Kidney Int. 86 (1), 162–167. doi:10.1038/ki.2013.460.

Moody, W.E., Ferro, C.J., Edwards, N.C., Chue, C.D., Lin, E.L.S., Taylor, R.J., Cockwell, P., Steeds, R.P., Townend, J.N., 2016. Cardiovascular effects of unilateral nephrectomy in living kidney donors. Hypertension 67 (2), 368–377. doi:10.1161/HYPERTENSIONAHA.115.06608.

Munch, P., Christiansen, C.F., Birn, H., Erikstrup, C., Nørgaard, M., 2021. Is the risk of cardiovascular disease increased in living kidney donors? A Danish population-based cohort study. Am. J. Transplant. 21 (5), 1857–1865. doi:10.1111/ajt.16384.

Muzaale, A.D., Massie, A.B., Wang, M.-C., Montgomery, R.A., McBride, M.A., Wainright, J.L., Segev, D.L., 2014. Risk of end-stage renal disease following live kidney donation. JAMA. 311 (6), 579–586. doi:10.1001/jama.2013.285141.

O'Brien, B., Mastoridis, S., Sabharwal, A., Hakim, N., Taube, D., Papalois, V., 2012. Expanding the donor pool: living donor nephrectomy in the elderly and the overweight. Transplantation 93 (11), 1158–1165. doi:10.1097/TP.0b013e31824ef1ae.

Ogata, M., Osako, K., Terashita, M., Miyauchi, T., Sakurai, Y., Shinoda, K., Sasaki, H., Shibagaki, Y., Yazawa, M., 2024. Consequences of kidney donation by age in Japanese living kidney donors: a single-center study. Clin. Exp. Nephrol. 28 (7), 664–673. doi:10.1007/s10157-024-02476-9.

Palzer, E.F., Vempati, S., Helgeson, E.S., Matas, A.J., 2020. Long-term living kidney donor risk: a web-based calculator. J. Am. Soc. Nephrol. 31 (12). doi:10.1681/ASN.2020081238.

Patel, K., Brotherton, A., Chaudhry, D., Evison, F., Nieto, T., Dabare, D., Sharif, A., 2024. Survival advantage comparing older living donor versus standard criteria donor kidney transplants. Transpl. Int. 37. doi:10.3389/ti.2024.12559

Poggio, E.D., Augustine, J.J., Arrigain, S., Brennan, D.C., Schold, J.D., 2021. Long-term kidney transplant graft survival—making progress when most needed. Am. J. Transplant. 21 (8), 2824–2832. doi:10.1111/ajt.16463.

Price, A.M., Moody, W.E., Stoll, V.M., Vijapurapu, R., Hayer, M.K., Biasiolli, L., Weston, C.J., Webster, R., Wesolowski, R., McGee, K.C., Liu, B., Baig, S., Pickup, L.C., Radhakrishnan, A., Law, J.P., Edwards, N.C., Steeds, R.P., Ferro, C.J., Townend, J.N., 2021. Cardiovascular effects of unilateral nephrectomy in living kidney donors at 5 years. Hypertension 77 (4), 1273–1284. doi:10.1161/HYPERTENSIONAHA.120.15398.

Reisæter, A.V., Røislien, J., Henriksen, T., Irgens, L.M., Hartmann, A., 2009. Pregnancy and birth after kidney donation: the Norwegian experience. Am. J. Transplant. 9 (4), 820–824. doi:10.1111/j.1600-6143.2008.02427.x.

Schoephoerster, J., Matas, A., Jackson, S., Pruett, T.L., Finger, E., Kandaswamy, R., Dunn, T., Kirchner, V., Anderson, J.K., Humphreville, V., 2022. Orchialgia after living donor nephrectomy: an underreported entity. Transplant. Direct. 8 (11). doi:10.1097/TXD.0000000000001383.

Timsit, M.-O., Nguyen, K.N., Rouach, Y., Elie, C., Loupy, A., Fournier, C., Legendre, C., Mejean, A., 2012. Kidney function following nephrectomy: similitude and discrepancies between kidney cancer and living donation. Urol. Oncol. 30 (4), 482–486. doi:10.1016/j.urolonc.2010.04.005.

Van Arendonk, K.J., James, N.T., Orandi, B.J., Garonzik-Wang, J.M., Smith, J.M., Colombani, P.M., Segev, D.L., 2013. Order of donor type in pediatric kidney transplant recipients requiring retransplantation. Transplantation 96 (5), 487–493. doi:10.1097/TP.0b013e31829acb10.

Vanhove, T., Elias, N., Safa, K., Cohen-Bucay, A., Schold, J.D., Riella, L.V., Gilligan, H., 2022. Long-term outcome reporting in older kidney transplant recipients and the limitations of conventional survival metrics. Kidney Int. Rep. 7 (11), 2397–2409. doi:10.1016/j.ekir.2022.08.010.

Vats, A., Gillingham, K., Matas, A., Chavers, B., 2002. Improved late graft survival and half-lives in pediatric kidney transplantation: a single center experience. Am. J. Transplant. 2 (10), 939–945. doi:10.1034/j.1600-6143.2002.21010.x.

Vella, I., Di Francesco, F., Accardo, C., Pagano, D., Petri, S.L., Boggi, U., Gruttadauria, S., 2024. Review of the history of living donor solid organ transplants. Eur. J. Transplant. Available from: https://www.eujtransplantation.com/article/view/403/380. doi:10.53388/EJT403.

Wang, S., Liu, Z., Zhang, D., Xiang, F., Zheng, W., 2022. The incidence and risk factors of chronic kidney disease after radical nephrectomy in patients with renal cell carcinoma. BMC Cancer 22 (1). doi:10.1186/s12885-022-10245-8.

Warren, P.H., Gifford, K.A., Hong, B.A., Merion, R.M., Ojo, A.O., 2014. Development of the National Living Donor Assistance Center: reducing financial disincentives to living organ donation. Prog. Transplant. 24 (1), 76–81. doi:10.7182/pit2014593.

Young, A., Hodsman, A.B., Boudville, N., Geddes, C., Gill, J., Goltzman, D., Jassal, S.V., Klarenbach, S., Knoll, G., Muirhead, N., Prasad, G.V.R., Treleaven, D., Garg, A.X., 2012. Bone and mineral metabolism and fibroblast growth factor 23 levels after kidney donation. Am. J. Kidney Dis. 59 (6), 761–769. doi:10.1053/j.ajkd.2011.09.019.

CHAPTER

23

CNS limitations in elderly kidney patients

Stephen Z. Fadem[a] *and Totini Sagorika Chatterjee*[b,c]

[a]Department of Medicine, Section of Nephrology, Baylor College of Medicine, Houston, TX, United States

[b]Division of Geriatrics, Department of Medicine, University of Texas Medical Branch, Galveston, TX, United States

[c]Division of Nephrology, Department of Medicine, University of Texas Medical Branch, Galveston, TX, United States

Introduction

Deteriorating kidney function contributes to factors that lead to cognitive decline in aging. Cognitive function declines by 30% to 60% in hemodialysis patients, which is double the percentage observed in age-matched controls (Bugnicourt et al., 2013). A study of cognitive function in 374 hemodialysis patients found mild impairment in 13.9% (95% CI 10.4–18.1), moderate impairment in 36.3% (95% CI 31.0%–41.5%), and severe impairment in 37.3% (95% CI 32.1–42.7). Only 12.7% scored normal (Murray et al., 2006). Its coexistence with hypertension, vascular calcification, inflammation, cardiovascular disorders, and diabetes also plays a role in causing dementia and stroke. The relationships between kidney disease and the brain have been established. Kidney damage has been documented to affect brain cortical structure in large-scale genetic studies using magnetic resonance imaging (Chen et al., 2021). This chapter aims to describe the cognitive landscape associated with advancing kidney disease, outlining when to suspect it, the simple tests currently available, and the principles of medical management. It subsequently reviews cognitive decline within the framework of the 12 hallmarks of aging, emphasizing how the hallmarks that impact the kidney secondarily affect the brain. Finally, the chapter reviews the major causes of stroke, along with their diagnosis and management in chronic kidney disease (CKD) patients.

Aging and the Kidney
https://doi.org/10.1016/B978-0-443-34069-7.00026-4

Cognitive impairment and its limitations in CKD

Neurocognitive decline progresses with age and is accelerated by chronic diseases like CKD. It may initially present as memory loss, sleep disturbances, depression, and confusion when attempting tasks that were once simple. It is associated with impaired judgment, confusion regarding medications, difficulty in communication, and repeated episodes of depression. Urinary incontinence is also a significant issue. Dementia increases the risk of falls (see Chapter 11), as forgetfulness can lead to clutter and obstacles on the floor. Patients with cognitive impairment are more likely to slip on wet surfaces or stumble over unexpected steps. Moreover, individuals with dementia often exhibit abnormal mobility, balance issues, and difficulties in depth and vision perception.

The socioeconomic environment of the patient is associated with symptoms and presents a subset of challenges to management. As dementia worsens, the patient is less likely to participate independently in daily living activities, more likely to have difficulty getting around, and may wander dangerously. Poor hygiene and soiled clothing, unkempt hair, frequent accidents, especially falls, and a change in socialization may be early warnings of dementia. The key indicator is a decrease in performing the activities of independent daily living. In the 1940s, a performance status scale was developed by David Karnofsky and colleagues (Timmermann, 2013). The Karnofsky Scale is offered as a free predictor app created by the author and is helpful in assessing patients who have lost their ability to function independently (https://zkidney.com/epi-sp).

There are six cognitive domains that describe decline: learning and memory, attention, executive function, language, perceptual-motor skills, and social cognition. Impairment in these domains has been demonstrated in systematic reviews and metaanalyses (Etgen et al., 2012). When adjusted for comorbidity-related risk factors, there is a significantly higher risk of impairment in scanning and tracking, as well as in visual-spatial organization and memory domains. The odds ratio for impaired function in the language domain is 2.65. The odds ratio for impaired executive functioning is 2.49 when compared to patients without kidney disease (Torres et al., 2017). By the time one reaches end-stage kidney disease, the prevalence of moderate or severe cognitive impairment is over 70% (Murray et al., 2006).

Assessing cognitive function starts with a patient history and physical examination. Certain signs that can alert family members and caregivers to early indicators of cognitive decline include sleep disturbances, obstructive sleep apnea, a history of falls, confusion about medications, forgetting appointments, and difficulty in memory retention. Focal signs, tremors, and gait and balance disorders may be associated with stroke. Patients with uncontrolled hypertension, atrial fibrillation, and peripheral vascular disease (indicated by an abnormal ankle-brachial index or amputations) are at high risk for stroke (Kolls et al., 2019). In a review by Franco et al., uremic toxins such as indoxyl sulfate, p-cresyl sulfate, uric acid, homocysteine, interleukin-1, interleukin-6, and parathyroid hormone were associated with abnormalities in cognitive testing (Franco et al., 2019).

As cognition declines, it becomes increasingly challenging and ultimately impossible for patients to perform activities of daily living. Memory decline, problem-solving difficulties, and diminished executive function can be assessed using screening tools.

1. The Mini-Mental State Examination (MMSE) is a 11-question screening tool that assesses five areas of cognitive function: language, attention and calculation, recall, orientation, and registration (Kay et al., 1985).

2. The Montreal Cognitive Assessment Test (MoCA) is a 30-point mental status examination. It measures visuospatial skills, executive function, short-term memory recall, attention and concentration, language, and orientation. A score of 26 or higher is considered normal, while a score between 19 and 25 suggests mild cognitive impairment. A score of 11 to 18 indicates moderate impairment, and a score of 10 or below signifies severe cognitive deficits (Nasreddine et al., 2005).
3. The Short Test of Mental Status is a 5 min, eight-question assessment with a total score of 38. It evaluates orientation, attention through digit span, immediate recall of four unrelated words, basic arithmetic calculations, abstraction through word similarities, figure copying, general information, and recall of those four words. A score of 29 or lower is a validated indicator of dementia.

Patients identified with potential cognitive impairment during screening should undergo a neurological assessment. This assessment includes a neurological examination, a review of medications, and brain imaging studies. An individualized therapy plan should be coordinated with the relatives or other responsible individuals caring for the patient. Managing cognitive decline requires social support, particularly when it is accompanied by CKD. This is especially challenging for patients who lack access to caregivers or health providers. A National Kidney Foundation survey utilizing the Dementia Knowledge Assessment Scale revealed that, despite the significant burden of dementia in dialysis patients, only 62% of providers have received training in dementia care, and many exhibited low DKA scores. Of the survey respondents, 67.5% were physicians. Subthemes from the study indicated that early diagnosis and treatment of cognitive impairment can enhance quality of life and that incorporating physical exercise, along with attention to mental and physical well-being, is crucial for managing the disease (Bender et al., 2024).

Besides exercise, patients on dialysis with cognitive impairment may benefit from addressing hearing and visual impairments, strengthening social connections, optimizing diabetes and heart disease management, correcting sleep disorders, quitting smoking, and obtaining social support. Each of these factors contributes to cognitive impairment in patients with CKD on dialysis (Crowe et al., 2021).

Improvements in cognitive function occur during the second hour of a dialysis session ($p < 0.001$) compared to the predialysis day; it is worse just before treatment (Karakizlis et al., 2021). Although this suggests that dialysis adequacy may also be a factor in cognitive impairment testing concerning timing, the Frequent Hemodialysis Network Daily Trial (FHN) demonstrated no benefit of frequent hemodialysis on cognitive function (Kurella Tamura et al., 2013).

A management strategy to reduce cognitive function decline involves the early detection of key factors contributing to its causes and, when possible, controlling or alleviating them. In this spirit, we will examine the hallmarks of aging.

The hallmarks of aging

The hallmarks of aging have been thoroughly explored, with nearly 700,000 articles published on the topic (Source: Pubmed). In this chapter, we will examine the potential impact

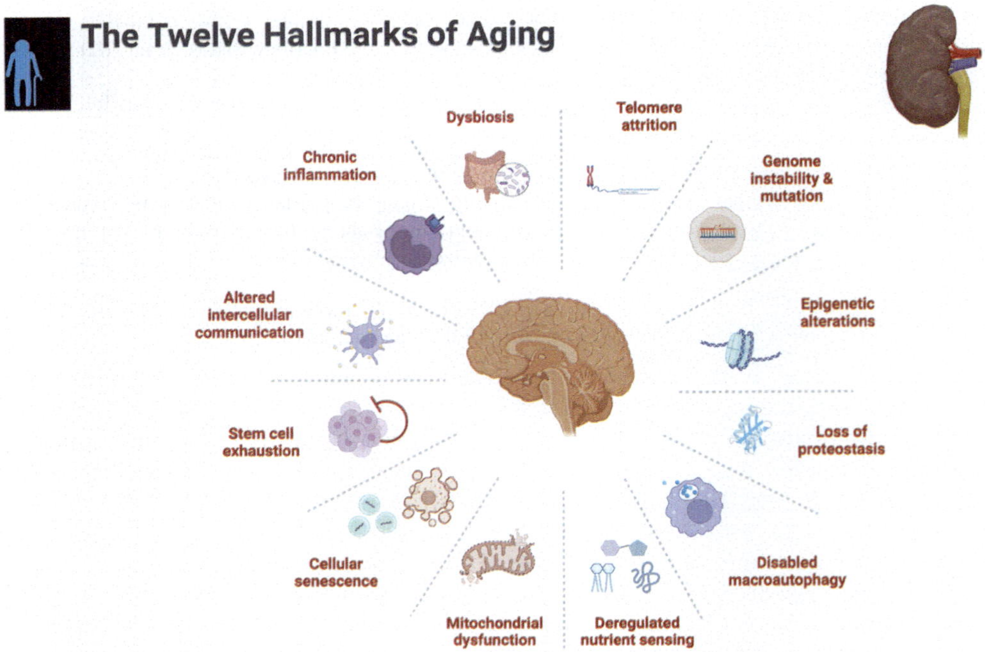

FIG. 23.1 The twelve hallmarks of aging. The classic hallmarks of aging. Kidney aging and poor function also influence aging in the brain and cognitive function. *Created in BioRender. Fadem, S., 2025. https://BioRender.com/hr9fzcs; From Lopez-Otin, C., Blasco, M.A., Partridge, L., Serrano, M., Kroemer, G., 2023. Hallmarks of aging: an expanding universe. Cell. 1097-4172. 186 (2), 243–278. Available from: https://www.sciencedirect.com/journal/cell. doi:10.1016/j.cell.2022.11.001.*

of CKD-related aging on cognitive decline within the context of the hallmarks of aging (López-Otín et al., 2023) (Fig. 23.1).

Genomic instability

Mutations in DNA, mitochondrial DNA, and RNA occur frequently, and as people age, the number of mutations increases. The cellular mechanisms that control these mutations in early life diminish with age. Genomic instability refers to the DNA changes that take place during the normal course of cell division. DNA replication is complex and consists of a series of phases. As the S phase is entered, the DNA complex opens and separates into two forks that travel to different locations. Challenges to DNA replication arise naturally with aging and also result from external factors such as radiation and environmental toxins. This replicative stress requires repair and activates a type 1 interferon response that induces inflammation (Técher and Pasero, 2021). CKD can worsen genomic damage both within and outside the body, and this instability may contribute to the inflammatory response linked to increased cognitive decline (Sartori et al., 2012). The consequences of unrepaired genetic mutations include not only inflammation but also cell dysfunction and carcinogenesis.

Studies on genomic instability using the micronucleus assay of buccal epithelial cells (MN-BEC) were conducted with predialysis, dialysis, and transplanted children suffering from

CKD. Abnormalities in MN-BEC for CKD were 5 to 7 times higher than those of controls ($p < 0.001$) (Aykanat et al., 2016). Loci of genomic instability in CKD were identified by examining polymorphisms in cells responsible for repair functions, such as base excision repair and nucleotide excision repair. Investigators also assessed genes related to metabolism and antioxidants. A significant relationship was found between the damaged genes and those involved in repair mechanisms, as well as with the genes encoding antioxidant enzymes. Genes associated with CKD showed oxidative DNA damage and genomic instability (Corredor et al., 2020).

Telomere attrition

The ends of DNA are capped with telomeres, which are repetitive nucleoprotein structures that protect against the loss of vital information during cell division. DNA polymerase is responsible for building nucleotides into DNA but cannot fully replicate the end of the strand. Telomeres start with a double strand and end with a single strand made up of six-nucleotide repeats of 5′TTAGGG-3′. This strand forms a loop to maintain its integrity and shield the chromosome from degradation, particularly by DNA repair machinery. Therefore telomeres must act as a buffer. Telomeres shorten with each cell division, and over time, this can compromise DNA functionality.

Telomerase, an enzyme that adds single-stranded nucleotide repeats (5′TTAGGG-3′) to the ends of the telomere, can counteract telomere shortening and extend its length. A telomerase deficiency is associated with DNA loss and the inability to produce essential cellular proteins and enzymes. This deficiency has been shown to cause age-related kidney fibrosis (Koh et al., 2020).

In addition to normal cell division, telomere shortening can occur as a consequence of oxidative stress, inflammation, and environmental toxins. It has been demonstrated that shorter leukocyte telomeres are associated with CKD. Leukocyte telomere length in single-nucleotide polymorphisms (SNPs) of 1628 patients with CKD and 3140 control subjects was assessed using Mendelian randomization. The genetically determined shortening of leukocyte telomeres was found to be associated with CKD and a risk factor (Odds Ratio 1.51, 95% CI 1.12–2.12, $p = 0.007$) (Gurung et al., 2021). In a 4 year study of 4926 patients, peripheral blood analysis of telomere length in CKD patients predicted all-cause mortality (Hazard Ratio 1.14, 95% CI 1.06–1.72) (Fazzini et al., 2020). Leukocyte telomere shortening is also associated with dementia. A UK study of 439,961 subjects evaluated peripheral blood leukocyte telomere length. During an 11.6 year follow-up period, 5820 cases of dementia were discovered. Shorter telomeres were significantly associated with a higher hazard ratio for dementia and Alzheimer's disease ($p < 0.05$) (Cao et al., 2023).

Telomere preservation can also occur with changes in lifestyle and the use of medications such as metformin or angiotensin receptor blockers. However, it is not clear whether the effects of these medications are direct or the result of better diabetes and blood pressure control. Exercise, smoking cessation, and a change to healthier diets may preserve telomeres in CKD. A telomerase activator, *Astragalus membrana*ceus telomerase activator-65, was shown to increase telomeres in animal models, but there is no direct evidence that this supplement is effective in either CKD or dementia (Alshinnawy et al., 2020). Glomerular mesangial cell senescence is a pathological consequence of diabetes. Tea phenols are beneficial in slowing factors related to mesangial senescence by lengthening telomeres (Cao et al., 2018; Hill et al., 2023).

Epigenetic alterations

Epigenetics is extensively discussed in Chapter 5. In this review, epigenetics encompasses gene activity that occurs independently of DNA sequence alterations. Epigenetic modification may involve the addition of a methyl (CH_3) group to DNA. This can occur as a gene-silencing mechanism, enabling successful DNA repair. DNA is wrapped around proteins known as histones, which can be modified by the epigenetic mechanisms outlined in Chapter 5. Transcription can be influenced by chromatin, a highly compact structure regulated by epigenetic factors. ATP-dependent chromatin remodeling may reveal genomic sequence regions, facilitating DNA repair, although the role of ATP-dependent chromatin remodeling in CKD and aging has yet to be clarified. A fourth epigenetic mechanism related to kidney disease is noncoding microRNAs (miRNAs), small RNA molecules that bind to messenger RNA (mRNA), disrupting its function and leading to its degradation. Like DNA, RNA can also undergo changes that alter its functionality when subjected to epigenetic mechanisms. These mechanisms have been studied as factors in kidney aging.

DNA methylation progresses as the kidney ages. DNA methylation progressively impacts vital proteins such as N-cadherin, the WNT/β-catenin pathway, Nrf2, and Klotho, worsening kidney cell senescence. As histone modification occurs, collagen increases, and fibrosis worsens. Noncoding RNAs associated with mitochondrial dysfunction, fibrosis, and senescence have been identified in rodents. In addition, rodent miR-181 downregulation has been identified; this upregulates the NF-κB pathway to increase inflammation. Epigenetic changes worsen inflammation, reduce protection against diabetes, and enhance fibrosis and oxidative stress. The aging process is exacerbated by oxidative stress, elevated advanced glycation end-products, and altered regulatory pathways, including Klotho, mTOR, NF-κB, and autophagy.

DNA methylation of memory-related genes in the hippocampus is part of the normal control of memory and learning. It also crosstalks with histone modification. DNA modification plays a role in memory storage through DNA methyltransferase. Disruptions in DNA methylation, histone protein modifications, chromatin remodeling, and long noncoding RNAs affect gene transcription in the brain. Alterations in DNA methylation are associated with neurodegenerative disorders such as Alzheimer's disease and age-related memory loss (Maity et al., 2021).

MiRNAs miR-125b, miR-145, and miR-155 decrease with CKD progression and, in the rat model, are associated with runt-related transcription factor-2 (RUNX2), angiotensin type II receptor 1, and myocardin, suggesting their role in vascular smooth muscle cell remodeling to an osteoblast phenotype and the formation of medial calcification. RUNX2 is also associated with atherosclerotic plaque. miR-126 is linked to the uremic toxins indoxyl-sulfate and p-cresyl glucuronide, which are increased in CKD models, and is associated with inflammation and endothelial dysfunction. Myofibrillar miR-30 inhibition is involved in cardiomyocyte pathology and occurs after nephrectomy, resulting in the development of ventricular hypertrophy. Urine miRNAs may also be markers for early diabetic nephropathy (Zou, 2023). Although miRNA dysregulation has been associated with tau proteins, amyloid, and synaptic plasticity, it has also been linked to the progression of Alzheimer's disease. However, the miRNAs associated with these neurological disorders have yet to be demonstrated in CKD (Ramakrishna and Muddashetty, 2019). On the other hand, atherosclerosis is associated with CKD through epigenetic mechanisms. Cerebral atherosclerosis results in vascular changes that are also associated with dementia (Wingo et al., 2020).

Loss of proteostasis

Proteomics is addressed elsewhere in this book. Proteostasis pertains to the complex networks that uphold normal protein function within the cell. Regarding health, these networks can detect stress and restore protein equilibrium. As diseases progress and with aging, stressors can surpass attempts to maintain protein balance, leading to protein dysfunction. For a protein to function properly, it must undergo three-dimensional folding. If misfolding happens, mechanisms may engage that allow the protein to be either refolded or directed for degradation. Proteins are synthesized on the ribosome, and folding starts as soon as they are released. Misfolded proteins can associate with chaperone proteins, which, in conjunction with ATP, refold the molecule (Guo et al., 2005). Other chaperones guide defective proteins to the proteasome. If the molecule cannot be refolded, or if there is chaperone depletion, aggregates of proteins can occur. Aggregates can be eliminated through autophagy. Misfolded proteins that are tagged for ubiquitination by proteasomes can also be eliminated from the cell as exosomes. Failure of proteostasis, either at the chaperone, ubiquitin, or autophagosome level, can lead to the accumulation of aggregates that damage the cell. The loss of proteostasis is seen as part of aging, impacting both CKD and dementia. Aging can lead to changes in chaperone type, particularly in the brain. Chaperone mutations can also appear with age. Impaired kidney function disrupts protein balance, which is crucial for brain health. Another age-related defect is the lack of crosstalk or harmony between the various components of the proteostasis network.

Proteasome damage occurs with age, and mutations in the ubiquitin-proteasome system can lead to many disorders, including frontotemporal dementia, amyotrophic lateral sclerosis, and Parkinson's disease. Defects in autophagy are likewise associated with AML, Alzheimer's disease, and Parkinson's disease (Kaushik and Cuervo, 2015). The mitochondrion and endoplasmic reticulum can preserve proteostasis but are vulnerable to the stresses related to aging. Conditions associated with endoplasmic reticulum stress include Alzheimer's disease, Parkinson's disease, metabolic syndrome/diabetes, atherosclerosis, and cardiovascular disease.

Deregulated nutrient sensing

Dysregulated nutrient sensing primarily refers to two kinases: adenosine monophosphate (AMP)-activated protein kinase (AMPK) and the mammalian or mechanistic target of rapamycin (mTOR). AMPK regulates energy homeostasis and is inhibited in the presence of glycogen. It can be activated by starvation, exercise, glycogen depletion, and metformin, switching off anabolic processes to conserve energy. Its downstream actions include increased glucose uptake, beta-oxidation of fatty acids, enhanced mitochondrial respiration, activation of the Forkhead box O transcription factor (FOXO), and increased autophagy. A reduction in

AMPK during excessive feeding may lead to increased cell damage and impaired repair mechanisms. AMPK may protect kidney cells and help maintain podocyte function (Banu et al., 2021). Randomized controlled clinical trials are currently in progress.

mTOR kinases can be inhibited by rapamycin, a medication with origins in the soil of Easter Island. Rapamycin has been used since 1999 to prevent organ transplant rejection. mTOR inhibits autophagy and promotes growth under various conditions. Amino acids, particularly leucine and arginine, activate sensing proteins that inhibit GATOR2, which in turn inhibits GATOR1. This process allows the mTOR complex to be recruited to the lysosomal membrane and become activated.

Skeletal muscle mass decreases with aging. While branched-chain amino acids and resistance exercise can activate mTOR to promote muscle synthesis, a diet rich in protein may be more beneficial for rebuilding and preserving muscle (Kaspy et al., 2024). The activation of mTOR occurs with all food intake, including lipids, fructose, glucose, and proteins. This stimulates the anabolic synthesis of lipids and nucleotides, in addition to proteins. It also inhibits autophagy. Furthermore, it can stimulate macrophage ingestion and promote atherosclerosis. While modulating mTOR is essential for balancing muscle growth and repair, the high energy demands and endoplasmic reticulum stresses that accompany diabetes, genetic mutations such as polycystic kidney disease, and glomerular hypertension lead to mTORC hyperactivation in podocytes and tubular cells, ultimately resulting in progressive kidney disease. Excess dietary intake of proteins, glucose, and lipids leads to the recruitment of lysosomes and activation of mTORC1 in podocytes and tubular cells. In type 1 diabetes, excess causes mTORC1 activity, while in type 2 diabetes, the elevated plasma insulin levels resulting from insulin resistance serve as potent activators. Studies have shown that this increased activity leads to podocyte hypertrophy, foot process effacement, mesangial expansion, and basement membrane thickening.

mTORC1 activity is implicated in various diseases, and maintaining its balance is necessary. In animal models of focal sclerosing glomerulonephritis, treatment with low-dose rapamycin offered a protective effect; however, higher doses resulted in albuminuria and sclerosis (Huynh et al., 2023). mTOR dysfunction is implicated in neurodegenerative disorders. It is involved in brain development and also in synaptic plasticity, which is essential for learning and storing information. It is also implicated in depression and cognitive behavior, as well as in feeding, circadian rhythm, and satiety. Increased mTOR has been associated with increased amyloid deposits and the presence of pathological forms of tau proteins. mTOR inhibition has shown a beneficial effect on clinical findings and behavior in mouse models (Lipton and Sahin, 2014). AMPK is an upstream inhibitor of mTOR and an initiator of autophagy. AMPK activators, such as adiporon, may be beneficial for both brain and kidney health. By stimulating adiponectin, AMPK and peroxisome proliferator-activated receptor alpha (PPARα) are activated. This process inhibits downstream mTORC activation and induces autophagy. Currently, there are no clinical trials for adiporon. So far, AMPK and adiponectin are best increased through caloric restriction and increased exercise. Excess caloric intake reduces adiponectin and AMPK levels and blocks cellular conservation mechanisms, such as autophagy.

Mitochondrial dysfunction

The kidneys are rich in mitochondria and, thus, sensitive to factors that disrupt the orderly process of oxidative phosphorylation. The balance between the generation of reactive oxygen species (ROS) and their dismutation helps keep excess ROS from damaging neighboring molecules. This balance deteriorates with time and, coupled with less efficient mitochondria, promotes cellular senescence, aging, and disease. An excess of ROS can further damage mitochondria, resulting in less ATP production and a further increase in ROS. Increased mitochondrial permeability causes the release of mitochondrial cytochromes, like cytochrome C. These induce inflammation and ultimately result in fibrosis. Oxidative stress is also associated with the overproduction of TGFβ and the imbalance of the renin-angiotensin system (Luo et al., 2015; Srivastava et al., 2023).

Neurons have a high energy demand; functioning mitochondria are essential for neuronal health. ATP powers neurotransmitter release at the synapse and is vital for learning (Devine and Kittler, 2018). With aging, mitochondrial function declines, leading to cognitive impairment (Ho and Shirakawa, 2023; Sorrentino et al., 2018). AMPK directs both the maintenance and genesis of mitochondria and is essential for mitochondrial health (Herzig and Shaw, 2018).

Adiponectin, a beneficial prohormone released by adipocytes, can restore and maintain mitochondrial dynamics and promote the formation of new mitochondria. It is valuable to the kidneys by reducing oxidative stress (Baldelli et al., 2024). Adiponectin levels increase during energy restriction, weight loss, and adherence to the Mediterranean diet, as well as with physical activity. Conversely, a high-fat diet suppresses adiponectin. Targeting mitochondria with adiponectin receptor activators has been shown to clear neurofibrillary tangles and tau proteins produced in the brain. These tangles further complicate the pathogenesis of Alzheimer's disease by obstructing mitochondrial function (McGregor et al., 2025).

Cellular senescence

Cellular senescence encompasses the aging process and occurs when cells can no longer grow or repair themselves in response to stressful insults. The accumulation of senescent cells leads to the pathological consequences of progressive kidney disease and dementia. The cell cycle is blocked by either shortened telomeres or the tumor suppressor gene p16. As the cell cycle withdraws and enters cycle arrest, ribosomes cease protein synthesis. Macromolecular damage occurs alongside dysregulated metabolism, and repair mechanisms fail to function adequately or not at all to mend the damage. The cells secrete bioactive molecules known as the senescence-associated secretory phenotype (SASP), sending a pathological message to neighboring cells and leading to chronic inflammation. Brain cells are particularly vulnerable to factors that lead to senescence, particularly protein aggregate accumulation, viruses, drugs, inflammation, radiation, and mutations. Senescent neurons are related to neurons that express tau pathology and neurofibrillary tangles. These cells have an abundance of inflammatory factors such as gamma interferon (IFN-γ).

CKD is widely recognized as a proinflammatory condition that promotes brain senescence by releasing factors that may impact cognitive function. During the senescence process, apoptosis is inhibited, leading to cell persistence. Senescent cells that accumulate in the aging or damaged kidney continue to secrete SASP, causing inflammation and ultimately affecting the entire organ. The direct role of SASP on distal organs remains unclear (Melo Dos Santos et al., 2024; Regulski, 2017; Rex et al., 2023).

Potential therapeutic approaches to reduce cellular senescence and SASP production include the use of agents like quercetin, metformin, rapamycin, MitoQ, resveratrol, and dasatinib (a medication used to treat chronic myelogenous leukemia). Caloric restriction, exercise, and angiotensin blockers are also potential approaches (Rex et al., 2023; Riessland et al., 2024).

Stem cell exhaustion

Adult stem cells have preserved some of the developmental pathways of embryonic stem cells and help maintain organ homeostasis, aiding in the repair and upkeep of somatic cells. Despite their ability to differentiate and self-renew, they also succumb to the same aging processes as other cells. Over time, they age, and their function declines. Systemic inflammation and environmental toxins can deplete stem cells. The relationships between the hallmarks of aging, including inflammation, oxidative stress, mitochondrial function, DNA damage and telomere shortening, proteostasis, epigenetic alterations, impaired autophagy, and cell senescence, affect stem cell function and may be targeted for intervention to reduce aging (Picerno et al., 2021).

Therapy using stem cell derivatives is being pursued for kidney disease. When administered to diabetic mice with a kidney failure model, extracellular vesicles (EVs) isolated from mesenchymal stem cells reduced renal fibrosis and improved kidney function by modulating the mTOR/autophagy pathway. Although not yet clinically feasible, stem cell therapy holds the potential to help patients with Alzheimer's disease (Liu et al., 2020).

Altered intercellular communication

Cell-to-cell communication is a vital function in health. Intercellular communication in the kidney is facilitated by EVs, which serve as important physiological messengers for other cells. These may be produced in glomerular tufts, proximal tubules, bladder cells, and interstitial cells. In the collecting duct, EVs may be regulated by vasopressin (Oosthuyzen et al., 2016). EVs can transfer proteins and RNA and play a significant role in both homeostasis and the progression of kidney disease. They are classified as microvesicles, exosomes, or apoptotic vesicles. Microvesicles arise from the budding of the cellular membrane, where they are pinched off and sealed. Vesicular bodies first fuse with the membrane and are then released into the extracellular space. Exosomes are vesicles that form inside the cell and are subsequently extruded. Apoptotic bodies form only during programmed cell death. All EVs can play a role in pathological processes.

EV release in hyperglycemia can transfer factors that cause podocyte dysfunction; mesangial cells can release EVs that stimulate p-AKT and TGF-β1. Podocytes injured by hyperglycemia release miR-221, which circulates and may be useful as a biomarker to monitor diabetic nephropathy (Carney, 2016).

Cell communication via exosomes, paracrine secretion, and nanotubules is crucial for brain function and contributes to the pathology of certain brain diseases. Nanotubules facilitate the transport of virions in infectious diseases such as herpes and HIV and aid in the transport of elevated Tau and toxic protein aggregates in neurodegenerative conditions. They are involved in repair, cargo trafficking, and even mitochondrial communication through tunneling nanotubules. These tunneling nanotubules increase during oxidative stress due to the activation of regulatory enzymes like Akt/PI3K/mTOR and are supported by the Wnt/Ca2 + pathway (Khattar et al., 2022).

Dysbiosis

Dysbiosis refers to a microbial imbalance in the gastrointestinal tract. Although microbes are important for digestion, disorders in the microbiome's composition can increase toxins in the bloodstream, causing low-grade inflammation and oxidative stress. The gut contains nearly 70% of the body's immune cells, helping provide a protective effect while enabling mutual coexistence with microbes. Yet, invasion is largely prevented by an intact gut-blood barrier. Uremic toxins both alter the GI tract's microbial composition and disrupt the intestinal epithelial barrier. Aging also disrupts the otherwise intact gut-blood barrier. Increased urea concentrations in rats with a 5/6 nephrectomy showed different bacterial taxa in their gut compared to controls. Serum uremic toxins correlate with Clostridia and Bacteroidia-affiliated species in the gut microbiome (Vaziri et al., 2013).

The modified microbiome increases tryptophan metabolism to indole, which is conjugated to indoxyl sulfate in the liver. Phenylalanine and tyrosine are metabolized to p-cresol, which the liver conjugates to p-cresol sulfate. These molecules are protein-bound and not removed with dialysis. They are associated with endothelial dysfunction, tubulointerstitial fibrosis, glomerulosclerosis, and atherosclerosis (Li et al., 2024). They also activate macrophages, promoting systemic inflammation. Uremic toxins derived from the gut impair cognitive function by affecting hippocampal function (Stadlbauer et al., 2020; Vallianou et al., 2023).

The diet plays an important role in regulating the gut microbiome. A diet rich in fermentable (soluble) fiber increases fecal elimination of protein derivatives by softening stools. Fermentable fiber is converted into short-chain fatty acids, which nourish beneficial gut bacteria. Foods containing fermentable fiber include apples, legumes, onions, and asparagus. Protein and animal products elevate the presence of D-amino acids such as tryptophan, phenylalanine, and tyrosine. Modifying the diet, along with the use of prebiotics, probiotics, and synbiotics, may reduce inflammatory mediators and uremic toxins like p-cresol and indoxyl sulfates (Yang et al., 2018). A systematic review of 82 articles reported positive effects on renal function with the use of probiotics containing the Lactobacillus and Bifidobacterium genera. In the three studies that examined inflammatory markers, C-reactive protein (CRP), TNF-α, interleukin-5 (IL-5), and interleukin-6 (IL-6) decreased, while IL-10 levels rose (Fagundes et al., 2018). In a meta-analysis of 931 hemodialysis patients, prebiotics, probiotics, and synbiotics decreased circulating levels of p-cresyl sulfate, C-reactive protein, and IL-6 compared to placebos (Nguyen et al., 2021).

Trimethylamine is derived from the gut through the bacterial breakdown of betaine, choline, and carnitine, and it is converted in the liver to trimethylamine N-oxide (TMAO), a promoter of oxidative stress and inflammation, particularly cardiac inflammation. Patients with elevated blood levels of TMAO and CKD who are not on dialysis have a higher risk of dying from a cardiac-related event, although the risk is not worsened by dialysis (Li et al., 2023). When TMAO levels are elevated, it is considered a risk factor for CKD, but limited research suggests that prebiotics may reduce the TMAO load. Other potential agents being evaluated include aspirin, finasteride, berberine, and black beans. It has been shown that a high-fat diet promotes TMAO production (Zixin et al., 2022). Although plasma TMAO is not associated with cognitive impairment in patients without CKD, it is a risk factor for dementia (HR 1.73, 95% CI 1.16–2.60) in those with impaired kidney function (Yaqub et al., 2024).

Chronic inflammation

Inflammaging refers to the role of inflammation in the aging process. The inflammation associated with uremia resembles "inflammaging" and can occur both systemically and locally due to (Lin et al., 2019) decreased kidney function and resulting diseases. The kidney is highly vulnerable to damage from inflammatory cytokines. The role of inflammation in causing senescence in the kidney is discussed in further detail elsewhere in this book. In summary, diabetes, diet, kidney diseases, uremia, and dialysis therapy all contribute to inflammation. Inflammation arises from uremic toxins such as indoxyl and cresyl sulfate, along with various other factors, including endoplasmic reticulum stress, oxidative stress, mitochondrial dysfunction, and dysbiosis. Senescent cells release SASP, the senescence-associated secretory phenotype, which consists of cytokines that affect nearby cells. Nonenzymatic glycation linked to diabetes triggers inflammation through NF-κB. Misfolded proteins that remain undegraded form aggregates, signaling cellular stress and inflammation. The protective mechanism of autophagy removes irreparable DNA, damaged and worn-out organelles, and misfolded protein aggregates, but this can decline with age and in CKD. Ubiquitin tags damaged proteins and transports them to a proteasome for degradation (Kooman et al., 2017).

CKD is known to upregulate IL-6, fibrinogen, TNF-α, IL-6, and IL-8 (Kadatane et al., 2023). A systematic review of 79 articles from the medical literature demonstrated increased serum levels of markers, including CRP, IL-6, and TNF-α in Alzheimer's disease. IL-1ß, IL-6, and TNF-α were elevated in patients with minimal cognitive impairment (Leonardo and Fregni, 2023).

Disabled macroautophagy

CKD can impair autophagy, which is critical for clearing damaged cell components in the brain (Lin et al., 2019). Neurons are particularly vulnerable to impaired autophagy. This impairment has been associated with Alzheimer's disease, ALS, and familial Parkinson's disease. Intracellular and extracellular tau aggregates are the result of disordered proteostasis. As discussed above, protein aggregates can be disposed of by chaperone-mediated autophagy. In neurodegenerative diseases, particularly during aging, chaperone-mediated autophagy (CMA) also declines. CMA differs from macroautophagy in that it delivers specific proteins to the lysosome. Macroautophagy involves larger structures and backs up CMA; there is crosstalk between them (Wu et al., 2015). Neurotoxic proteins that result from brain metabolism rely on intact autophagy systems. The combination of increased oxidative stress in later life compromises the networks that incorporate endosomes, lysosomes, and autophagy. Impaired lysosomal function, in addition to decreased and defective autophagy, coupled with an increase in misfolded protein aggregation, are key factors in neurodegeneration. Therapeutic regimens aim to maintain autophagy, preserve lysosomal function, and reduce stressors that compromise proteostasis (Nixon and Rubinsztein, 2024).

Stroke

Strokes are more prevalent in the CKD population; the risk of stroke is 5–30 times higher in patients with CKD (Nayak-Rao and Shenoy, 2017). Mortality from these strokes is also higher, and may reach 40% at one year (Wetmore et al., 2020). Several traditional risk factors can increase the risk of stroke in patients with CKD, including older age, diabetes, heart failure, obesity, dyslipidemia, carotid artery disease, male gender, ethnicity, and a positive family history. While these risk factors can also be found in other patients, there are several mechanisms by which kidney disease itself confers a higher risk of stroke, including accelerated atherosclerosis, vascular calcification (especially if the calcium-phosphorus product exceeds 55), uremic toxins, prothrombotic tendency, and impaired cerebral autoregulation. When comparing patients on maintenance hemodialysis to the general population, hemorrhagic strokes are more common in the South Asian population, while ischemic strokes are more prevalent among the Caucasian population. Patients on hemodialysis are also younger (Toyoda and Ninomiya, 2014).

Strokes can either be ischemic or hemorrhagic. Ischemic strokes can be classified as large vessel, cardioembolic, or small vessel. Atrial fibrillation and carotid disease both increase with advancing CKD. There is an inverse relationship between GFR and carotid total plaque area; patients with advanced CKD have been shown to have larger plaque areas (Porta et al., 2025). Chronic hypertension is a cause of chronic vascular damage and contributes to both stroke and vascular dementia. Atrial fibrillation is a major stroke risk factor in the CKD population.

Proteinuria is independent of blood pressure and can occur with or without diabetes. In several studies composed of 46,638 patients, there were 1479 stroke incidents. The relative risk was 2.65 (95% CI 2.25–3.14) with overt proteinuria and 1.58 (95% CI 1.39–1.80) with microalbuminuria ($p < 0.001$) (Lee et al., 2010).

The high incidence of stroke in CKD can be tied to stages 4 and 5, particularly in the 30-day period before and after commencing dialysis. Hemodialysis patients have a higher incidence. The incidence is higher after the weekend. Transplant patients are also at high risk of having an ischemic stroke (Kelly et al., 2021).

Atrial fibrillation

Atrial fibrillation is one of many etiologies that confer a higher stroke risk to patients with CKD. In CKD stages III to V, the rate of AF is 14.4%. CKD and atrial fibrillation propagate each other, as AF leads to further renal dysfunction mediated hemodynamically, which, in turn, leads to further AF (Gadde et al., 2022). One of the many reasons patients with CKD are more likely to have AF is the increase in inflammation, as evidenced by increases in CRP, IL-6, and fibrinogen (Mihai et al., 2018). Another pathway through which patients with CKD can develop AF is anemia. The mechanisms involved include increases in circulating volume by decreasing afterload and increasing preload due to a reduction in oxygen supply to tissues. Volume overload potentiates the dilation of the left ventricle, which then leads to left ventricular hypertrophy and heart failure. Many patients with CKD also have hypertension, which can lead to LVH. This LVH and HF, in turn, increase end-diastolic pressure, causing enlargement of the left atrium and resulting in increased AF burden.

Hypertension

Hypertension is a well-known risk factor for stroke, and there is strong evidence that controlling blood pressure helps with its prevention. In a list of 19 clinical trials that included

162,341 patients, treatment with RAS blockade lowered stroke risk compared with placebo. Diuretics, beta blockers, and calcium channel blockers did not reach significance when compared with ACEI. More recent trial reviews suggest ARB therapy may be superior to ACEI in reducing stroke risks.

Hypertension is another etiology that may increase the stroke risk in patients with CKD. Hypertension is similar to AF in that elevated blood pressure is both a cause and a result of kidney disease. For every 20/10 mmHg a person's blood pressure is elevated over 115/75 mmHg, the stroke risk is thought to double (Saeed et al., 2009). The evidence is mixed regarding whether hypertension is part of the reason why patients with CKD have a higher stroke risk. The interplay between CKD, hypertension, and stroke was recently studied using a Mendelian randomization analysis. Even when controlling for systolic blood pressure, an independent causal effect existed between CKD and stroke risk, particularly large-artery stroke (Kelly et al., 2023). In a randomized controlled study of CKD stage III patients in China, patients who achieved an SBP of <135 mmHg experienced a lower incidence of total first stroke and ischemic stroke (Li et al., 2018). Therefore the stroke risk conferred by hypertension in the CKD population may depend on the stage of CKD.

Atherosclerotic disease

Atherosclerosis is another well-known risk factor for stroke, described well over 40 years ago. Recently, the risk of stroke due to atherosclerosis has been found to develop in the early stages of CKD and thereafter remains stable (Valdivielso et al., 2019). The NEFRONA study showed that this atherosclerosis increases in magnitude as CKD progresses. A total of 2,455 patients with eGFR < 60 mL/min were enrolled alongside those with normal kidney function. Other factors that increased a patient's risk of atherosclerosis included smoking status and triglyceride level, both of which were independently associated with the presence of plaque and both of which are present in patients with CKD. In more advanced CKD, hyperphosphatemia and hsCRP levels also had a significant association with atherosclerosis (Betriu et al., 2014). In a cohort of 455 patients with a mean eGFR of 68 mL/min, the intima-media thickness was significantly higher in patients with CKD compared to those without. After adjusting for other factors, eGFR was a negative determinant of symptomatic ischemic stroke (Kajitani et al., 2018).

Management considerations

Dementia

A management strategy to reduce cognitive function decline involves early detection of key factors contributing to its causes and, when possible, controlling or alleviating them. Prevention of dementia may entail better blood pressure control, the use of prebiotics, and avoiding a proinflammatory lifestyle by refraining from cigarette smoking, addressing an elevated body mass index (BMI) > 30, and adopting healthy eating habits. If dementia is already present, kidney disease patients may be offered a trial of cholinesterase inhibitors. Donepezil and rivastigmine do not require adjustment in renal patients. However, medications such as memantine are not indicated in dialysis patients. Exercise has been demonstrated to improve cognitive function in clinical trials, although the results are modest (Liu et al., 2022). Besides exercise, patients on dialysis with cognitive impairment may benefit from addressing hearing and visual impairments, strengthening social connections, optimizing diabetes and heart disease management, correcting sleep disorders, quitting smoking, and obtaining social support. Each of these factors contributes to cognitive impairment in patients with CKD on dialysis (Crowe et al., 2021; Liu et al., 2025).

Improvements in cognitive function occur during the second hour of a dialysis session ($p < 0.001$) compared to the predialysis day; it is worse just before treatment (Karakizlis et al., 2021). Although this suggests that dialysis adequacy may also be a factor in cognitive impairment testing concerning timing, the Frequent Hemodialysis Network Daily Trial (FHN) demonstrated no benefit of frequent hemodialysis on cognitive function (Kurella Tamura et al., 2013).

Stroke

Stroke prevention centers around blood pressure control, anticoagulation for atrial fibrillation, and statin therapy. However, in the CKD population, evidence may be insufficient.

Anticoagulation—Although there is an evidence gap, most nephrologists anticoagulate atrial fibrillation patients with direct oral anticoagulants, particularly apixaban. In the general population, anticoagulation reduces the risk of an embolic stroke by 65%. Since CKD patients were excluded, there is a lack of evidence for the use of DOACs. Warfarin did not reduce the risk of stroke or mortality but increased major bleeding when evaluated in dialysis patients, in contrast to nondialysis patients. DOACs have similar benefits in nondialysis patients as warfarin but a lower risk of major bleeding (HR 0.72, 95% CI 0.59–0.87).

Hypertension targets to prevent stroke in CKD patients vary. ARB therapy is recommended, and a target of < 130/80 mmHg is advised for patients with proteinuria or diabetes. Other targets are < 140/90 mmHg. The SPRINT trial demonstrated that intensively treating systolic blood pressure to < 120 mmHg reduced cardiovascular outcomes and mortality in patients with CKD, but the GFR was slightly worse in the intensively treated group. There was no difference in the incidence of stroke between intensively treated patients and those receiving standard treatment, but the study was stopped early (Cheung et al., 2017). The current KDIGO Guideline recommends a target SBP <120 mmHg using standardized office measurement, but it does not specify a diastolic target.

Statin therapy has been recommended for CKD patients. The SHARP trial revealed a 25% reduction in nonhemorrhagic stroke in patients with CKD on cholesterol-lowering therapy.

Carotid intervention has been effective in treating CKD patients not on dialysis with advanced carotid lesions, but outcomes in dialysis patients are poor. Regardless, patients undergoing carotid procedures must undergo a careful perioperative assessment and be closely managed in the postoperative period due to the high risk of procedural complications.

First steps in the management of a stroke in a patient without CKD include the emergent use of intravenous thrombolysis within the first 4.5 h of symptoms. However, older CKD patients are more likely to have a large infarct due to atrial fibrillation, as well as underlying cerebrovascular disease, and may experience reduced therapeutic benefits from the use of intravenous thrombolysis. There is an evidence-gap because clinical trials often excluded CKD patients, and the results of small studies have been conflicting. Other management steps include minimizing the risk of hemodynamic shifts by employing gentle dialysis, avoiding excessive anticoagulation, and preventing excess fluid removal (Kelly et al., 2021).

Stroke prevention centers around blood pressure control, anticoagulation for atrial fibrillation, and statin therapy. However, in the CKD population, evidence may be insufficient.

Anticoagulation—Although there is an evidence gap, most nephrologists anticoagulate atrial fibrillation patients with direct oral anticoagulants, particularly apixaban. In the general population, anticoagulation reduces the risk of an embolic stroke by 65%. Since CKD patients were excluded, there is a lack of evidence for the use of DOACs. Warfarin did not reduce the risk of stroke or mortality but increased major bleeding when evaluated in dialysis patients, in contrast to nondialysis patients. DOACs have similar benefits in nondialysis patients as warfarin but a lower risk of major bleeding (HR 0.72, 95% CI 0.59–0.87).

Hypertension targets to prevent stroke in CKD patients vary. ARB therapy is recommended, and a target of < 130/80 mmHg is advised for patients with proteinuria or diabetes. Other targets are < 140/90 mmHg. The SPRINT trial demonstrated that intensively treating the systolic blood pressure to < 120 mmHg reduced cardiovascular outcomes and mortality in patients with CKD, but the GFR was slightly worse in the group that was intensively treated. There was no difference in the incidence of stroke between intensively treated patients and those receiving standard treatment, but the study was stopped early (Cheung et al., 2017). The current KDIGO Guideline recommends a target SBP <120 mmHg using standardized office measurement, but it does not specify a diastolic target.

Statin therapy has been recommended for CKD patients. The SHARP trial revealed a 25% reduction in nonhemorrhagic stroke among patients on cholesterol-lowering therapy with CKD.

Carotid intervention has been effective in treating CKD patients not on dialysis with advanced carotid lesions, but outcomes in dialysis patients are poor. Regardless, patients undergoing carotid procedures must undergo a careful perioperative assessment and be closely managed in the postoperative period due to the high risk of procedural complications.

First steps in the management of a stroke in a patient without CKD include the emergent use of intravenous thrombolysis within the first 4.5 h of symptoms. However, older CKD patients are more likely to have a large infarct due to atrial fibrillation, as well as underlying cerebrovascular disease, and may experience reduced therapeutic benefits from the use of intravenous thrombolysis. There is an evidence-gap because clinical trials often excluded CKD patients, and the results of small studies have been conflicting.

Other management steps include minimizing the risk of hemodynamic shifts by employing gentle dialysis, avoiding excessive anticoagulation, and preventing excess fluid removal (Kelly et al., 2021).

Conclusion

CKD is a cause of cognitive impairment. Over 80% of hemodialysis patients have some degree of decreased cognitive function. As this disorder progresses, it limits the patient's ability to function and creates risk factors that require specialized management. Established hallmarks that characterize the aging process also play a role in progressive kidney disease. The consequence of this is an increase in stressors and inflammation that interfere with cognitive function.

Cerebrovascular disease is also more common in kidney patients, namely as a result of hypertension, carotid atherosclerosis, or atrial fibrillation.

The identification of patients with cognitive dysfunction requires a comprehensive evaluation, but simple tests can quickly demonstrate its presence. Early detection is valuable, as it can alert caregivers to prepare for the future. Other than the management of the underlying conditions that cause CKD and lifestyle modifications, which include changes in diet and lifestyle, there is currently no therapy or medication shown to reverse or slow progressive dementia in CKD patients, although research projects on medications that can arrest inflammation show promise for the future.

AI disclosure

During the preparation of this work, the author(s) used Grammarly to check grammar. After using this tool/service, the author(s) reviewed and edited the content as needed and take(s) full responsibility for the content of the publication.

References

Alshinnawy, A.S., El-Sayed, W.M., Taha, A.M., Sayed, A.A., Salem, A.M., 2020. Astragalus membranaceus and punica granatum alleviate infertility and kidney dysfunction induced by aging in male rats. Turk. J. Biol. 1303-6092. 44 (4), 166–175. Available from: http://journals.tubitak.gov.tr/biology/issues/biy-20-44-4/biy-44-4-5-2001-5.pdf. doi:10.3906/biy-2001-5.

Aykanat, B., Demircigil, G.C., Buyan, N., Baskin, E., Gulleroglu, K., Fidan, K., Bayrakci, U.S., Dalgic, A., Karakayali, H., Haberal, M., Burgaz, S., 2016. Micronuclei and other nuclear anomalies in buccal epithelial cells of children with chronic kidney disease. Arh Hig Rada Toksikol. 0004-1254. 67 (4), 317–325. Available from: http://www.degruyter.com/view/j/aiht. doi:10.1515/aiht-2016-67-2851.

Baldelli, S., Aiello, G., Mansilla di Martino, E., Campaci, D., Muthanna, F.M.S., Lombardo, M., 2024. The role of adipose tissue and nutrition in the regulation of adiponectin. Nutrients. 2072-6643. 16 (15). Available from: http://www.mdpi.com/journal/nutrients/. doi:10.3390/nu16152436.

Banu, K., Lin, Q., Basgen, J.M., Planoutene, M., Wei, C., Reghuvaran, A.C., Tian, X., Shi, H., Garzon, F., Garzia, A., Chun, N., Cumpelik, A., Santeusanio, A.D., Zhang, W., Das, B., Salem, F., Li, L., Ishibe, S., Cantley, L.G., Kaufman, L., Lemley, K.V., Ni, Z., He, J.C., Murphy, B., Menon, M.C., 2021. AMPK mediates regulation of glomerular volume and podocyte survival. JCI Insight. 2379-3708. 6 (19). Available from: https://insight.jci.org/articles/view/150004/pdf. doi:10.1172/jci.insight.150004.

Bender, A.A., Urbanski, M., Morgan, J.C., Hoge, C., Joseph, J., Damron, K.C., Douglas-Ajayi, C., Rickenbach, F., Jaar, B.G., Sheshadri, A., Plantinga, L.C., 2024. Dementia care among United States dialysis providers: a mixed methods study evaluating clinician comfort and knowledge. Kidney Med. 2590-0595. 6 (10). Available from: https://www.sciencedirect.com/science/journal/25900595. doi:10.1016/j.xkme.2024.100884.

Betriu, A., Martinez-Alonso, M., Arcidiacono, M.V., Cannata-Andia, J., Pascual, J., Valdivielso, J.M., Fernandez, E., 2014. Prevalence of subclinical atheromatosis and associated risk factors in chronic kidney disease: the NEFRONA study. Nephrol. Dial. Transplant. 0931-0509. 29 (7), 1415–1422. doi:10.1093/ndt/gfu038.

Bugnicourt, J.M., Godefroy, O., Chillon, J.M., Choukroun, G., Massy, Z.A., 2013. Cognitive disorders and dementia in CKD: the neglected kidney-brain axis. J. Am. Soc. Nephrol. 1533-3450. 24 (3), 353–363. Available from: http://jasn.asnjournals.org/content/24/3/353.full.pdf+html. doi:10.1681/ASN.2012050536.

Cao, D.W., Han, W.B., He, J.S., Zhao, M., Jiang, C.M., Zhang, Q.Y., Wan, C., Liu, J., Feng, Y., Jin, B., Yang, B., Zhu, D.L., Han, X., 2018. Tea polyphenols delays human glomerular mesangial cells senescence induced by high glucose via regulating STAT3/miR-126/telomere signaling pathway activation. Zhongguo Zhongyao Zazhi.

1001-5302. 43 (23), 4678–4684. Available from: http://zgzye.cbpt.cnki.net/WKE/WebPublication/wkTextContent.aspx?colType=4&yt=2017&tp=gklb.

Cao, Z., Hou, Y., Xu, C., 2023. Leucocyte telomere length, brain volume and risk of dementia: a prospective cohort study. Gen. Psychiatry. 2517-729X. 36 (4), e101120. doi:10.1136/gpsych-2023-101120.

Carney, E.F., 2016. Intercellular communication in the kidney. Nat. Rev. Nephrol. 1759-5061. 12 (6), 314. doi:10.1038/nrneph.2016.50.

Chen, X., Kong, J., Pan, J., Huang, K., Zhou, W., Diao, X., Cai, J., Zheng, J., Yang, X., Xie, W., Yu, H., Li, J., Pei, L., Dong, W., Qin, H., Huang, J., Lin, T., 2021. Kidney damage causally affects the brain cortical structure: a Mendelian randomization study. eBioMedicine. 2352-3964. 72, 103592. doi:10.1016/j.ebiom.2021.103592.

Cheung, A.K., Rahman, M., Reboussin, D.M., Craven, T.E., Greene, T., Kimmel, P.L., Cushman, W.C., Hawfield, A.T., Johnson, K.C., Lewis, C.E., Oparil, S., Rocco, M.V., Sink, K.M., Whelton, P.K., Wright, J.T., Basile, J., Beddhu, S., Bhatt, U., Chang, T.I., Chertow, G.M., Chonchol, M., Freedman, B.I., Haley, W., Ix, J.H., Katz, L.A., Killeen, A.A., Papademetriou, V., Ricardo, A.C., Servilla, K., Wall, B., Wolfgram, D., Yee, J., 2017. Effects of intensive BP control in CKD. J. Am. Soc. Nephrol. 1533-3450. 28 (9), 2812–2823. Available from: http://jasn.asnjournals.org/content/28/9/2812.full.pdf. doi:10.1681/ASN.2017020148.

Corredor, Z., da Silva Filho, M.I., Rodríguez-Ribera, L., Catalano, C., Hemminki, K., Coll, E., Silva, I., Diaz, J.M., Ballarin, J.A., Henández, A., Försti, A., Marcos, R., Pastor, S., 2020. Loci associated with genomic damage levels in chronic kidney disease patients and controls. Mutat. Res. Genet. Toxicol. Environ. Mutagen. 1879-3592. 852. Available from: http://www.elsevier.com/wps/find/journaldescription.cws_home/522820/description#description. doi:10.1016/j.mrgentox.2020.503167.

Crowe, K., Quinn, T.J., Mark, P.B., Findlay, M.D., 2021. Is it removed during dialysis? Cognitive dysfunction in advanced kidney failure-a review article. Front. Neurol. 12, 787370.

Devine, M.J., Kittler, J.T., 2018. Mitochondria at the neuronal presynapse in health and disease. Nat. Rev. Neurosci. 1471-0048. 19 (2), 63–80. Available from: http://www.nature.com/nrn/. doi:10.1038/nrn.2017.170.

Etgen, T., Chonchol, M., Förstl, H., Sander, D., 2012. Chronic kidney disease and cognitive impairment: a systematic review and meta-analysis. Am. J. Nephrol. 0250-8095. 35 (5), 474–482. doi:10.1159/000338135.

Fagundes, R.A.B., Soder, T.F., Grokoski, K.C., Benetti, F., Mendes, R.H., 2018. Probiotics in the treatment of chronic kidney disease: a systematic review. J. Bras. Nefrol. 2175-8239. 40 (3), 278–286. doi:10.1590/2175-8239-JBN-3931.

Fazzini, F., Lamina, C., Raschenberger, J., Schultheiss, U.T., Kotsis, F., Schönherr, S., Weissensteiner, H., Forer, L., Steinbrenner, I., Meiselbach, H., Bärthlein, B., Wanner, C., Eckardt, K.-U., Köttgen, A., Kronenberg, F., Eckardt, K.-U., Meiselbach, H., Schneider, M., Dienemann, T., Prokosch, H.-U., Bärthlein, B., Beck, A., Ganslandt, T., Reis, A., Ekici, A.B., Avendaño, S., Becker-Grosspitsch, D., Alberth-Schmidt, U., Hausknecht, B., Zitzmann, R., Weigel, A., Walz, G., Köttgen, A., Schultheiß, U.T., Kotsis, F., Meder, S., Mitsch, E., Reinhard, U., Floege, J., Schlieper, G., Saritas, T., Ernst, S., Beaujean, N., Schaeffner, E., Baid-Agrawal, S., Theisen, K., Haller, H., Menne, J., Zeier, M., Sommerer, C., Woitke, R., Wolf, G., Busch, M., Fuß, R., Sitter, T., Blank, C., Wanner, C., Krane, V., Börner-Klein, A., Bauer, B., Kronenberg, F., Raschenberger, J., Kollerits, B., Forer, L., Schönherr, S., Weissensteiner, H., Oefner, P., Gronwald, W., Zacharias, H., Schmid, M., Nadal, J., 2020. Results from the German Chronic Kidney Disease (GCKD) study support association of relative telomere length with mortality in a large cohort of patients with moderate chronic kidney disease. Kidney Int. 0085-2538. 98 (2), 488–497. doi:10.1016/j.kint.2020.02.034.

Franco, Á.O., Starosta, R.T., Roriz-Cruz, M., Jan-Mar. 2019. The specific impact of uremic toxins upon cognitive domains: a review. J. Bras. Nefrol. 41 (1), 103–111. Epub 2018 Aug 9. PMID: 30095142; PMCID: PMC6534037. doi:10.1590/2175-8239-JBN-2018-0033.

Gadde, S., Kalluru, R., Cherukuri, S.P., Chikatimalla, R., Dasaradhan, T., Koneti, J., 2022. Atrial fibrillation in chronic kidney disease: an overview. Cureus. 2168-8184. 14 (8). doi:10.7759/cureus.27753.

Guo, W., Shea, J.E., Berry, R.S., Dec. 2005. The physics of the interactions governing folding and association of proteins. Ann. N Y Acad. Sci. 1066, 34–53. PMID: 16533917. doi:10.1196/annals.1363.025.

Gurung, R.L., Dorajoo, R., Yiamunaa, M., Wang, L., Liu, S., Liu, J.J., Shao, Y.M., Chen, Y., Sim, X., Ang, K., Subramaniam, T., Tang, W.E., Sum, C.F., Liu, J.J., Lim, S.C., 2021. Association of leukocyte telomere length with chronic kidney disease in East Asians with type 2 diabetes: a Mendelian randomization study. Clin. Kidney J. 2048-8513. 14 (11), 2371–2376. Available from: http://ckj.oxfordjournals.org/. doi:10.1093/ckj/sfab067.

Herzig, S., Shaw, R.J., 2018. AMPK: guardian of metabolism and mitochondrial homeostasis. Nat. Rev. Mol. Cell Biol. 1471-0080. 19 (2), 121–135. Available from: http://www.nature.com/molcellbio. doi:10.1038/nrm.2017.95.

Hill, C., Duffy, S., Coulter, T., Maxwell, A.P., McKnight, A.J., 2023. Harnessing genomic analysis to explore the role of telomeres in the pathogenesis and progression of diabetic kidney disease. Genes. 2073-4425. 14 (3). Available from: http://www.mdpi.com/journal/genes/. doi:10.3390/genes14030609.

Ho, H.J., Shirakawa, H., 2023. Oxidative stress and mitochondrial dysfunction in chronic kidney disease. Cells 12 (1). Accession Number: 36611880. PMCID: PMC9818928. doi:10.3390/cells12010088.

Huynh, C., Ryu, J., Lee, J., Inoki, A., Inoki, K., 2023. Nutrient-sensing mTORC1 and AMPK pathways in chronic kidney diseases. Nat. Rev. Nephrol. 1759-5061. 19 (2), 102–122. doi:10.1038/s41581-022-00648-y.

Kadatane, S.P., Satariano, M., Massey, M., Mongan, K., Raina, R., 2023. The role of inflammation in CKD. Cells. 2073-4409. 12 (12). Available from: https://www.mdpi.com/journal/cells. doi:10.3390/cells12121581.

Kajitani, N., Uchida, H.A., Suminoe, I., Kakio, Y., Kitagawa, M., Sato, H., Wada, J., 2018. Chronic kidney disease is associated with carotid atherosclerosis and symptomatic ischaemic stroke. J. Int. Med. Res. 1473-2300. 46 (9), 3873–3883. Available from: http://imr.sagepub.com/content/by/year. doi:10.1177/0300060518781619.

Karakizlis, H., Thiele, S., Greene, B., Hoyer, J., 2021. Cognitive performance in dialysis patients—"when is the right time to test?". BMC Nephrol. 1471-2369. 22 (1). doi:10.1186/s12882-021-02333-x.

Kaspy, M.S., Hannaian, S.J., Bell, Z.W., Churchward-Venne, T.A., 2024. The effects of branched-chain amino acids on muscle protein synthesis, muscle protein breakdown and associated molecular signalling responses in humans: an update. Nutr. Res. Rev. 0954-4224. 37 (2), 273–286. doi:10.1017/s0954422423000197.

Kaushik, S., Cuervo, A.M., 2015. Proteostasis and aging. Nat. Med. 1546-170X. 21 (12), 1406–1415. Available from: http://www.nature.com/nm/index.html. doi:10.1038/nm.4001.

Kay, D.W., Henderson, A.S., Scott, R., Wilson, J., Rickwood, D., Grayson, D.A., Nov. 1985. Dementia and depression among the elderly living in the Hobart community: the effect of the diagnostic criteria on the prevalence rates. Psychol. Med. 15 (4), 771–788. PMID: 4080881. doi:10.1017/s0033291700005006.

Kelly, D.M., Ademi, Z., Doehner, W., Lip, G.Y.H., Mark, P., Toyoda, K., Wong, C.X., Sarnak, M., Cheung, M., Herzog, C.A., Johansen, K.L., Reinecke, H., Sood, M.M., 2021. Chronic kidney disease and cerebrovascular disease. Stroke. 0039-2499. 52 (7). doi:10.1161/strokeaha.120.029680.

Kelly, D.M., Georgakis, M.K., Franceschini, N., Blacker, D., Viswanathan, A., Anderson, C.D., 2023. Interplay between chronic kidney disease, hypertension, and stroke: insights from a multivariable mendelian randomization analysis. Neurology. 1526-632X. 101 (20), E1960. Available from: http://www.neurology.org. doi:10.1212/WNL.0000000000207852.

Khattar, K.E., Safi, J., Rodriguez, A.M., Vignais, M.L., 2022. Intercellular communication in the brain through tunneling nanotubes. Cancers. 2072-6694. 14 (5). Available from: https://www.mdpi.com/2072-6694/14/5/1207/pdf. doi:10.3390/cancers14051207.

Koh, S.H., Choi, S.H., Jeong, J.H., Jang, J.W., Park, K.W., Kim, E.J., Kim, H.J., Hong, J.Y., Yoon, S.J., Yoon, B., Kang, J.H., Lee, J.M., Park, H.H., Ha, J., Suh, Y.J., Kang, S., 2020. Telomere shortening reflecting physical aging is associated with cognitive decline and dementia conversion in mild cognitive impairment due to Alzheimer's disease. Aging. 1945-4589. 12 (5), 4407–4423. Available from: https://s3-us-west-1.amazonaws.com/paperchase-aging/pdf/brg6G3nZE6ya7Qoma.pdf. doi:10.18632/aging.102893.

Kolls, B.J., Sapp, S., Rockhold, F.W., Jordan, J.D., Dombrowski, K.E., Fowkes, F.G.R., Mahaffey, K.W., Berger, J.S., Katona, B.G., Blomster, J.I., Norgren, L., Abramson, B.L., Leiva-Pons, J.L., Prieto, J.C., Sokurenko, G., Hiatt, W.R., Jones, W.S., Patel, M.R., 2019. Stroke in patients with peripheral artery disease: insights from the euclid study. Stroke. 1524-4628. 50 (6), 1356–1363. Available from: http://stroke.ahajournals.org/. doi:10.1161/STROKEAHA.118.023534.

Kooman, J.P., Dekker, M.J., Usvyat, L.A., Kotanko, P., van der Sande, F.M., Schalkwijk, C.G., Shiels, P.G., Stenvinkel, P., 2017. Inflammation and premature aging in advanced chronic kidney disease. Am. J. Physiol. Renal Physiol. 1522-1466. 313 (4), F938. Available from: http://ajprenal.physiology.org/content/313/4/F938.full.pdf. doi:10.1152/ajprenal.00256.2017.

Kurella Tamura, M., Unruh, M.L., Nissenson, A.R., Larive, B., Eggers, P.W., Gassman, J., Mehta, R.L., Kliger, A.S., Stokes, J.B., 2013. Effect of more frequent hemodialysis on cognitive function in the frequent hemodialysis network trials. Am. J. Kidney Dis. 1523-6838. 61 (2), 228–237. doi:10.1053/j.ajkd.2012.09.009.

Lee, M., Saver, J.L., Chang, K.H., Ovbiagele, B., 2010. Level of albuminuria and risk of stroke: systematic review and meta-analysis. Cerebrovasc. Dis. 1015-9770. 30 (5), 464–469. doi:10.1159/000317069.

Leonardo, S., Fregni, F., 2023. Association of inflammation and cognition in the elderly: a systematic review and meta-analysis. Front. Aging Neurosci. 1663-4365. 15. doi:10.3389/fnagi.2023.1069439.

Li, X.J., Shan, Q.Y., Wu, X., Miao, H., Zhao, Y.Y., 2024. Gut microbiota regulates oxidative stress and inflammation: a double-edged sword in renal fibrosis. Cell. Mol. Life Sci. 1420-9071. 81 (1). Available from: https://www.springer.com/journal/18. doi:10.1007/s00018-024-05532-5.

Li, Y., Liang, M., Jiang, C., Wang, G., Li, J., Zhang, Y., Fan, F., Sun, N., Cui, Y., He, M., Tang, G., Yin, D., Cheng, X., Wang, B., Huo, Y., Xu, X., Hou, F.F., Xu, X., Qin, X., 2018. Impact of achieved blood pressure on renal function decline and first stroke in hypertensive patients with chronic kidney disease. Nephrol. Dial. Transplant. 1460-2385. 33 (3), 409–417. Available from: http://ndt.oxfordjournals.org/. doi:10.1093/ndt/gfx267.

Li, Y., Lu, H., Guo, J., Zhang, M., Zheng, H., Liu, Y., Liu, W., 2023. Gut microbiota-derived trimethylamine N-oxide is associated with the risk of all-cause and cardiovascular mortality in patients with chronic kidney disease: a systematic review and dose-response meta-analysis. Ann. Med. 55 (1). doi:10.1080/07853890.2023.2215542.

Lin, T.A., Wu, V.C., Wang, C.Y., 2019. Autophagy in chronic kidney diseases. Cells 8 (1). Accession Number: 30654583. PMCID: PMC6357204. doi:10.3390/cells8010061.

Lipton, J.O., Sahin, M., 2014. The neurology of mTOR. Neuron. 1097-4199. 84 (2), 275–291. Available from: http://www.cell.com/neuron/home. doi:10.1016/j.neuron.2014.09.034.

Liu, C.K., Cheung, K.L., Tamura, M.K., 2025. Diagnosis and management of dementia for the nephrology clinician: a review. Am. J. Kidney Dis. 0272-6386. doi:10.1053/j.ajkd.2025.01.007.

Liu, H., Song, Y., Zhao, D., Zhan, M., 2022. Effect of exercise on cognitive impairment in patients undergoing haemodialyses: a systematic review and meta-analysis of randomised controlled trials. J. Ren. Care. 1755-6678. 48 (4), 243–252. doi:10.1111/jorc.12420.

Liu, X., Yang, L., Zhao, L., 2020. Stem cell therapy for Alzheimer's disease. World J. Stem Cells 12 (8), 787–802. doi:10.4252/wjsc.v12.i8.787.

López-Otín, C., Blasco, M.A., Partridge, L., Serrano, M., Kroemer, G., 2023. Hallmarks of aging: an expanding universe. Cell. 1097-4172. 186 (2), 243–278. Available from: https://www.sciencedirect.com/journal/cell. doi:10.1016/j.cell.2022.11.001.

Luo, H., Wang, X., Chen, C., Wang, J., Zou, X., Li, C., Xu, Z., Yang, X., Shi, W., Zeng, C., 2015. Oxidative stress causes imbalance of renal renin angiotensin system (RAS) components and hypertension in obese zucker rats. J. Am. Heart Assoc. 2047-9980. 4 (2). doi:10.1161/jaha.114.001559.

Maity, S., Farrell, K., Navabpour, S., Narayanan, S.N., Jarome, T.J., 2021. Epigenetic mechanisms in memory and cognitive decline associated with aging and Alzheimer's disease. Int. J. Mol. Sci. 1422-0067. 22 (22). Available from: https://www.mdpi.com/1422-0067/22/22/12280/pdf. doi:10.3390/ijms222212280.

McGregor, E.R., Lasky, D.J., Rippentrop, O.J., Clark, J.P., Wright, S., Jones, M.V., Anderson, R.M., 2025. Reversal of neuronal tau pathology via adiponectin receptor activation. Commun. Biol. 2399-3642. 8 (1). Available from: https://www.springer.com/journal/42003. doi:10.1038/s42003-024-07391-z.

Melo dos Santos, L.S., Trombetta-Lima, M., Eggen, B.J.L., Demaria, M., 2024. Cellular senescence in brain aging and neurodegeneration. Ageing Res. Rev. 1568-1637. 93, 102141. doi:10.1016/j.arr.2023.102141.

Mihai, S., Codrici, E., Popescu, I.D., Enciu, A.M., Albulescu, L., Necula, L.G., Mambet, C., Anton, G., Tanase, C., 2018. Inflammation-related mechanisms in chronic kidney disease prediction, progression, and outcome. J. Immunol. Res. 2314-7156. 2018. Available from: http://www.hindawi.com/journals/jir/. doi:10.1155/2018/2180373.

Murray, A.M., Tupper, D.E., Knopman, D.S., Gilbertson, D.T., Pederson, S.L., Li, S., Smith, G.E., Hochhalter, A.K., Collins, A.J., Kane, R.L., 2006. Cognitive impairment in hemodialysis patients is common. Neurology. 0028-3878. 67 (2), 216–223. doi:10.1212/01.wnl.0000225182.15532.40.

Nasreddine, Z.S., Phillips, N.A., Bédirian, V., Charbonneau, S., Whitehead, V., Collin, I., Cummings, J.L., Chertkow, H., 2005. The montreal cognitive assessment, MoCA: a brief screening tool for mild cognitive impairment. J. Am. Geriatr. Soc. 1532-5415. 53 (4), 695–699. Available from: http://onlinelibrary.wiley.com/journal/10.1111/(ISSN)1532-5415. doi:10.1111/j.1532-5415.2005.53221.x.

Nayak-Rao, S., Shenoy, M., 2017. Stroke in patients with chronic kidney disease: how do we approach and manage it? Indian J. Nephrol. 1998-3662. 27 (3), 167–171. Available from: http://www.indianjnephrol.org. doi:10.4103/0971-4065.202405.

Nguyen, T.T., Kim, H.W., Kim, W., 2021. Effects of probiotics, prebiotics, and synbiotics on uremic toxins, inflammation, and oxidative stress in hemodialysis patients: a systematic review and meta-analysis of randomized controlled trials. J Clin. Med. 10 (19), 4456. doi:10.3390/jcm10194456.

Nixon, R.A., Rubinsztein, D.C., 2024. Mechanisms of autophagy–lysosome dysfunction in neurodegenerative diseases. Nat. Rev. Mol. Cell Biol. 1471-0080. 25 (11), 926–946. Available from: https://www.nature.com/molcellbio. doi:10.1038/s41580-024-00757-5.

Oosthuyzen, W., Scullion, K.M., Ivy, J.R., Morrison, E.E., Hunter, R.W., Lewis, P.J.S., O'Duibhir, E., Street, J.M., Caporali, A., Gregory, C.D., Forbes, S.J., Webb, D.J., Bailey, M.A., Dear, J.W., 2016. Vasopressin regulates extracellular vesicle uptake by kidney collecting duct cells. J. Am. Soc. Nephrol. 1533-3450. 27 (11), 3345–3355. Available from: http://jasn.asnjournals.org/content/27/11/3345.full.pdf+html. doi:10.1681/ASN.2015050568.

Picerno, A., Stasi, A., Franzin, R., Curci, C., di Bari, I., Gesualdo, L., Sallustio, F., 2021. Why stem/progenitor cells lose their regenerative potential. World J. Stem Cells. 1948-0210. 13 (11), 1714–1732. doi:10.4252/wjsc.v13.i11.1714.

Porta, D.J., Carrillo, M.N., Pérez, H.A., Rivoira, M.A., Ledesma, G.N., Muñoz, S.E., Aballay, L.R., Armando, L.J., Schelling, J.R., Spence, J.D., García, N.H., 2025. Assessment of total carotid plaque area progression in patients with chronic kidney disease. Good practices for decision-making. J. Nephrol. 1724-6059. 38 (1), 207–214. Available from: https://www.springer.com/journal/40620. doi:10.1007/s40620-024-02146-9.

Ramakrishna, S., Muddashetty, R.S., 2019. Emerging role of microRNAs in dementia. J. Mol. Biol. 1089-8638. 431 (9), 1743–1762. Available from: https://www.journals.elsevier.com/journal-of-molecular-biology. doi:10.1016/j.jmb.2019.01.046.

Regulski, M.J., 2017. Cellular senescence: what, why, and how. Wounds. 1943-2704. 29 (6), 168–174. Available from: http://www.woundsresearch.com.

Rex, N., Melk, A., Schmitt, R., 2023. Cellular senescence and kidney aging. Clin. Sci. (Lond.) 137 (24), 1805–1821. doi:10.1042/CS20230140.

Riessland, M., Ximerakis, M., Jarjour, A.A., Zhang, B., Orr, M.E., 2024. Therapeutic targeting of senescent cells in the CNS. Nat. Rev. Drug Discov. 1474-1784. 23 (11), 817–837. Available from: https://www.nature.com/nrd/. doi:10.1038/s41573-024-01033-z.

Saeed, F., Kousar, N., Qureshi, K., Laurence, T.N., 2009. A review of risk factors for stroke in patients with chronic kidney disease. J. Vasc. Interv. Neurol. 2 (1), 126–131.

Sartori, A.C., Vance, D.E., Slater, L.Z., Crowe, M., 2012. The impact of inflammation on cognitive function in older adults: implications for healthcare practice and research. J. Neurosci. Nurs. 0888-0395. 44 (4), 206–217. doi:10.1097/JNN.0b013e3182527690.

Sorrentino, V., Menzies, K.J., Auwerx, J., 2018. Repairing mitochondrial dysfunction in disease. Annu. Rev. Pharmacol. Toxicol. 58, 353–389. Accession Number: 28961065. doi:10.1146/annurev-pharmtox-010716-104908

Srivastava, A., Tomar, B., Sharma, D., Rath, S.K., 2023. Mitochondrial dysfunction and oxidative stress: role in chronic kidney disease. Life Sci. 0024-3205. 319, 121432. doi:10.1016/j.lfs.2023.121432.

Stadlbauer, V., Engertsberger, L., Komarova, I., Feldbacher, N., Leber, B., Pichler, G., Fink, N., Scarpatetti, M., Schippinger, W., Schmidt, R., Horvath, A., 2020. Dysbiosis, gut barrier dysfunction and inflammation in dementia: a pilot study. BMC Geriatr. 1471-2318. 20 (1). doi:10.1186/s12877-020-01644-2.

Técher, H., Pasero, P., 2021. The replication stress response on a narrow path between genomic instability and inflammation. Front. Cell Dev. Biol. 2296-634X. 9. doi:10.3389/fcell.2021.702584.

Timmermann, C., 2013. Just give me the best quality of life questionnaire': the Karnofsky scale and the history of quality of life measurements in cancer trials. Chronic Illn. 9, 179–190.

Torres, R.V., Elias, M.F., Seliger, S., Davey, A., Robbins, M.A., 2017. Risk for cognitive impairment across 22 measures of cognitive ability in early-stage chronic kidney disease. Nephrol. Dial. Transplant. 1460-2385. 32 (2), 299–306. Available from: http://ndt.oxfordjournals.org/. doi:10.1093/ndt/gfw005.

Toyoda, K., Ninomiya, T., 2014. Stroke and cerebrovascular diseases in patients with chronic kidney disease. Lancet Neurol. 1474-4422. 13 (8), 823–833. doi:10.1016/s1474-4422(14)70026-2.

Valdivielso, J.M., Rodríguez-Puyol, D., Pascual, J., Barrios, C., Bermúdez-López, M., Sánchez-Niño, M.D., Pérez-Fernández, M., Ortiz, A., 2019. Atherosclerosis in chronic kidney disease: more, less, or just different? Arterioscler. Thromb. Vasc. Biol. 1524-4636. 39 (10), 1938–1966. Available from: http://atvb.ahajournals.org/. doi:10.1161/ATVBAHA.119.312705.

Vallianou, N.G., Kounatidis, D., Panagopoulos, F., Evangelopoulos, A., Stamatopoulos, V., Papagiorgos, A., Geladari, E., Dalamaga, M., 2023. Gut Microbiota and its role in the brain-gut-kidney axis in hypertension. Curr. Hypertens. Rep. 1534-3111. 25 (11), 367–376. Available from: https://www.springer.com/journal/11906. doi:10.1007/s11906-023-01263-3.

Vaziri, N.D., Wong, J., Pahl, M., Piceno, Y.M., Yuan, J., Desantis, T.Z., Ni, Z., Nguyen, T.H., Andersen, G.L., 2013. Chronic kidney disease alters intestinal microbial flora. Kidney Int. 1523-1755. 83 (2), 308–315. Available from: https://www.journals.elsevier.com/kidney-international. doi:10.1038/ki.2012.345.

Wetmore, J.B., Herzog, C.A., Sexter, A., Gilbertson, D.T., Liu, J., Kasner, S.E., 2020. Outcomes Following Ischemic Stroke in Older Patients With CKD Stages 4 and 5: A Retrospective Cohort Study. Am J Kidney Dis. 76 (6), 784–793. doi:10.1053/j.ajkd.2020.03.021. Epub 2020 May 28. PMID: 32474166; PMCID: PMC8218249.

Wingo, A.P., Fan, W., Duong, D.M., Gerasimov, E.S., Dammer, E.B., Liu, Y., Harerimana, N.V., White, B., Thambisetty, M., Troncoso, J.C., Kim, N., Schneider, J.A., Hajjar, I.M., Lah, J.J., Bennett, D.A., Seyfried, N.T., Levey, A.I., Wingo, T.S., 2020. Shared proteomic effects of cerebral atherosclerosis and Alzheimer's disease on the human brain. Nat. Neurosci. 1546-1726. 23 (6), 696–700. Available from: http://www.nature.com/neuro/index.html. doi:10.1038/s41593-020-0635-5.

Wu, H., Chen, S., Ammar, A.B., Xu, J., Wu, Q., Pan, K., Zhang, J., Hong, Y., 2015. Crosstalk between macroautophagy and chaperone-mediated autophagy: implications for the treatment of neurological diseases. Mol. Neurobiol. 1559-1182. 52 (3), 1284–1296. Available from: http://www.springer.com/biomed/neuroscience/journal/12035. doi:10.1007/s12035-014-8933-0.

Yang, T., Richards, E.M., Pepine, C.J., Raizada, M.K., 2018. The gut microbiota and the brain-gut-kidney axis in hypertension and chronic kidney disease. Nat. Rev. Nephrol. 1759-507X. 14 (7), 442–456. Available from: http://www.nature.com/nrneph/archive/index.html. doi:10.1038/s41581-018-0018-2.

Yaqub, A., Vojinovic, D., Vernooij, M.W., Slagboom, P.E., Ghanbari, M., Beekman, M., van der Grond, J., Hankemeier, T., van Duijn, C.M., Ikram, M.A., Ahmad, S., 2024. Plasma trimethylamine N-oxide (TMAO): associations with cognition, neuroimaging, and dementia. Alzheimers Res. Ther. 1758-9193. 16 (1), 113. doi:10.1186/s13195-024-01480-1.

Zixin, Y., Lulu, C., Xiangchang, Z., Qing, F., Binjie, Z., Chunyang, L., Tai, R., Dongsheng, O., 2022. TMAO as a potential biomarker and therapeutic target for chronic kidney disease: a review. Front. Pharmacol. 1663-9812. 13. Available from: http://www.frontiersin.org/Pharmacology. doi:10.3389/fphar.2022.929262.

Zou, C., 2023. Advances in the study of miRNAs in chronic kidney disease with cardiovascular complications. Front. Physiol. 1664-042X. 14. doi:10.3389/fphys.2023.1283597.

CHAPTER

24

Cancer and the kidney in an elderly individual

Raad Chowdhury[a] *and Si Yuan Khor*[b]

[a]BWH-MGH Combined Renal Fellowship, Medical Director of Onconephrology, Dana-Farber Cancer Institute, Harvard Medical School, Brigham and Women's Hospital, Boston, MA, United States

[b]Renal Division, Department of Medicine, Brigham and Women's Hospital, Boston, MA, United States

Epidemiology of patients with cancer and kidney disease

Patients with cancer are at an increased risk of developing kidney disease, in particular acute kidney injury (AKI) and chronic kidney disease (CKD). The increased incidence of AKI can be attributed to the effects of cancer itself, cancer therapy, and related complications. A Danish observational study by Christiansen et al., involving a cohort of 1.2 million people with 37,267 individuals diagnosed with incident cancer, found that 27% of patients developed AKI and 7.6% of patients required renal replacement therapy over a 5-year period. The risk of developing AKI was highest in the first year after a cancer diagnosis was made, particularly in the elderly population and those with metastatic disease. The type of malignancy also influences the risk, with the incidence of AKI being higher in patients with kidney cancer, liver cancer, and multiple myeloma (Christiansen et al., 2011). Another Canadian population-based study by Kitchlu et al. found that the rate of AKI was 27 per 1000 person-years in 163,071 cancer patients who initiated systemic therapy, with an overall cumulative incidence of 9.3% (Kitchlu et al., 2019). Risk factors associated with AKI included advanced cancer stage, CKD, diabetes mellitus, and patients aged 66 years or older.

The prevalence of CKD is also widespread in patients with cancer. CKD may preexist in this vulnerable population mainly due to comorbidities such as hypertension and diabetes, which are highly prevalent in the general population with aging, highlighting that both CKD and cancer share some common risk factors. In general, CKD prevalence in the cancer population ranges from 12% to 25% (Rosner et al., 2021). A French study, the Renal Insufficiency

https://doi.org/10.1016/B978-0-443-34069-7.00024-0

and Cancer Medications (IRMA) study, found that the prevalence of CKD was 12% and 19.8%, respectively, using the Modification of Diet in Renal Disease (MDRD) and Cockcroft-Gault (C–G) formulas (Launay-Vacher et al., 2007). An observational study in Romania by Ciorcan et al. found that the prevalence of advanced CKD (stage 4 and 5) was as high as 22.2%. Patients with kidney cancer have the highest prevalence of CKD (50%), followed by malignancy of the urinary tract (33.6%) and pancreatic cancer (19.6%) (Ciorcan et al., 2022). It is also worth noting that cancer has a higher incidence in the elderly population; thus it is unclear whether the association with milder stage CKD is directly related to the cancer or simply due to age-related decreases in GFR.

Kidney disease and cancer

The relationship between kidney disease and cancer is bidirectional. Risk factors for developing kidney disease in cancer patients can be grouped into three main categories, namely patient-specific, disease-specific, and therapy-specific factors. Patient-specific factors include age, baseline renal function, and underlying comorbid diseases. Comorbidities such as pre-existing CKD, diabetes mellitus, congestive heart failure, and liver cirrhosis all predispose individuals to the risk of developing AKI and CKD. In addition, modifiable risk factors such as smoking, poor diet, and obesity, as well as healthcare literacy and environmental and occupational exposures (e.g., pesticides, asbestos, and other pollutants), are all potential shared risk factors for both kidney disease and cancer (Rosner et al., 2021). Disease-specific factors include certain diseases with the tendency to affect the kidneys and how different malignancies can manifest with related kidney diseases. Chronic infections with hepatitis B and C, human immunodeficiency virus, Epstein-Barr virus, cytomegalovirus, and human papillomavirus can cause cancer via their oncogenic effects and, at the same time, can cause kidney disease on their own as well. The severity of AKI is a strong predictor of progression to CKD (Chawla et al., 2011). Patients who have had severe AKI and required renal replacement therapy are at substantial risk of developing CKD. Kidney disease treatment predisposes patients to cancer and vice versa.

Aging, kidney disease and cancer

Aging has been a well-known risk factor for the development of both kidney disease and cancer. It significantly impacts renal function and increases the risk of kidney disease through a combination of structural, functional, and physiological changes. The number of functioning nephrons declines with age, along with increased glomerulosclerosis and age-related vascular changes, ultimately resulting in a reduced glomerular filtration rate even in the absence of overt disease (Glassock and Rule, 2016). The rate of decline may accelerate with the superimposition of age-related diseases such as hypertension, diabetes, and cardiovascular disease. Aging is a major risk factor for CKD, and the elderly are also more prone to AKI due to reduced renal reserve (Denic et al., 2016).

Aging impacts cancer risk via a combination of biological, genetic, and environmental factors. Aging is associated with a decline in DNA repair mechanisms, resulting in an increased risk of mutations in oncogenes and tumor suppressor genes, which disrupt the balance of cellular proliferation that can drive cancer development (López-Otín et al., 2013).

In addition, aging is linked with a decline in immune surveillance and a chronic low-grade inflammatory state, which promotes a pro-oncogenic microenvironment (Franceschi et al., 2018). Key mechanisms, such as epigenetic changes and genomic instability, which are critical to cancer development, also become more prevalent with age.

As individuals age, hematopoietic stem cells face a higher risk of developing mutations in leukemia-associated oncogenes, which can lead to the formation of mutant clones. If these mutant clones expand to a clinically significant size, it can ultimately result in clonal hematopoiesis of indeterminate potential (CHIP). The occurrence of CHIP is rare, affecting less than 1% of individuals under 40 years old. However, its prevalence rises dramatically with age, reaching about 10% by the age of 70 and 20% by the age of 90 (Jaiswal and Ebert, 2019). Interestingly, CHIP has also been described as being linked to poor renal outcomes. Dawoud et al. reported the association between myeloid CHIP and adverse outcomes in CKD, which was hypothesized to be driven by the accumulation of inflammatory cells in the tubulointerstitium, ultimately leading to tubulointerstitial fibrosis, a hallmark of CKD (Dawoud et al., 2022). In addition, Vlasschaert et al. found that CHIP was associated with an increased incidence of AKI, even among the non-CKD population. In particular, mutations TET2 and ASXL1 were associated with a higher risk of AKI (Vlasschaert et al., 2024).

Outcomes

AKI and CKD have been associated with poor outcomes in the cancer population. A single-center ICU study in Brazil showed that cancer patients with severe AKI requiring renal replacement therapy had inferior outcomes, with a mortality rate of 87% compared to patients without AKI, who had a mortality rate of 14% (Libório et al., 2011). In addition, a cross-sectional analysis by MD Anderson Cancer Center involving 3558 patients over 3 months showed that AKI was also associated with a longer duration of hospital stay (2 times) and higher costs (2.1 times) (Salahudeen et al., 2013).

Similar to AKI, cancer patients with CKD are associated with poor survival as well. A few studies have demonstrated an increased risk of mortality (12%–27%) in cancer patients with stage 3 and stage 4 CKD compared to patients without CKD (Na et al., 2011; Launay-Vacher et al., 2007). This might be explained by the limited access to clinical trials, limited options for therapies, and challenges in dosing therapies, which may eventually result in reduced efficacy or toxicity.

How can malignancy affect the kidneys?

Direct tumor infiltration of kidneys

The kidney is the most common extra-hematopoietic organ infiltrated by leukemia and lymphoma, with the incidence reported to be approximately 60% of patients (Richmond et al., 1962). Only about 1% of cases might result in clinically apparent AKI due to the massive degree of infiltration, while in the majority of cases, the infiltration is only found during autopsy. Barcos et al. examined 1206 autopsies in patients with leukemia and found that the prevalence of renal infiltration was the highest in chronic lymphocytic leukemia (63%), followed by acute lymphoblastic leukemia (54%), chronic myeloid leukemia (34%), and acute myeloid leukemia (33%) (Barcos et al., 1987).

The mechanism of AKI from direct infiltration is thought to be due to the compression of renal parenchyma and the disruption of microvasculature and tubules, leading to acute tubular necrosis. Recovery in kidney function is dependent on the treatment of the underlying malignancy, and renal function improvement is fairly drastic after the initiation of chemotherapy, sometimes seen within 2–3 days of chemotherapy (Obrador et al., 1997).

Primary kidney lymphoma is an uncommon disease entity, which constitutes only 0.7% of all extra-nodal lymphomas; this might be partly explained by the lack of significant lymphoid tissue in the kidney itself (Da'as et al., 2001). Although rare, the prognosis is extremely poor.

Urinary tract obstruction

Tumors can cause local compression effects, and such clinical courses are usually more indolent and gradual in nature. Intratubular obstruction can also occur in the setting of tumor lysis syndrome due to the precipitation of uric acid. High-dose methotrexate and intravenous acyclovir also have the potential to cause intratubular crystal formation and subsequent obstruction (Rosner et al., 2021). Malignant urinary tract obstruction is associated with poor outcomes. A case series examined 102 patients with malignant ureteral obstruction and found that two-thirds of the patients (68%) had bilateral obstruction, with a 95% success rate in initial decompression interventions such as percutaneous nephrostomy and ureteral stent placement. However, urinary tract infection and compression of ureteral stents and nephrostomy tubes later occurred in 53% of patients, with a median survival of only seven months (Wong et al., 2007).

Renal cancer and nephrectomy

Renal cell carcinoma (RCC) is the most common primary renal neoplasm, accounting for up to 80%–85%, followed by transitional cell carcinoma (8%) (Znaor et al., 2015). The majority of RCCs are found incidentally on abdominal imaging. Fortunately, the 5-year survival rate has increased tremendously in recent years due to early detection and available curative surgical interventions (Hollingsworth et al., 2006). However, nephrectomy is associated with an elevated risk of AKI, with rates as high as 60%, depending on the individual's preexisting risk factors or underlying CKD (Schmid et al., 2014). Given this, emphasis on preoperative risk assessment and nephron-preserving surgery is highly recommended. Partial nephrectomy has been shown to achieve noninferior oncologic outcomes compared to radical nephrectomy, and with the higher AKI rate observed in radical nephrectomy, partial nephrectomy is recommended with the goal of preserving nephron mass (Kim et al., 2012). Collaboration between surgeons and nephrologists is crucial in preventing the development of AKI or the worsening of CKD in this setting.

Tumor lysis syndrome

Tumor lysis syndrome (TLS) is an oncologic emergency caused by the massive breakdown of cancer cells, leading to the release of intracellular constituents such as potassium, phosphate, and uric acid into the systemic circulation. Uric acid accumulation results in crystallization within the renal tubules, causing tubular obstruction. It also induces renal vasoconstriction, impaired autoregulation, and decreased renal blood flow, ultimately resulting in AKI. TLS can occur either spontaneously or after the initiation of chemotherapy in patients with high-grade lymphomas, acute lymphoblastic leukemia, and cancers with significant tumor burden (Criscuolo et al., 2016). Due to the various associated complications—such as cardiac arrhythmias, acute respiratory failure, seizures, and the need for renal replacement therapy—the reported mortality rate was as high as 70% in patients who experienced these complications (Garimella et al., 2017). Risk stratification for TLS should be carried out prior to the initiation of cytotoxic therapy. Unfortunately, due to the lack of a validated scoring system, clinicians must rely on their own clinical judgment. Oral hydration and the avoidance of nephrotoxic drugs are recommended for low-risk patients. For high-risk patients, intravenous crystalloid fluid hydration is recommended prior to and during chemotherapy. Allopurinol or febuxostat can be used to block the formation of uric acid. For patients with hyperuricemia, rasburicase can be administered to rapidly lower the uric acid level. Although the effect of uric acid lowering is often clinically apparent, evidence and data supporting its utility in promoting AKI recovery are lacking (Alakel et al., 2017; Martens et al., 2020).

Paraneoplastic glomerulopathies

Malignancy can exert an indirect, distant effect on the kidneys via paraneoplastic manifestations. This can present prior to a cancer diagnosis and is associated with both solid and hematological malignancies. Definitive treatment is primarily directed at the underlying cancer driving the pathological process. The most commonly reported glomerulopathy associated with solid tumors is membranous nephropathy. Lefaucheur et al. studied a cohort of 240 patients with membranous nephropathy and found that approximately 10% of patients were diagnosed with cancer at the time of renal biopsy or within a year thereafter (Lefaucheur et al., 2006). Lung and gastric cancers are the malignancies most commonly associated with membranous nephropathy. Specific forms of membranous nephropathy, such as THSD7A-associated membranous nephropathy, have been found to have an association with malignancies (Beck, 2017). Age-appropriate screening for cancer should be strictly implemented in cases of membranous nephropathy. Other glomerulopathies associated with solid malignancies include minimal change disease, IgA nephropathy, and crescentic glomerulonephritis. Minimal change disease has been reported to have an association with Hodgkin lymphoma. In Waldenström macroglobulinemia, common glomerular diseases observed include immunoglobulin AL amyloidosis and cryoglobulinemic glomerulopathies (Uppal et al., 2019).

Paraprotein-mediated kidney diseases

Another interesting intersection between aging, renal disease, and cancer is paraprotein-mediated kidney disease. Monoclonal gammopathy of undetermined significance and CKD both increase with age. B-cell or plasma cell proliferative disorders can manifest as kidney disease via the production of nephrotoxic monoclonal immunoglobulins. Such a condition is termed monoclonal gammopathy of renal significance (MGRS). MGRS encompasses a wide spectrum of kidney diseases due to the deposition of monoclonal proteins in various locations in the kidney, including tubules, glomeruli, interstitium, and vessels. Organized diseases include fibrillary glomerulonephritis, AL amyloidosis, cryoglobulinemic glomerulopathy, and immunotactoid glomerulopathy. Light chain cast nephropathy and proximal tubulopathy belong to another subgroup involving crystal inclusions. On the other hand, MGRS lesions with nonorganized deposits include monoclonal immunoglobulin deposition diseases (MIDD), proliferative glomerulonephritis with monoclonal immunoglobulin deposits (PGNMID), and C3 glomerulopathy. Patients with high suspicion for MGRS require a renal biopsy with expert review of light microscopy, immunofluorescence, electron microscopy, and potentially even mass spectrometry. The next step after diagnosis is determining the clonal cell line responsible for the production of monoclonal immunoglobulins by utilizing monoclonal protein testing and bone marrow biopsy. The treatment is primarily directed at the underlying B-cell or plasma cell clones, with expected improvement in renal outcomes if the clones are eradicated (Gumber et al., 2018).

Cancer screening in ESKD

Introduction

The overall incidence of cancer is higher in patients with end-stage kidney disease (ESKD) compared to the general population. Cancer screening in the general population is based on the proposition that early detection of cancer in a precancerous or early stage, with subsequent early treatment, results in improved outcomes and survival. However, the cancer screening recommendations for the general population are not generalizable or applicable to the ESKD population, especially those on maintenance dialysis, due to differences in life expectancy, inaccuracy of screening tests, efficacy of therapy, and increased risks associated with treatment. In this section, we will discuss the prevalence and risk factors for cancer in the ESKD population, the accuracy of cancer screening tests, and specific groups of patients who may benefit from cancer screening.

Cancer risk in patients with ESKD

It is well established that patients with ESKD are associated with an increased risk of various malignancies, especially those on maintenance dialysis (Stengel, 2010). A cohort study by Lin et al. in Taiwan showed that patients on dialysis were associated with an increased risk for all malignancies, with a hazard ratio of 3.43 (Lin et al., 2015). Another retrospective cohort study in the United States found that dialysis patients had an increased 5-year cumulative incidence of 9.48% for any cancer, compared to 4.4% in renal transplant patients. In this study, out of all malignancies, kidney cancer was the highest, with a standardized incidence rate of 4.03 (Butler et al., 2015). The higher incidence of cancer observed in this population may be due to an immunocompromised state, chronic infections, a proinflammatory state, nutritional deficiencies, and altered DNA repair (Maisonneuve et al., 1999).

Accuracy of cancer screening tests

The accuracy of cancer screening tests remains questionable when applied to the ESKD population on maintenance dialysis. Unlike in the general population, the sensitivity and specificity of cancer screening tests cannot be directly extrapolated to the ESKD population. Due to their high molecular weight, tumor markers can be elevated as they are not removed effectively via hemodialysis, thus limiting their role as cancer screening or monitoring tools (Odagiri et al., 1991). Total Prostate-Specific Antigen (PSA), which is the sum of complex and free PSA, is commonly used to screen for prostate cancer. However, free PSA levels will be elevated and are not as valuable as a tool for screening in dialysis patients (Bruun et al., 2003). Cancer antigen 125 (CA-125) can be falsely elevated in patients on peritoneal dialysis due to peritoneal irrigation or peritonitis (Bastani and Chu, 1995). On the other hand, α-fetoprotein and β-human chorionic gonadotropin are valid tumor markers in the dialysis population. The high positive rate of fecal occult blood tests is confounded by several factors, including a higher rate of subclinical mucosal bleeding due to uremic platelet dysfunction and anticoagulant use. Mammograms should be interpreted with caution due to the higher incidence of benign breast tissue microcalcifications in dialysis patients (Evans et al., 1992).

Approach to cancer screening in the ESKD population

Previous studies suggested that although cancer screening is generally not effective in the ESKD population, certain subgroups of patients may still benefit from cancer screening, particularly populations with increased cancer risk and patients with longer-than-expected life expectancy. Rather than using a "one-size-fits-all" approach, emphasis on individualization is of utmost importance due to the heterogeneity of this population. The ultimate decision relies on answers to several important questions, including: (1) estimation of life expectancy, (2) risk stratification for cancer, (3) weighing potential benefits and related harm, (4) considering patient preferences and values, and (5) transplant candidacy (Rosner, 2020). Life expectancy is one of the most crucial factors to consider, in part due to the lag time that precedes the observation of benefits. There are no validated tools to assess the 10-year survival for patients on maintenance dialysis. Several risk factors are associated with poor prognosis: age 75 years or older, high comorbidity score (Charlson Comorbidity Index), poor functional status, and poor nutritional status (Cohen et al., 2010). Age-appropriate cancer screening would benefit those with longer life expectancy and good functional status. Patients who are active on the transplant waiting list should undergo cancer screening similar to the general population, with the ultimate goal of achieving successful outcomes following transplantation rather than directly decreasing the risk of mortality from cancers. Patients who are at high risk of developing cancer may benefit from cancer screening. These include patients with acquired cystic kidney disease, a history of high-dose cyclophosphamide exposure, and those with a genetic predisposition to cancer. Acquired cystic kidney disease predisposes individuals to the development of renal cell carcinoma, typically seen in 2%–7% of these patients (Fick and Gabow, 1994). Exposure to high-dose cyclophosphamide is associated with a higher risk of developing bladder cancer. Patients with genetic syndromes such as Von Hippel-Lindau syndrome, Wiskott-Aldrich syndrome, and Denys-Drash syndrome require regular protocolized cancer screening due to their high risk of cancer development.

Lastly, patients' preferences and a shared decision-making model should be applied in every roadmap for determining cancer screening interventions.

Renal replacement therapy (RRT) in cancer patients

Although there is interindividual variability and factors involved, including age, functional capacity, and comorbidities, the survival rate of patients on maintenance renal replacement therapy remains poor, with a reported 5-year survival rate of 46.9% (Wachterman et al., 2013). Besides, it is well known that with the initiation of dialysis, individuals experience a sudden decline in functional status and quality of life, especially in the elderly population (Tamura et al., 2009). The mortality rate is highest during the first year after patients with ESKD are initiated on maintenance renal replacement therapy, reaching up to 25%, with the risk of death peaking in the first 90 days, estimated to be over 40 deaths per 100 patient-years (Wingard et al., 2009). The outcomes are even more dismal for patients affected by malignancy. In the French Renal Epidemiology and Information Network (FREIN) study, it was found that dialysis patients with active malignancy had higher odds of mortality at 6 months (Couchoud et al., 2009). Metastatic disease predicts survival of less than 1 year in patients with ESKD (Scherer and Swidler, 2014).

Despite the poor outcomes associated with dialysis, decision-making regarding the initiation and termination of renal replacement therapy in patients with cancer is often not as straightforward as it seems; it can be an extremely complex and daunting experience for both the patient/family as well as healthcare providers, partly due to the sparsity of clinical data in the literature, as this specific population is not well represented in clinical trials. Collaboration between nephrologists, oncologists, and geriatricians is imperative in the decision-making roadmap, utilizing several available prognostication tools so that an informed decision can be made. A systematic approach includes disease prognostication, discussing available treatment options, effectively communicating overall prognosis and illness trajectory, while weighing the patient's preferences, specific goals, and values. An individualized treatment strategy and shared decision-making are crucial in achieving an informed decision.

The Eastern Cooperative Oncology Group (ECOG) and Karnofsky Performance Scale (KPS) are two validated clinical tools commonly utilized by oncologists to determine if a patient is a candidate for cytotoxic cancer treatment. Patients with KPS < 50 and ECOG ≥ 2 are generally poor candidates for aggressive cancer therapies. On the other hand, the Charlston Comorbidity Index (CCI) is often used in the nephrology literature to predict 1-year survival for ESKD patients at the initiation of dialysis. Metastatic solid tumor carries the highest weightage in CCI scoring system. However, it is important to note that CCI was derived >40 years ago and may have limited utility now due to the improvement in therapies over the years (Latcha, 2019). Due to the lack of validated tools to prognosticate a patient's tolerance for renal replacement therapy, patients who are precluded from cancer treatments based on KPS and ECOG, with no foreseeable improvement in functional status, will most likely be poor candidates for renal replacement therapy. Elderly cancer patients with kidney disease are often complicated by multiple comorbidities and geriatric syndromes, which confer a risk for poor outcomes with dialysis (Scherer and Swidler, 2014). The Comprehensive

Geriatric Assessment (CGA) is a multidimensional method used in geriatric oncology to prognosticate older patients. Frailty is associated with increased mortality in cancer and dialysis patients. Johansen et al. reported that incident dialysis patients who met frailty criteria had an increased hazard ratio of 2.24 for death within one year (Johansen et al., 2007). Another study found that frailty was associated with an increased risk of death in elderly patients with breast cancer receiving chemotherapy (Aaldriks et al., 2013). All in all, it is important to assess patients by utilizing available prognostic tools from oncology, nephrology, and a geriatric perspective to determine a patient's candidacy for renal replacement therapy.

Expected quality of life (QOL) is a critical component in decision-making for RRT initiation. Although dialysis can be lifesaving, it can also be viewed as a life-prolonging intervention that worsens quality of life while increasing the burden of care (Sprangers et al., 2021). However, perception of QOL differs from individual to individual. Certain patients are willing to endure the discomfort of going through RRT as long as it prolongs their life expectancy to reach a personal milestone or experience important life events (e.g., the birth of a grandchild, attending the wedding of a loved one). On the other hand, for patients with an unclear prognosis and potentially reversible AKI, a time-limited trial of dialysis can be offered with clearly defined personal goals and clinical objectives.

For patients who are poor candidates for RRT, palliative care should be involved early in the discussion of treatment strategy to guide conservative kidney management. A randomized controlled trial by Temel et al. found that early palliative care led to improvements in quality of life and mood among patients with metastatic non-small cell lung cancer. In addition, the median survival was longer among those patients compared to patients who received aggressive end-of-life care (Temel et al., 2010). Nondialysis medical therapy (NDMT) is an alternative approach to dialysis and may be better suited to help patients achieve their goals of care in parallel with palliative care; this involves advance care planning, symptom management, psychosocial support, and hospice referral when prognosis is <6 months (Scherer and Swidler, 2014).

Kidney transplantation and cancer

Introduction

The first kidney transplantation was successfully performed at Peter Bent Brigham Hospital in Boston, Massachusetts, in 1954. Since then, kidney transplantation has undergone tremendous development and revolutionized the landscape of therapies for patients with kidney diseases. It has now become the most effective treatment for advanced kidney diseases, with more than 25,000 kidney transplants performed annually in the United States since 2022 (Network, 2025). Despite this, cancer is the leading cause of morbidity and mortality in kidney transplant recipients, especially with better long-term immunosuppressive therapy to prevent transplant rejection, resulting in longer life expectancy in this population (Howard et al., 2002). Compared with the general population, kidney transplant recipients are at a 2- to 4-fold greater risk of developing malignancies (Engels et al., 2011). In addition, with advancements in cancer therapies, there is an increasing number of cancer survivors who later develop kidney diseases during their lifespan, requiring kidney transplantation. Furthermore, there are variable approaches to managing kidney transplant patients who develop cancer and require immune checkpoint inhibitors, as the risk of rejection is high (Murakami et al., 2021). This specific population is at particular risk of developing posttransplant malignancies (Acuna et al., 2016). In this section, we will discuss kidney transplant wait times for patients with a history of malignancies, immunosuppression and cancer risk post-transplant, and recommendations on cancer screening after kidney transplantation.

Kidney transplant wait times for patients with malignancies

The ideal timing for renal transplantation for patients with a history of cancer is debatable. Most clinical practice guidelines recommend a waiting time of 2–5 years from the time of complete remission from cancer to transplantation, primarily determined by the cancer's location and initial stage of the disease (Acuna et al., 2018). The American Society of Transplantation released a report of recommended guidelines in 2021, based on expert opinion consensus, with the goal of aiding transplant providers in determining the candidacy and timing of transplantation for patients with a history of cancer. Several caveats should be considered when interpreting the recommended guidelines: (1) Cancer outcomes are based on the general population due to the sparsity of data in the transplant population, and (2) The evidence underpinning the recommendations is not graded, as it was based on a consensus report from expert opinions. In this report, tumor, node, and metastasis (TNM) staging, tumor markers, and epigenetics are used to risk-stratify different types of cancers. The recommended wait times are based on a benchmark of a 5-year cancer survival rate of 80% or more. Proposed pretransplant wait times vary from no wait time to 2 years for low-grade diseases and up to 5 years for high-grade diseases (Al-Adra et al., 2021b; Al-Adra et al., 2021a). Aging is a critical factor in this context, as older patients may have reduced life expectancy and increased comorbidities, which could influence the risk-benefit analysis of transplantation. In addition, aging is associated with a higher risk of cancer recurrence and poorer outcomes, further complicating the timing of transplantation in this population (Table 24.1).

Immunosuppression and cancer risk posttransplantation

Immunosuppression remains one of the major risk factors for cancer in patients who have undergone transplantation. There are different mechanisms through which immunosuppression can predispose individuals to the risk of developing cancers: (1) decreased immune surveillance, (2) impaired defense mechanisms against oncogenic viruses, and (3) drug-specific pathways (Kasiske et al., 2004). The overall level of immunosuppression appears to be the principal factor that increases the risk of posttransplant cancer. This was highlighted by the multicenter study by Opelz et al., who found that the incidence of posttransplant lymphoproliferative disorder (PTLD) was the highest in the first year posttransplant, which is the period of most intense immunosuppression. Furthermore, the incidence of PTLD was found to be significantly higher in heart transplant recipients compared to kidney transplant recipients, explained by the greater degree of immunosuppression (Opelz and Henderson,

TABLE 24.1 Recommended wait times for transplantation.

Cancer type	Cancer stages/groups/features/risks	Recommended wait times
Breast	Ductal carcinoma in situ Stage 1	None
	Stage 2	1–2 years
	Stage 3	3–5 years
	Stage 4 Inflammatory type	Not recommended for transplantation
Colorectal	Stage 1	1 year
	Stage 2 T3 T4	2 years 3–5 years
	Stage 3	5 years
	Stage 4 (special consideration) With liver metastasis in the absence of extra-hepatic involvement	5 years
Prostate	Localized disease	None
	High-volume intermediate-risk and high-risk diseases PSA > 20 ng/mL, high-volume Gleason 7, or any Gleason > 7, T3	None Treatment is recommended prior to transplant.
	Metastatic castration-sensitive	2 years
	Metastatic castration-resistant	Not recommended for transplantation
Renal cell carcinoma	Stage 1 T1a T1b with Fuhrman grade 1–2 T1b with Fuhrman grade 3–4 T2, T3, T4	None None 1–2 years Minimum of 2 years
	Nodal or metastatic diseases	Not recommended for transplantation
Gynecologic	Low risk diseases	None
	Intermediate risk diseases	2-3 years
	High risk diseases	5 years
	Very high risk diseases	Not recommended for transplantation
Non-small cell lung cancer	Stage < 1b	3 years
	Stage 1b-3a	Minimum of 5 years
	Beyond stage 3a	Not recommended for transplantation

1993). In the next section, we will briefly discuss the commonly used transplant immunosuppressive therapies and the cancers associated with transplantation.

Immunosuppressive therapies in transplant

Calcineurin inhibitors, such as tacrolimus and cyclosporine, are the cornerstone of immunosuppressive therapy in kidney transplantation and are known to promote carcinogenesis via upregulation of cytokines such as transforming growth factor (TGF)-beta, vascular endothelial growth factor (VEGF), and IL-6, as well as impaired DNA repair mechanisms, especially with high-dose use (Kasiske et al., 2004). Mycophenolate use is associated with a decreased incidence of posttransplant malignancy (Robson et al., 2005). Azathioprine has been implicated in the development of posttransplant malignancy, in particular, cutaneous squamous cell carcinoma (Buell et al., 2005). Mammalian target of rapamycin (mTOR) inhibitors, such as sirolimus and everolimus, have a direct antitumor effect by inhibiting the mTOR pathway and decreasing VEGF signaling. Knoll et al. found that sirolimus was associated with a 40% reduction in the risk of malignancy and a 56% reduction in the risk of nonmelanoma skin cancer compared to controls in kidney and combined pancreatic-renal transplant recipients (Knoll et al., 2014). Belatacept increases the risk of EBV-associated PTLD and should not be used in patients who are EBV-seronegative and received a transplant from an EBV-seropositive donor (Vincenti et al., 2010).

Skin cancer

The most common cancer in kidney transplant recipients is skin cancer. Garrett et al. reported that approximately 8% of transplant recipients are affected by skin cancer, with squamous cell carcinoma being the most common type (Garrett et al., 2017). Compared to the general population, cutaneous squamous cell carcinoma occurs 250 times more frequently in transplant recipients. Pathogenesis involves the interplay of multiple risk factors (old age, race, UV radiation exposure, and history of skin cancer), aggravated by immunosuppressive therapy, which promotes carcinogenic processes. Kidney transplant recipients should be educated on the risk of developing skin cancer, as well as preventative strategies, which include minimizing sun exposure, using sunscreen, and undergoing annual skin examinations by dermatologists. Definitive therapy for cutaneous squamous cell carcinoma is Mohs microscopic surgery, with cure rates of 95%–100% (Mittal and Colegio, 2017). However, systemic chemotherapy and/or immunotherapy is recommended for metastatic disease. Kidney transplant recipients have a five to eight times higher risk of developing melanoma compared to the general population. Melanoma has the worst prognosis and highest mortality among all types of skin cancers (Robbins et al., 2015). Treatment involves wide local excision based on Breslow depth. For disease without complete surgical resection and advanced stages, immune checkpoint inhibitors and/or targeted combination therapy are recommended for patients with BRAF mutations. Patients treated with calcineurin inhibitors are predisposed to the risk of developing Kaposi sarcoma. The mainstay of therapy involves immunosuppression reduction and switching from calcineurin inhibitors to mTOR inhibitors (Al-Adra et al., 2022).

PTLD

PTLD is a well-recognized complication of chronic immunosuppression in kidney transplant recipients. It comprises a spectrum of lymphoproliferative disorders that range from low-grade polyclonal lymphoid proliferations to aggressive monomorphic clonal lesions. The prevalence of PTLD in kidney transplant recipients is around 0.8%–2.5%, with the majority occurring in the first year posttransplant (Opelz and Döhler, 2004). The incidence of PTLD follows a bimodal curve, with an initial peak during the first year of transplant and a second peak occurring 5–15 years posttransplantation (Morton et al., 2013). Risk factors for PTLD include the intensity of immunosuppression, duration of maintenance therapy, use of lymphocyte-depleting agents, transplantation involving an EBV-seropositive donor and an EBV-seronegative recipient, and pretransplant malignancy. PTLD has a heterogeneous clinical presentation, ranging from nonspecific constitutional symptoms to organ failure. Most PTLD patients present with extra-nodal masses and involvement of organs, including the gastrointestinal tract, lungs, skin, liver, central nervous system, and the allograft itself (Nalesnik et al., 1988). Most cases of PTLD are caused by EBV-positive B cell proliferation. In the setting of immunosuppression, T cell immunity wanes, rendering it unable to eliminate the infected B cells. This subsequently leads to the outgrowth of EBV-positive B cell proliferation, giving rise to the development of PTLD. On the other hand, EBV-negative PTLD is observed in up to 30% of PTLD cases, though its exact etiology has not been elucidated (Leblond et al., 1998). PTLD is categorized based on the WHO 2017 Classification of Tumors of Hematopoietic and Lymphoid Tissues into four subclasses: nondestructive PTLD (plasmacytic hyperplasia, infectious mononucleosis, florid follicular hyperplasia), polymorphic PTLD, monomorphic PTLD, and classic Hodgkin lymphoma PTLD. Management of PTLD largely depends on the type of PTLD. The main goals of treatment are the eradication of PTLD and the preservation of graft function. The cornerstone of therapy is a reduction in immunosuppression, with a response rate of 30%–40%, though this predisposes patients to the risk of acute rejection (Reshef et al., 2011). Unfortunately, there are no randomized trials to guide the optimal reduction of immunosuppression. Reducing calcineurin inhibitors or discontinuing antimetabolites are common initial approaches. Rituximab is the next line of therapy after the reduction of immunosuppression, but it is only effective for PTLD that expresses CD20. This can be administered in combination with chemotherapy, either concurrently or sequentially. The prognosis for PTLD varies depending on the type and extent of the disease. Outcomes have improved with the use of rituximab and newer therapies compared to historical data. The PTLD-1 trial by Trappe et al. reported a complete remission rate of 70%, with a median overall survival of 6.6 years (Trappe et al., 2017).

Cancer screening posttransplantation

Kidney transplant recipients are three times more likely to develop malignancy than the general population. Thus cancer screening is an integral part of the care for this specific population (Vajdic et al., 2006). In general, kidney transplant recipients follow the same routine age-appropriate cancer screenings as the general population. This applies to screening for breast, colon, cervical, and lung cancer. Due to the increased incidence of skin cancer in kidney transplant recipients, an annual total body skin examination is recommended to be performed by dermatologists or expert physicians. Routine screening for renal cell carcinoma (RCC) is not recommended except in high-risk individuals (history of acquired cystic disease, history of RCC, heavy smoking, chronic analgesia use), in which screening with ultrasound every 1–2 years is suggested (Wong et al., 2011).

Conclusion

This chapter highlights how aging serves as a critical link between cancer and kidney disease, creating a complex interplay that significantly impacts patient outcomes. As individuals age, the risk of both cancer and kidney disease increases. It also becomes imperative to screen for certain cancers in elderly patients with ESKD. This adds an additional layer of complexity and challenge to the decision-making process and treatment management when caring for these groups of patients, underscoring the need for a tailored and individualized approach. Overall, a multidisciplinary approach is essential for optimizing care and improving outcomes in this vulnerable population.

References

Aaldriks, A.A., Giltay, E.J., le Cessie, S., van der Geest, L.G.M., Portielje, J.E.A., Tanis, B.C., Nortier, J.W.R., Maartense, E., 2013. Prognostic value of geriatric assessment in older patients with advanced breast cancer receiving chemotherapy. Breast. 09609776. 22 (5), 753–760. doi:10.1016/j.breast.2013.01.011.

Acuna, S.A., Fernandes, K.A., Daly, C., Hicks, L.K., Sutradhar, R., Kim, S.J., Baxter, N.N., 2016. Cancer mortality among recipients of solid-organ transplantation in Ontario, Canada. JAMA Oncol. 23742445. 2 (4), 463–469. Available from: http://oncology.jamanetwork.com/journal.aspx. doi:10.1001/jamaoncol.2015.5137.

Acuna, S.A., Lam, W., Daly, C., Kim, S.J., Baxter, N.N., 2018. Cancer evaluation in the assessment of solid organ transplant candidates: a systematic review of clinical practice guidelines. Transplant. Rev. 15579816. 32 (1), 29–35. Available from: http://www.elsevier.com/inca/publications/store/6/2/3/2/0/1/index.htt. doi:10.1016/j.trre.2017.10.002.

Al-Adra, D., Al-Qaoud, T., Fowler, K., Wong, G., 2022. De novo malignancies after kidney transplantation. Clin. J. Am. Soc. Nephrol. 1555-9041. 17 (3), 434–443. doi:10.2215/cjn.14570920.

Al-Adra, D.P., Hammel, L., Roberts, J., et al., 2021a, Preexisting melanoma and hematological malignancies, prognosis, and timing to solid organ transplantation: A consensus expert opinion statement. Am. J. Transplant. 21 (2), 475-483. doi:10.1111/ajt.16324.

Al-Adra, D.P., Hammel, L., Roberts, J., et al., 2021b. Pretransplant solid organ malignancy and organ transplant candidacy: A consensus expert opinion statement Am. J. Transplant. 21 (2), 460-474. doi:10.1111/ajt.16318.

Alakel, N., Middeke, J.M., Schetelig, J., Bornhäuser, M., 2017. Prevention and treatment of tumor lysis syndrome, and the efficacy and role of rasburicase. OncoTargets Ther. 11786930. 10, 597–605. Available from: https://www.dovepress.com/getfile.php?fileID=34722. doi:10.2147/OTT.S103864.

Barcos, M., Lane, W., Gomez, G.A., Han, T., Freeman, A., Preisler, H., Henderson, E., 1987. An autopsy study of 1206 acute and chronic leukemias (1958 to 1982). Cancer. 10970142. 60 (4), 827–837. doi:10.1002/1097-0142(19870815)60:4<827: :AID-CNCR2820600419>3.0.CO;2-A.

Bastani, B., Chu, N., 1995. Serum CA-125 level in end-stage renal disease patients maintained on chronic peritoneal dialysis or hemodialysis: the effect of continuous presence of peritoneal fluid, peritonitis, and peritoneal catheter implantation. Am. J. Nephrol. 1421-9670. 15 (6), 468–472. doi:10.1159/000168888.

Beck, L.H., 2017. PLA2R and THSD7A: disparate paths to the same disease? J. Am. Soc. Nephrol. 15333450. 28 (9), 2579–2589. Available from: http://jasn.asnjournals.org/content/28/9/2579.full.pdf. doi:10.1681/ASN.2017020178.

Bruun, L., Björk, T., Lilja, H., Becker, C., Gustafsson, O., Christensson, A., 2003. Percent-free prostate specific antigen is elevated in men on haemodialysis or peritoneal dialysis treatment. Nephrol. Dial. Transplant. 09310509. 18 (3), 598–602. Available from: http://ndt.oxfordjournals.org/. doi:10.1093/ndt/18.3.598.

Buell, J.F., Gross, T.G., Woodle, E.S., 2005. Malignancy after transplantation. Transplantation 80 (2 Suppl), 254–264. doi:10.1097/01.tp.0000186382.81130.ba.

Butler, A.M., Olshan, A.F., Kshirsagar, A.V., Edwards, J.K., Nielsen, M.E., Wheeler, S.B., Brookhart, M.A., 2015. Cancer incidence among US Medicare ESRD patients receiving hemodialysis, 1996-2009. Am. J. Kidney Dis. 15236838. 65 (5), 763–772. Available from: http://www.elsevier.com/inca/publications/store/6/2/3/2/7/6/index.htt. doi:10.1053/j.ajkd.2014.12.013.

Chawla, L.S., Amdur, R.L., Amodeo, S., Kimmel, P.L., Palant, C.E., 2011. The severity of acute kidney injury predicts progression to chronic kidney disease. Kidney Int. 15231755. 79 (12), 1361–1369. Available from: https://www.journals.elsevier.com/kidney-international. doi:10.1038/ki.2011.42.

Christiansen, C.F., Johansen, M.B., Langeberg, W.J., Fryzek, J.P., Sørensen, H.T., 2011. Incidence of acute kidney injury in cancer patients: a Danish population-based cohort study. Eur. J. Intern. Med. 18790828. 22 (4), 399–406. doi:10.1016/j.ejim.2011.05.005.

Ciorcan, M., Chisavu, L., Mihaescu, A., Gadalean, F., Bob, F.R., Negru, S., Schiller, O.M., Grosu, I.D., Marc, L., Chisavu, F., Pascota, R.D., Apostol, A., Ivan, V., Schiller, A., 2022. Chronic kidney disease in cancer patients, the analysis of a large oncology database from Eastern Europe. PLoS One. 19326203. 17 (6). Available from: https://journals.plos.org/plosone/article/file?id=10.1371/journal.pone.0265930&type=printable. doi:10.1371/journal.pone.0265930.

Cohen, L.M., Ruthazer, R., Moss, A.H., Germain, M.J., 2010. Predicting six-month mortality for patients who are on maintenance hemodialysis. Clin. J. Am. Soc. Nephrol. 1555905X. 5 (1), 72–79. Available from: http://cjasn.asnjournals.org/cgi/reprint/5/1/72. doi:10.2215/CJN.03860609.

Couchoud, C., Labeeuw, M., Moranne, O., Allot, V., Esnault, V., Frimat, L., Stengel, B., 2009. A clinical score to predict 6-month prognosis in elderly patients starting dialysis for end-stage renal disease. Nephrol. Dial. Transplant. 0931-0509. 24 (5), 1553–1561. doi:10.1093/ndt/gfn698.

Criscuolo, M., Fianchi, L., Dragonetti, G., Pagano, L., 2016. Tumor lysis syndrome: review of pathogenesis, risk factors and management of a medical emergency. Expert Rev. Hematol. 1747-4086. 9 (2), 197–208. doi:10.1586/17474086.2016.1127156.

Da'as, N., Polliack, A., Cohen, Y., Amir, G., Darmon, D., Kleinman, Y., Goldfarb, A.W., Ben-Yehuda, D., 2001. Kidney involvement and renal manifestations in non-Hodgkin's lymphoma and lymphocytic leukemia: a retrospective study in 700 patients. Eur. J. Haematol. 0936-6555. 67 (3), 158-164. doi:10.1034/j.1600-0609.2001.5790493.x.

Dawoud, A.A.Z., Gilbert, R.D., Tapper, W.J., Cross, N.C.P., 2022. Clonal myelopoiesis promotes adverse outcomes in chronic kidney disease. Leukemia. 14765551. 36 (2), 507–515. Available from: https://www.nature.com/leu/. doi:10.1038/s41375-021-01382-3.

Denic, A., Glassock, R.J., Rule, A.D., 2016. Structural and Functional Changes With the Aging Kidney. Adv. Chronic Kidney Dis. 23 (1). 19-28. doi:10.1053/j.ackd.2015.08.004.

Engels, E.A., Pfeiffer, R.M., Fraumeni, J.F., Kasiske, B.L., Israni, A.K., Snyder, J.J., Wolfe, R.A., Goodrich, N.P., Bayakly, A.R., Clarke, C.A., Copeland, G., Finch, J.L., Fleissner, M.L., Goodman, M.T., Kahn, A., Koch, L., Lynch, C.F., Madeleine, M.M., Pawlish, K., Rao, C., Williams, M.A., Castenson, D., Curry, M., Parsons, R., Fant, G., Lin, M., 2011. Spectrum of cancer risk among US solid organ transplant recipients. JAMA 15383598. 306 (17), 1891–1901. Available from: http://jama.ama-assn.org/content/306/17/1891.full.pdf+html. doi:10.1001/jama.2011.1592.

Evans, A.J., Cohen, M.E., Cohen, G.F., 1992. Patterns of breast calcification in patients on renal dialysis. Clin. Radiol. 0009-9260. 45 (5), 343-344. doi:10.1016/s0009-9260(05)80090-x.

Fick, G.M., Gabow, P.A., 1994. Hereditary and acquired cystic disease of the kidney. Kidney Int. 00852538. 46 (4), 951–964. Available from: https://www.journals.elsevier.com/kidney-international. doi:10.1038/ki.1994.354.

Franceschi, C., Garagnani, P., Parini, P., Giuliani, C., Santoro, A., 2018. Inflammaging: a new immune–metabolic viewpoint for age-related diseases. Nat. Rev. Endocrinol. 1759-5029. 14 (10), 576–590. doi:10.1038/s41574-018-0059-4.

Garimella, P.S., Balakrishnan, P., Ammakkanavar, N.R., Patel, S., Patel, A., Konstantinidis, I., Annapureddy, N., Nadkarni, G.N., 2017. Impact of dialysis requirement on outcomes in tumor lysis syndrome. Nephrology. 14401797. 22 (1), 85–88. Available from: http://onlinelibrary.wiley.com/journal/10.1111/(ISSN)1440-1797. doi:10.1111/nep.12806.

Garrett, G.L., Blanc, P.D., Boscardin, J., Lloyd, A.A., Ahmed, R.L., Anthony, T., Bibee, K., Breithaupt, A., Cannon, J., Chen, A., Cheng, J.Y., Chiesa-Fuxench, Z., Colegio, O.R., Curiel-Lewandrowski, C., Guzzo, C.A.D., Disse, M., Dowd, M., Eilers, R., Ortiz, A.E., Morris, C., Golden, S.K., Graves, M.S., Griffin, J.R., Hopkins, R.S., Huang, C.C., Bae, G.H., Jambusaria, A., Jennings, T.A., Jiang, S.I.B., Karia, P.S., Khetarpal, S., Kim, C., Klintmalm, G., Konicke,

K., Koyfman, S.A., Lam, C., Lee, P., Leitenberger, J.J., Loh, T., Lowenstein, S., Madankumar, R., Moreau, J.F., Nijhawan, R.I., Ochoa, S., Olasz, E.B., Otchere, E., Otley, C., Oulton, J., Patel, P.H., Patel, V.A., Prabhu, A.V., Pugliano-Mauro, M., Schmults, C.D., Schram, S., Shih, A.F., Shin, T., Soon, S., Soriano, T., Srivastava, D., Stein, J.A., Sternhell-Blackwell, K., Taylor, S., Vidimos, A., Wu, P., Zajdel, N., Zelac, D., Arron, S.T., 2017. Incidence of and risk factors for skin cancer in organ transplant recipients in the United States. JAMA Dermatol. 21686068. 153 (3), 296–303. Available from: http://jamanetwork.com/pdfaccess.ashx?url=/data/journals/derm/936062/jamadermatology_garrett_2017_oi_160068.pdf&routename=jamadermatology. doi:10.1001/jamadermatol.2016.4920.

Glassock, R.J., Rule, A.D., 2016. Aging and the kidneys: anatomy, physiology and consequences for defining chronic kidney disease. Nephron. 22353186. 134 (1), 25–29. Available from: http://www.karger.com/Journal/Home/223854. doi:10.1159/000445450.

Gumber, R., Cohen, J.B., Palmer, M.B., Kobrin, S.M., Vogl, D.T., Wasserstein, A.G., Nasta, S.D., Bleicher, M.B., Bloom, R.D., Dember, L., Cohen, A., Weiss, B.M., Hogan, J.J., 2018. A clone-directed approach may improve diagnosis and treatment of proliferative glomerulonephritis with monoclonal immunoglobulin deposits. Kidney Int. 15231755. 94 (1), 199–205. Available from: https://www.journals.elsevier.com/kidney-international. doi:10.1016/j.kint.2018.02.020.

Hollingsworth, J.M., Miller, D.C., Daignault, S., Hollenbeck, B.K., 2006. Rising incidence of small renal masses: a need to reassess treatment effect. J. Natl. Cancer Inst. 14602105. 98 (18), 1331–1334. doi:10.1093/jnci/djj362.

Howard, R.J., Patton, P.R., Reed, A.I., Hemming, A.W., Werf, W.J.V.D., Pfaff, W.W., Srinivas, T.R., Scornik, J.C., 2002. The changing causes of graft loss and death after kidney transplantation. Transplantation. 00411337. 73 (12), 1923–1928. Available from: https://journals.lww.com/transplantjournal/pages/default.aspx. doi:10.1097/00007890-200206270-00013.

Jaiswal, S., Ebert, B.L., 2019. Clonal hematopoiesis in human aging and disease. Science 10959203. 366 (6465). Available from: https://science.sciencemag.org/content/366/6465/eaan4673/tab-pdf. doi:10.1126/science.aan4673.

Johansen, K.L., Chertow, G.M., Jin, C., Kutner, N.G., 2007. Significance of frailty among dialysis patients. J. Am. Soc. Nephrol. 10466673. 18 (11), 2960–2967. Available from: https://journals.lww.com/jasn/pages/default.aspx. doi:10.1681/ASN.2007020221.

Kasiske, B.L., Snyder, J.J., Gilbertson, D.T., Wang, C., 2004. Cancer after kidney transplantation in the United States. Am. J. Transplant. 4 (6), 905–913. doi:10.1111/j.1600-6143.2004.00450.x.

Kim, S.P., Thompson, R.H., Boorjian, S.A., Weight, C.J., Han, L.C., Murad, M.H., Shippee, N.D., Erwin, P.J., Costello, B.A., Chow, G.K., Leibovich, B.C., 2012. Comparative effectiveness for survival and renal function of partial and radical nephrectomy for localized renal tumors: a systematic review and meta-analysis. J. Urol. 15273792. 188 (1), 51–57. Available from: http://www.sciencedirect.com/science?_ob=Publication. doi:10.1016/j.juro.2012.03.006.

Kitchlu, A., McArthur, E., Amir, E., Booth, C.M., Sutradhar, R., Majeed, H., Nash, D.M., Silver, S.A., Garg, A.X., Chan, C.T., Kim, S.J., Wald, R., 2019. Acute kidney injury in patients receiving systemic treatment for cancer: a population-based cohort study. J. Natl. Cancer Inst. 14602105. 111 (7), 727–736. Available from: http://jnci.oxfordjournals.org/. doi:10.1093/jnci/djy167.

Knoll, G.A., Kokolo, M.B., Mallick, R., Beck, A., Buenaventura, C.D., Ducharme, R., Barsoum, R., Bernasconi, C., Blydt-Hansen, T.D., Ekberg, H., Felipe, C.R., Firth, J., Gallon, L., Gelens, M., Glotz, D., Gossmann, J., Guba, M., Morsy, A.A., Salgo, R., Scheuermann, E.H., Tedesco-Silva, H., Vitko, S., Watson, C., Fergusson, D.A., 2014. Effect of sirolimus on malignancy and survival after kidney transplantation: systematic review and meta-analysis of individual patient data. BMJ. 1756-1833. 349 (nov24 1), g6679. doi:10.1136/bmj.g6679.

Latcha, S., 2019. Decision making for the initiation and termination of dialysis in patients with advanced cancer. Semin. Dial. 0894-0959. 32 (3), 215–218. doi:10.1111/sdi.12780.

Launay-Vacher, V., Oudard, S., Janus, N., Gligorov, J., Pourrat, X., Rixe, O., Morere, J.F., Beuzeboc, P., Deray, G., 2007. Prevalence of renal insufficiency in cancer patients and implications for anticancer drug management: the renal insufficiency and anticancer medications (IRMA) study. Cancer. 10970142. 110 (6), 1376–1384. doi:10.1002/cncr.22904.

Leblond, V., Davi, F., Charlotte, F., Dorent, R., Bitker, M.O., Sutton, L., Gandjbakhch, I., Binet, J.L., Raphael, M., 1998. Posttransplant lymphoproliferative disorders not associated with Epstein-Barr virus: a distinct entity? J. Clin. Oncol. 0732183X. 16 (6), 2052–2059. Available from: http://jco.ascopubs.org/content/by/year. doi:10.1200/JCO.1998.16.6.2052.

Lefaucheur, C., Stengel, B., Nochy, D., Martel, P., Hill, G.S., Jacquot, C., Rossert, J., for the GN-PROGRESS Study Group, 2006. Membranous nephropathy and cancer: epidemiologic evidence and determinants of high-risk cancer association. Kidney Int. 00852538. 70 (8), 1510–1517. doi:10.1038/sj.ki.5001790.

Libório, A.B., Abreu, K.L.S., Silva, G.B., Lima, R.S.A., Barreto, A.G.C., Barbosa, O.A., Daher, E.F., 2011. Predicting hospital mortality in critically ill cancer patients according to acute kidney injury severity. Oncology. 14230232. 80 (3-4), 160–166. doi:10.1159/000329042.

Lin, M.Y., Kuo, M.C., Hung, C.C., Wu, W.J., Chen, L.T., Yu, M.L., Hsu, C.C., Lee, C.H., Chen, H.C., Hwang, S.J., 2015. Association of dialysis with the risks of cancers. PLoS One 19326203. 10 (4). Available from: http://www.plosone.org/article/fetchObject.action?uri=info:doi/10.1371/journal.pone.0122856&representation=PDF. doi:10.1371/journal.pone.0122856.

López-Otín, C., Blasco, M.A., Partridge, L., Serrano, M., Kroemer, G., 2013. The hallmarks of aging. Cell. 10974172. 153 (6), 1194. Available from: https://www.cell.com. doi:10.1016/j.cell.2013.05.039.

Maisonneuve, P., Agodoa, L., Gellert, R., Stewart, J.H., Buccianti, G., Lowenfels, A.B., Wolfe, R.A., Jones, E., Disney, A.P.S., Briggs, D., McCredie, M., Boyle, P., 1999. Cancer in patients on dialysis for end-stage renal disease: an international collaborative study. Lancet. 01406736. 354 (9173), 93–99. Available from: http://www.journals.elsevier.com/the-lancet/. doi:10.1016/S0140-6736(99)06154-1.

Martens, K.L., Khalighi, P.R., Li, S., White, A.A., Silgard, E., Frieze, D., Estey, E., Garcia, D.A., Hingorani, S., Li, A., 2020. Comparative effectiveness of rasburicase versus allopurinol for cancer patients with renal dysfunction and hyperuricemia. Leuk. Res. 18735835. 89. Available from: https://www.elsevier.com/locate/leukres. doi:10.1016/j.leukres.2020.106298.

Mittal, A., Colegio, O.R., 2017. Skin cancers in organ transplant recipients. Am. J. Transplant. 16006135. 17 (10), 2509–2530. doi:10.1111/ajt.14382.

Morton, M., Coupes, B., Roberts, S.A., Klapper, P.E., Byers, R.J., Vallely, P.J., Ryan, K., Picton, M.L., 2013. Epidemiology of posttransplantation lymphoproliferative disorder in adult renal transplant recipients. Transplantation. 00411337. 95 (3), 470–478. doi:10.1097/TP.0b013e318276a237.

Murakami, N., Mulvaney, P., Danesh, M., Abudayyeh, A., Diab, A., Abdel-Wahab, N., Abdelrahim, M., Khairallah, P., Shirazian, S., Kukla, A., Owoyemi, I.O., Alhamad, T., Husami, S., Menon, M., Santeusanio, A., Blosser, C.D., Zuniga, S.C., Soler, M.J., Moreso, F., Mithani, Z., Ortiz-Melo, D., Jaimes, E.A., Gutgarts, V., Lum, E., Danovitch, G.M., Cardarelli, F., Drews, R.E., Bassil, C., Swank, J.L., Westphal, S., Mannon, R.B., Shirai, K., Kitchlu, A., Ong, S., Machado, S.M., Mothi, S.S., Ott, P.A., Rahma, O., Hodi, F.S., Sise, M.E., Gupta, S., Leaf, D.E., Devoe, C.E., Wanchoo, R., Nair, V.V., Schmults, C.D., Hanna, G.J., Sprangers, B., Riella, L.V., Jhaveri, K.D., 2021. A multi-center study on safety and efficacy of immune checkpoint inhibitors in cancer patients with kidney transplant. Kidney Int. 15231755. 100 (1), 196–205. Available from: https://www.journals.elsevier.com/kidney-international. doi:10.1016/j.kint.2020.12.015.

Na, S.Y., Sung, J.Y., Chang, J.H., Kim, S., Lee, H.H., Park, Y.H., Chung, W., Oh, K.H., Jung, J.Y., 2011. Chronic kidney disease in cancer patients: an independent predictor of cancer-specific mortality. Am. J. Nephrol. 02508095. 33 (2), 121–130. doi:10.1159/000323740.

Nalesnik, M.A., Jaffe, R., Starzl, T.E., Demetris, A.J., Porter, J.A.B., Makowka, L., Ho, M., Locker, J., 1988. The pathology of posttransplant lymphoproliferative disorders occurring in the setting of cyclosporine A-prednisone immunosuppression. Am. J. Pathol. 133 (1), 173–192. PMID: 2831927.

Obrador, G.T., Price, B., O'Meara, Y., Salant, D.J., 1997. Acute renal failure due to lymphomatous infiltration of the kidneys. J. Am. Soc. Nephrol. 1046-6673. 8 (8), 1348–1354. doi:10.1681/asn.v881348.

Odagiri, E., Jibiki, K., Takeda, M., Sugimura, H., Wachika, C., Abe, Y., Kihara, K., Kihara, Y., Itou, M., Nomura, T., Demura, R., Demura, H., Kubo, K., Sugino, N., Ohta, K., 1991. Effect of hemodialysis on the concentration of the seven tumor markers carcinoembryonic antigen, alpha-fetoprotein, squamous cell carcinoma-related antigen, neuron-specific enolase, CA 125, CA 19-9 and CA 15-3 in uremic patients. Am. J. Nephrol. 14219670. 11 (5), 363–368. doi:10.1159/000168339.

Opelz, G., Döhler, B., 2004. Lymphomas after solid organ transplantation: a collaborative transplant study report. Am. J. Transplant. 16006135. 4 (2), 222–230. doi:10.1046/j.1600-6143.2003.00325.x.

Opelz, G., Henderson, R., 1993. Incidence of non-hodgkin lymphoma in kidney and heart transplant recipients. The Lancet. 01406736. 342 (8886-8887), 1514–1516. doi:10.1016/s0140-6736(05)80084-4.

Reshef, R., Vardhanabhuti, S., Luskin, M.R., Heitjan, D.F., Hadjiliadis, D., Goral, S., Krok, K.L., Goldberg, L.R., Porter, D.L., Stadtmauer, E.A., Tsai, D.E., 2011. Reduction of immunosuppression as initial therapy for posttransplantation lymphoproliferative disorder. Am. J. Transplant. 16006135. 11 (2), 336–347. doi:10.1111/j.1600-6143.2010.03387.x.

Richmond, J., Sherman, R.S., Diamond, H.D., Craver, L.F., 1962. Renal lesions associated with malignant lymphomas. Am. J. Med. 00029343. 32 (2), 184–207. doi:10.1016/0002-9343(62)90289-9.

Robbins, H.A., Clarke, C.A., Arron, S.T., Tatalovich, Z., Kahn, A.R., Hernandez, B.Y., Paddock, L., Yanik, E.L., Lynch, C.F., Kasiske, B.L., Snyder, J., Engels, E.A., 2015. Melanoma risk and survival among organ transplant recipients.

J. Invest. Dermatol. 15231747. 135 (11), 2657–2665. Available from: http://www.nature.com/jid/index.html. doi:10.1038/jid.2015.312.

Robson, R., Cecka, J.M., Opelz, G., Budde, M., Sacks, S., 2005. Prospective registry-based observational cohort study of the long-term risk of malignancies in renal transplant patients treated with mycophenolate mofetil. Am. J. Transplant. 16006135. 5 (12), 2954–2960. doi:10.1111/j.1600-6143.2005.01125.x.

Rosner, M.H., 2020. Cancer screening in patients undergoing maintenance dialysis: who, what, and when. Am. J. Kidney Dis. 15236838. 76 (4), 558–566. Available from: http://www.elsevier.com/inca/publications/store/6/2/3/2/7/6/index.htt. doi:10.1053/j.ajkd.2019.12.018.

Rosner, M.H., Jhaveri, K.D., McMahon, B.A., Perazella, M.A., 2021. Onconephrology: the intersections between the kidney and cancer. CA Cancer J. Clin. 15424863. 71 (1), 47–77. Available from: http://onlinelibrary.wiley.com/journal/10.3322/(ISSN)1542-4863. doi:10.3322/caac.21636.

Salahudeen, A.K., Doshi, S.M., Pawar, T., Nowshad, G., Lahoti, A., Shah, P., 2013. Incidence rate, clinical correlates, and outcomes of AKI in patients admitted to a comprehensive cancer center. Clin. J. Am. Soc. Nephrol. 1555905X. 8 (3), 347–354. Available from: http://cjasn.asnjournals.org/content/8/3/347.full.pdf+html. doi:10.2215/CJN.03530412.

Scherer, J.S., Swidler, M.A., 2014. Decision-making in patients with cancer and kidney disease. Adv. Chronic Kidney Dis. 15485609. 21 (1), 72–80. doi:10.1053/j.ackd.2013.07.005.

Schmid, M., Abd-El-Barr, A.E.R., Gandaglia, G., Sood, A., Olugbade, K., Ruhotina, N., Sammon, J.D., Varda, B., Chang, S.L., Kibel, A.S., Chun, F.K., Menon, M., Fisch, M., Trinh, Q.D., 2014. Predictors of 30-day acute kidney injury following radical and partial nephrectomy for renal cell carcinoma. Urol. Oncol. 18732496. 32 (8), 1259–1266. Available from: http://www.elsevier.com/locate/issn/10781439. doi:10.1016/j.urolonc.2014.05.002.

Sprangers, B., Van der Veen, A., Hamaker, M.E., Rostoft, S., Latcha, S., Lichtman, S.M., de Moor, B., Wildiers, H., 2021. Initiation and termination of dialysis in older patients with advanced cancer: providing guidance in a complicated situation. Lancet Healthy Longev. 26667568. 2 (1), e42. Available from: https://www.thelancet.com/lanhl/about. doi:10.1016/S2666-7568(20)30060-X.

Stengel, B., 2010. Chronic kidney disease and cancer: a troubling connection. J. Nephrol. 17246059. 23 (3), 253–262. Available from: http://www.jnephrol.com/public/JN/Article/Attach.action?cmd=Download&uid=9CA86AA6-BA54-4B07-9183-95E18BD64E2D.

Tamura, M.K., Covinsky, K.E., Chertow, G.M., Yaffe, K., Landefeld, C.S., McCulloch, C.E., 2009. Functional status of elderly adults before and after initiation of dialysis. N. Engl. J. Med. 15334406. 361 (16), 1539–1547. Available from: http://content.nejm.org/cgi/reprint/361/16/1539.pdf. doi:10.1056/NEJMoa0904655.

Temel, J.S., Greer, J.A., Muzikansky, A., Gallagher, E.R., Admane, S., Jackson, V.A., Dahlin, C.M., Blinderman, C.D., Jacobsen, J., Pirl, W.F., Billings, J.A., Lynch, T.J., 2010. Early palliative care for patients with metastatic non-small-cell lung cancer. N. Engl. J. Med. 15334406. 363 (8), 733–742. Available from: http://www.nejm.org/doi/pdf/10.1056/NEJMoa1000678. doi:10.1056/NEJMoa1000678.

Trappe, R.U., Dierickx, D., Zimmermann, H., Morschhauser, F., Mollee, P., Zaucha, J.M., Dreyling, M.H., Dührsen, U., Reinke, P., Verhoef, G., Subklewe, M., Hüttmann, A., Tousseyn, T., Salles, G., Kliem, V., Hauser, I.A., Tarella, C., Van den Neste, E., Gheysens, O., Anagnostopoulos, I., Leblond, V., Riess, H., Choquet, S., 2017. Response to rituximab induction is a predictive marker in B-cell post-transplant lymphoproliferative disorder and allows successful stratification into rituximab or r-chop consolidation in an international, prospective, multicenter Phase II trial. J. Clin. Oncol. 15277755. 35 (5), 536–543. http://ascopubs.org/doi/pdf/10.1200/JCO.2016.69.3564. doi:10.1200/JCO.2016.69.3564.

Uppal, N.N., Monga, D., Vernace, M.A., Mehtabdin, K., Shah, H.H., Bijol, V., Jhaveri, K.D., 2019. Kidney diseases associated with *Waldenström macroglobulinemia*. Nephrol. Dial. Transplant. 14602385. 34 (10), 1644–1652. Available from: http://ndt.oxfordjournals.org/. doi:10.1093/ndt/gfy320.

Vajdic, C.M., McDonald, S.P., McCredie, M.R.E., Van Leeuwen, M.T., Stewart, J.H., Law, M., Chapman, J.R., Webster, A.C., Kaldor, J.M., Grulich, A.E., 2006. Cancer incidence before and after kidney transplantation. JAMA. 15383598. 296 (23), 2823–2831. Available from: http://jama.ama-assn.org/cgi/reprint/296/23/2823. doi:10.1001/jama.296.23.2823.

Vincenti, F., Charpentier, B., Vanrenterghem, Y., Rostaing, L., Bresnahan, B., Darji, P., Massari, P., Mondragon-Ramirez, G.A., Agarwal, M., Di Russo, G., Lin, C.-S., Garg, P., Larsen, C.P., 2010. A phase III study of belatacept-based immunosuppression regimens versus cyclosporine in renal transplant recipients (BENEFIT study). Am. J. Transplant. 16006135. 10 (3), 535–546. doi:10.1111/j.1600-6143.2009.03005.x.

Vlasschaert, C., Robinson-Cohen, C., Chen, J., Akwo, E., Parker, A.C., Silver, S.A., Bhatraju, P.K., Poisner, H., Cao, S., Jiang, M., Wang, Y., Niu, A., Siew, E., Van Amburg, J.C., Kramer, H.J., Kottgen, A., Franceschini, N., Psaty, B.M., Tracy, R.P., Alonso, A., Arking, D.E., Coresh, J., Ballantyne, C.M., Boerwinkle, E., Grams, M., Zhang, M.Z., Kestenbaum, B., Lanktree, M.B., Rauh, M.J., Harris, R.C., Bick, A.G., 2024. Clonal hematopoiesis of indeterminate potential is associated with acute kidney injury. Nat. Med. 1546170X. 30 (3), 810–817. Available from: https://www.nature.com/nm/. doi:10.1038/s41591-024-02854-6.

Wachterman, M.W., Marcantonio, E.R., Davis, R.B., Cohen, R.A., Waikar, S.S., Phillips, R.S., McCarthy, E.P., 2013. Relationship between the prognostic expectations of seriously Ill patients undergoing hemodialysis and their nephrologists. JAMA Intern. Med. 21686106. 173(13), 1206–1214. Available from: http://archinte.jamanetwork.com/data/Journals/INTEMED/927256/ioi130038.pdf. doi:10.1001/jamainternmed.2013.6036.

Wingard, R.L., Chan, K.E., Lazarus, J.M., Hakim, R.M., 2009. The "right" of passage: surviving the first year of dialysis. Clin. J. Am. Soc. Nephrol. 1555905X. 4 (Supplement 1), S114–S120. http://cjasn.asnjournals.org/cgi/reprint/4/Supplement_1/S114. doi:10.2215/CJN.04360709.

Wong, G., Howard, K., Webster, A.C., Chapman, J.R., Craig, J.C., 2011. Screening for renal cancer in recipients of kidney transplants. Nephrol. Dial. Transplant. 0931-0509. 26 (5), 1729–1739. doi:10.1093/ndt/gfq627.

Wong, L.M., Cleeve, L.K., Milner, A.D., Pitman, A.G., 2007. Malignant ureteral obstruction: outcomes after intervention. Have things changed? J. Urol. 00225347. 178 (1), 178–183. doi:10.1016/j.juro.2007.03.026.

Znaor, A., Lortet-Tieulent, J., Laversanne, M., Jemal, A., Bray, F., 2015. International variations and trends in renal cell carcinoma incidence and mortality. Eur. Urol. 03022838. 67 (3), 519–530. doi:10.1016/j.eururo.2014.10.002.

CHAPTER

25

Cardiovascular disease in aging kidney

Ahmad Armoghan Yousuf Awan[a], *Muhammad Rizwan*[b], *Rameesha Awan*[c], *and Carl Peter Walther*[d]

[a]Memorial Heart and Vascular Center, Interventional and Endovascular Cardiologist, Lake Charles, LA, United States

[b]Medstar Washington Hospital Center, Washington, DC, United States

[c]Hull York Medical School, York, United Kingdom

[d]Department of Nephrology, Baylor St. Luke's Medical Center, Houston, TX, United States

Introduction

As the population ages, the incidence of cardiovascular disease (CVD) increases. Similarly, as renal function declines, the incidence of coronary artery disease (CAD) also increases. In addition, aging itself predisposes individuals to kidney function decline. Chronic kidney disease (CKD) is an independent risk factor for CAD (Ohtake et al., 2005; Cai et al., 2014), with the incidence of CAD more than doubling in people with CKD compared to those without CKD. The incidence of CVD is markedly elevated in patients with CKD compared to the general population. CKD and CVD share several common risk factors, including hypertension and diabetes mellitus, which contribute to the increased prevalence of CVD among individuals with CKD. Furthermore, systemic complications associated with CKD exacerbate the risk of developing CVD in this vulnerable population.

CKD affects approximately 14% of adults in the United States, equating to an estimated 37 million individuals (Centers for Disease Control and Prevention [CDC], 2021). Patients with CKD experience accelerated cardiovascular aging, which significantly increases their risk for conditions such as CAD, congestive heart failure, arrhythmias, and sudden cardiac death. The prevalence of CVD escalates with the progression of CKD, particularly in stages 4 and 5. Notably, cardiovascular mortality accounts for approximately 40% to 50% of all deaths in patients with end-stage kidney disease (ESKD), compared to only 26% in individuals with normal kidney function (Go et al., 2004).

https://doi.org/10.1016/B978-0-443-34069-7.00029-X

The relationship between CKD and CVD is complex and bidirectional; each condition can exacerbate the other. For instance, people with advanced stages of CKD have a significantly higher mortality rate from cardiovascular causes—ranging from 58% to 71%—compared to those without CKD, whose rates are between 22% and 27.5% (Foley et al., 1998). This heightened risk underscores the critical need for early detection and proactive management of CVD in individuals with CKD. Implementing strategies that target modifiable risk factors—such as blood pressure control, glycemic management, and lipid profile monitoring—can substantially improve morbidity and mortality outcomes in this high-risk group.

The interplay between CKD and CVD necessitates a comprehensive approach to patient care that prioritizes cardiovascular health to mitigate risks associated with these interconnected conditions.

Pathophysiology

CKD significantly elevates the risk of CVD through a combination of atheromatous and non-atheromatous mechanisms. Atheromatous conditions, such as CAD, arise from accelerated plaque formation, while non-atheromatous conditions, including heart failure and arrhythmias, stem from structural and functional changes in the heart. The multifactorial nature of cardiovascular risk in CKD is underscored by shared risk factors, including hypertension and diabetes mellitus, as well as CKD-specific contributors such as chronic inflammation, uremia, endothelial dysfunction, dyslipidemia, mineral metabolism disturbances, anemia, and autonomic dysfunction (Kovesdy et al., 2017; Cai et al., 2014). Recognizing these interrelated pathways is critical to mitigating CVD risk in CKD patients.

Hypertension

Hypertension is pervasive in CKD and results from multiple overlapping mechanisms. Impaired renal sodium and water excretion, overactivation of the renin-angiotensin-aldosterone system (RAAS), vascular calcification, and reduced nitric oxide (NO) bioavailability are key drivers of elevated blood pressure (Vaziri, 2004; Raj and Safar, 2007). The RAAS plays a central role by increasing levels of angiotensin II, a potent vasoconstrictor, which raises blood pressure directly and stimulates aldosterone secretion. Aldosterone, in turn, promotes sodium and water retention, exacerbating hypertension (Vaziri, 2004). Sympathetic overactivity in CKD further contributes to vasoconstriction and vascular remodeling, compounding blood pressure elevation (Vaziri, 2004).

Endothelial dysfunction is another significant factor in CKD-associated hypertension. Uremic toxins, such as indoxyl sulfate and p-cresyl sulfate, impair vascular function by promoting oxidative stress and vascular smooth muscle proliferation, leading to arterial stiffness and diminished vasodilation (Stenvinkel et al., 2008; Mehta et al., 2015). These complex mechanisms result in persistent hypertension despite interventions such as pharmacotherapy and dietary modifications. Chronic hypertension contributes to endothelial damage, accelerating atherosclerotic plaque formation and increasing the risk of CAD. Over time, sustained elevated blood pressure leads to myocardial hypertrophy, diastolic dysfunction, and heart failure (Cai et al., 2014; London et al., 1995).

Fluid and sodium retention

Impaired kidney function leads to fluid and sodium retention, which causes fluid overload and elevated blood pressure. As CKD advances, the kidneys' ability to excrete sodium and water worsens, exacerbating hypertension. This fluid overload and hypertension contribute to left ventricular hypertrophy (LVH) and subsequently heart failure. Hypertension also increases the risk of CAD by promoting atherosclerotic processes. An increase in RAAS activity is a key phenomenon in CKD, further exacerbating hypertension. This leads to myocardial hypertrophy and contributes to endothelial dysfunction and vascular remodeling (Nishimoto et al., 2024).

Endothelial dysfunction and accelerated atherosclerosis

Endothelial dysfunction refers to structural and functional abnormalities in the vascular endothelium, increasing the risk of CAD and hypertension. In CKD patients, endothelial dysfunction is mediated by oxidative stress, chronic inflammation, and uremic toxins, which directly damage the endothelium and accelerate atherosclerosis (Baaten et al., 2023; Harlacher et al., 2022). Endothelial progenitor cells (EPCs), responsible for endothelial repair, are reduced in number and function due to oxidative stress, inflammation, and uremic toxins in CKD. This reduction further contributes to endothelial dysfunction. In addition, uremic toxins decrease endothelial-derived nitric oxide, impairing vasodilation and increasing the risk of atherosclerosis (Roumeliotis et al., 2020; Cuenca et al., 2020). Vasoconstriction in CKD is multifactorial and mediated by endothelin-1 and angiotensin II. Chronic elevation of inflammatory cytokines, such as TNF-α, IL-6, and CRP, disrupts endothelial cell function and promotes atherogenesis (Baaten et al., 2023; Six et al., 2012).

Myocardial remodeling

Hypertension, fluid overload, aldosterone-mediated cardiac remodeling, and chronic anemia are factors in CKD that lead to LVH, increasing myocardial oxygen demand and ischemia. Microvascular dysfunction in CKD patients also contributes to myocardial ischemia. Uremic toxins, like indoxyl sulfate and p-cresyl sulfate, promote myocardial fibrosis and impaired cardiac function (Wu et al., 2011; Moradi et al., 2013). Aldosterone contributes to myocardial collagen deposition, inflammation, and oxidative stress, driving myocardial remodeling through its profibrotic and pro-hypertrophic effects (Al-Hashedi and Abdu, 2024; Young and Funder, 2002).

Uremic toxins and chronic inflammation

Uremic toxins, such as advanced glycation end products (AGEs) and phosphate, potentiate inflammation and atherosclerosis. Pro-inflammatory cytokines, such as TNF-α and IL-6, intensify atherosclerotic processes in CKD (Chamieh et al., 2022). Chronic uremia also increases platelet activation and aggregation, heightening the risk of thrombosis and plaque rupture, which can lead to myocardial infarction. Elevated trimethylamine-N-oxide (TMAO) levels in CKD reduce nitric oxide production by increasing vascular oxidative stress and inflammation, exacerbating endothelial dysfunction (Li et al., 2018; Chamieh et al., 2022).

Vascular calcification and bone-mineral disorders

Vascular calcification, a significant complication in CKD, involves the pathological accumulation of calcium phosphate crystals in the intima and media layers of arterial walls. Compared to non-CKD patients, vascular calcification in CKD is more severe and contributes to CAD through plaque formation and instability (Chen and Moe, 2012). Hyperparathyroidism, hypercalcemia, and hyperphosphatemia—key components of bone-mineral disorders in CKD—accelerate vascular calcification. This calcification is associated with arterial stiffness and a higher risk of CVD events, including ischemia and LVH (Dube et al., 2021; Six et al., 2012).

Vascular calcification is mediated by oxidative stress, chronic inflammation, and signaling pathways in vascular smooth muscle cells (VSMCs), macrophages, and endothelial cells. Calcium and phosphate imbalances lead to the differentiation of VSMCs into osteoblast-like cells, increasing hydroxyapatite deposition in the vessel walls. Promoters of vascular calcification include bone morphogenetic proteins (BMP-2, BMP-4, BMP-6), osteocalcin, alkaline phosphatase, SOX9, osterix, matrix metalloproteinases (MMP-2, MMP-3, MMP-7), Runx2, oxidized low-density lipoproteins, collagen I, and receptor activator of nuclear factor-κB ligand (RANKL) (Nakanishi et al., 2020). Elevated fibroblast growth factor 23 (FGF-23) levels in CKD contribute to endothelial dysfunction and increased CAD risk (Chen and Moe, 2012).

Deposition of calcium in the aortic valve leads to aortic stenosis, and calcification of small blood vessels disrupts microvascular function, causing ischemia. These processes collectively highlight the complexity of vascular calcification and its profound impact on cardiovascular health in CKD patients.

Dyslipidemia

Impaired lipid metabolism in CKD leads to hypertriglyceridemia, low HDL cholesterol, and increased LDL cholesterol, all of which accelerate atherosclerosis and CAD (Schwarz et al., 2000; Hager et al., 2017). Key factors contributing to dyslipidemia in CKD include chronic inflammation, oxidative stress, and endothelial dysfunction. Below are the critical changes observed in lipid metabolism in CKD patients:

- Reduced Lipoprotein Lipase (LPL) Activity: LPL, responsible for hydrolyzing triglycerides in chylomicrons and very-low-density lipoproteins (VLDL), is inhibited in CKD, leading to hypertriglyceridemia (Schwarz et al., 2000).
- Increased Hepatic Lipogenesis and VLDL Secretion: CKD promotes enhanced production and secretion of VLDL by the liver (Hager et al., 2017).
- Altered Apolipoproteins: Levels of ApoC-II, an activator of LPL, are reduced, whereas levels of ApoC-III, an inhibitor of LPL, are elevated. This imbalance slows VLDL and chylomicron clearance (Suh and Kim, 2023).

- Decreased HDL Cholesterol: Chronic inflammation increases HDL catabolism and decreases ApoA synthesis, reducing protective HDL levels (Suh and Kim, 2023).
- Oxidized LDL Particles: Uremic toxins and oxidative stress increase the oxidation of atherogenic LDL particles, exacerbating vascular damage (Schwarz et al., 2000; Suh and Kim, 2023).
- Impact of Pro-inflammatory Cytokines: Elevated levels of TNF-α and IL-6 suppress LPL activity and promote LDL oxidation (Hager et al., 2017).
- Oxidative Stress: Increased production of reactive oxygen species (ROS) oxidizes LDL and HDL, impairing their function and promoting endothelial injury (Suh and Kim, 2023).

Anemia and myocardial ischemia

Anemia in CKD results from reduced erythropoietin production, chronic inflammation, and dietary iron deficiency. As CKD progresses, anemia becomes nearly universal, leading to myocardial ischemia. The combination of CKD, anemia, and heart failure significantly increases morbidity and mortality (Virani et al., 2008; Al-Ahmad et al., 2001). Early identification and management of anemia in this population are critical to improving cardiovascular outcomes.

Autonomic dysfunction

CKD, particularly in advanced stages, is frequently associated with autonomic dysfunction. This results from chronic overactivation of the sympathetic nervous system, which desensitizes baroreceptors and contributes to vascular stiffness. Impaired baroreceptor sensitivity exacerbates hypertension, which can lead to CAD and congestive heart failure (Salman, 2015).

Hyperuricemia

Impaired uric acid excretion in CKD leads to hyperuricemia, which is associated with endothelial dysfunction, further contributing to vascular injury and cardiovascular complications (Nishizawa et al., 2022).

ESKD and dialysis

As CKD progresses to end-stage kidney disease (ESKD), requiring renal replacement therapy, the aforementioned pathological processes worsen. Dialysis, while lifesaving, negatively impacts cardiovascular outcomes due to fluctuations in blood pressure, which increase myocardial stress and worsen myocardial ischemia (Cozzolino et al., 2018). Effective management of cardiovascular risk factors is crucial in this patient population to reduce mortality.

Congestive heart failure with an emphasis on cardiorenal syndrome (CRS)

Introduction

Congestive heart failure (CHF) and CKD frequently coexist, creating a complex and bidirectional interplay known as cardiorenal syndrome (CRS). In CRS, heart failure exacerbates kidney dysfunction, while impaired kidney function further deteriorates cardiac performance, forming a vicious cycle. This section focuses on understanding the mechanisms underlying CRS, recognizing early signs of worsening kidney function in CHF patients, and reviewing evidence-based management strategies.

Definition and impact

Cardiorenal syndrome is characterized by the interdependent dysfunction of the heart and kidneys, where acute or chronic dysfunction of one organ induces or worsens the dysfunction of the other. The presence of CRS signifies advanced disease in either system and is associated with increased morbidity and mortality. Studies indicate a 15% increase in mortality for every 10 ml/min decrease in estimated glomerular filtration rate (eGFR) in CHF patients (Rangaswami et al., 2019; Mullens et al., 2009).

Classification of CRS

See Table 25.1.

TABLE 25.1 Types of cardiorenal syndrome.

Type	Primary mechanism	Key features	Examples
Type 1 (acute cardiorenal syndrome)	Acute heart failure (HF) causing acute kidney injury (AKI)	Decreased cardiac output (CO), venous congestion, renin-angiotensin-aldosterone System (RAAS) activation	Acute decompensated HF, cardiogenic shock
Type 2 (chronic cardiorenal syndrome)	Chronic HF leading to progressive chronic kidney disease (CKD)	Chronic low CO, neurohormonal activation, renal hypoperfusion	Long-standing HF with CKD progression
Type 3 (acute renocardiac syndrome)	AKI causing acute cardiac dysfunction	Volume overload, uremic toxins, arrhythmias	AKI from sepsis causing acute HF
Type 4 (chronic renocardiac syndrome)	CKD leading to chronic cardiac dysfunction	Chronic uremia, volume overload, hypertension	CKD-induced left ventricular hypertrophy and HF
Type 5 (secondary CRS)	Systemic illness affecting both the heart and kidneys	Multisystem dysfunction	Sepsis, systemic lupus erythematosus (SLE), and cirrhosis-induced cardiorenal failure

Pathophysiology

The pathophysiology of CRS revolves around complex hemodynamic changes and maladaptive neurohormonal responses. Key mechanisms include:

- Decreased cardiac output (CO): In type 1 CRS, reduced CO leads to renal hypoperfusion, triggering the activation of the renin-angiotensin-aldosterone system (RAAS), the sympathetic nervous system, and arginine vasopressin secretion. These responses exacerbate fluid retention, increase preload, and worsen heart failure (Winton, 1931).
- Elevated central venous pressure (CVP): Elevated CVP in CHF (both reduced and preserved ejection fraction) results in renal venous congestion, compromising glomerular filtration, and increasing renal resistance (Ichikawa et al., 1984).
- Neurohormonal dysregulation: Persistent activation of the RAAS and sympathetic nervous system leads to preglomerular vasoconstriction and enhanced sodium/water reabsorption, worsening congestion and oliguria (Ronco et al., 2008).
- Venous congestion: Studies have highlighted the role of venous congestion as a critical determinant of renal dysfunction in CRS, independent of CO (Hillege et al., 2006).
- Oxidative stress and inflammation: In CRS, oxidative stress and systemic inflammation further contribute to endothelial dysfunction and vascular remodeling in both the heart and kidneys (Tang and Mullens, 2010).

Diagnosis

The diagnosis of CRS is multifaceted, requiring clinical assessment, laboratory tests, and imaging studies:

- Clinical history and physical examination: Symptoms of CHF (dyspnea, edema), reduced urine output, or worsening CKD.
- Laboratory tests: Elevated serum creatinine, blood urea nitrogen (BUN), and brain natriuretic peptide (BNP); proteinuria or hematuria on urinalysis.
- Imaging: Echocardiography showing evidence of CHF; Doppler studies for renal perfusion; chest X-ray for pulmonary congestion (Damman and Testani, 2015).

Management strategies

The management of CRS requires an integrated approach involving cardiology, nephrology, and critical care teams. The goals are to optimize hemodynamics, achieve euvolemia, and prevent further decline in renal and cardiac function.

- Type 1 CRS (acute cardiorenal syndrome): Loop diuretics (furosemide, bumetanide, torsemide) are first-line therapy to relieve fluid overload. High-dose diuretics are favored over home doses in acute decompensation. Adding thiazides (e.g., metolazone) can help overcome diuretic resistance (Costanzo et al., 2005). Continuous infusion versus bolus dosing provides similar outcomes in terms of symptom relief and renal function (Felker et al., 2011). Close monitoring of renal function is critical, as diuretic use may transiently worsen kidney function. In severe left ventricular dysfunction, inotropes like dobutamine or milrinone may be required to maintain renal perfusion (Neuberg et al., 2002). Dialysis is reserved for severe diuretic resistance, volume overload, or complications of AKI (Bart et al., 2012).

- Type 2 CRS (chronic cardiorenal syndrome): ACE inhibitors/ARBs/ARNIs are used for reducing afterload and improving survival in CHF with reduced ejection fraction (HFrEF). Beta-blockers are recommended to reduce mortality and slow the progression of CHF. Aldosterone antagonists have been shown to improve outcomes in CHF but require careful monitoring of potassium and renal function (McAlister et al., 2004). Lifestyle interventions are recommended, including salt and fluid restriction, physical activity, and weight management. Regular assessment of renal function and potassium levels may be needed as medications are adjusted.
- Type 3 CRS (acute renocardiac syndrome) and Type 4 CRS (chronic renocardiac syndrome): Management focuses on addressing and treating acute kidney injury and mitigating its effects on cardiac function. Management includes volume optimization, electrolyte management, and treating underlying causes.
- Type 5 CRS: Secondary cardiorenal syndrome: Treatments target the underlying secondary systemic disease, along with the simultaneous treatment and protection of the underlying cardiac and renal diseases.

Conclusion

Cardiorenal syndrome represents a complex interplay between cardiac and renal dysfunction, significantly increasing morbidity and mortality. A thorough understanding of the classification, pathophysiology, and tailored management strategies is essential for optimizing outcomes in this high-risk population.

CAD in the aging kidney

A decline in glomerular filtration rate (GFR) is strongly associated with adverse outcomes in patients with CAD. The risk of CAD progression and complications increases significantly as GFR declines. Patients with CKD often present with multivessel and heavily calcified coronary artery disease, posing unique diagnostic and therapeutic challenges. In this population, CAD manifests in several forms, including asymptomatic coronary artery disease, stable angina, and acute coronary syndromes (ACS). The management strategies for CAD vary depending on its clinical presentation. This review aims to comprehensively address the pathophysiology, diagnostic modalities, and management strategies for CAD in patients with CKD.

Asymptomatic coronary artery disease

Advances in computed tomography (CT) technology have significantly enhanced the detection of asymptomatic coronary artery disease, facilitating early intervention to slow disease progression. Coronary artery calcium (CAC) scoring has emerged as a vital tool for quantifying atherosclerotic burden and guiding therapy. The 2018 American Heart Association/American College of Cardiology (AHA/ACC) guidelines on hyperlipidemia emphasize the importance of CAC in risk stratification (Grundy et al., 2018). Management of asymptomatic CAD focuses on aggressive medical therapy and risk factor control. Hyperlipidemia management is particularly critical to reducing the risk of symptomatic CAD. Statins, recognized for their lipid-lowering and antiinflammatory properties, form the cornerstone of therapy and have shown efficacy in patients with CKD (Scarpioni, 2012). A target low-density lipoprotein cholesterol (LDL-C) level of <70 mg/dL is recommended. For patients unable to achieve LDL-C targets with statins or those intolerant to them, PCSK9 inhibitors are indicated. The FOURIER trial demonstrated a 59% reduction in LDL-C levels with evolocumab, irrespective of kidney function, with a safety profile comparable to non-CKD patients (Charytan et al., 2019). Bempedoic acid is another lipid-lowering agent approved by the ACC/AHA guidelines. However, its use in CKD requires caution due to the potential risk of worsening renal function. Comprehensive management of other risk factors, such as hypertension, diabetes mellitus, and peripheral artery disease, is also essential.

Stable angina

Stable angina arises from myocardial ischemia caused by fixed coronary obstructions and is typically triggered by physical or emotional stress. The diagnostic evaluation of CAD in CKD patients involves multiple modalities, each with distinct strengths and limitations. Exercise stress testing is widely used but has limited sensitivity (60%–70%) and specificity (40%) in detecting CAD, especially in intermediate-risk populations (Singh et al., 2003). To improve diagnostic accuracy, imaging-based stress tests, such as stress echocardiography and nuclear stress testing, are recommended. Stress echocardiography provides a sensitivity of 75%–85% and specificity of 80%–90% due to its ability to identify wall motion abnormalities. It is particularly advantageous for CKD patients as it avoids radiation exposure. Conversely, nuclear stress testing offers higher sensitivity (85%–90%) but lower specificity (70%–80%), with the added benefit of localizing ischemia and detecting perfusion defects in multivessel disease (Wang et al., 2015). Coronary computed tomography angiography (CCTA) provides direct visualization of coronary arteries. However, its utility in CKD is limited by the need for iodinated contrast and reduced accuracy in heavily calcified vessels. The ISCHEMIA-CKD trial demonstrated that an initial invasive strategy is not superior to optimal medical therapy in stable CAD patients with CKD (Bangalore et al., 2020). Current guidelines recommend optimizing guideline-directed medical therapy (GDMT) and reserving invasive angiography for patients with left ventricular dysfunction or those unresponsive to medical therapy.

Acute coronary syndrome

Acute coronary syndrome (ACS) encompasses unstable angina, non-ST elevation myocardial infarction (NSTEMI), and ST elevation myocardial infarction (STEMI). CKD patients with ACS often present with advanced Killip class heart failure and multivessel CAD, leading to worse outcomes. Invasive angiography is recommended for ACS patients. For single-vessel disease, percutaneous coronary intervention (PCI) is the preferred strategy. However, in multivessel disease, evidence is limited due to the underrepresentation of CKD patients in randomized trials. Observational studies suggest that coronary artery bypass grafting (CABG) is superior to PCI in end-stage renal disease (ESRD) patients with triple-vessel disease, left main coronary artery disease, or proximal left anterior descending artery disease (Luo et al., 2023). New-generation drug-eluting stents may improve PCI outcomes in this population, though evidence is still evolving.

Revascularization in CKD

Both PCI and CABG present unique risks and benefits for CKD patients. PCI is associated with lower periprocedural morbidity, shorter hospital stays, and reduced risk of AKI. However, it carries higher rates of restenosis and repeat revascularization. In contrast, CABG offers superior long-term outcomes due to improved graft patency and reduced need for repeat interventions, despite higher early mortality and perioperative complications (e.g., stroke, myocardial infarction, AKI) (Li et al., 2021). Strategies to mitigate PCI-related complications include limiting contrast exposure, using the radial approach, and adjusting medications for renal function. Ultra-low contrast PCI techniques can further reduce the risk of contrast-induced nephropathy (Tobe et al., 2023). The choice between PCI and CABG should involve a multidisciplinary heart team, considering CAD severity, CKD stage, and patient preferences.

Arrhythmias in CKD

Arrhythmias are frequently encountered in patients with CKD, often arising from structural myocardial disease or electrolyte imbalances. Managing arrhythmias in this population is uniquely challenging.

Management of atrial arrhythmias

Atrial fibrillation (AF) and atrial flutter are more common in CKD patients and are associated with increased risks of thromboembolism and bleeding (Wyse et al., 2002). Rate control, using beta-blockers and calcium channel blockers, is typically the initial management strategy. A heart rate target of < 110 beats per minute is associated with better outcomes compared to stricter control targets. Trials such as AFFIRM and RACE found no significant benefit of rhythm control over rate control. However, the CASTLE-AF trial showed improved outcomes with catheter ablation, while the CABANA trial demonstrated improved quality of life and symptom control with rhythm control strategies (Van Gelder et al., 2002; Marrouche et al., 2018). Anticoagulation is critical to reducing thromboembolic risk. CHADS2-VASc scoring guides therapy, with scores > 3 in females and > 2 in males warranting anticoagulation. Direct oral anticoagulants (DOACs) and warfarin are commonly used, with dose adjustments based on renal function to minimize bleeding risks (Packer et al., 2019).

Ventricular arrhythmias

Ventricular arrhythmias, including sudden cardiac death, are the leading causes of mortality in dialysis patients. Risk factors include structural heart disease, electrolyte imbalances, and the arrhythmogenic effects of certain medications (Bonato et al., 2013). Early diagnosis using ECG and Holter monitoring is critical. Management involves treating ischemia and correcting electrolyte disturbances. Identifying repolarization abnormalities and QT interval defects is crucial, as dialysis patients are prone to acquired long QT syndrome, which increases the risk of sudden cardiac death. Implantable cardioverter-defibrillators (ICDs) are indicated for secondary prevention in patients with ventricular tachycardia (VT) or ventricular fibrillation, and for primary prevention in those with left ventricular dysfunction.

CKD and valvular heart disease (VHD)

CKD is recognized as a major risk factor for the development of VHD. In particular, aortic and mitral valve calcifications are prevalent in CKD patients and frequently result in valvular stenosis and regurgitation. These valvular abnormalities are strongly associated with a significantly elevated risk of mortality in this population. The five-year mortality rate for CKD patients with aortic stenosis (AS) or mitral regurgitation (MR) is >50% higher than that observed in non-CKD patients. Even in the absence of clinically significant valvular dysfunction, echocardiographic evidence of valvular abnormalities in CKD patients is linked to adverse cardiovascular outcomes (Chen et al., 2019; Thaden et al., 2020). In addition to valvular calcifications, CKD-related volume overload can lead to ventricular enlargement, contributing to secondary mitral and tricuspid regurgitation. Among patients with end-stage kidney disease (ESKD), valvular calcifications are identified in 35% to 40% of cases and are independently associated with poor cardiovascular outcomes. Risk stratification during pre-procedural evaluation is therefore critical in this high-risk population. Importantly, the number of calcified valves in dialysis patients correlates directly with cardiovascular mortality. For instance, the one-year all-cause mortality rate is approximately 57% in patients with calcifications of both the aortic and mitral valves, 40% in those with calcification of either valve, and 15% in patients without valvular calcification. Although left-sided valvular involvement predominates in CKD, right-sided valve disease, particularly tricuspid regurgitation, is also observed and is primarily attributed to chronic volume overload (Vahanian et al., 2021).

Management of stenotic valvular lesions in CKD

The management of aortic stenosis (AS) in CKD generally follows standard guidelines as outlined for the general population. However, a multidisciplinary approach is strongly recommended due to the elevated procedural risks in CKD patients. Medical management is limited for severe AS, but optimal volume control and risk factor modification remain crucial components of care. Decisions regarding transcatheter aortic valve replacement (TAVR) and surgical aortic valve replacement (SAVR) should be individualized, taking into account the patient's overall risk profile, functional status, age, comorbidities, and life expectancy. For patients undergoing TAVR, strategies to mitigate the risk of contrast-induced nephropathy (CIN), such as hydration protocols and minimization of contrast use, should be implemented.

Mitral stenosis (MS) in patients with CKD is primarily attributable to mitral annular calcification (MAC) or, less commonly, rheumatic heart disease. Management typically focuses on symptom control through volume optimization and medical therapy. In cases of severe mitral stenosis, percutaneous mitral balloon valvuloplasty (PMBV) or mitral valve replacement (MVR) should be considered, guided by the severity of symptoms and overall clinical status (Vahanian et al., 2021).

Management of regurgitant valvular lesions in CKD

Valvular regurgitation in CKD is frequently secondary to left ventricular dysfunction, volume overload, or annular dilation. Management strategies are centered on achieving optimal volume control, often requiring diuretics or ultrafiltration in dialysis patients. In the presence of left ventricular dysfunction, guideline-directed medical therapy (GDMT) for heart failure should be employed to mitigate symptoms and improve outcomes. For patients with severe aortic or mitral regurgitation, surgical or transcatheter valve replacement should be considered. These decisions require careful evaluation of procedural risk, long-term prognosis, and the patient's overall health status (Vahanian et al., 2021).

Conclusion

As populations age, CKD and CVD increasingly intersect. CKD independently doubles the risk of CAD, and both conditions are driven by shared factors such as hypertension, diabetes, oxidative stress, inflammation, and endothelial injury. CKD adds unique insults, including the accumulation of uremic toxins such as indoxyl sulfate and p-cresyl sulfate, impaired nitric oxide signaling with reduced endothelial repair, and profound lipid abnormalities—high triglycerides, low HDL cholesterol, oxidized LDL cholesterol, diminished lipoprotein lipase activity, reduced apolipoprotein C-II, and elevated apolipoprotein C-III.

Disruptions in mineral and bone metabolism accelerate vascular and valvular calcification through bone morphogenetic protein signaling, RUNX2 activation, and the RANKL pathway. Additional contributors—anemia, autonomic imbalance, and hyperuricemia—further damage the heart. Collectively, these mechanisms produce diffuse, calcified multivessel coronary disease and non-atherosclerotic complications such as left ventricular hypertrophy, heart failure, arrhythmias, and sudden cardiac death. Dialysis compounds the burden by imposing hemodynamic stress, which worsens ischemia and vascular injury.

Optimal management requires an integrated heart–kidney approach. Priorities include early detection of renal decline, rigorous control of blood pressure with modulation of the renin–angiotensin–aldosterone system, careful management of sodium and fluid balance, targeted lipid lowering, correction of anemia, and control of mineral and bone disease to slow calcification. Reducing the burden of uremic toxins through dietary measures and microbiome-directed strategies is also essential. Decisions regarding revascularization and valve interventions should be made by a multidisciplinary team, with ultra-low-contrast percutaneous coronary intervention via the radial artery favored when feasible.

Coronary artery bypass grafting should be chosen for long-term durability, and transcatheter or surgical valve replacement should be selected according to the overall risk and goals of care. Continuous rhythm surveillance, anticoagulation adjusted for kidney function, and consideration of implantable cardioverter–defibrillators address leading causes of mortality.

Future progress will depend on clinical trials that fully include patients with CKD and on precision therapies that target inflammation, oxidative stress, and calcification biology.

AI disclosure

During the preparation of this work, the author(s) used ChatGPT for refinement. After using this tool/service, the author(s) reviewed and edited the content as needed and take(s) full responsibility for the content of the publication.

References

Al-Ahmad, A., Rand, W.M., Manjunath, G., Konstam, M.A., Salem, D.N., Levey, A.S., Sarnak, M.J., 2001. Reduced kidney function and anemia as risk factors for mortality in patients with left ventricular dysfunction. J. Am. Coll. Cardiol. 07351097. 38 (4), 955–962. doi:10.1016/S0735-1097(01)01470-X.

Al-Hashedi, E.M., Abdu, F.A., 2024. Aldosterone effect on cardiac structure and function. Curr. Cardiol. Rev. 18756557. 20 (4), 60–67. Available from: https://www.eurekaselect.com/article/138876. doi:10.2174/0115734 03X281390240219063817.

Baaten, C.C.F.M.J., Vondenhoff, S., Noels, H., 2023. Endothelial cell dysfunction and increased cardiovascular risk in patients with chronic kidney disease. Circ. Res. 15244571. 132 (8), 970–992. Available from: https://www.ovid.com/product-details.454.html. doi:10.1161/CIRCRESAHA.123.321752.

Bangalore, S., Maron, D.J., Stone, G.W., 2020. Outcomes with invasive vs. conservative management of coronary disease and chronic kidney disease: ISCHEMIA-CKD Trial. N. Engl. J. Med. 382, 1519–1530. doi:10.1056/NEJMoa1915925.

Bart, B.A., Goldsmith, S.R., Lee, K.L., Givertz, M.M., O'Connor, C.M., Bull, D.A., Redfield, M.M., Deswal, A., Rouleau, J.L., LeWinter, M.M., Ofili, E.O., Stevenson, L.W., Semigran, M.J., Felker, G.M., Chen, H.H., Hernandez, A.F., Anstrom, K.J., McNulty, S.E., Velazquez, E.J., Ibarra, J.C., Mascette, A.M., Braunwald, E., 2012. Ultrafiltration in decompensated heart failure with cardiorenal syndrome. N. Engl. J. Med. 15334406. 367 (24), 2296–2304. Available from: http://www.nejm.org/doi/pdf/10.1056/NEJMoa1210357. doi:10.1056/NEJMoa1210357.

Bonato, F.O.B., Lemos, M.M., Cassiolato, J.L., Canziani, M.E.F., 2013. Prevalence of ventricular arrhythmia and its associated factors in nondialyzed chronic kidney disease patients. PLoS One. 19326203. 8 (6). Available from: http://www.plosone.org/article/fetchObject.action?uri=info%3Adoi%2F10.1371%2Fjournal.pone.0066036&representation=PDF. doi:10.1371/journal.pone.0066036Brazil.

Cai, Q., Mukku, V., Ahmad, M., 2014. Coronary artery disease in patients with chronic kidney disease: a clinical update. Curr. Cardiol. Rev. 1573403X. 9 (4), 331–339. doi:10.2174/1573403X10666140214122234.

Centers for Disease Control and Prevention (CDC), 2021. Chronic kidney disease in the United States. Atlanta (GA): U.S. Department of Health and Human Services, Centers for Disease Control and Prevention; 2021.

Chamieh, C.E., Liabeuf, S., Massy, Z., 2022. Uremic toxins and cardiovascular risk in chronic kidney disease: what have we learned recently beyond the past findings? Toxins. 2072-6651. 14 (4), 280. doi:10.3390/toxins14040280.

Charytan, D.M., Sabatine, M.S., Pedersen, T.R., Im, K.A., Park, J.G., Pineda, A.L., Wasserman, S.M., Deedwania, P., Olsson, A.G., Sever, P.S., Keech, A.C., Giugliano, R.P., 2019. Efficacy and safety of evolocumab in chronic kidney disease in the fourier trial. J. Am. Coll. Cardiol. 15583597. 73 (23), 2961–2970. Available from: https://www.elsevier.com/locate/jacc.. doi:10.1016/j.jacc.2019.03.513.

Chen, J., Budoff, M.J., Reilly, M.P., 2019. Valvular heart disease in chronic kidney disease: epidemiology and outcomes. Kidney Int. Rep. 4, 572–582.

Chen, N.X., Moe, S.M., 2012. Vascular calcification: pathophysiology and risk factors. Curr. Hypertens. Rep. 15343111. 14 (3), 228–237. doi:10.1007/s11906-012-0265-8.

Costanzo, M.R., Saltzberg, M., O'Sullivan, J., Sobotka, P., 2005. Early ultrafiltration in patients with decompensated heart failure and diuretic resistance. J. Am. Coll. Cardiol. 07351097. 46 (11), 2047–2051. doi:10.1016/j.jacc.2005.05.099.

Cozzolino, M., Mangano, M., Stucchi, A., Ciceri, P., Conte, F., Galassi, A., 2018. Cardiovascular disease in dialysis patients. Nephrol. Dial. Transplant. 0931-0509. 33 (suppl_3), iii28. doi:10.1093/ndt/gfy174.

Cuenca, M.V., Hordijk, P.L., Vervloet, M.G., 2020. Most exposed: the endothelium in chronic kidney disease. Nephrol. Dial. Transplant. 14602385. 35 (9), 1478–1487. Available from: http://ndt.oxfordjournals.org/. doi:10.1093/ndt/gfz055.

Damman, K., Testani, J.M., 2015. The kidney in heart failure: an update. Eur. Heart J. 15229645. 36 (23), 1437–1444. Available from: http://eurheartj.oxfordjournals.org/. doi:10.1093/eurheartj/ehv010.

Dube, P., DeRiso, A., Patel, M., Battepati, D., Khatib-Shahidi, B., Sharma, H., Gupta, R., Malhotra, D., Dworkin, L., Haller, S., Kennedy, D., 2021. Vascular calcification in chronic kidney disease: diversity in the vessel wall. Biomedicines. 2227-9059. 9 (4), 404. doi:10.3390/biomedicines9040404.

Felker, G.M., Lee, K.L., Bull, D.A., Redfield, M.M., Stevenson, L.W., Goldsmith, S.R., LeWinter, M.M., Deswal, A., Rouleau, J.L., Ofili, E.O., Anstrom, K.J., Hernandez, A.F., McNulty, S.E., Velazquez, E.J., Kfoury, A.G., Chen, H.H., Givertz, M.M., Semigran, M.J., Bart, B.A., Mascette, A.M., Braunwald, E., O'Connor, C.M., 2011. Diuretic strategies in patients with acute decompensated heart failure. N. Engl. J. Med. 0028-4793. 364 (9), 797–805. doi:10.1056/NEJMoa1005419.

Foley, R.N., Parfrey, P.S., Sarnak, M.J., 1998. Clinical epidemiology of cardiovascular disease in chronic renal disease. Am. J. Kidney Dis. 02726386. 32 (5), S112. Available from: http://www.elsevier.com/inca/publications/store/6/2/3/2/7/6/index.htt. doi:10.1053/ajkd.1998.v32.pm9820470.

Go, A.S., Chertow, G.M., Fan, D., McCulloch, C.E., Hsu, C.Y., 2004. Chronic kidney disease and the risks of death, cardiovascular events, and hospitalization. N. Engl. J. Med. 351 (13), 1296–1305. doi:10.1056/NEJMoa041031.

Grundy, S.M., Stone, N.J., Bailey, A.L., 2018. AHA/ACC/AACVPR/AAPA/ABC/ACPM/ADA/AGS/APhA/ASPC/NLA/PCNA guideline on the management of blood cholesterol: a report of the American College of Cardiology/American Heart Association task force on clinical practice guidelines. J. Am. Coll. Cardiol. 73 (24), e285–e350.

Hager, M.R., Narla, A.D., Tannock, L.R., 2017. Dyslipidemia in patients with chronic kidney disease. Rev. Endocr. Metab. Disord. 15732606. 18 (1), 29–40. doi:10.1007/s11154-016-9402-z.

Harlacher, E., Wollenhaupt, J., Baaten, C.C.F.M.J., Noels, H., 2022. Impact of uremic toxins on endothelial dysfunction in chronic kidney disease: a systematic review. Int. J. Mol. Sci. 14220067. 23 (1). Available from: https://www.mdpi.com/1422-0067/23/1/531/pdf. doi:10.3390/ijms23010531.

Hillege, H.L., Nitsch, D., Pfeffer, M.A., Swedberg, K., McMurray, J.J.V., Yusuf, S., Granger, C.B., Michelson, E.L., Östergren, J., Cornel, J.H., De Zeeuw, D., Pocock, S., Van Veldhuisen, D.J., 2006. Renal function as a predictor of outcome in a broad spectrum of patients with heart failure. Circulation. 00097322. 113 (5), 671–678. doi:10.1161/CIRCULATIONAHA.105.580506.

Ichikawa, I., Pfeffer, J.M., Pfeffer, M.A., Hostetter, T.H., Brenner, B.M., 1984. Role of angiotensin II in the altered renal function of congestive heart failure. Circ. Res. 0009-7330. 55 (5), 669–675. doi:10.1161/01.res.55.5.669.

Kovesdy, C.P., Furth, S.L., Zoccali, C., Li, P.K.T., Garcia-Garcia, G., Benghanem-Gharbi, M., Bollaert, R., Dupuis, S., Erk, T., Kalantar-Zadeh, K., Kovesdy, C., Osafo, C., Riella, M.C., Zakharova, E., 2017. Obesity and kidney disease: hidden consequences of the epidemic. Kidney Int. 15231755. 91 (2), 260–262. Available from: https://www.journals.elsevier.com/kidney-international. doi:10.1016/j.kint.2016.10.019.

Li, T., Gua, C., Wu, B., Chen, Y., 2018. Increased circulating trimethylamine N-oxide contributes to endothelial dysfunction in a rat model of chronic kidney disease. Biochem. Biophys. Res. Commun. 10902104. 495 (2), 2071–2077. Available from: http://www.sciencedirect.com/science/journal/0006291X. doi:10.1016/j.bbrc.2017.12.069.

Li, X., Xiao, F., Zhang, S., 2021. Coronary revascularisation in patients with chronic kidney disease and end-stage renal disease: a meta-analysis. Int. J. Clin. Pract. 17421241. 75 (11). Available from: http://onlinelibrary.wiley.com/journal/10.1111/(ISSN)1742-1241. doi:10.1111/ijcp.14506.

London, G.M., Guerin, A.P., Sj, M., 1995. Pathophysiology of left ventricular dysfunction in end-stage renal disease. Nephrol. Dial. Transplant. 10, 36–39.

Luo, C., wang, Q., Nong, S., Chen, Y., Longchang, L., Gui, C., 2023. Meta-analysis of clinical adverse events after CABG vs. PCI in patients with chronic kidney disease and coronary artery disease. BMC Cardiovasc. Disord. 1471-2261. 23 (1). doi:10.1186/s12872-023-03560-w.

Marrouche, N.F., Brachmann, J., Andresen, D., Siebels, J., Boersma, L., Jordaens, L., Merkely, B., Pokushalov, E., Sanders, P., Proff, J., Schunkert, H., Christ, H., Vogt, J., Bänsch, D., 2018. Catheter ablation for atrial fibrillation with heart failure. N. Engl. J. Med. 15334406. 378 (5), 417–427. Available from: http://www.nejm.org/medical-index. doi:10.1056/NEJMoa1707855.

Mehta, R., Cai, X., Sood, M.M., 2015. Uremic toxins and cardiovascular disease: pathogenesis and risk factors. Clin. Nephrol. 83 (4), 223–235. doi:10.5414/CN108054.

Moradi, H., Sica, D.A., Kalantar-Zadeh, K., 2013. Cardiovascular burden associated with uremic toxins in patients with chronic kidney disease. Am J. Nephrol. 38 (2), 136–148.

Mullens, W., Abrahams, Z., Francis, G.S., Sokos, G., Taylor, D.O., Starling, R.C., Young, J.B., Tang, W.H.W., 2009. Importance of venous congestion for worsening of renal function in advanced decompensated heart failure. J. Am. Coll. Cardiol. 07351097. 53 (7), 589–596. doi:10.1016/j.jacc.2008.05.068.

Nakanishi, T., Nanami, M., Kuragano, T., 2020. The pathogenesis of CKD complications; Attack of dysregulated iron and phosphate metabolism. Free Radic. Biol. Med. 18734596. 157, 55–62. Available from: https://www.elsevier.com/locate/freeradbiomed.. doi:10.1016/j.freeradbiomed.2020.01.024.

Neuberg, G.W., Miller, A.B., O'Connor, C.M., Belkin, R.N., Carson, P.E., Cropp, A.B., Frid, D.J., Nye, R.G., Pressler, M.L., Wertheimer, J.H., Packer, M., PRAISE Investigators, 2002. Diuretic resistance predicts mortality in patients with advanced heart failure. Am. Heart J. 144 (1), 31–38. doi:10.1067/mhj.2002.123456.

Nishimoto, M., Griffin, K.A., Wynne, B.M., Fujita, T., 2024. Salt-sensitive hypertension and the kidney. Hypertension. 15244563. 81 (6), 1206–1217. Available from: https://www.ahajournals.org/journal/hyp. doi:10.1161/HYPERTENSIONAHA.123.21369.

Nishizawa, H., Maeda, N., Shimomura, I., 2022. Impact of hyperuricemia on chronic kidney disease and atherosclerotic cardiovascular disease. Hypertens. Res. 13484214. 45 (4), 635–640. Available from: http://www.nature.com/hr/archive/index.html. doi:10.1038/s41440-021-00840-w.

Ohtake, T., Kobayashi, S., Moriya, H., Negishi, K., Okamoto, K., Maesato, K., Saito, S., 2005. High prevalence of occult coronary artery stenosis in patients with chronic kidney disease at the initiation of renal replacement therapy: an angiographic examination. J. Am. Soc. Nephrol. 10466673. 16 (4), 1141–1148. Available from: https://journals.lww.com/jasn/pages/default.aspx. doi:10.1681/ASN.2004090765.

Packer, D.L., Mark, D.B., Robb, R.A., 2019. Catheter ablation versus antiarrhythmic drug therapy for atrial fibrillation: the CABANA trial. J. Am. Coll. Cardiol. 74 (3), 292–303.

Raj, D.S., Safar, M.E., 2007. Hypertension in chronic kidney disease: role of arterial stiffness. Am. J. Nephrol. 28 (6), 891–899. doi:10.1159/000108941.

Rangaswami, J., Bhalla, V., Blair, J.E.A., Chang, T.I., Costa, S., Lentine, K.L., Lerma, E.V., Mezue, K., Molitch, M., Mullens, W., Ronco, C., Tang, W.H.W., Mccullough, P.A., 2019. Cardiorenal syndrome: classification, pathophysiology, diagnosis, and treatment strategies: a scientific statement from the American Heart Association. Circulation 15244539. 139 (16), E840. Available from: http://circ.ahajournals.org. doi:10.1161/CIR.0000000000000664.

Ronco, C., Haapio, M., House, A.A., Anavekar, N., Bellomo, R., 2008. Cardiorenal Syndrome. J. Am. Coll. Cardiol. 07351097. 52 (19), 1527–1539. Available from: https://www.elsevier.com/locate/jacc.. doi:10.1016/j.jacc.2008.07.051.

Roumeliotis, S., Mallamaci, F., Zoccali, C., 2020. Endothelial dysfunction in chronic kidney disease, from biology to clinical outcomes: a 2020 update. J. Clin. Med. 2077-0383. 9 (8), 2359. doi:10.3390/jcm9082359.

Salman, I.M., 2015. Cardiovascular autonomic dysfunction in chronic kidney disease: a comprehensive review. Curr. Hypertens. Rep. 15343111. 17 (8). Available from: https://www.springer.com.. doi:10.1007/s11906-015-0571-z.

Scarpioni, R., 2012. Treatment of dyslipidemia in chronic kidney disease: effectiveness and safety of statins. World J. Nephrol. 2220-6124. 1 (6), 184. doi:10.5527/wjn.v1.i6.184.

Schwarz, U., Buzello, M., Ritz, E., Stein, G., Raabe, G., Wiest, G., Mall, G., Amann, K., 2000. Morphology of coronary atherosclerotic lesions in patients with end-stage renal failure. Nephrol. Dial. Transplant. 1460-2385. 15 (2), 218–223. doi:10.1093/ndt/15.2.218.

Singh, A.K., Kari, J.A., Metry, G., 2003. Limitations of the exercise stress test in end-stage renal disease. Nephrol. Dial. Transplant. 18 (7), 1375–1378.

Sligl, W., McAlister, F.A., Ezekowitz, J., Armstrong, P.W., 2004. Usefulness of spironolactone in a specialized heart failure clinic. Am. J. Cardiol. 94 (4), 443–447. doi:10.1016/j.amjcard.2004.04.059.

Six, I., Maizel, J., Barreto, F.C., Rangrez, A.Y., Dupont, S., Slama, M., Tribouilloy, C., Choukroun, G., Mazière, J.C., Bode-Boeger, S., Kielstein, J.T., Drüeke, T.B., Massy, Z.A., 2012. Effects of phosphate on vascular function under normal conditions and influence of the uraemic state. Cardiovasc. Res. 17553245. 96 (1), 130–139. doi:10.1093/cvr/cvs240.

Stenvinkel, P., Carrero, J.J., Axelsson, J., Lindholm, B., Heimbürger, O., Massy, Z., 2008. Emerging biomarkers for evaluating cardiovascular risk in the chronic kidney disease patient: how do new pieces fit into the uremic puzzle? Clin. J. Am. Soc. Nephrol. 1555905X. 3 (2), 505–521. doi:10.2215/CJN.03670807.

Suh, S.H., Kim, S.W., 2023. Dyslipidemia in patients with chronic kidney disease: an updated overview. Diabetes Metab. J. 22336087. 47 (5), 612–629. Available from: https://www.e-dmj.org/upload/pdf/dmj-2023-0067.pdf. doi:10.4093/dmj.2023.0067.

Tang, W.H.W., Mullens, W., 2010. Cardiorenal syndrome in decompensated heart failure. Heart. 1355-6037. 96 (4), 255–260. doi:10.1136/hrt.2009.166256.

Thaden, J.J., Nkomo, V.T., Enriquez-Sarano, M., 2020. Aortic stenosis in CKD: multidisciplinary perspectives. J. Am. Coll. Cardiol. 75 (12), 1529–1539.

Tobe, A., Sawano, M., Kohsaka, S., Ishii, H., Tanaka, A., Numasawa, Y., Amano, T., Nakamura, M., Ikari, Y., Murohara, T., 2023. Ischemic and bleeding outcomes in patients who underwent percutaneous coronary intervention with chronic kidney disease or dialysis (from a Japanese nationwide registry). Am. J. Cardiol. 18791913. 195, 37–44. Available from: https://www.elsevier.com/locate/amjcard.. doi:10.1016/j.amjcard.2023.02.027.

Vahanian, A., Beyersdorf, F., Praz, F., Milojevic, M., Baldus, S., Bauersachs, J., Capodanno, D., Conradi, L., De Bonis, M., De Paulis, R., Delgado, V., Freemantle, N., Gilard, M., Haugaa, K.H., Jeppsson, A., Jüni, P., Pierard, L., Prendergast, B.D., Sádaba, J.R., Tribouilloy, C., Wojakowski, W., Neumann, F.-J., Myers, P., Abdelhamid, M., Achenbach, S., Asteggiano, R., Barili, F., Borger, M.A., Carrel, T., Collet, J.-P., Foldager, D., Habib, G., Hassager, C., Irs, A., Iung, B., Jahangiri, M., Katus, H.A., Koskinas, K.C., Massberg, S., Mueller, C.E., Nielsen, J.C., Pibarot, P., Rakisheva, A., Roffi, M., Rubboli, A., Shlyakhto, E., Siepe, M., Sitges, M., Sondergaard, L., Sousa-Uva, M., Tarantini, G., Zamorano, J.L., Praz, F., Milojevic, M., Baldus, S., Bauersachs, J., Capodanno, D., Conradi, L., De Bonis, M., De Paulis, R., Delgado, V., Freemantle, N., Gilard, M., Haugaa, K.H., Jeppsson, A., Jüni, P., Pierard, L., Prendergast, B.D., Sádaba, J.R., Tribouilloy, C., Wojakowski, W., Benchabi, Y., Chilingaryan, A., Metzler, B., Rustamova, Y., Shumavets, V., Lancellotti, P., Smajic, E., Trendafilova-Lazarova, D., Samardzic, J., Karakyriou, M., Palecek, T., Dahl, J.S., Meshaal, M.S., Palm, K., Virtanen, M., Bouleti, C., Bakhutashvili, Z., Achenbach, S., Boutsikou, M., Béla Kertész, A., Danielsen, R., Topilsky, Y., Golino, P., Tuleutayev, R., Elezi, S., Kerimkulov, A., Rudzitis, A., Glaveckaite, S., Sow, R., Demarco, D.C., Bulatovic, N., Aouad, A., van den Brink, R., Antova, E., Beitnes, J.O., Ochala, A., Ribeiras, R., Vinereanu, D., Irtyuga, O., Ivanovic, B., Simkova, I., González Gómez, A., Sarno, G., Pedrazzini, G.B., Bsata, W., Zakhama, L., Korkmaz, L., Cherniuk, S., Khanji, M.Y., Sharipov, I., 2021. ESC/EACTS Guidelines for the management of valvular heart disease. Eur. Heart J. 0195-668X. 43 (7), 561–632. doi:10.1093/eurheartj/ehab395.

Van Gelder, I.C., Hagens, V.E., Bosker, H.A., Kingma, J.H., Kamp, O., Kingma, T., Said, S.A., Darmanata, J.I., Timmermans, A.J.M., Tijssen, J.G.P., Crijns, H.J.G.M., 2002. A comparison of rate control and rhythm control in patients with recurrent persistent atrial fibrillation. N. Engl. J. Med. 00284793. 347 (23), 1834–1840. doi:10.1056/NEJMoa021375.

Vaziri, N.D., 2004. Role of oxidative stress in the pathogenesis of hypertension. Korean J Nephrol. 23 (Suppl), 420-424.

Virani, S.A., Khosla, A., Levin, A., 2008. Chronic kidney disease, heart failure and anemia. Can. J. Cardiol. 0828282X. 24, 22B. doi:10.1016/s0828-282x(08)71026-2.

Wang, L.W., Fahim, M.A., Hayen, A., 2015. Cardiac testing for coronary artery disease in potential kidney transplant recipients. Am. J. Kidney Dis. 66 (5), 782–791.

Winton, F.R., 1931. The influence of venous pressure on the isolated mammalian kidney. J. Physiol. 0022-3751. 72 (1), 49–61. doi:10.1113/jphysiol.1931.sp002761.

Wu, I.W., Hsu, K.H., Hsu, H.J., Lee, C.C., Sun, C.Y., Tsai, C.J., et al., 2011. Serum free p-cresyl sulfate levels predict cardiovascular and all-cause mortality in elderly hemodialysis patients. Nephrol. Dial. Transplant. 26 (3), 938–947.

Wyse, D.G., Waldo, A.L., DiMarco, J.P., Domanski, M.J., Rosenberg, Y., Schron, E.B., Kellen, J.C., Greene, H.L., Mickel, M.C., Dalquist, J.E., Corley, S.D., 2002. A comparison of rate control and rhythm control in patients with atrial fibrillation. N. Engl. J. Med. 00284793. 347 (23), 1825–1833. Available from: http://www.nejm.org/medical-index. doi:10.1056/NEJMoa021328.

Young, M.J., Funder, J.W., 2002. Mineralocorticoid receptors and pathophysiological roles for aldosterone in the cardiovascular system. J. Hypertens. 02636352. 20 (8), 1465–1468. Available from: http://journals.lww.com/jhypertension. doi:10.1097/00004872-200208000-00002.

CHAPTER

26

Benefits of renin angiotensin aldosterone system blockage

Faruk Hilmi Turgut[a] *and Emaad M. Abdel-Rahman*[b]

[a]**Department of Internal Medicine, Division of Nephrology, Hatay Mustafa Kemal University, Hatay, Turkey**

[b]**Division of Nephrology, University of Virginia, Charlottesville, VA, United States**

Introduction

The renin-angiotensin-aldosterone system (RAAS) is a hormonal cascade that regulates blood pressure (BP) and sodium and water balance (Fig. 26.1).

Chronic activation of the RAAS can lead to pathological remodeling of the heart and blood vessels (Forrester et al., 2018). The RAAS plays an important role in the pathophysiology of hypertension, heart failure, and chronic kidney disease (CKD) (Forrester et al., 2018). Inhibition of this system results in decreased circulating levels and biological activity of angiotensin II, leading to vasodilation, reduced aldosterone secretion, and diminished sympathetic nervous system activity. Pharmacological blockade of the RAAS is an effective therapeutic strategy for hypertension, cardiovascular disease, and CKD. However, the older adult population has specific physiological changes that render them particularly susceptible to complications from RAAS blockade.

Components and effects of the RAAS

The RAAS includes three significant compounds: renin, angiotensin II, and aldosterone. The cascade of RAAS initiates the production of renin, an acid protease, by the juxtaglomerular apparatus in the kidney.

Renin release is triggered by low BP, sympathetic nervous system activity, and various hormones, including angiotensin II, endothelin, prostaglandins, vasopressin, dopamine, and nitric oxide. Renin then converts angiotensinogen, produced by the liver, to angiotensin I,

https://doi.org/10.1016/B978-0-443-34069-7.00030-6

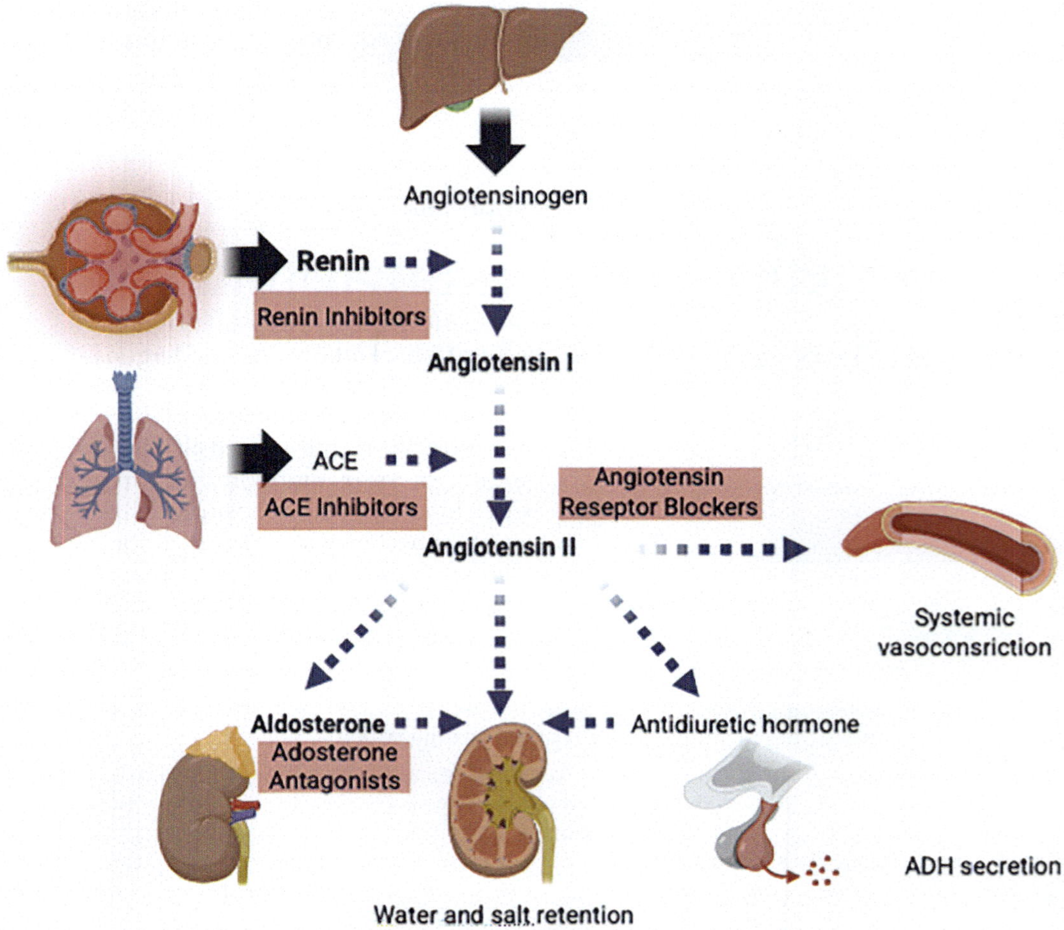

FIG. 26.1 The renin–angiotensin–aldosterone system (RAAS) pathway and sites of pharmacological intervention. The RAAS regulates blood pressure and fluid balance. Angiotensinogen from the liver is converted by renin (from the kidney) into angiotensin I, which is then converted by ACE (from the lungs) into angiotensin II. Angiotensin II causes vasoconstriction, aldosterone release, and ADH secretion, leading to sodium and water retention. Key drug classes—renin inhibitors, ACE inhibitors, ARBs, and aldosterone antagonists—block this cascade at different steps.

the rate-limiting step in this cascade. Subsequently, angiotensin-converting enzyme (ACE) transforms angiotensin I into angiotensin II.

Angiotensin II, the key effector of the RAAS, acts through two distinct G protein-coupled receptors: AT_1 and AT_2. The AT_1 receptor is strongly associated with the adverse pathological effects of the RAAS. AT_1 receptors are expressed in a wide variety of organs. The AT_1 receptor mediates vasoconstriction, cellular growth and proliferation, oxidative stress, and inflammation (Colin et al., 2023). Activation of AT_1 receptor directly promotes vasoconstriction of the vessels and sodium reabsorption in the proximal tubule of the kidney. In contrast to the AT_1 receptor, the AT_2 receptor mediates opposing physiological effects. The activation of the AT2 receptor leads to vasodilation, antiproliferative, and pro-apoptotic effects (Steckelings et al., 2022).

Angiotensin II, primarily through activation of the AT_1 receptor, stimulates the adrenal cortex to release aldosterone. Aldosterone acts on the distal nephron (the distal tubules and collecting ducts of the kidneys) to regulate sodium and potassium homeostasis. It increases sodium reabsorption and potassium excretion. In addition to its established role in the physiological regulation of water, sodium, and potassium homeostasis, aldosterone modulates a spectrum of physiological and pathological processes within the cardiovascular system. It promotes end-organ fibrosis in the vasculature, heart, and kidneys (Buffolo et al., 2022). This contributes to vascular stiffening and atherosclerosis, cardiac remodeling and heart failure, and renal fibrosis and progression of CKD (Forrester et al., 2018; Colin et al., 2023). As a result, elevated plasma aldosterone is a recognized risk factor for the development of cardiovascular disease.

Besides the systemic effects of RAAS, there is evidence for the existence of local and tissue-specific RAAS, including localized RAAS effects on the kidney (Yang and Xu, 2017). Local RAAS performs organ-specific functions and can function independently or in close interaction with the systemic RAAS components. Local RAAS activation can occur even when the systemic RAAS is suppressed, potentially leading to organ damage.

The RAAS can be inhibited by four different drug classes: direct renin inhibitors, ACE inhibitors, angiotensin receptor blockers (ARBs), and aldosterone receptor antagonists. ACE inhibitors were the first RAAS inhibitors, and numerous ACE inhibitors are currently synthesized and used clinically. ACE inhibitors competitively inhibit the ACE enzyme, thereby preventing the conversion of angiotensin I to angiotensin II and effectively blocking the downstream effects of angiotensin II. They also reduce aldosterone and vasopressin secretion. ACE inhibitors lower BP in a dose-dependent manner and promote vasodilation in vital organs, including the kidneys. Chronic use of ACE inhibitors triggers ACE escape pathways, and angiotensin II is produced despite the blockage of ACE. ACE inhibitors not only prevent the formation of angiotensin II but also increase bradykinin, which contributes to vasodilation through the kinin-kallikrein system. However, elevated bradykinin may cause the development of cough and angioedema in some patients taking ACE inhibitors.

Over a decade after the initial use of ACE inhibitors, ARBs were discovered. ARBs work by directly blocking angiotensin II from binding to AT_1 receptors, preserving the potential beneficial effects of angiotensin II via the AT_2 receptor pathway. ARBs reduce blood pressure by decreasing systemic vascular resistance. ARBs have minimal impact on bradykinin levels, thereby significantly lowering the risk of cough and angioedema compared to ACE inhibitors. Moreover, direct receptor blockade eliminates the angiotensin II escape phenomenon.

The efficacy of ACE inhibitors and ARBs in blocking the RAAS for various diseases is now widely recognized. Despite their proven benefits, they do not completely inhibit RAAS activity, possibly due to angiotensin and aldosterone escape phenomena. The occurrence of these feedback effects highlights the need for alternative approaches to achieve more effective RAAS blockade. Prolonged use of ACE inhibitors or ARBs leads to increased renin activity, suggesting that direct renin inhibition may offer superior benefits. Renin inhibitors prevent the formation of renin, thereby blocking the synthesis of all angiotensin peptides downstream. Aliskiren is the first in a new class of oral direct renin inhibitors. The U.S. Food and Drug Administration (FDA) approved it for hypertension in 2007. Aliskiren provides effective blockade, resulting in beneficial effects such as reduced blood pressure, decreased proteinuria, and improvement in kidney fibrosis and inflammation (Feldman et al., 2008). The safety and tolerability of aliskiren in older adults have been evaluated through multiple trials (Verdecchia et al., 2007).

Aldosterone represents a critical component of the RAAS system. It regulates fluid volume by increasing sodium reabsorption via the mineralocorticoid receptor (MR) in the distal nephron's collecting duct cells. ACE inhibitors and ARBs can initially lower aldosterone, but it may return to normal levels subsequently, a phenomenon known as aldosterone escape. Overactivation of MR is another critical factor in the pathogenesis of hypertension, cardiovascular disease, and kidney disease (Buffolo et al., 2022). The development of selective aldosterone antagonists is highly anticipated due to their potential to protect the heart and kidneys beyond their diuretic properties. Spironolactone, the first steroidal aldosterone antagonist developed in 1960, has been widely used to treat primary hyperaldosteronism, edema, hypertension, and low potassium. However, its side effects often lead to poor tolerability. Eplerenone was developed in 1987 as a modified version of spironolactone. The higher selectivity of eplerenone for the aldosterone receptor results in a lower likelihood of adverse effects compared to spironolactone. The efficacy of aldosterone antagonists in improving cardiovascular outcomes is well documented (Pitt et al., 1999). However, they remain underutilized due to the associated risk of inducing hyperkalemia, impotence, and gynecomastia.

Finerenone, a novel, highly selective, nonsteroidal MR antagonist, was developed to address the limitations of steroidal MR antagonists. The FDA approved finerenone in 2021, making it the first nonsteroidal MR antagonist (MRA) available commercially. Finerenone shows greater potency than eplerenone, equivalent potency to spironolactone, and superior selectivity over both in MR inhibition. Beyond finerenone, additional MRAs (ocedurenone, esaxerenone) are undergoing preclinical and clinical evaluation for their potential therapeutic utility in the management of hypertension and CKD (Bakris et al., 2021; Ito et al., 2020). MRAs exhibit significant therapeutic potential in the management of cardiorenal disease (Shah et al., 2023).

Changes in RAAS with aging

The RAAS plays a crucial role in the functional, structural, and mechanical alterations of the vasculature that accompany hypertension and cardiovascular events. The RAAS is identified as a major contributor to vascular changes in both aging individuals and hypertensive patients.

Pathophysiological and mechanistic changes with aging

The chronic stimulation of RAAS is implicated in the pathogenesis of age-associated end-organ damage (Musso and Jauregui, 2014). Angiotensin II modulates energy metabolism and influences the initiation and progression of cellular senescence. Accumulating evidence suggests that angiotensin II serves as a pivotal mediator in both physiological and pathological processes within the heart, kidney, and brain. It induces inflammation, cellular proliferation, and reactive oxygen species generation at both cellular and mitochondrial levels, leading to cell senescence and accelerating the process of vascular aging and arterial stiffness (Conti et al., 2012; Feng et al., 2011; Neves et al., 2018). Preclinical studies provide evidence that RAAS blockers exert a beneficial effect on cellular senescence (Feng et al., 2011).

There is a gradual decline in mean plasma renin activity and plasma renin levels during each decade of life from puberty onward (Bauer, 1993). The influence of age on plasma renin activity and aldosterone becomes more evident under stimulated conditions, such as upright posture and dietary sodium restriction, compared to basal states. Age-related nephrosclerosis is thought to cause a decrease in plasma renin activity in older adults (Messerli et al., 1983). In the same manner, both plasma aldosterone levels and its excretion in urine decrease progressively with advancing age (Bauer, 1993). Similarly, age-related reductions in hepatic angiotensinogen synthesis may contribute to the observed decline in RAAS activity (Belmin et al., 1994). A compensatory upregulation of angiotensin II receptor density in older adults partially mitigates this reduction (Wray et al., 2008). The age-related changes in the RAAS are also observed in the kidney and disrupt fluid and electrolyte balance, leading to increased risks of hyponatremia due to impaired sodium conservation and reduced tubular concentrating ability. Additionally, the risk of hyperkalemia increases as the transtubular potassium gradient is reduced in older adults (Musso and Jauregui, 2014; Yoon and Choi, 2014). This modest decrease in renin and aldosterone activity raises concerns about the risk-benefit profile of RAAS blocker use in older adults.

Benefits of RAAS blockers

Experimental and clinical studies consistently show that blocking the RAAS protects the heart, kidneys, and brain from age-related damage, beyond just lowering BP (Feng et al., 2011; Benigni et al., 2011). RAAS blockade represents a cornerstone of cardiovascular and renal protection, offering significant clinical benefits through various mechanisms (Table 26.1). All classes of RAAS blockers are primarily used in a variety of clinical conditions, including hypertension, coronary artery disease, heart failure, and CKD.

Cardiovascular benefits

ACE inhibitors and ARBs are largely similarly effective in lowering BP and preventing major cardiovascular events in essential hypertension, yet ARBs are generally better tolerated

TABLE 26.1 Beneficial physiological effects of RAAS inhibitors.

Effect	Main mechanism
Antihypertensive	Attenuate vasoconstriction, reduction in peripheral vascular resistance
Renoprotection	Reduction in glomerular capillary pressure, antifibrotic effects
Cardioprotection	Reduction in cardiac afterload and preload, improvement in ventricular remodeling
Endothelial function	Reduction in vascular remodeling

and considered valuable alternatives, particularly for those who experience cough or angioedema.

The evidence base for RAAS blocker use in older adults is limited. Multiple clinical trials have found that RAAS blockers effectively lower BP compared to other drugs and demonstrate lower morbidity and mortality in this population (Turgut et al., 2010). Starting BP medication with ACE inhibitors seems to lead to better results in older adults, especially men, compared to starting with diuretics, even when both lower BP by the same amount (Wing et al., 2003). The Hypertension in the Very Elderly (HYVET) trial further emphasized the efficacy of the ACE inhibitor perindopril in reducing heart failure events in patients aged 80 years and older (Beckett et al., 2008). The Second Australian National Blood Pressure Study (ANBP2) demonstrated that ACE inhibitors, compared to diuretics, led to fewer adverse events and improved cardiovascular outcomes in older adults aged 65–84 with hypertension, especially in men (Wing et al., 2003).

ARBs exhibit beneficial effects in many clinical studies involving older adult patients (Turgut et al., 2010). The Study on Cognition and Prognosis in the Elderly (SCOPE) trial found that candesartan, an ARB, significantly lowered systolic and diastolic BP and reduced cardiovascular events by 11% compared to placebo in hypertensive adults aged 70–89 (Lithell et al., 2003). A meta-analysis of 25 studies (N = 4487, ages 60–79) found that olmesartan was more effective than active control in reducing BP and achieving BP goals in older adult patients with hypertension. This benefit was also observed in older adult patients with impaired renal function (Redon et al., 2018). Olmesartan was well tolerated in older hypertensive patients (Redon et al., 2018). In addition, olmesartan provided a greater 24-h blood pressure effect than ramipril in patients aged 65–89 (Omboni et al., 2012).

ACE inhibitors and ARBs are associated with a reduced risk of mortality in older adult patients with atrial fibrillation (Menichelli et al., 2024). A metaanalysis of heart failure with reduced ejection fraction trials showed benefits in younger patients but inconclusive results in those over 75 due to limitations in sample size (Flather et al., 2000). Conversely, observational studies, such as the Euro Heart Failure Survey II and the US National Heart Care Project, suggest RAAS blockers may improve survival in older and very old adult patients (Komajda et al., 2009; Masoudi et al., 2004). RAAS blockers seem to be most effective in patients with comorbidities, such as congestive heart failure and diabetes.

There were minimal to no differences noted between ACE inhibitors and ARBs in systolic and diastolic BP control across the studies. According to Cochrane analyses, ARBs and ACE inhibitors are equally effective in preventing death and cardiovascular events in the general population (Li et al., 2014). The Ongoing Telmisartan Alone and in Combination with Ramipril Global Endpoint Trial (ONTARGET) trial showed that telmisartan was as effective as ramipril in lowering BP in patients with vascular disease or diabetes (Yusuf et al., 2008). This study also found no difference in myocardial infarction and cardiovascular mortality rates between the two treatments. While specific studies comparing ACE inhibitors and ARBs in older adult patients are not available, the available data show that both these groups reduce BP, improve cardiovascular outcomes, and are well tolerated in older adults.

The renin inhibitor aliskiren demonstrated a dose-dependent reduction in both systolic and diastolic BP, with the BP-lowering effect being similar to ACE inhibitors and ARBs in older adults (Verdecchia et al., 2007; Musini et al., 2017). The older adult population with systolic hypertension experienced better BP control and overall treatment outcomes with aliskiren compared to ramipril (Duprez et al., 2010).

Conflicting results arose regarding the clinical benefits of aliskiren in managing cardiovascular diseases. While some studies suggest positive outcomes in managing cardiovascular diseases, a larger number of studies and meta-analyses have found no significant benefits and even reported an increased risk of hypotension, without any reduction in major cardiovascular events (MACE) or death (Zhao et al., 2020; Bjerre et al., 2019). Current evidence suggests that renin inhibitors and ACE inhibitors may have comparable effects on mortality and heart attack risk, though this remains uncertain. They also appear to have similar rates of adverse events (Wang et al., 2020). Based on the limited data, aliskiren appears to be effective at lowering BP and is also well tolerated by older patients with hypertension, but with uncertain benefits on MACE.

A number of previous studies have shown that blockage of the MR prevents cardiovascular diseases. The Randomized Aldactone Evaluation Study (RALES) study revealed that spironolactone significantly improved survival outcomes in patients with severe heart failure (Pitt et al., 1999). Eplerenone, when added to standard therapy, further decreased overall and cardiovascular mortality (Pitt et al., 2003).

The Finerenone in Reducing Cardiovascular Mortality and Morbidity in Diabetic Kidney Disease (FIGARO-DKD) trial revealed that finerenone, relative to placebo, yielded a 13% reduction in the primary composite cardiovascular outcome, encompassing cardiovascular death, nonfatal myocardial infarction, nonfatal stroke, or hospitalization for heart failure (HR: 0.87; 95% CI: 0.76–0.98) (Pitt et al., 2021). Finerenone administration in patients with heart failure improved cardiovascular risks, including deaths from any cause, cardiovascular events, and renal outcomes (Vardeny et al., 2025; Vaduganathan et al., 2024). There are limited dedicated, prospective clinical trials designed to investigate the effects of finerenone in older adults. In a prespecified analysis of phase III trials, finerenone demonstrated improvements in cardiovascular and renal composite outcomes across all age groups (Bansal et al., 2024).

Cerebrovascular benefits

Prospective clinical studies consistently show a strong, continuous, and increasing link between BP (especially systolic BP) and the risk of both ischemic and hemorrhagic stroke (Bushnell et al., 2024). Effective BP control is vital for preventing primary (and secondary) strokes. Generally, most types of BP-lowering medications are similarly effective in reducing the risk of both fatal and nonfatal cardiovascular events, with equivalent BP lowering (Thomopoulos et al., 2018). In adults with hypertension, diuretics, calcium channel blockers, ACE inhibitors, and ARBs are recommended as initial antihypertensive drug therapies to prevent stroke (Bushnell et al., 2024).

The RAAS seems to play a role in causing acute ischemic stroke and interacts with other stroke risk factors. Both ACE inhibitors and ARBs have shown positive therapeutic potential in managing stroke, independent of their ability to reduce BP. When comparing different antihypertensive drug classes, ACE inhibitors and ARBs are superior to placebo but inferior to diuretics and calcium channel blockers in preventing strokes (Thomopoulos et al., 2018). The HYVET trial, in patients aged > 80 years, demonstrated a reduction in both fatal and nonfatal strokes (Beckett et al., 2008). The combination of both ACE inhibitors and calcium channel blockers may provide enhanced protection against stroke compared to ACE inhibitors or ARBs monotherapy (Yu et al., 2025). Ramipril showed benefits in secondary stroke prevention in a subgroup analysis of the HOPE study (Bosch et al., 2002). On the other hand, the ONTARGET study found no difference between telmisartan and ramipril in primary stroke prevention (Yusuf et al., 2008). Direct comparisons of ACE inhibitors versus ARBs for stroke prevention are lacking, but based on existing data, they are generally considered to be equally effective.

It is well demonstrated that older adult patients have an increased risk of dementia and cognitive dysfunction related to hypertension. Clinical studies on RAAS blocker use in older adults have yielded conflicting results regarding their potential role in reducing dementia risk or slowing the progression from mild cognitive impairment to dementia, with some studies suggesting a benefit, while others have not been able to establish any clear association (Hajjar et al., 2020; Lennon et al., 2023; Anderson et al., 2011; Orchard et al., n.d.). Studies have also suggested that ARBs may be more effective than ACE inhibitors in reducing the risk of dementia (Hajjar et al., 2020; Orchard et al., n.d.; Deng et al., 2022).

Renal benefits

RAAS blockade offers benefits to the kidneys beyond lowering systemic BP. These benefits include reducing intraglomerular pressure and proteinuria, thus delaying CKD progression (Abdel-Rahman and Reeves, 2012). For diabetic patients with early or established kidney disease (microalbuminuria or CKD), both ACE inhibitors and ARBs are effective in reducing proteinuria, slowing kidney disease progression, and delaying end-stage kidney disease (Abdel-Rahman and Reeves, 2012; Parving et al., 2001; Brenner et al., 2001). Consequently, current guidelines recommend RAAS blockers as first-line treatment for high BP in patients with diabetic and nondiabetic kidney disease, especially those with proteinuria (Kidney Disease: Improving Global Outcomes CKDWG, 2024).

A subgroup analysis of the Reduction of Endpoints in NIDDM with the Angiotensin II Antagonist Losartan (RENAAL) trial showed that losartan provided the same kidney protection in patients over 65 with type 2 diabetes and macroalbuminuria as it did in the entire study group when compared to placebo, indicating its equal effectiveness in older adult patients with albuminuria (Winkelmayer et al., 2006). In a retrospective study of patients aged ≥ 70 years, ACEIs and ARBs were found to be equally effective in terms of the risks of MACE as well as the side effects of acute kidney injury (AKI) and hyperkalemia (Forrester et al., 2018). ACE inhibitors and ARBs provide similar renal benefits in CKD. Renal benefits with RAAS blockers extend beyond diabetic patients to nondiabetic CKD patients with proteinuria; ACE inhibitors have shown renal benefits, but ARB studies are scarce. Aliskiren demonstrated beneficial effects in older adult hypertensive patients with CKD by lowering BP and albuminuria, and preserving kidney function (Morishita et al., 2012).

Aldosterone receptor antagonists, spironolactone and eplerenone, effectively reduce BP and proteinuria and enhance this effect when used in conjunction with ACE inhibitors or ARBs (Chung et al., 2020). In the phase III clinical trial program, the Finerenone in Reducing Kidney Failure and Disease Progression in Diabetic Kidney Disease (FIDELIO-DKD) trial showed that finerenone, compared to placebo, reduced the occurrence of the primary composite kidney endpoint, defined as the time to onset of kidney failure, a sustained ≥ 40% decline in estimated glomerular filtration rate from baseline, or death from renal causes, by 18% (HR 0.82; 95% CI 0.73–0.93) (Bakris et al., 2020). Finerenone also improved cardiovascular outcomes and reduced albuminuria in diabetic patients with CKD stage 4 (Sarafidis et al., 2023).

The benefit of RAAS blockers in slowing CKD progression may be limited in older adult patients. In a small, randomized controlled clinical trial, RAAS blockers did not demonstrate a reduction in CKD progression in older adult patients with CKD but without diabetes, heart disease, or proteinuria (García-Prieto et al., 2024).

Conflicting clinical studies exist regarding the impact of RAAS blocker discontinuation on renal and cardiovascular outcomes. Stopping RAAS blockers in advanced CKD may even delay the progression of CKD to end-stage kidney disease in older adults (Ahmed et al., 2010). However, the potential benefits, particularly in high-proteinuria cases, sustain the debate regarding their use. Therefore additional data are necessary to understand how RAAS blockers affect CKD progression in older adult patients, particularly in the absence of proteinuria.

Concerns with RAAS blocking in older adults

The most significant potential complications of RAAS-blocking medications are AKI, hyperkalemia, and low BP.

Hyperkalemia

Hyperkalemia is a common clinical problem among patients prescribed RAAS blockers (Adelborg et al., 2019). Hyperkalemia causes cardiac conduction disturbances and can lead to cardiac arrhythmias, cardiac arrest, and sudden death. RAAS blockers can either reduce the production of aldosterone or diminish aldosterone action at the distal nephron, leading to hyperkalemia. Among patients with normal kidney function prescribed RAAS blockers, the increase in serum potassium is generally mild, and severe hyperkalemia is rare. The risk of hyperkalemia increases with concurrent risk factors like diabetes, heart failure, older age, high doses, or taking medications such as beta-blockers, potassium supplements, heparin, or potassium-sparing diuretics. The incidence progressively increases in patients with advancing stages of kidney disease (Sriperumbuduri et al., 2021). The incidence is also higher in patients using a combination of RAAS blockers (Yusuf et al., 2008). The older adult population experiences a higher incidence of hypertension, diabetes, CKD, and heart failure. While RAAS blockers are effective treatments for these conditions, they also independently increase the risk of hyperkalemia.

Hyperkalemia is a limiting factor in the use of RAAS blockers. The development of hyperkalemia should be carefully monitored in patients receiving RAAS blockers. Guidelines advise checking serum potassium 2–4 weeks after starting or increasing the dose of a RAAS inhibitor (Kidney Disease: Improving Global Outcomes CKDWG, 2024).

Management of mild hyperkalemia typically involves restriction of dietary potassium intake, discontinuation or reduced dosing of RAAS blockers, initiation or increased dosing of potassium-wasting diuretics, or administration of oral potassium binders such as sodium polystyrene sulfonate, patiromer, or zirconium cyclosilicate. Hyperkalemia from RAAS blockers can often be managed by lowering potassium levels rather than reducing the dose or stopping the medication. Discontinuing or reducing the dose of RAAS blockers in response to hyperkalemia may lead to suboptimal management of conditions like CKD and congestive heart failure, where the evidence supporting their use is substantial (Qiao et al., 2020). Therefore the decision to discontinue or reduce RAAS blockers after hyperkalemia requires a tailored approach, carefully balancing the potential benefits and harms for each patient.

Acute kidney injury

AKI is a sudden decline in kidney function. The Kidney Disease Improving Global Outcomes (KDIGO) guidelines define AKI using the following criteria: an absolute increase in serum creatinine of ≥ 0.3 mg/dl within 48 h, a relative increase in serum creatinine to ≥ 1.5 times baseline within the preceding 7 days, or a urine output of < 0.5 ml/kg/h for a minimum of 6 h (Kellum and Lameire, 2013). The older adult population is more susceptible to AKI. Several factors contribute to AKI in older adults, including renal hypoperfusion, underlying kidney diseases such as diabetes and hypertension, polypharmacy, and the potential need for more invasive procedures. Older adult patients, particularly those with advanced CKD, face a significantly higher risk of further kidney function decline. ACE inhibitors and ARBs dilate the kidney afferent arterioles and lower the filtration pressure. This can reduce glomerular filtration. It has been recommended to maintain RAAS blocker treatment unless serum creatinine exceeds a 30% increase within four weeks of initiation or dose escalation (Belmin et al., 1994). However, these drugs may potentially cause AKI, particularly during certain clinical conditions (Table 26.2). Dehydration and sepsis increase the risk of AKI associated with RAAS blockers, particularly at high doses of ACE inhibitors (Redon et al., 2018). Arteriosclerosis contributes to reduced renal blood flow and makes older patients highly susceptible to hypovolemia-causing AKI. The combination therapy of RAAS blockers with an NSAID or a diuretic also increases the risk of AKI, especially in older adults with preexisting renal impairment (Chaumont et al., 2016; Lapi et al., 2013).

Despite the limited evidence, there is a growing consensus that ACE inhibitors and ARBs should be withheld during acute illness. In cases of new or progressive AKI without another clear cause, a trial discontinuation of RAAS blockers is a justifiable therapeutic approach.

TABLE 26.2 Conditions increasing the risk of AKI.

Renal hypoperfusion	Hypotension Congestive heart failure (poor cardiac output) Sepsis
Volume depletion	Diuretic use Diarrhea
Renal vascular disease	Bilateral renal artery stenosis Renal artery stenosis of a solitary kidney Diffuse atherosclerosis in small renal vessels.
Afferent arteriolar narrowing	NSAIDs, Cyclosporine
Decreased number of nephrons	Chronic kidney disease

Hypotension

The older adult population has a higher risk of hypotension and subsequent syncope, including those receiving hypertension treatment. There is no universally accepted definition of hypertension specifically for older adults. Hypotension may be symptomatic or asymptomatic, and the clinical significance and implications differ. Some well-known risk factors for hypotension include diabetes, stroke history, severe heart failure, CKD, frailty, and aggressive BP control (Frey et al., 2019). In older adults, it is crucial to avoid hypotension, as RAAS blockers can exacerbate this condition and increase the risk of falls. Careful monitoring of BP, along with modifications in diuretic strategies, can help minimize the risk.

Cough and angioedema

Dry cough is the most frequent side effect of ACE inhibitors. It is likely caused by increased bradykinin levels due to the suppression of kininase II activity by ACE inhibition. It can appear not only soon after starting the medication but also months or even a year later. The reported cough incidence varies widely in different studies and ranges from 5% to 20% (Israili and Hall, 1992). Cough is a class effect occurring with all ACE inhibitors; therefore replacement by another ACE inhibitor should not be tried. It typically resolves within a few days after stopping the medication.

Angioedema, though less common than cough, is a significantly more serious and potentially life-threatening complication. It usually manifests as swelling of the lips, tongue, mouth, larynx, pharynx, or periorbital regions. Angioedema is mediated by vasoactive mediators, particularly bradykinin. ACE inhibitors have a higher incidence of angioedema (0.3%) compared to ARBs (0.13%) (Makani et al., 2012). While some cases occur after a long period (over a year), the highest risk is during the initial period of treatment.

Practical considerations using RAAS blockers for older adults

Starting with lower doses

The use of RAAS blockers is mandated by guidelines due to evidence from randomized clinical trial findings that establish their effectiveness in cardiovascular disease compared to other antihypertensive classes (Kidney Disease: Improving Global Outcomes CKDWG, 2024). In general, RAAS blockers should be administered at the highest approved dose. Hypotension is a common limiting factor in the optimal use of RAAS blockers, more so in older adults. Therapy should be resumed or titrated upwards as quickly as safety permits following a temporary interruption. ACE inhibitor or ARB dose reduction or discontinuation should be considered in cases of symptomatic hypotension, refractory hyperkalemia, or to alleviate uremic symptoms in advanced kidney failure (eGFR < 15 ml/min/1.73 m^2) (Kidney Disease: Improving Global Outcomes CKDWG, 2024).

Regular monitoring

The older adult population can develop life-threatening complications from RAAS blockers. Better monitoring and careful use of these drugs can lower the risk. Blood pressure (BP), serum creatinine, and potassium levels should be monitored 2–4 weeks following RAAS blocker initiation or dose increase, with the timing determined by current GFR and potassium levels (Kidney Disease: Improving Global Outcomes CKDWG, 2024).

Adherence to guideline-recommended monitoring among patients initiating RAAS blocker therapy is low (Schmidt et al., 2017); RAAS blockers should be continued in patients with CKD even when eGFR falls below 30 ml/min per 1.73 m^2. Checking potassium levels regularly reduces the risk of high potassium caused by RAAS blockers, particularly in patients with both diabetes and CKD (Raebel et al., 2010).

Dual RAAS blockade

In theory, the combination of RAAS blockers provides a more complete RAAS blockade, suggesting greater protection. Expectedly, combination therapy demonstrates greater efficacy in reducing BP compared to monotherapy (Izzo et al., 2004). Dual RAAS blockade (ACE inhibitor and ARB) in the ONTARGET trial failed to demonstrate superiority in reducing hard cardiovascular endpoints compared to monotherapy (Yusuf et al., 2008). Aliskiren added to RAAS blockers showed no benefit in type 2 diabetes (Parving et al., 2012). In the Aliskiren Trial on Acute Heart Failure Outcomes (ASTRONAUT) trial, the combination of aliskiren and ARB did not demonstrate a significant improvement in post-discharge mortality and heart failure readmissions. While dual therapy modestly reduced hospitalizations for heart failure, it did not significantly improve overall cardiovascular mortality, even though it did significantly decrease NT-proBNP levels (Gheorghiade et al., 2013). With limited additive efficacy, dual therapy significantly increased the risk of several side effects, including hyperkalemia, hypotension, renal failure, and adverse events leading to treatment withdrawal (Parving et al., 2012; Makani et al., 2013). Due to the clear risk of harm, avoiding any combination of ACE inhibitor, ARB, and direct renin inhibitor therapy is recommended (Kidney Disease: Improving Global Outcomes CKDWG, 2024).

Conclusion

Drug selection for older patients must be tailored to the specific physiological and pathological changes that come with age and any existing comorbidities. The primary focus should be on achieving BP reduction, regardless of the specific drug used. The risk/benefit ratio of RAAS blockers must be considered in older adults, particularly in patients with CKD. Before initiating RAAS blockers in an older adult patient with CKD, the clinician should evaluate the presence of proteinuria, assess the progression risk of CKD, and consider any other health concerns or priorities that might favor an alternative antihypertensive agent.

References

Abdel-Rahman, A., Reeves, A., 2012. Management of diabetic nephropathy in the elderly: special considerations. J. Nephrol. Ther. 2 (5), 124.

Adelborg, K., Nicolaisen, S.K., Hasvold, P., Palaka, E., Pedersen, L., Thomsen, R.W., Shearer, G., 2019. Predictors for repeated hyperkalemia and potassium trajectories in high-risk patients — a population-based cohort study. PLOS One. 1932-6203. 14 (6), e0218739. doi:10.1371/journal.pone.0218739.

Ahmed, A.K., Kamath, N.S., Kossi, M.E., Nahas, A.M.E., 2010. The impact of stopping inhibitors of the renin-angiotensin system in patients with advanced chronic kidney disease. Nephrol. Dial. Transplant. 14602385. 25 (12), 3977–3982. doi:10.1093/ndt/gfp511.

Anderson, C., Teo, K., Gao, P., Arima, H., Dans, A., Unger, T., Commerford, P., Dyal, L., Schumacher, H., Pogue, J., Paolasso, E., Holwerda, N., Chazova, I., Binbrek, A., Young, J., Yusuf, S., 2011. Renin-angiotensin system blockade and cognitive function in patients at high risk of cardiovascular disease: analysis of data from the ONTARGET and TRANSCEND studies. Lancet Neurol. 14744422. 10 (1), 43–53. doi:10.1016/s1474-4422(10)70250-7.

Bakris, G.L., Agarwal, R., Anker, S.D., Pitt, B., Ruilope, L.M., Rossing, P., Kolkhof, P., Nowack, C., Schloemer, P., Joseph, A., Filippatos, G., 2020. Effect of finerenone on chronic kidney disease outcomes in type 2 diabetes. N. Engl. J. Med. 15334406. 383 (23), 2219–2229. Available from: http://www.nejm.org/medical-index. doi:10.1056/NEJMoa2025845.

Bakris, G., Pergola, P.E., Delgado, B., Genov, D., Doliashvili, T., Vo, N., Yang, Y.F., McCabe, J., Benn, V., Pitt, B., 2021. Effect of KBP-5074 on blood pressure in advanced chronic kidney disease: results of the BLOCK-CKD study. Hypertension. 15244563. 78 (1), 74–81. Available from: https://www.ahajournals.org/journal/hyp. doi:10.1161/HYPERTENSIONAHA.121.17073.

Bansal, S., Canziani, M.E.F., Birne, R., Anker, S.D., Bakris, G.L., Filippatos, G., Rossing, P., Ruilope, L.M., Farjat, A.E., Kolkhof, P., Lage, A., Brinker, M., Pitt, B., 2024. Finerenone cardiovascular and kidney outcomes by age and sex: FIDELITY post hoc analysis of two phase 3, multicentre, double-blind trials. BMJ Open. 20446055. 14 (3). Available from: http://bmjopen.bmj.com/content/early/by/section. doi:10.1136/bmjopen-2023-076444.

Bauer, J.H., 1993. Age-related changes in the renin-aldosterone system: physiological effects and clinical implications. Drugs Aging. 11791969. 3 (3), 238–245. doi:10.2165/00002512-199303030-00005.

Beckett, N.S., Peters, R., Fletcher, A.E., Staessen, J.A., Liu, L., Dumitrascu, D., Stoyanovsky, V., Antikainen, R.L., Nikitin, Y., Anderson, C., Belhani, A., Forette, F., Rajkumar, C., Thijs, L., Banya, W., Bulpitt, C.J., 2008. Treatment of hypertension in patients 80 years of age or older. N. Engl. J. Med. 15334406. 358 (18), 1887–1898. Available from: http://content.nejm.org/cgi/reprint/358/18/1887.pdf. doi:10.1056/NEJMoa0801369.

Belmin, J., Lévy, B.I., Michel, J.B., 1994. Changes in the renin-angiotensin-aldosterone axis in later life. Drugs Aging. 11791969. 5 (5), 391–400. doi:10.2165/00002512-199405050-00007.

Benigni, A., Morigi, M., Rizzo, P., Gagliardini, E., Rota, C., Abbate, M., Ghezzi, S., Remuzzi, A., Remuzzi, G., 2011. Inhibiting angiotensin-converting enzyme promotes renal repair by limiting progenitor cell proliferation and restoring the glomerular architecture. Am. J. Pathol. 00029440. 179 (2), 628–638. doi:10.1016/j.ajpath.2011.04.003.

Bjerre, H.L., Christensen, J.B., Buus, N.H., Simonsen, U., Su, J., 2019. The role of aliskiren in the management of hypertension and major cardiovascular outcomes: a systematic review and meta-analysis. J. Hum. Hypertens. 14765527. 33 (11), 795–806. Available from: http://www.nature.com/jhh/index.html. doi:10.1038/s41371-018-0149-8.

Bosch, J., Yusuf, S., Pogue, J., Sleight, P., Lonn, E., Rangoonwala, B., Davies, R., Ostergren, J., Probstfield, J., 2002. Use of ramipril in preventing stroke: double blind randomised trial. BMJ. 09598146. 324 (7339), 699–702.

Brenner, B.M., Cooper, M.E., De Zeeuw, D., Keane, W.F., Mitch, W.E., Parving, H.H., Remuzzi, G., Snapinn, S.M., Zhang, Z., Shahinfar, S., 2001. Effects of losartan on renal and cardiovascular outcomes in patients with type 2 diabetes and nephropathy. N. Engl. J. Med. 00284793. 345 (12), 861–869. doi:10.1056/NEJMoa011161.

Buffolo, F., Tetti, M., Mulatero, P., Monticone, S., 2022. Aldosterone as a mediator of cardiovascular damage. Hypertension. 0194-911X. 79 (9), 1899–1911. doi:10.1161/hypertensionaha.122.17964.

Bushnell, C., Kernan, W.N., Sharrief, A.Z., Chaturvedi, S., Cole, J.W., Cornwell 3rd, W.K., et al., 2024. Guideline for the primary prevention of stroke: a guideline from the american heart association/american stroke association. Stroke 55 (12), e344–e424.

Chaumont, M., Pourcelet, A., van Nuffelen, M., Racapé, J., Leeman, M., Hougardy, J.M., 2016. Acute kidney injury in elderly patients with chronic kidney disease: do angiotensin-converting enzyme inhibitors carry a risk? J. Clin. Hypertens. 17517176. 18 (6), 514–521. Available from: http://onlinelibrary.wiley.com/journal/10.1111/(ISSN)1751-7176. doi:10.1111/jch.12795.

Chung, E.Y.M., Ruospo, M., Natale, P., Bolignano, D., Navaneethan, S.D., Palmer, S.C., Strippoli, G.F.M., 2020. Aldosterone antagonists in addition to renin angiotensin system antagonists for preventing the progression of chronic kidney disease. Cochrane Database Syst. Rev. 14651858. 2020 (10). Available from: https://www.cochranelibrary.com/cdsr/table-of-contents. doi:10.1002/14651858.CD007004.pub4.

Colin, M., Delaitre, C., Foulquier, S., Dupuis, F., 2023. The AT(1)/AT(2) receptor equilibrium is a cornerstone of the regulation of the renin angiotensin system beyond the cardiovascular system. Molecules 28 (14), 5481.

Conti, S., Cassis, P., Benigni, A., 2012. Aging and the renin-angiotensin system. Hypertension. 0194-911X. 60 (4), 878–883. doi:10.1161/hypertensionaha.110.155895.

Deng, Z., Jiang, J., Wang, J., Pan, D., Zhu, Y., Honghong, L., Zhang, X., Liu, X., Yongteng, X., Li, Y., Tang, Y., 2022. Angiotensin receptor blockers are associated with a lower risk of progression from mild cognitive impairment to dementia. Hypertension. 0194-911X. 79 (10), 2159–2169. doi:10.1161/hypertensionaha.122.19378.

Duprez, D.A., Munger, M.A., Botha, J., Keefe, D.L., Charney, A.N., 2010. Aliskiren for geriatric lowering of systolic hypertension: a randomized controlled trial. J. Hum. Hypertens. 14765527. 24 (9), 600–608. doi:10.1038/jhh.2009.107.

Feldman, D.L., Jin, L., Xuan, H., Contrepas, A., Zhou, Y., Webb, R.L., Mueller, D.N., Feldt, S., Cumin, F., Maniara, W., Persohn, E., Schuetz, H., Danser, A.H.J., Nguyen, G., 2008. Effects of aliskiren on blood pressure, albuminuria, and (Pro)renin receptor expression in diabetic TG(mRen-2)27 Rats. Hypertension. 0194911X. 52 (1), 130–136. doi:10.1161/HYPERTENSIONAHA.107.108845.

Feng, X., Wang, L., Li, Y., 2011. Change of telomere length in angiotensin II-induced human glomerular mesangial cell senescence and the protective role of losartan. Mol. Med. Rep. 17913004. 4 (2), 255–260. Available from: http://www.spandidos-publications.com/serveFile/mmr_4_2_255_PDF.pdf?type=article&article_id=mmr_4_2_255&item=PDF. doi:10.3892/mmr.2011.436China.

Flather, M.D., Yusuf, S., Køber, L., Pfeffer, M., Hall, A., Murray, G., Torp-Pedersen, C., Ball, S., Pogue, J., Moyé, L., Braunwald, E., 2000. Long-term ACE-inhibitor therapy in patients with heart failure or left-ventricular dysfunction: a systematic overview of data from individual patients. Lancet. 01406736. 355 (9215), 1575–1581. Available from: http://www.journals.elsevier.com/the-lancet/. doi:10.1016/S0140-6736(00)02212-1.

Forrester, S.J., Booz, G.W., Sigmund, C.D., Coffman, T.M., Kawai, T., Rizzo, V., Scalia, R., Eguchi, S., 2018. Angiotensin II signal transduction: an update on mechanisms of physiology and pathophysiology. Physiol. Rev. 15221210. 98 (3), 1627–1738. Available from: https://www.physiology.org/doi/pdf/10.1152/physrev.00038.2017. doi:10.1152/physrev.00038.2017.

Frey, L., Gravestock, I., Pichierri, G., Steurer, J., Burgstaller, J.M., 2019. Serious adverse events in patients with target-oriented blood pressure management: a systematic review. J. Hypertens. 14735598. 37 (11), 2135–2144. Available from: http://journals.lww.com/jhypertension. doi:10.1097/HJH.0000000000002176.

García-Prieto, A.M., Verdalles, Ú., de José, A.P., Arroyo, D., Aragoncillo, I., Barbieri, D., Camacho, R.E., Goicoechea, M., 2024. Renin–angiotensin–aldosterone system blockers effect in chronic kidney disease progression in hypertensive elderly patients without proteinuria: PROERCAN trial. Hipertensión Y Riesgo Vascular. 18891837. 41 (2), 95–103. doi:10.1016/j.hipert.2023.11.005.

Gheorghiade, M., Böhm, M., Greene, S.J., Fonarow, G.C., Lewis, E.F., Zannad, F., Solomon, S.D., Baschiera, F., Botha, J., Hua, T.A., Gimpelewicz, C.R., Jaumont, X., Lesogor, A., Maggioni, A.P., 2013. Effect of aliskiren on postdischarge mortality and heart failure readmissions among patients hospitalized for heart failure: the ASTRONAUT randomized trial. JAMA 15383598. 309 (11), 1125–1135. Available from: http://jama.jamanetwork.com/data/Journals/JAMA/926606/joc130023_1125_1135.pdf. doi:10.1001/jama.2013.1954.

Hajjar, I., Okafor, M., McDaniel, D., Obideen, M., Dee, E., Shokouhi, M., Quyyumi, A.A., Levey, A., Goldstein, F., 2020. Effects of candesartan vs lisinopril on neurocognitive function in older adults with executive mild cognitive impairment: a randomized clinical trial. JAMA Netw. Open. 25743805. 3 (8). Available from: https://jamanetwork.com/journals/jamanetworkopen. doi:10.1001/jamanetworkopen.2020.12252.

Israili, Z.H., Hall, W.D., 1992. Cough and angioneurotic edema associated with angiotensin-converting enzyme inhibitor therapy: a review of the literature and pathophysiology. Ann. Intern. Med. 00034819. 117 (3), 234–242. Available from: http://annals.org/issues.aspx. doi:10.7326/0003-4819-117-3-234.

Ito, S., Kashihara, N., Shikata, K., Nangaku, M., Wada, T., Okuda, Y., Sawanobori, T., 2020. Esaxerenone (CS-3150) in patients with type 2 diabetes and microalbuminuria (ESAX-DN): phase 3 randomized controlled clinical trial. Clin. J. Am. Soc. Nephrol. 1555905X. 15 (12), 1715–1727. Available from: https://cjasn.asnjournals.org/content/15/12/1715/full-text.pdf?with-ds=yes. doi:10.2215/CJN.06870520.

Izzo, J.L., Weinberg, M.S., Hainer, J.W., Kerkering, J., Tou, C.K.P., 2004. Antihypertensive efficacy of candesartan-lisinopril in combination vs. up-titration of lisinopril: the AMAZE trials. J. Clin. Hypertens. 15246175. 6 (9), 485–493. doi:10.1111/j.1524-6175.2004.03511.x.

Kellum, J.A., Lameire, N., 2013. Diagnosis, evaluation, and management of acute kidney injury: a KDIGO summary (Part 1). Crit Care. 1364-8535. 17 (1), 204. doi:10.1186/cc11454.

Kidney Disease: Improving Global Outcomes CKDWG, 2024. KDIGO 2024 clinical practice guideline for the evaluation and management of chronic kidney disease. Kidney Int. 105 (4S), 117.

Komajda, M., Hanon, O., Hochadel, M., Lopez-Sendon, J.L., Follath, F., Ponikowski, P., Harjola, V.P., Drexler, H., Dickstein, K., Tavazzi, L., Nieminen, M., 2009. Contemporary management of octogenarians hospitalized for heart failure in Europe: euro Heart Failure Survey II. European Heart Journal. 15229645. 30 (4), 478–486. doi:10.1093/eurheartj/ehn539.

Lapi, F., Azoulay, L., Yin, H., Nessim, S.J., Suissa, S., 2013. Concurrent use of diuretics, angiotensin converting enzyme inhibitors, and angiotensin receptor blockers with non-steroidal anti-inflammatory drugs and risk of acute kidney injury: nested case-control study. BMJ. 1756-1833. 346 (jan08 12), e8525. doi:10.1136/bmj.e8525.

Lennon, M.J., Lam, B.C.P., Lipnicki, D.M., Crawford, J.D., Peters, R., Schutte, A.E., Brodaty, H., Thalamuthu, A., Rydberg-Sterner, T., Najar, J., Skoog, I., Riedel-Heller, S.G., Röhr, S., Pabst, A., Lobo, A., De-La-Cámara, C., Lobo, E., Bello, T., Gureje, O., Ojagbemi, A., Lipton, R.B., Katz, M.J., Derby, C.A., Kim, K.W., Han, J.W., Oh, D.J., Rolandi, E., Davin, A., Rossi, M., Scarmeas, N., Yannakoulia, M., Dardiotis, T., Hendrie, H.C., Gao, S., Carrière, I., Ritchie, K., Anstey, K.J., Cherbuin, N., Xiao, S., Yue, L., Li, W., Guerchet, M.M., Preux, P.M., Aboyans, V., Haan, M.N., Aiello, A.E., Ng, T.P., Nyunt, M.S.Z., Gao, Q., Scazufca, M., Sachdev, P.S.S., 2023. Use of antihypertensives, blood pressure, and estimated risk of dementia in late life: an individual participant data meta-analysis. JAMA Netw. Open. 25743805. 6 (9). Available from: https://jamanetwork.com/journals/jamanetworkopen/issue/6/9. doi:10.1001/jamanetworkopen.2023.33353.

Li, E.C.K., Heran, B.S., Wright, J.M., 2014. Angiotensin converting enzyme (ACE) inhibitors versus angiotensin receptor blockers for primary hypertension. Cochrane Database Syst. Rev. 14651858. 2014 (8). doi:10.1002/14651858.cd009096.pub2.

Lithell, H., Hansson, L., Skoog, I., Elmfeldt, D., Hofman, A., Olofsson, B., Trenkwalder, P., Zanchetti, A., 2003. The study on cognition and prognosis in the elderly (SCOPE): principal results of a randomized double-blind intervention trial. J. Hypertens. 02636352. 21 (5), 875–886. Available from: http://journals.lww.com/jhypertension. doi:10.1097/00004872-200305000-00011.

Makani, H., Bangalore, S., Desouza, K.A., Shah, A., Messerli, F.H., 2013. Efficacy and safety of dual blockade of the renin-angiotensin system: meta-analysis of randomised trials. BMJ 17561833. 346 (7896). Available from: http://www.bmj.com/highwire/filestream/627585/field_highwire_article_pdf/0/bmj.f360. doi:10.1136/bmj.f360.

Makani, H., Messerli, F.H., Romero, J., Wever-Pinzon, O., Korniyenko, A., Berrios, R.S., Bangalore, S., 2012. Meta-analysis of randomized trials of angioedema as an adverse event of renin-angiotensin system inhibitors. Am. J. Cardiol. 18791913. 110 (3), 383–391. doi:10.1016/j.amjcard.2012.03.034.

Masoudi, F.A., Rathore, S.S., Wang, Y., Havranek, E.P., Curtis, J.P., Foody, J.A.M., Krumholz, H.M., 2004. National patterns of use and effectiveness of angiotensin-converting enzyme inhibitors in older patients with heart failure and left ventricular systolic dysfunction. Circulation. 00097322. 110 (6), 724–731. doi:10.1161/01.CIR.0000138934.28340.ED.

Menichelli, D., Poli, D., Antonucci, E., Palareti, G., Pignatelli, P., Pastori, D., 2024. Renin-angiotensin-aldosterone system inhibitors and mortality risk in elderly patients with atrial fibrillation. Insights from the nationwide START registry. Eur. J. Intern. Med. 18790828. 119, 84–92. Available from: https://www.sciencedirect.com/science/journal/09536205. doi:10.1016/j.ejim.2023.08.019.

Messerli, F.H., Ventura, H.O., Glade, L.B., Sundgaard-Riise, K., Dunn, F.G., Frohlich, E.D., 1983. Essential hypertension in the elderly: haemodynamics, intravascular volume, plasma renin activity, and circulating catecholamine levels. Lancet. 01406736. 322 (8357), 983–986. doi:10.1016/S0140-6736(83)90977-7.

Morishita, Y., Yasui, T., Numata, A., Onishi, A., Ishibashi, K., Kusano, E., 2012. Aliskiren suppresses the renin-angiotensin-aldosterone system and reduces blood pressure and albuminuria in elderly chronic kidney disease patients with hypertension. Int. J. Nephrol. Renovasc. Dis. 11787058. 5, 125–133. Available from: http://www.dovepress.com/getfile.php?fileID=14026. doi:10.2147/IJNRD.S36451Japan.

Musini, V.M., Lawrence, K.A., Fortin, P.M., Bassett, K., Wright, J.M., 2017. Blood pressure lowering efficacy of renin inhibitors for primary hypertension. Cochrane Database Syst. Rev. 14651858. 2017 (4). Available from: https://www.cochranelibrary.com/cdsr/table-of-contents. doi:10.1002/14651858.CD007066.pub3.

Musso, C.G., Jauregui, J.R., 2014. Renin-angiotensin-aldosterone system and the aging kidney. Expert. Rev Endocrinol. Metab. 17448417. 9 (6), 543–546. Available from: http://www.tandfonline.com/loi/iere20#.V6Qca01f1Fo. doi:10.1586/17446651.2014.956723.

Neves, C., Cunha, G., Oigman, W., 2018. The role of renin-angiotensin-aldosterone system and its new components in arterial stiffness and vascular aging. High Blood Press. Cardiovasc. Prev. 25 (2), 137–145.

Omboni, S., Malacco, E., Mallion, J.M., Volpe, M., Zanchetti, A., Baghestanian, M., Eber, B., Zweiker, R., Riegelnik, V., Van Mieghem, W., DuCailar, G., Panzer, P.K., Kresse, W.R., Carewicz, O., Iserloh, J., Krause, K.H., Prechtel,

E., Naudts, I.F.K., Schmidt, A., Zimmermann, U., Borbas, E., Kremastinos, D., Triantafyllidi, H., Stefanadis, C., Barton, J., Ambrosio, G.B., Anastasio, L., Antonelli, B., Antonucci, G., Aurelio, G., Auteri, A., Baldi, F., Battistello, L., Baule, G.M., Bellazzi, R., Blasio, A., Bonollo, V., Borello, L., Campanini, M., Candido, R., Capobianco, G., Capuano, V., Caruso, D., Corbara, F., Casanova, R., Cerasola, G., Cianflone, D., Ciconte, V., Cipriani, M., Cocchi, R., Cucchini, F., Dallemule, J., D'Amico, F., De Cesaris, R., De Curtis, G., Defeo, G.D., Cas, L.D., Carratore, G.D., Demartino, M., Desideri, G., Destro, M., Di Biase, M., Di Somma, S., Donadon, V., Doronzo, B., Fariello, R., Feraco, E., Ferri, C., Fiorini, F., Fogari, R., Foresti, A., Galasso, D., Gargiulo, A., Gaudio, G.V., Gavazzi, A., Giannatempo, C., Guzzardi, G., Iaconelli, G., Lacchè, A., Laghi, F., Lechi, A., Lembo, G., Lettica, G.V., Licata, G., Locatelli, F., Maimone, I., Manfrè, M., Manfredini, R., Marracci, G., Mauro, G.F., Mazzuca, L., Melandri, F., Meloni, L., Mezzetti, A., Minutiello, L., Mondillo, S., Montereggi, A., Mos, L., Musca, R.N., Nigro, P., Novo, S., Noto, R., Olivieri, O., Palasciano, G., Palatini, P., Panettieri, M.I., Pedrinelli, R., Perticone, F., Pini, C., Pirrone, G.T., Portaluppi, F., Prinzi, D., Pulitanò, G., Pupilella, T., Puzzolante, V., Radaeli, A., Raisaro, A., Rappelli, A., Ricciardi, B., Fanelli, F.R., Rovero, E., Russo, F., Uriarte, J.S., Santonastaso, M., Scala, A., Schipani, F., Sechi, L., Serviddio, G., Sganzerla, P., Spadola, V., Sprovieri, M., Stornello, M.G.R., Tamburino, C., Totaro, G., Turiel, M., Varì, N., Venco, A., Ventrella, F., Villa, G., Uguccioni, M., Narkiewicz, K., Chrostowska, M., Napora, P., Gornikiewicz-Brzezicka, B., Graczak, I., Klimkiewicz, J., Jesewska, M., Gamiz, J.L.P., Olivan, J., Puig, J.G., Extremera, B.G., Lopez, P.J., Martinez, J.S., Adrian, M.J., Coca, A., Doménech, M., 2012. Twenty-four hour and early morning blood pressure control of olmesartan vs. ramipril in elderly hypertensive patients: pooled individual data analysis of two randomized, double-blind, parallel-group studies. J. Hypertens. 14735598. 30 (7), 1468–1477. Available from: http://journals.lww.com/jhypertension. doi:10.1097/HJH.0b013e32835466ac.

Orchard, S.G., Zhou, Z., Fravel, M., Ryan, J., Woods, R.L., Wolfe, R., Shah, R.C., Murray, A., Sood, A., Reid, C.M., Nelson, M.R., Bellin, L., Polkinghorne, K.R., Stocks, N., Ernst, M.E., 2024. Antihypertensive medications and dementia in older adults with hypertension. medRxiv [Preprint]. doi:10.1101/2024.08.28.24312754.

Parving, H.H., Brenner, B.M., McMurray, J.J.V., De Zeeuw, D., Haffner, S.M., Solomon, S.D., Chaturvedi, N., Persson, F., Desai, A.S., Nicolaides, M., Richard, A., Xiang, Z., Brunel, P., Pfeffer, M.A., 2012. Cardiorenal end points in a trial of aliskiren for type 2 diabetes. N. Engl. J. Med. 15334406. 367 (23), 2204–2213. Available from: http://www.nejm.org/doi/pdf/10.1056/NEJMoa1208799. doi:10.1056/NEJMoa1208799.

Parving, H.H., Lehnert, H., Brochner-Mortensen, J., Gomis, R., Andersen, S., Arner, P., 2001. The effect of irbesartan on the development of diabetic nephropathy in patients with type 2 diabetes. N. Engl. J. Med. 00284793. 345 (12), 870–878. doi:10.1056/NEJMoa011489.

Pitt, B., Filippatos, G., Agarwal, R., Anker, S.D., Bakris, G.L., Rossing, P., Joseph, A., Kolkhof, P., Nowack, C., Schloemer, P., Ruilope, L.M., 2021. Cardiovascular events with finerenone in kidney disease and type 2 diabetes. N. Engl. J. Med. 15334406. 385 (24), 2252–2263. Available from: http://www.nejm.org/medical-index. doi:10.1056/NEJMoa2110956.

Pitt, B., Remme, W., Zannad, F., Neaton, J., Martinez, F., Roniker, B., Bittman, R., Hurley, S., Kleiman, J., Gatlin, M., 2003. Eplerenone, a selective aldosterone blocker, in patients with left ventricular dysfunction after myocardial infarction. N. Engl. J. Med. 00284793. 348 (14), 1309–1321. Available from: http://www.nejm.org/medical-index. doi:10.1056/NEJMoa030207.

Pitt, B., Zannad, F., Remme, W.J., Cody, R., Castaigne, A., Perez, A., Palensky, J., Wittes, J., 1999. The effect of spironolactone on morbidity and mortality in patients with severe heart failure. N. Engl. J. Med. 00284793. 341 (10), 709–717. doi:10.1056/NEJM199909023411001.

Qiao, Y., Shin, J.I., Chen, T.K., Inker, L.A., Coresh, J., Alexander, G.C., Jackson, J.W., Chang, A.R., Grams, M.E., 2020. Association between renin-angiotensin system blockade discontinuation and all-cause mortality among persons with low estimated glomerular filtration rate. JAMA Intern. Med. 21686114. 180 (5), 718–726. Available from: http://archinte.jamanetwork.com/issues.aspx. doi:10.1001/jamainternmed.2020.0193.

Raebel, M.A., Ross, C., Xu, S., Roblin, D.W., Cheetham, C., Blanchette, C.M., Saylor, G., Smith, D.H., 2010. Diabetes and drug-associated hyperkalemia: effect of potassium monitoring. J. Gen. Intern. Med. 15251497. 25 (4), 326–333. doi:10.1007/s11606-009-1228-x.

Redon, J., Weber, M.A., Reimitz, P.E., Wang, J.G., 2018. Comparative effectiveness of an angiotensin receptor blocker, olmesartan medoxomil, in older hypertensive patients. J. Clin. Hypertens. 17517176. 20 (2), 356–365. Available from: http://onlinelibrary.wiley.com/journal/10.1111/(ISSN)1751-7176. doi:10.1111/jch.13183.

Sarafidis, P., Agarwal, R., Pitt, B., Wanner, C., Filippatos, G., Boletis, J., Tuttle, K.R., Ruilope, L.M., Rossing, P., Toto, R., Anker, S.D., Liu, Z.H., Joseph, A., Ahlers, C., Brinker, M., Lawatscheck, R., Bakris, G., 2023. Outcomes with finerenone in participants with stage 4 CKD and type 2 diabetes: a FIDELITY subgroup analysis. Clin. J. Am.

Soc. Nephrol. 1555905X. 18 (5), 602–612. Available from: http://cjasn.asnjournals.org/content/by/year. doi:10.2215/CJN.0000000000000149.

Schmidt, M., Mansfield, K.E., Bhaskaran, K., Nitsch, D., Sørensen, H.T., Smeeth, L., Tomlinson, L.A., 2017. Adherence to guidelines for creatinine and potassium monitoring and discontinuation following renin–angiotensin system blockade: a UK general practice-based cohort study. BMJ Open. 2044-6055. 7 (1), e012818. doi:10.1136/bmjopen-2016-012818.

Shah, M., Awad, A.S., Abdel- Rahman, E.M., 2023. Nonsteroidal mineralocorticoid receptor antagonist (finerenone) in cardiorenal disease. J. Clin. Med. 12, 6285. doi:https://doi.org/10.3390/jcm12196285.

Sriperumbuduri, S., McArthur, E., Hundemer, G.L., Canney, M., Tangri, N., Leon, S.J., Bota, S., Bugeja, A., Akbari, A., Knoll, G., Sood, M.M., 2021. Initial and recurrent hyperkalemia events in patients with ckd in older adults: a population-based cohort study. Can. J. Kidney Health Dis. 2054-3581. 8. doi:10.1177/20543581211017408.

Steckelings, U.M., Widdop, E.D.S., Lubbe, T.H., Kaschina, E., et al., 2022. The angiotensin at(2) receptor: from a binding site to a novel therapeutic target. Pharmacol. Rev. 74, 1051–1135.

Thomopoulos, C., Parati, G., Zanchetti, A., 2018. Effects of blood pressure-lowering treatment on cardiovascular outcomes and mortality: 14-effects of different classes of antihypertensive drugs in older and younger patients: overview and meta-analysis. J. Hypertens. 14735598. 36 (8), 1637–1647. Available from: http://journals.lww.com/jhypertension. doi:10.1097/HJH.0000000000001777.

Turgut, F., Balogun, R.A., Abdel-Rahman, E.M., 2010. Renin-angiotensin-aldosterone system blockade effects on the kidney in the elderly: benefits and limitations. Clin. J. Am. Soc. Nephrol. 1555905X. 5 (7), 1330–1339. Available from: http://cjasn.asnjournals.org/cgi/reprint/5/7/1330. doi:10.2215/CJN.08611209.

Vaduganathan, M., Filippatos, G., Claggett, B.L., Desai, A.S., Jhund, P.S., Henderson, A., Brinker, M., Kolkhof, P., Schloemer, P., Lay-Flurrie, J., Viswanathan, P., Lam, C.S.P., Senni, M., Shah, S.J., Voors, A.A., Zannad, F., Rossing, P., Ruilope, L.M., Anker, S.D., Pitt, B., Agarwal, R., McMurray, J.J.V., Solomon, S.D., 2024. Finerenone in heart failure and chronic kidney disease with type 2 diabetes: FINE-HEART pooled analysis of cardiovascular, kidney and mortality outcomes. Nat. Med. 1546170X. 30 (12), 3758–3764. Available from: https://www.nature.com/nm/. doi:10.1038/s41591-024-03264-4.

Vardeny, O., Vaduganathan, M., Claggett, B.L., Desai, A.S., Jhund, P.S., et al., 2025. Finerenone, Serum potassium, and clinical outcomes in heart failure with mildly reduced or preserved ejection fraction. JAMA Cardiol. 10 (1), 42–48.

Verdecchia, P., Calvo, C., Möckel, V., Keeling, L., Satlin, A., 2007. Safety and efficacy of the oral direct renin inhibitor aliskiren in elderly patients with hypertension. Blood Press. 0803-7051. 16 (6), 381–391. doi:10.1080/08037050701717014.

Wang, G.M., Li, L.J., Tang, W.L., Wright, J.M., 2020. Renin inhibitors versus angiotensin converting enzyme (ACE) inhibitors for primary hypertension. Cochrane Database Syst. Rev. 14651858. 2020 (10). Available from: https://www.cochranelibrary.com/cdsr/table-of-contents. doi:10.1002/14651858.CD012569.pub2.

Wing, L.M., Reid, C.M., Ryan, P., et al., 2003. A comparison of outcomes with angiotensin-converting–enzyme inhibitors and diuretics for hypertension in the elderly. N. Engl. J. Med. 348 (7), 583–592.

Winkelmayer, W.C., Zhang, Z., Shahinfar, S., Cooper, M.E., Avorn, J., Brenner, B.M., 2006. Efficacy and safety of angiotensin II receptor blockade in elderly patients with diabetes. Diabetes Care 01495992. 29 (10), 2210–2217. Available from: http://care.diabetesjournals.org/cgi/reprint/29/10/2210.pdf. doi:10.2337/dc06-0570.

Wray, D.W., Nishiyama, S.K., Harris, R.A., Richardson, R.S., 2008. Angiotensin II in the elderly: impact of angiotensin II type 1 receptor sensitivity on peripheral hemodynamics. Hypertension. 0194911X. 51 (6), 1611–1616. doi:10.1161/HYPERTENSIONAHA.108.111294.

Yang, T., Xu, C., 2017. Physiology and pathophysiology of the intrarenal renin-angiotensin system: an update. J. Am. Soc. Nephrol. 1046-6673. 28 (4), 1040–1049. doi:10.1681/asn.2016070734.

Yoon, H.E., Choi, B.S., 2014. The renin-angiotensin system and aging in the kidney. Korean J. Intern. Med. 20056648. 29 (3), 291–295. Available from: http://www.ncbi.nlm.nih.gov/pmc/articles/PMC4028516/pdf/kjim-29-291.pdf. doi:10.3904/kjim.2014.29.3.291.

Yu, D., Li, J.X., Cheng, Y., Wang, H.D., Ma, X.D., Ding, T., Zhu, Z., 2025. Comparative efficacy of different antihypertensive drug classes for stroke prevention: a network meta-analysis of randomized controlled trials. PLoS One 19326203. 20 (2). Available from: https://journals.plos.org/plosone/article?id=10.1371/journal.pone.0313309. doi:10.1371/journal.pone.0313309.

Yusuf, S., Teo, K.K., Pogue, J., Dyal, L., Copland, I., Schumacher, H., Dagenais, G., Sleight, P., Anderson, C., Ramos, B., Richardson, L., Murphy, J., Haehl, M., Hilbrich, L., Svaerd, R., Martin, K., Murwin, D., Meinicke, T., Schlosser, A., Schmidt, G., Creek, R., Schumacher, H., Distel, M., Aubert, B., Pogue, J., Dyal, L., Schmieder, R., Unger, T., Asmar, R., Mancia, G., Diaz, R., Paolasso, E., Piegas, L., Avezum, A., Munoz, E.C., Probstfield, J., Weber, M., Young, J., Fagard, R., Jansky, P., Mallion, J., Mann, J., Böhm, M., Eber, B., Karatzas, N.B., Keltai, M., Trimarco, B., Verdecchia,

P., Maggioni, A., Verheugt, F.W.A., Holwerda, N.J., Ceremuzynski, L., Budaj, A., Ferreira, R., Chazova, I., Rydén, L., Svendsen, T.L., Metsärinne, K., Dickstein, K., Fodor, G., Commerford, P., Redon, J., Luescher, T.R., Oto, A., Binbrek, A., Parkhomenko, A., Jennings, G., Liu, L.S., Yu, C.M., Dans, A.L., Shah, R., Kim, J.H., Chen, J.H., Chaithiraphan, S., Cairns, J., Wilhelmsen, L., Chalmers, J., Wittes, J., Gent, M., Hennekens, C.H., Anderson, N., Yusoff, K., Auger, P., Bernstein, V., Panju, A., Anand, I., Bigger, J.T., Linz, P., Healey, J., Held, C., McGorrian, C., Rokoss, M., Villar, J., Anderson, C., Dans, A., Yusuf, S., McDonald, A., Pogue, J., Dyal, L., Afzal, R., Zhao, F., Sleight, P., Richardson, L., Anderson, C., Murphy, J., Paolasso, E., Guerrero, R.A.A., Amuchastegui, M., Baglivo, H.P., Bendersky, M., Bono, J., Bustos, B., Caccavo, A., Cartasegna, L.R., Castellanos, C.R., Cipullo, M.A., Crunger, P., Cuneo, C.A., Focaccia, M., Fuselli, J.J., Hasbani, E., Hominal, M.A., Humphreys, J., Inserra, F., Killinger, C.R., Kuschnir, E., Majul, C.R., Manuale, O.D., Martinez, G., Marzetti, E.M., Nordaby, R., Orlandini, A.D., Pomposiello, J.C., Rodríguez, G.M., Salas, J., Salomone, O.A., Sanchez, R.A., Serra, C., Vico, M.L., Jennings, G.L.R., Amerena, J.V., Arnolda, L.F., Aroney, G.M., Aylward, P.E., Bladin, C.F., Bridgeman, J.C., Chambers, B.R., Corbett, A.J., Crimmins, D.S., Cross, D.B., Davies, L., Davis, S.M., Donnan, G.A., Eccleston, D.S., Frayne, J.H., Hendriks, R., Herkes, G.K., Hill, A.T., Jeffery, I.M., Karrasch, J.A., Koshy, G., Marwick, T.H., Owensby, D.A., Parsons, M.W., Rees, D.M., Russell, A., Schwartz, R., Singh, B., Thompson, P.L., Waites, J.H., Walsh, W.F., Walters, D.L., Watts, R.W., Whelan, A.P., Böhm, M., Eber, B.E., Bonelli, J.B., Dolliner, P., Hohenecker, J.H., Steurer, G.S., Weihs, W.W., Bekaert, I., Brohet, C., Chaumont, P., Cheron, P., Crasset, V., Degaute, J.P., Dendale, P., Dujardin, K., Elshot, S., Hellemans, S., Herssens, M., Heyndrickx, G., Laloux, P., Lesseliers, H., Noyens, P., Quinonez, M., Stammen, F., Striekwold, H., Thoeng, J., Van Mieghem, W., Vanhooren, G., Vervoort, G., Vrolix, M., Wollaert, B., Piegas, L., Avezum, A., Abrantes, J.A.M., Armaganijan, D., Ayoub, J.C., Bodanese, L.C., Carvalho, A.C., Coutinho, M., Esteves, J.P., Franco, R.J.S., Jardim, P.C.B.V., Saraiva, J.F.K., Leães, P.E., Maia, L.N., Marin-Neto, J.A., Marino, R.L., Mion, D., Moreira, J.R., Oigman, W., Pedrosa, R.C., Pelloso, E.A., Plavnik, F.L., Polanczyk, C.A., Rabelo, S.R., Reis, G., Ribeiro, A.B., Ribeiro, J.M., Rocha, J.C., Rossi, P.R.F., Santos, R.D., Tarastchuk, J.C.E., Villalón, M.N., Abramson, B., Arnold, M., Ashton, T., Auger, P., Bata, I., Bayly, K., Beauchef, J., Bélanger, A., Bernstein, V., Bhargava, R., Booth, A.W., Bose, S., Boulianne, M., Cameron, M., Chan, Y.K., Constance, C., Costi, P., Dion, D., Douketis, J., Fell, D., Giannoccaro, J.P., Glanz, A., Gosselin, G., Gould, D., Goulet, S., Grondin, F., Gupta, M., Gyenes, G., Heath, J.W., Heath, V.A., Hess, A., Hiscock, J.G., Hoag, G., Honos, G., Imrie, J., Kuritzky, R., Lai, C., Lalani, A., Lamy, A., LeBouthillier, P., Lochnan, H., Lonn, E., Lubelsky, B., Mackey, A., Meunier, M., Milot, A., Mitchell, L.B., Nawaz, S., Omichinski, M., Panju, A., Pilon, C., Pilon, D., Polasek, P., Proulx, G., Rebane, T., Ricci, A.J., Rupka, D.W., Sabbah, D.S., Sharma, N.K., Shu, D., Hilaire, R.S., Maurice, F.S., Starra, R., Sussex, B., Szaky, T., Talbot, P., Tan, K.W., To, T.B., Tobe, S., Tytus, R., Vexler, R., Whitsitt, P., Woo, V., Liu, L., Bai, X., Chen, X., Feng, J., Fu, S., Ge, Y., Gong, L., He, Z., Huang, J., Jiang, Y., Li, L., Li, Q.H., Liao, Y., Lu, Z., Lu, F., Ma, S., Niu, F., Pan, C., Qian, F., Shi, X., Sun, N., Sun, M., Sun, G., Wang, J., Wang, S., Wang, Y., Wu, Z., Yan, X., Yang, X., Yang, H., Ye, X., Yuan, S., Zhang, T., Zhang, C., Zhang, F., Zhang, S., Zhao, D., Zheng, B., Zhou, H.Y., Zhou, S., Zhu, J., Janský, P., Dedek, V., Dvorák, J., Holaj, R., Kotouš, J., Pederzoliová, E., Polák, M., Povolný, J., Smetana, K., Špác, J., Svendsen, T.L., Götzsche, L., Juhl, H.F., Koelendorf, K., Lund, P., Pedersen, F., Perdersen, O.L., Pindborg, T., Rasmussen, L.H., Rasmussen, S.L., Thygesen, K., Tuxen, C., Metsärinne, K., Antikainen, R., Jääskivi, M., Kantola, I., Kastarinen, M., Kohonen-Jalonen, P., Koistinen, A., Lehmus, E., Nuuttila, R., Tuominen, M.L., Ylihärsilä, H., Mallion, J., Abenhaim, N., Allix, J., Boucher, L., Bourgoin, M., Boye, A., Breton, N., Cadinot, D., Campagne, A., Churet, J., Constantin, G., Lorette, E.D.S., Sawy, A.E., Etchegarray, G., Farhat, S., Lacoin, F., Latte, T., Magnani, C., Pineau-Valenciennes, D., Pithon, M., Quéguiner, A., Sicard, J., Sorbe, G., Taminau, D., Vilarem, H., Vogel, J.Y., Ebert, H.H., Genth-Zotz, S., Hermanns, N., Holzer, C., Minnich, J., Schimkus, D., Boehm, M., Brado, B., Claus, G., Dietz, U., Griebenow, R., Haak, T., Hahn, K., Hampel, R., Heitzer, H., Holle, G., Horacek, T., Jordan, J., Klein, C., Kolloch, R., Ludewig, S., Motz, W., Muenzel, T., Nast, H.P., Nauck, M., Nebelsieck, H., Rybak, K., Samer, H., Schaefer, T., Scholze, J., Schulze, B., Schleppinghoff, R., Schmieder, E., Schwaab, B., Sechtem, U., Sehnert, W., Steinhagen-Thiessen, E., Stenzel, G., Trenkwalder, P., Wedler, B., Zippel, J., Karatzas, N., Achimastos, A., Diamantopoulos, E., Efstratopoulos, A., Elisaf, M., Karvounis, H., Mentzikof, D., Mytas, D., Papadogiannis, D., Pyrgakis, V., Stefanadis, C., Symeonidis, D., Tsoukas, A., Vogiatzis, I., Voyaki, S., Zamboulis, C., Yu, C.M., Chan, C.K.H., Lam, L., Lau, Y.K., Sanderson, J., Wong, J., Wu, E.B., Yue, C.S., Keltai, M., Czuriga, I., Édes, I., Farsang, C.S., Kalina, K.K., Keltai, K., Kozma, M., László, Z., Nagy, V., Papp, A., Polák, G.Y., Préda, I., Rónaszéki, A., Sereg, M., Simon, K., Sonkodi, S., Szegedi, J., Timár, S., Tóth, K., Vándorfi, G.Y., Vértes, A., Feely, J., Maher, V.M.G., Stanton, A.V., Sullivan, P., Trimarco, B., Verdecchia, P., Rosei, E.A., Ambrosio, G.B., Bentivoglio, M., Branzi, A., Perin, P.C., Chiariello, M., Cirrincione, V., Ferrari, R., Gattobigio, R., Giovannini, E., Giugliano, D., Lacchè, A., Lauro, R., Lembo, G., Marchetti, G., Moretti, L., Pancaldi, L., Partemi, L., Pede, S., Pettinati, G., Reboldi, G., Ricci, R., Rosiello, G., Rozza, F., Sardone, M.G., Scabbia, E.V., Selvetella, G., Tavazzi, L., Terrosu, P., Venco, A., Vetrano, A., Volpe, M., Zilio, G., Ismail, T., Shah, R.P., Singaraveloo, M., Ahmad,

W.A.W., Yusof, Z., Yusoff, K., Abidin, I.Z., Zambahari, R., Munoz, E.C., Diaz, L.A., Pascoe-Gonzalez, S., Nava, R.A., De La Peña Topete, G., Sifuentes, L.A.E., Hernández García, H.R., Illescas-Diaz, J., Macías Islas, M.A., Arellano, J.A.N., Ruiz, R.O., Carrillo, J.Z.P., Sánchez, G.V., Velásquez, M.V., Verheugt, F.W.A., Holwerda, N.J., Basart, D.C.G., Boermans, A.J.M., Bosker, H.A., Bouter, K.P., Buiks, C.P., de Backer, W.A., de Graaf, J.J., Deppenbroek, J.H.M., Eefting, F.D., Gunneweg, F.C.N.M., Michels, H.R., Poldermans, D., Schrijver, G., Sedney, M.I., Slagboom, T., Smilde, J.G., Storms, G.E.M.G., Tjon, R.M., van Bergen, P.F.M.M., van Doesburg, G.J.M., van Kempen, L.H.J., van Mierlo, H.F.C.M., Veerman, A., Vermetten, F.A.A.M., Wester, A., Bagg, W., Benatar, J., Coxon, R.J., Doughty, R.N., Friedlander, D.H., Luke, R.A., Nairn, P.L., Ratnasabapathy, Y., Richards, A.M., Singh, G.P., Stewart, R.A.H., Troughton, R.W., White, H.D., Williams, M., Wong, S.P., Dickstein, K., Bogale, N., Lier, J.O., Otterstad, J.E., Rønnevik, P.K., Skeie, S., Walle, P.O., Dans, A.L., Abola, M.T.B., Añonuevo, J.C., Jaro, J.M., Marañon, D.R., Mendoza, V.L., Morales, D.R., Pacheco, E.P., Reyes, E.B., Roxas, A.A., Sedurante, M.B., Ceremuzynski, L., Budaj, A., Binio, Z., Bronisz, M., Buszman, P., Czerski, T., Dalkowski, M., Gessek, J., Gieroba, A., Janik, K., Janion, M., Kawka-Urbanek, T., Klabisz, R., Krauze-Wielicka, M., Malinowski, S., Miekus, P., Mormul, J., Ogorek, M., Opolski, G., Skura, M., Szpajer, M., Tendera, M., Waszyrowski, T., Wierzchowiecki, M., Zalska, B., Ferreira, R., Capucho, R., Correia, C., Cunha, L., Ferro, J.M., Ribeiro, V.G., Gil, V., da Silva, P.M., Carrageta, M.O., Gomes, R.S., Gomes, M.V., Chazova, I., Ageev, F., Belenkov, Y., Ivleva, A., Karpov, Y., Shestakova, M., Shlyakhto, E., Shustov, S., Sidorenko, B., Chang, H.M., Kwok, B., Fodor, G., Dukát, A., Gonsorcík, J., Hranai, M., Lietava, J., Pella, D., Rybar, R., Ruffini, L., Commerford, P., Bonnici, F., Brown, B., Dalby, A.J., Gibson, G.J., Herbst, L., King, J., Klug, E., Middle, M., Naidoo, D.P., Pretorius, M., Podgorski, G., Ranjith, N., Silwa-Hahnle, K., Theron, H., Kim, J.H., Chae, S.C., Chung, N.S., Hong, K.P., Jeong, M.H., Kang, H.J., Kim, J.J., Kim, M.H., Seo, H.S., Shin, E.K., Redón, J., Abellán, J., Aranda, P., Barrios, V., Calvo, C., Figuera, M.D.L., De Teresa, E., Durá, R., Escobar, F., Fernandez-Cruz, F., Galve, E., Garcia-Puig, J., Gil-Extremera, B., Gomis, R., Gonzalez-Albarran, O., González-Juanatey, J.R., Llacer, A., López-Bescós, L., Oliván, J., Picó, A., Pose, A., Roca-Cusachs, A., Ruilope, L.M., Rydén, L., Alvång, A., Boström, P., Dellborg, M., Ericsson, U.B., Herlitz, J., Juhlin, T., Pedersen, K., Sträng, B., Sundqvist, B., Tengmark, B.O., Ulvenstam, G., Westerdahl, B., Winberg, L., Luescher, T.R., Baumgartner, I., Dubach, P., Gallino, A., Moccetti, T., Noll, G., Nordmann, A., Rickli, H., Schläpfer, H., Weber, K., Chen, J.H., Chao, T.H., Chen, C.Y., Cheng, J.J., Chiou, H.C., Fu, C.C., Fu, M., Lai, W.T., Li, Y.H., Lien, L.M., Tsai, C.D., Wang, J.H., Yeh, P.S., Chaithiraphan, S., Chantadansuwan, T., Jirasirirojanakorn, K., Krittayaphong, R., Laothavorn, P., Mahanonda, N., Sitthisook, S., Tanomsup, S., Tansuphaswadikul, S., Tatsanavivat, P., Yamwong, S., Oto, A., Akin, M., Caglar, N.T., Ergin, A., Müderrisoglu, H., Oguz, A., Ongen, Z., Sansoy, V., Tetiker, T., Uysal, A., Amosova, E., Cherkasova, O., Dykun, Y., Dzyak, G., Galystska, A., Grishyna, O., Jaremenko, O., Kononenko, L., Koval, E., Kovalenko, V., Netyazhenko, V., Pertseva, T., Prokhorov, A., Radchenko, G., Rudyk, Y.U., Sirenko, Y., Skarzhevsky, A., Binbrek, A.S., Hajiri, A.A.R.A., Hatou, E.A., Al-Sousi, A.A.S., Alomairi, M., Wajib, I.M., Sleight, P., Adgey, A.A.J., Andrews, R., Ball, S.G., Barer, D.H., Barnett, A.H., Bridges, A.B., Bryson, V., Cowie, A.S., De Belder, A.J., Donnelly, R., Francis, C.M., Furnace, J., Glen, S.K., Gough, N., Heagerty, A.M., Jackson, P.R., Jackson, S.H.D., Joyce, E., McEneaney, D.J., Moriarty, A.J., Murdoch, D.L., O'Hare, J.P., Penny, W.J., Reid, C.J., Tilley, J., Vora, J.P., Webster, J., Williams, B., Weber, M., Young, J., Ahmed, I., Anand, I.S., Anderson, J.L., Pagán, J.S.A., Barzilay, J., Basile, J.N., Bass, P.F., Blumenthal, S.S., Bommer, W.J., Brautigam, D.F., Brown, C.D., Brown, N., Byrum, J.D., Carr, A.A., Chinn, J., Chiu, D., Cho, N.R., Ciocon, J.O., Colón-Ortíz, P.J., Cruz, J.B., Dachman, W.D., Dolson, G.M., Dorfman, S.G., Drummond, W., East, C., Eelani, F., Ellison, H.S., Felicetta, J.V., Fishbach, M.H., Force, R.W., Giddings, S.J., Goldberg, M.C., Goldman, S., Adrover, R.G., Goss, S.L., Graham, S.P., Granger, C.B., Greenspan, M.M., Grimm, R.H., Habib, G.B., Hagen, M.R., Hart, P.D., Hartney, T.J., Henriquez, M.A., Holland, J.J., Hoogwerf, B.J., Hossfeld, M., Jacobson, A.K., Jelley, M.J., Jones, T.V., Kaplan, R.A., Karalis, D.G., Katz, L.A., Kereiakes, D.J., Khan, M., Kipperman, R.M., Kozinn, M.J., Kozlowski, J.G., Lader, E.W., Landau, C., Landzberg, J.S., Laughrun, D., Lewis, S.J., Liang, C.S., Limacher, M.C., Linz, P.E., Lo, T.S., Lopez-Arostegui, F., Maddox, R.R., Mahrer, P.R., Maurer, M.S., McGuire, D.K., Mercando, A.D., Mersey, J.H., Meyer, M., Mooss, A.N., Narayan, P., Oparil, S., Padhiar, D.N., Phillips, A.L., Prisant, M., Qureshi, N., Raghuwanshi, M.P., Randall, R.R., Retta, T.M., Ringrose, R.E., Rizvi, A.A., Rizvi, M.D., Saklayen, M.G., Sastrasinh, S., Savani, I.K., Schlau, A., Schultz, H.S., Schweiger, M.J., Smith, R.D., Sosa-Padilla, M., Streja, D., Stuver, T.P., Subich, D.C., Sulak, F.C., Swagler, W.A., Taitano, M., Tavarez-Valle, J.A., Taylor, E.M., Tuck, M.L., White, W.B., Wickemeyer, W.J., Wiegmann, T.B., Zee, P.A., Zhao, X.Q., 2008. Telmisartan, ramipril, or both in patients at high risk for vascular events. N. Engl. J. Med. 15334406. 358 (15), 1547–1559. Available from http://content.nejm.org/cgi/reprint/358/15/1547.pdf. doi:10.1056/NEJMoa0801317.

Zhao, Q., Shen, J., Jingya, L., Fan, L., Jiang, Q., Wang, Y., 2020. Clinical efficacy, safety and tolerability of aliskiren monotherapy: a protocol for an umbrella review. BMJ Open. 2044-6055. 10 (1), e033448. doi:10.1136/bmjopen-2019-033448.

CHAPTER

27

Active medical care without dialysis

Ojaswi Singh Tomar[a], Rebecca J. Schmidt[a], and Alvin Howard Moss[b]

[a]Department of Medicine, Division of Nephrology, West Virginia University School of Medicine, Morgantown, WV, United States

[b]Department of Medicine, Division of Geriatrics, Palliative Medicine and Hospice, West Virginia University School of Medicine, Morgantown, WV, United States

Case Example: Mr. D

The nephrology clinician sees Mr. D for the first time: a frail 78-year-old man with stage G5 CKD (estimated glomerular filtration rate [eGFR] 15 mL/min) from diabetes, who lives with his wife of 52 years. His short-term memory is poor, and he is thought to have early vascular dementia. Two years ago, he had a massive heart attack, resulting in heart failure with a reduced ejection fraction and the subsequent placement of an internal cardiac defibrillator. He is weak, with limited exercise tolerance. He requires assistance with dressing and showering. For the past three months, he has been too weak to attend church or his grandchildren's events. For activities outside his home, he uses a wheelchair.

When asked what is most important to him, he says he wants to live for his spouse. He has avoided thinking about kidney failure and has not had a conversation with a nephrology clinician about it. He knows it is getting worse. When asked if there was anything he would want to avoid in treatment, he stated he would not want to be put on a breathing machine. He has not completed a medical order form for life-sustaining measures. He has not discussed preferences with his spouse, but he suspects that she knows them. Some days, he does not think he will be able to make it through the day. He would like to know his kidney failure treatment options in case his kidneys get worse.

Introduction

The realization that dialysis may not benefit all patients with kidney failure is not new. In 1977, nephrologist Belding Scribner, inventor of the arteriovenous shunt that made chronic dialysis possible, and his colleagues were concerned about "how not to dialyze" certain

Aging and the Kidney
https://doi.org/10.1016/B978-0-443-34069-7.00032-X

patients. They started a "deselection committee" to back up a nephrologist's decision not to put a patient on dialysis (Fox and Swazey, 1991, p. 370). In 1991, the Institute of Medicine (IOM) Committee to Study the Medicare End-Stage Renal Disease (ESRD) Program, in their report *Kidney Failure and the Federal Government*, noted that since the enactment of the Medicare ESRD entitlement, an increasing number of patients with limited survival possibilities and relatively poor quality of life were starting dialysis. The committee questioned the appropriateness of dialysis for patients with kidney failure who have limited life expectancy and major comorbidities such as atherosclerotic, cardiac, and peripheral vascular disease, chronic pulmonary disease, cancer, or severe dementia. They recommended the development of clinical practice guidelines that could identify patients for whom the burdens of treatment with dialysis might outweigh the benefits. They foresaw guidelines that would support nephrologists in not offering dialysis to patients for whom it would be disproportionately burdensome (Rettig and Levinsky, 1991).

In 2000, recognizing that an increasing number of older patients suffering from substantial comorbid conditions were initiating KRT and heeding the suggestion of the IOM committee, the American Society of Nephrology (ASN) and the Renal Physicians Association (RPA) conducted a systematic review of the nephrology literature and published the clinical practice guideline *Shared Decision-Making in the Appropriate Initiation of and Withdrawal from Dialysis*. The guideline identified age as a powerful and consistent risk factor for death, with the oldest patients having the shortest survival as a group. Indeed, the oldest patients, those 75–84 years old, had the greatest increase in incident treatment rate, the most comorbid conditions, and were at the greatest risk for deciding to stop dialysis and die. It explicitly identified AMCWD as a treatment option for ESKD (Renal Physicians Association and American Society of Nephrology, 2000).

In the second edition of the guideline, the term "active medical care without dialysis (AMCWD)" was introduced. Patients preferred this term over "conservative management" (Renal Physicians Association and American Society of Nephrology, 2010; p. 157). The guideline explained that AMCWD consists of active treatment to preserve kidney function and to treat acidosis, anemia, bone disease, fluid imbalance, hypertension, pain, and symptoms for a patient with stage 5 CKD who does not want dialysis. In addition, it recommended advance care planning (ACP) with documentation of the patient's goals of care in an advance directive and medical order, such as a Portable Order for Life-Sustaining Treatment (POLST) form (or a comparable form depending on the state).

Over the next decade, AMCWD was increasingly noted to be a treatment choice desired by some patients; yet, it was not utilized systematically and was poorly integrated with dialysis in many countries, especially those with low and middle incomes. In 2020, another major step occurred regarding AMCWD when the International Society of Nephrology (ISN) developed a Strategic Plan for Integrated Care of Patients with Kidney Failure to improve the quality of and access to care for these patients and included AMCWD (the ISN chose to call it CKM) as a key component of its strategy (Harris et al., 2020). As a result, the ISN formed a CKM Working Group. Recognizing that patients with kidney disease have many kidney supportive care (KSC) needs throughout their illness trajectory, in 2024, the ISN CKM Working Group renamed itself the CKM/KSC Working Group and, in its report, explicitly defined CKM and KSC and promoted acceptance of CKM as a treatment option for kidney failure and KSC as a core component of nephrology (Davison et al., 2024). Defining CKM as "care for people with kidney failure that focuses predominantly on providing KSC to promote quality of life but does not include KRT" (Davison et al., 2024; p. 39), the group further clarified the guiding principle in CKM: that all active treatment be aligned with an individual's values, preferences, and goals. Optimal CKM was noted to require the full integration of KSC, defined as "an approach that aims to improve the quality of life for people for whom kidney disease, either directly or indirectly, substantially impacts their well-being, treatment options, or access to care, and their families, through the prevention and relief of suffering by means of early identification and impeccable assessment and treatment of pain and other problems, physical, psychosocial, and spiritual" (Davison et al., 2024; p. 37).

Implementation of active medical care without dialysis for older patients

Patients who might be appropriate for active medical care without dialysis

Drawing on work from the IOM Committee and recommendations from the RPA/ASN clinical practice guideline, the ISN CKM/KSC Working Group sought to identify patients for whom dialysis might be overly burdensome because of their comorbidities, a debilitated or malnourished state, and/or their inability to comply with treatment. Prognostic predictors to help identify such patients, and for whom AMCWD might be appropriate, are shown in Table 27.1. The Figure presents a decision tree for how a patient with advanced CKD might approach a kidney failure treatment decision (Fig. 27.1).

Outcomes of patients who chose active medical care without dialysis

Not surprisingly, patients with two or more prognostic predictors may experience little or no survival benefit from dialysis compared to AMCWD. A systematic review of the

TABLE 27.1 Prognostic predictors to identify persons with kidney failure potentially appropriate for AMCWD.

Experiencing another life-limiting illness (e.g., advanced-stage cancer)
Poor quality of life with irremediable suffering, where dialysis may extend life but prolong suffering
Frailty, the geriatric syndrome associated with cognitive and physical declines, and poor functional status
High comorbidity, especially in cases of severe heart failure, multiple comorbidities, and/or advanced age (>80 years)
Severe malnutrition
Clinician's response of "No, I would not be surprised" to the question ("Would I be surprised if this patient died in the next year?")
Those whose medical condition precludes the technical process of dialysis because the patient is: • Unable to cooperate (e.g., advanced dementia) • Unstable medically (e.g., profound hypotension) • Experiencing another life-limiting illness (e.g., advanced-stage cancer)

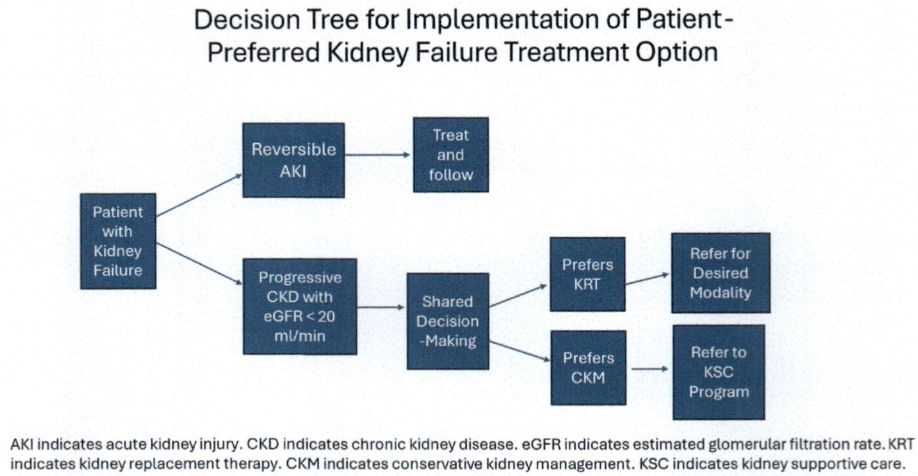

FIG. 27.1 Approach to decision-making for a patient with progressive kidney failure. A provider's guide to the shared decision-making process in advanced kidney disease.

survival of patients treated with AMCWD showed considerable heterogeneity in study designs and outcome measures, which limited comparability. The median survival of AMCWD patient cohorts varied widely, from 1 to 41 months, with baseline mean eGFR ranging from 7 to 19 mL/min/1.73 m^2. There was substantial variability among studies in the percentage of patients treated with AMCWD who were enrolled in hospice (20%–76%) and those dying at home (12%–71%) (O'Hare et al. 2018; Wong et al., 2022). In the largest observational prospective study, Australian researchers compared outcomes of 510 stage 4 and 5 CKD patients aged 65 years or older, 280 of whom chose AMCWD and 230 chose dialysis. Those choosing AMCWD were older (median age 84 versus 74) and more often had three or more comorbidities than those who chose dialysis (43% versus 25%), both $P < .001$. The median survival after the point in time when the eGFR was ≤ 15 mL/min/1.73 for the AMCWD patients was lower compared with dialysis patients (15 months [IQR 7–34] versus 64 months [IQR 30–103], $P < .001$). However, AMCWD patients followed in the KSC clinic had fewer days per year of hospitalization (9 versus 20, $P < .03$) and a lower symptom score than the dialysis patients by their third KSC clinic visit ($P < .001$). Confounding the comparison of survival between those choosing AMCWD and those choosing dialysis (a weakness of this study) is that the patients choosing AMCWD were older and had higher comorbidity (Chou et al., 2023). In a target trial emulation study of 20,440 patients aged 65 years or older with an eGFR below 12 mL/min/1.73 who were not transplant candidates, over 3 years, the group starting dialysis survived on average 11 weeks longer than those choosing AMCWD but had 2 weeks fewer days at home. Thus dialysis provided modest gains in life expectancy but at the expense of less time at home (Montez-Rath et al., 2024).

TABLE 27.2 Reasons why patients choose active medical care without dialysis instead of dialysis (Jongejan et al., 2024; Morton et al., 2012; Saeed et al., 2020).

Willing to trade off longer survival for independence
Quality of life is more important than quantity
Symptoms are better controlled, and no symptoms are caused by dialysis
More time to themselves—don't want to go to dialysis three times a week
Less of a burden on family and friends, including no need for transport to dialysis
Not long to live, and I don't want to go through the bother
Saw the high dialysis treatment burden on a family member or a friend
Had a fulfilling life and want a peaceful death
Freedom to travel, not being tied down to a schedule

Reasons why patients choose active medical care without dialysis

Patient values significantly influence decisions about kidney failure treatments (Table 27.2). Research shows that CKD patients prioritize independence over longevity; in a study of 271 patients with a median age of 77, 49% ranked independence as their top priority, while only 35% prioritized survival. Many viewed staying alive as a lower priority (Ramer et al., 2018). A scoping review revealed that quality of life, treatment burdens, cost, and not wanting to burden family were primary reasons for choosing AMCWD (Jongejan et al., 2024). Other factors included poor prognosis and a desire for dignified life closure (Saeed et al., 2020). Studies indicate CKD patients might trade up to 15 months of survival for a perceived better quality of life with AMCWD (Morton et al., 2012; Davison et al., 2024; Hole et al., 2024).

Recommended best practices for providing active medical care without dialysis

Articles describing AMCWD care have come primarily from nephrologists, often collaborating with palliative care clinicians in Australia and Canada, who have established KSC programs. In the United States, only a few programs offer KSC to support patients who have opted for AMCWD (Lam et al., 2019). In New South Wales, Australia, the KSC program is well developed, and outcomes of patients treated with AMCWD are well-described (Chou et al., 2023; Li and Brown, 2023). Their findings highlight the complex decision-making process for older or seriously ill patients with kidney failure and the necessity of SDM. They note that nephrology clinicians must present balanced treatment options—dialysis should not be the default—and develop an individualized plan based on the patient's values and goals. When discussing options, relevant prognostic information is needed, including estimates of survival and anticipated symptom burden, functional trajectory, and quality of life with dialysis and with AMCWD. Brown and colleagues describe AMCWD as a holistic, proactive, and multidisciplinary treatment for kidney failure that ideally is co-managed with a dedicated KSC service throughout the continuum of the patient's life (Li and Brown, 2023).

In Alberta, Canada, AMCWD is offered through the CKM Clinical Working Group, led by the Kidney Supportive Care Research Group. Their guidelines for AMCWD include recommendations for the management of symptoms and metabolic complications of advanced CKD. On their website, they provide five distinct, freely accessible algorithms specific to the end of life for the following symptoms: breathlessness, pain, nausea and vomiting, respiratory secretions, and agitation and restlessness (Davison et al., 2019). They observe that there is great variation in Canada and around the world in how patients choosing AMCWD are treated. The publication of their recommendations and algorithms is a step toward standardizing an approach to AMCWD care that is based on evidence and knowledge of best practices.

In its 2024 report, the ISN CKM/KSC Working Group described the key components of KSC, which provide the framework for CKM: SDM, symptom management, crisis planning, ACP, spiritual care, integration with community services, end-of-life care, and bereavement support for the family. In addition, AMCWD care involves management of CKD progression insofar as doing so aligns with the individual's priorities, preservation of kidney function, and management of medical complications of CKD to the extent the patient desires (Davison et al., 2024). The above Australian and Canadian publications provide excellent resources for those wishing to implement an AMCWD program.

Barriers to advocating for active medical care without dialysis

Patient perspective

The decision to pursue AMCWD is a personal one, likely influenced by family or caregivers, the treating physician, and the patient's life circumstances. Barriers to choosing AMCWD include patient uncertainties and unrealistic views on prognosis. Fear of the unknown and a lack of knowledge about the dying process can significantly impact a patient's considerations. Patients may fear that choosing to forgo dialysis will be seen as unacceptable by their families, akin to "giving up," religiously unacceptable (a sin), or suicide (Elliott et al., 2012). Patients may also worry that this choice indicates a lack of hope, leading physicians to provide less care (Davison and Simpson, 2006). In addition, the anticipation of distressing symptoms, should they forgo dialysis, may compel patients to decide against AMCWD (Weisbord et al., 2005). Patients may be concerned about what they anticipate as an undue burden falling upon family members providing care. The presence of depression (P.L, 2002) or cognitive decline (Murray et al., 2006) should be considered a potential contributing factor to a patient's decision-making. Information about the potential benefits, risks, and burdens of dialysis is a key element of the dialog as are the individual patient's values and preferences (Morton et al., 2012) and a one-size-fits-all approach to this conversation may fail to uncover patient-specific concerns.

Delaying ACP discussions risks the development of kidney failure symptoms. If treatment decisions are postponed, symptoms may impair a patient's objectivity, pushing them toward dialysis as a rescue option. Acknowledging that dialysis is life-sustaining but not life-restoring can be challenging and may hinder acceptance of nondialytic approaches.

Family and caregiver perspective

Family members may feel unequipped to deal with their loved one's end-of-life needs at home, and the intricacies, magnitude, and type of care that is anticipated may outweigh what they can reasonably or realistically provide (Maddalena et al., 2018). Hospice offers a wide range of services for patients who meet the criteria (Medicare, 2020a) though often these services are provided at a frequency that is insufficient to meet the needs of either the patient or their caregiver.

Family members may share the patient's fears regarding spiritual or ethical issues, symptom burden, or witnessing the dying experience. They might also feel guilty for not pursuing life-saving treatment or have unrealistic expectations of dialysis. Discussing these matters can be challenging, especially for those who rely on the patient for emotional or financial support. Terminology is crucial; patients and caregivers might associate "palliative" with dying, and the term "nondialysis" can suggest that dialysis is the focus rather than care specific to the patient.

Physician perspective

Historically, physicians have not received significant training in end-of-life care or ACP (Holley et al., 2003; Davison et al., 2006; Combs et al., 2015) and thus may feel ill-prepared or uncomfortable initiating conversations about AMCWD. The recognition that AMCWD, as well as KSC, are key components of nephrology care (Davison et al., 2024) along with a much-needed national focus on SDM as the "pinnacle" of patient-centered care (Barry and Edgman-Levitan, 2012) has fueled efforts to include experiences and skills in ACP and end-of-life care in nephrology training programs (Schell et al., 2013). The question of who should assume the responsibility for ACP has also been raised (Hamroun et al., 2022; O'Hare et al., 2016).

A notable barrier continues to be the difficulty of estimating a patient's prognosis and predicting their course (with and without dialysis), the symptoms to be expected, and the time frame over which they may suffer these symptoms before death. Although patients may wish to discuss these issues with their nephrologists (Levy et al., 1996; Davison, 2010) they may wait for their nephrologist to raise the topic, underscoring the importance of being proactive as the appropriate time for such discussions nears. Furthermore, these conversations can be emotionally challenging (Wachterman et al., 2019a; Ladin et al., 2017) and logistically difficult.

Setting aside a specific time for these conversations, separate from times that deal with medical concerns, may be appropriate; the time needed for these discussions can be significant, but they warrant sufficient time to allow for questions to be raised, scenarios to be explored, and a patient's personal goals to be identified.

Dialysis, due to its effectiveness and low risk, has become the default treatment for many ESKD patients. Some nephrologists believe that not choosing dialysis goes against their ethical responsibility under the Hippocratic Oath to do no harm (Ladin et al., 2018a). Others may consider forgoing life-sustaining treatment spiritually and ethically unacceptable, leading them to hesitate or refuse to offer such care (Wachterman et al., 2019a).

Coverage/regulatory perspective

Since the passage of entitlement legislation in 1972, the availability and effectiveness of dialysis have hampered the development of a coordinated and meaningful system for ACP for patients with advanced CKD (Tamura et al., 2018). In contrast to patients who choose to forgo dialysis, patients who choose to pursue dialysis benefit from structured operations and the embedded support system of the dialysis staff.

Patients who choose AMCWD often have an unpredictable prognosis, rendering them unable to meet the criteria for some hospices. Although hospice may be an option for many of these patients, the frequency with which specific services can be provided by a given hospice entity may not be sufficient to meet the patient's needs. Indeed, the inability to garner support for home care was cited as a major barrier to proceeding with conservative care for patients with advanced CKD who chose to forgo dialysis (Tam-Tham et al., 2016). Regional differences in hospice practices also exist (O'Hare et al., 2010). By contrast, the support system offered by the dialysis facility for patients initiating dialysis therapy may exceed that available to a patient with advanced CKD in an interdisciplinary palliative care program (Grubbs et al., 2017). Finally, reimbursement for outpatient palliative care programs is lacking; thus the profitability of starting a patient on dialysis disincentivizes the alternative of proceeding with outpatient palliative care (Tamura et al., 2018).

Role of the nephrologist in providing active medical care without dialysis

Identifying patients with a poor prognosis

Individuals with advanced CKD face substantial coexisting health problems, as well as the emotional burden of a life-limiting illness and the need to make complex treatment choices (Heyland et al., 2009) (Table 27.1). It is the responsibility of nephrologists to identify such patients and discuss prognosis (Michel and Moss, 2005). Sensitive discussions with patients and their families will include comprehensive information and facilitate patient education about survival benefits associated with both AMCWD and dialysis, which may be comparable but, in the case of dialysis, come with significant impairments in quality of life (Heyland et al., 2009; Lopez Revuelta et al., 2004).

Nephrologists may overestimate how well patients will do, feel uncomfortable discussing what the future holds for them, and find it simpler, quicker, and more financially beneficial to start dialysis (Ladin et al., 2017; Ladin et al., 2018a). The quality of physician-patient communication significantly influences how patients cope and prepare themselves for the future. Indeed, it is well-accepted that effective communication improves patient comprehension, satisfaction, and optimism (Davison and Simpson, 2006).

Comorbidities that have been associated with a prognosis of less than one year in CKD patients include metastatic cancer, severe chronic obstructive pulmonary disease (COPD), severe peripheral vascular disease (PVD), advanced dementia, severe heart failure (New York Heart Association class IV), disruptive behavioral disorders, and acquired immunodeficiency syndrome (AIDS) (Lopez Revuelta et al., 2004; Kurella et al., 2006; Postorino et al., 2007; Rakowski et al., 2006).

Clinical and functional parameters

Initiating dialysis in patients aged 80 and above often leads to functional decline, with about 30% requiring caregiver support or long-term care within 6 months. Those starting dialysis from a nursing facility have a particularly poor prognosis, typically living less than a year (Tamura et al., 2009). This population has a high mortality rate, especially within the first 30–120 days of treatment (Wachterman et al., 2019b).

Worsening functional status among CKD and ESKD patients correlates with increased mortality, as indicated by a higher incidence of falls and decreased transfer ability (Lopez Revuelta et al., 2004). Serum albumin levels below 3.5 g/dL predict approximately 50% 1-year mortality in dialysis patients (Bleyer et al., 1996).

Use of the surprise question

The "surprise" question—"Would I be surprised if this patient died within the next year?"—is a recognized tool for improving end-of-life care. It helps identify patients with a poor prognosis who could benefit from palliative care. The surprise question encourages clinicians to consider if death within a year is a realistic possibility, rather than simply asking if they believe death will occur (Moss et al., 2008; Pattison and Romer, 2001). The "surprise" question has been validated in several patient populations—cancer, heart failure, chronic obstructive pulmonary disease, and sepsis (White et al., 2017)—in addition to hemodialysis patients (Moss et al., 2008). In a study of 147 dialysis patients, the "No, I would not be surprised" response to the "surprise question" flagged a sicker subgroup of dialysis patients (Moss et al., 2008) at high risk for early mortality. These patients were older, had a higher comorbidity score, and a lower performance status score. The surprise question is available for free through TouchCalc (Caberto, 2025).

Use of integrated prognostic models

Utilizing prognostic models is an important clinical practice so that patients and their families can understand their prognosis and have time for important end-of-life discussions. Recognizing a poor prognosis can also lead to palliative care and hospice, depending on the patient's symptoms and wishes (Cohen et al., 2010).

An integrated prognostic model for 12-month mortality in advanced CKD patients was developed and validated to assist nephrologists in guiding patients on whether to initiate dialysis or pursue AMCWD. The model found that the surprise question, Karnofsky performance status, and age were most predictive of 12-month mortality, with odds ratios (ORs) [95% confidence interval (CI)] of 3.29 (1.87–5.78) for a "No" response to the SQ, 2.09 (95% CI 1.19–3.66) for fair KPS, and 1.41 (95% CI 1.15–1.74) per 10-year increase in age (Schmidt et al., 2019).

Davison and Rathwell (2024) explored the real-world effectiveness of the Cohen prognostic model in predicting survival in a study of hemodialysis patients. This model combines patient data with a clinician's intuitive assessment of prognosis (the "Surprise Question") to forecast survival at 6, 12, and 18 months. Analyzing data from over 1300 patients in a Canadian dialysis program between 2010 and 2019, researchers compared the model's predictions with observed survival outcomes. The model overestimated mortality at the twelve- and eighteen-month marks, but it did successfully stratify patients into risk categories, offering a practical approach to identifying high-risk dialysis patients, thereby enabling more effective targeting of KSC interventions.

Developing a treatment plan

Conservative kidney management and KSC are now considered core components of integrated kidney care (Davison et al., 2024) with AMCWD accepted as appropriate for certain patients. Central to the nephrologist's role in providing AMCWD is the obligation to learn about a patient's preferences, goals, and values in the context of their life and illness. At the outset, it is important to clarify that choosing to forgo dialysis does not mean one is forgoing care.

With this shared understanding, a treatment plan can be developed that reflects a patient's true wishes and constitutes an informed choice. ACP improves the likelihood that dialysis will not be initiated under emergent circumstances or because options were not presented. A proactive and deliberate decision to forgo dialysis requires ongoing conversation. Such a dialog will help inform a treatment plan that is specific to a patient's values, needs, hopes, and desires (Davison and Simpson, 2006).

Developing a treatment plan requires a strategy that prioritizes patient comfort and daily quality of life (Li and Brown, 2023). While the nephrologist leads this effort, a multidisciplinary approach involving palliative care specialists, social workers, mental health professionals, and pain specialists is essential to meet the patient's needs. Palliative care specialists can effectively manage end-of-life symptoms and tailor interventions (Quill and Abernethy, 2013). Patients may experience fear, anxiety, or depression (Levy et al., 1996; P.L, 2002; Blumenfield et al., 1997), making counseling or spiritual care beneficial. Ongoing monitoring of physical and emotional symptoms is vital to ensure medical and psychosocial care remains comprehensive and compassionate (Fletcher et al., 2022; Speyer et al., 2024).

Educating patients and their families about active medical care without dialysis

Process, care options and expectations

Patients and families deserve clear, cogent, and individually focused education about their decision to forgo dialysis and the care that may be offered within the realm of AMCWD. Patients must be reassured that they will receive care that meets their needs and that different degrees of palliative care are available irrespective of their choice to pursue or forgo dialysis. Expectations should be discussed and clarified in the context of each patient's clinical scenario and with their prognosis in mind, including the likelihood that functional status will deteriorate (Tamura et al., 2009; Holley and Schmidt, 2014; Murtagh et al., 2011).

Recommendations emphasize that a plan should be comfort-focused rather than disease-focused. A key part of the treatment plan involves educating patients and families about the prognosis and symptom burden (Speyer et al., 2024; Abdel-Kader et al., 2009).

Use of data to support the dialog

Providing data that verifies poor kidney function to the discussion may instill confidence in patients who voice no symptoms or have a normal physical exam and may question the need for ACP. The use of 24-hour urine collection to assess creatinine clearance, a record of output volumes, and the presentation of other lab values, such as the eGFR, may be helpful tools for nephrologists to utilize in presenting expectations to patients who are worried that they will suffer unimaginable symptoms after forgoing dialysis.

Managing symptoms and addressing crisis events

Establishing a patient-specific plan for preventing and managing symptoms (Chou et al., 2023; Davison et al., 2019) includes proactively addressing "heat-of-the-moment" events. Setting the stage with the expectation that symptoms will be addressed is key to helping patients accept the possibility that acute symptoms, such as respiratory distress, involuntary jerking, or worsening of chronic pain (Barakzoy and Moss, 2006) will occur.

Symptom management should be prioritized and may include medical management of hypertension and fluid balance, as well as treatment of acid-base imbalance, mineral metabolism abnormalities, anemia (if symptomatic), nausea and vomiting, pain (Barakzoy and Moss, 2006), and itching. Depending on a patient's prognosis and anticipated life expectancy, blood tests may be discontinued. Recommendations include the implementation of POLST, POST, or MOST, depending on the state (Citko et al., 2011), determination of the patient's preferred site of death, and whether it is a feasible location. The plan should include the patient's wishes for pain control in the form of palliative sedation, should symptoms become unbearable.

Importance of a structured kidney supportive care

A structured KSC program is essential for ensuring comprehensive patient care. Emotional, psychosocial, and spiritual support are also vital components of any KSC program (Davison et al., 2024). Patients should be offered plans for hospice and other care for support based on their specific needs.

Shared decision-making

From 2000 to 2012, the number of new dialysis patients in the United States grew by almost 60%, with the largest increase seen in those aged 75 and older (United States Renal Data System, 2014). For some older adults, especially those aged 75 and above with comorbidities, survival rates may be similar whether they undergo dialysis or receive AMCWD (Ladin et al., 2017). However, quality-of-life outcomes differ significantly between these two approaches (Frazier et al., 2022).

Importance of shared decision-making

Shared decision-making (SDM) is the gold standard in patient care, promoting collaboration between physicians and patients to develop treatment plans based on mutual goals, risks, benefits, and alternatives. This approach values patient preferences alongside medical expertise, resulting in personalized care and fostering a supportive healthcare environment (Ladin et al., 2017).

To better understand the extent to which older patients experience SDM, a cross-sectional analysis was conducted among 350 older individuals with CKD using a nine-item SDM Questionnaire (SDM-Q-9), which was derived and found to be reliable (Kriston et al., 2010) (Table 27.3). The findings revealed a suboptimal level of SDM, with only 22% of patients scoring above 80%, (indicating strong or complete agreement with the statements (Frazier et al., 2022). A survey of 295 dialysis patients found that over half (60.7%) regretted starting dialysis, and nearly 14% said they chose dialysis due to family influence rather than personal choice (Davison, 2010).

Many patients initiating dialysis reported that, despite the often-predictable nature of progressive CKD, they received insufficient or incomprehensible information or initiated dialysis without fully understanding the long-term implications it may have on their quality of life (Ladin et al., 2017). Many older patients felt they did not have a choice about dialysis, were not actively involved in decisions about their care, and were unaware of nondialysis management options. This lack of preparedness and autonomy frequently leads to regret among older patients who start dialysis (Ladin et al., 2017). These reports suggest that, despite established guidelines, shared decision-making is underutilized in clinical encounters among older adults with advanced CKD (Frazier et al., 2022).

Shared decision-making can empower patients with knowledge and reduce their anxiety about treatment outcomes, ultimately leading to greater confidence in their choices (Frazier et al., 2022). As patient complexity increases, effective communication, characterized by transparency, plain language, sensitivity, and encouragement of open dialog, becomes paramount for optimal care and informed decision-making.

TABLE 27.3 Elements of shared decision-making.

Patient is aware of the choice and the decision to be made
Opportunity to express needs, values, and preferences
Informed of prognosis and *all* options
• Benefits and risks of each
• Patient decision aid to standardize information and facilitate understanding
Adequate time for decision (not rushed)
Active participant
• Co-equal in decision with physician
• Co-equal in developing a plan of care with the physician.

Adapted from Kriston, L., Scholl, I., Hölzel, L., Simon, D., Loh, A., Härter, M., 2010. The 9-item shared decision making questionnaire (SDM-Q-9). Development and psychometric properties in a primary care sample. Patient Educ. Couns. 07383991. 80 (1), 94–99. doi:10.1016/j.pec.2009.09.034.

SDM is a continuous process that should begin early in CKD and continue as it progresses to ESKD. Familiarity with these discussions can reduce patient anxiety and encourage active participation. Repetitive conversations not only benefit patients but also ease the discomfort of providers in initiating these discussions. Considered the ideal approach to patient-centered care, SDM enhances patient satisfaction and upholds the ethical principles of autonomy, beneficence, and nonmaleficence (Barry and Edgman-Levitan, 2012; Ladin et al., 2017).

Studies show that well-informed patients who attend educational classes are more likely to engage in SDM. Specifically, knowledge of treatment options, participation in classes, use of decision aids, and high self-reported information levels about KRT correlate with greater SDM (Frazier et al., 2022; Ladin et al., 2023).

Care partners play a crucial but complex role in SDM and patient satisfaction. Support from care partners can be beneficial if it aligns with the patient's desires, but it can be detrimental if their preferences clash with the patient's (Davison, 2010; Frazier et al., 2022).

Use of patient decision aids to promote shared decision-making

Patient decision aids support SDM by standardizing information about treatment options' benefits, risks, and uncertainties in a patient-friendly format. They help patients make informed choices when multiple reasonable options exist and when personal values are crucial. Research shows that patients are better informed, more involved in decision-making, more aligned with their values, have accurate risk perceptions, and experience less decisional conflict (Stacey et al., 2024).

Because kidney disease education in the past has not emphasized, and often omitted, mention of AMCWD, older patients with advanced CKD participating in SDM and facing a decision about initiation of dialysis versus AMCWD are particularly likely to benefit from high-quality patient decision aids that present accurate, balanced, comprehensive, and accessible kidney failure treatment options education, including AMCWD. Only recently have patient decision aids describing AMCWD become available (Ladin et al., 2023; Wong et al., 2022). Their impact on patients' kidney failure treatment decisions has yet to be determined.

Consequences of suboptimal shared decision-making for patients with advanced CKD

Despite ethical arguments for the importance of SDM, studies indicate that it is not implemented effectively in dialysis settings (Frazier et al., 2022). Surveys reveal that many dialysis patients report a lack of information about treatment options, with over a third unaware of alternatives to in-center hemodialysis. Patients often struggle to understand their choices, feel coerced into quick decisions, and experience increased anxiety regarding their prognosis (Frazier et al., 2022; Morton et al., 2012; Song et al., 2013; Wong et al., 2019; Kaufman et al., 2006). While most patients desire better communication about their options, a significant gap remains in physician-patient discussions, particularly about end-of-life care (Shared Decision-Making in the Appropriate Initiation of and Withdrawal from Dialysis, second ed., 2010b).

Conflict in the conservative kidney care decision-making

Difference in values between patients and nephrology clinicians or caregivers

A difference in values between nephrologists and patients can lead to conflict in kidney failure treatment options decision-making. In a qualitative study of 851 adults with CKD receiving treatment in the US Veterans Health Administration health care system who had chosen not to start dialysis, researchers found that nephrologists did not accept patients' decisions to forgo dialysis and repeatedly questioned them about their choice during subsequent clinic visits. In reviewing electronic health record documentation, researchers observed that patients who did not wish to start dialysis had to resist immense pressure from nephrologists to do so. The researchers noted that nephrologists seemed to take "an all-or-nothing" approach to caring for these patients, with dialysis being a powerful default in the absence of other options for the nephrologist to offer (Wong et al., 2019; p. 312). In agreement with these findings, a qualitative study using semi-structured interviews with 35 purposively sampled nephrologists showed that only about one-third would offer AMCWD. Those not so inclined valued active, life-prolonging interventions, promoted their perception of the patient's well-being irrespective of patients' preferences, and adhered to an institutional culture in which the norm was starting dialysis (Ladin et al., 2018a). Nephrologists who would not offer AMCWD perceived it as "no care," favored offering active treatments (dialysis) to instill hope and avoid upsetting patients, and sensed a lack of institutional support for AMCWD. Those who offered AMCWD felt that they took a more patient-centered approach in which they accepted patient preferences not to start dialysis (Ladin et al., 2018b; p. 630).

Also, conflict regarding the decision to start dialysis or AMCWD often arises between patients and their families. A study involving 393 American Nephrology Nurses Association nurses indicated that 15% of dialysis patients aged 65 and older may have been on dialysis inappropriately, as the burdens outweighed the benefits. Frequently, patients were influenced by family members to start dialysis against their wishes (Badzek et al., 2000).

Recommendations for resolving conflict

Whether it is a nephrologist-patient or patient-family conflict, the second edition of the *Shared Decision-Making in the Appropriate Initiation of and Withdrawal from Dialysis* clinical practice guideline recommends resolving conflicts over treatment decisions. It recommends, "Establish a systematic due process approach for conflict resolution if there is disagreement about what decision should be made with regard to dialysis" (p. 61) and observes that conflicts may occur between the patient (or their legal decision-maker if the patient lacks decision-making capacity) and the kidney care team about whether dialysis will benefit the patient. In addition, they may occur within the kidney care team or between the kidney care team and other health care providers. The recommendation urges that nephrology clinicians seek to understand others' views, cite data to provide more informed decision-making, and seek to correct any misunderstandings of the benefits and burdens of the kidney failure treatment options. The guideline specifically identifies the following potential sources of conflict: (1) miscommunication or misunderstanding about prognosis; (2) intrapersonal or interpersonal issues; or (3) special values. If dialysis is indicated emergently and requested by the patient or legal decision-maker, it urges that it be provided while pursuing conflict resolution. To resolve conflict, it recommends potentially involving another physician for a second opinion, an ethics consult, or a palliative care consult.

The time-limited trial and deciding not to decide: Additional approaches to resolve conflict

A time-limited trial of dialysis is highlighted in the guidelines as another way to resolve conflicts about choosing between dialysis and AMCWD. It can help reduce uncertainty regarding how patients with an unclear prognosis will tolerate dialysis. If dialysis is not needed immediately, nephrologists and clinicians may agree on a "decide-not-to-decide" approach, which allows patients more time to consider their options (Saeed et al., 2022). This method respects patients' ambivalence and enables them to delay decisions about treatment and dialysis access until they feel ready. Research shows that many older patients with CKD prefer a "wait and-see" strategy, focusing on living well in the present rather than planning for the future (House et al., 2022).

Clinical application: Return to Mr. D

Mr. D presents several poor prognostic indicators, including frailty, dementia, functional impairment, and comorbidities, leading to an expected unfavorable outcome with dialysis. Consequently, his nephrologist has initiated a discussion about his prognosis and recommended AMCWD as part of KSC. Mr. D can reasonably be predicted to do poorly with dialysis. He is grateful for his nephrologist's recommendation because he did not feel up to dialysis access surgery and the intensive change in his life that starting dialysis would entail once he developed an indication for it. Though he wanted to live for his wife, he did not think he had the energy to prepare for and undergo dialysis. Together, through SDM, they agreed to proceed with AMCWD.

Summary

Though palliative care, including end-of-life care, has received attention for its important role in comprehensive health care for chronically ill patients, it has yet to be entrenched in the national health care system at all levels and for all patients.

Prognostic predictors that identify patients for whom the burdens of dialysis might exceed the benefits have been identified. Patients with two or more of these predictors may experience little or no survival benefit from dialysis as compared to AMCWD. Barriers to advocating for AMCWD are multifaceted and include those posed by the patient, family, or caregiver, those harbored by many nephrologists, and others that are widespread in our healthcare system and culture. Attention to patients' values, preferences, and goals, along with clear communication and systematic due process in the management of conflicts and decision inertia, are key to the SDM that patients need, want, and deserve.

Integration of clinical guidelines for the delivery of AMCWD as a component of integrated kidney care, and their alignment with national and international palliative care initiatives, continues to evolve (Tamura et al 2013). Inherent to this movement is the acceptance that dialysis will not improve the quality of life for every patient. Treating our patients with kindness, respect, and support as they strive to retain their dignity throughout the continuum of kidney care will always be of paramount importance.

References

Abdel-Kader, K., Unruh, M.L., Weisbord, S.D., 2009. Symptom burden, depression, and quality of life in chronic and end-stage kidney disease. Clin. J. Am. Soc. Nephrol. 1555905X. 4 (6), 1057–1064. Available from: http://cjasn.asnjournals.org/cgi/reprint/4/6/1057. doi:10.2215/CJN.00430109.

Badzek, L.A., Cline, H.S., Moss, A.H., Hines, S.C., 2000. Inappropriate use of dialysis for some elderly patients: nephrology nurses' perceptions and concerns. Nephrol. Nurs. J. 1526744X. 27 (5), 462–472.

Barakzoy, A.S., Moss, A.H., 2006. Efficacy of the World Health Organization analgesic ladder to treat pain in end-stage renal disease. J. Am. Soc. Nephrol. 10466673. 17 (11), 3198–3203. Available from: https://journals.lww.com/jasn/pages/default.aspx. doi:10.1681/ASN.2006050477.

Barry, M.J., Edgman-Levitan, S., 2012. Shared decision making—the pinnacle of patient-centered care. N. Engl. J. Med. 15334406. 366 (9), 780–781. Available from: http://www.nejm.org/doi/pdf/10.1056/NEJMp1109283. doi:10.1056/NEJMp1109283.

Bleyer, A.J., Tell, G.S., Evans, G.W., Ettinger, W.H., Burkart, J.M., 1996. Survival of patients undergoing renal replacement therapy in one center with special emphasis on racial differences. Am. J. Kidney Dis. 02726386. 28 (1), 72–81. Available from: http://www.elsevier.com/inca/publications/store/6/2/3/2/7/6/index.htt. doi:10.1016/S0272-6386(96)90133-X.

Blumenfield, M., Levy, N.B., Spinowitz, B., Charytan, C., Beasley Jr, C.M., Dubey, A.K., Solomon, R.J., Todd, R., Goodman, A., Bergstrom, R.F., 1997. Fluoxetine in depressed patients on dialysis. Int. J. Psychiatry Med. 27 (1), 71–80.

Caberto, S.C., 2025. Surprise Question Smartphone', zkidney.com. Available from: https://www.zkidney.com/sq-sp (Accessed: 19 June 2026).

Centers for Medicare & Medicaid Services, 2020. Medicare Hospice Benefits. U.S. Department of Health and Human Services, Baltimore, MD. Available from: https://www.medicare.gov/Pubs/pdf/02154-Medicare-Hospice-Benefits.pdf (Accessed: 4 June 2020).

Chou, A., Li, C., Farshid, S., Hoffman, A., Brown, M., 2023. Survival, symptoms and hospitalization of older patients with advanced chronic kidney disease managed without dialysis. Nephrol. Dial. Transplant. 14602385. 38 (2), 405–413. Available from: http://ndt.oxfordjournals.org/. doi:10.1093/ndt/gfac154.

Citko, J., Moss, A.H., Carley, M., Tolle, S., 2011. The national POLST paradigm initiative, 2nd Edition #178. J. Palliat. Med. 10966218. 14 (2), 241–242. doi:10.1089/jpm.2010.9730.

Cohen, L.M., Ruthazer, R., Moss, A.H., Germain, M.J., 2010. Predicting six-month mortality for patients who are on maintenance hemodialysis. Clin. J. Am. Soc. Nephrol. 1555905X. 5 (1), 72–79. Available from: http://cjasn.asnjournals.org/cgi/reprint/5/1/72. doi:10.2215/CJN.03860609.

Combs, S.A., Culp, S., Matlock, D.D., Kutner, J.S., Holley, J.L., Moss, A.H., 2015. Update on end-of-life care training during nephrology fellowship: a cross-sectional national survey of fellows. Am. J. Kidney Dis. 15236838. 65 (2), 233–239. Available from: http://www.elsevier.com/inca/publications/store/6/2/3/2/7/6/index.htt. doi:10.1053/j.ajkd.2014.07.018.

Dartmouth Atlas of Health Care, 2007. Preference-sensitive care. Dartmouth Institute for Health Policy and Clinical Practice, Lebanon, NH.

Davison, S.N., 2010. End-of-life care preferences and needs: perceptions of patients with chronic kidney disease. Clin. J. Am. Soc. Nephrol. 1555905X. 5 (2), 195–204. Available from: http://cjasn.asnjournals.org/cgi/reprint/5/2/195. doi:10.2215/CJN.05960809Canada.

Davison, S.N., Levin, A., Moss, A.H., Jha, V., Brown, E.A., Brennan, F., Murtagh, F.E., Naicker, S., Germain, M.J., O'Donoghue, D.J., Morton, R.L., 2015. Executive summary of the KDIGO controversies conference on supportive care in chronic kidney disease: developing a roadmap to improving quality care. Kidney Int. 88 (3), 447–459.

Davison, S.N., Pommer, W., Brown, M.A., Douglas, C.A., Gelfand, S.L., Gueco, I.P., Hole, B.D., Homma, S., Kazancıoğlu, R.T., Kitamura, H., Koubar, S.H., Krause, R., Li, K.C., Lowney, A.C., Nagaraju, S.P., Niang, A., Obrador, G.T., Ohtake, Y., Schell, J.O., Scherer, J.S., Smyth, B., Tamba, K., Vallath, N., Wearne, N., Zakharova, E., Zúñiga, C., Brennan, F.P., 2024. Conservative kidney management and kidney supportive care: core components of integrated care for people with kidney failure. Kidney Int. 15231755. 105 (1), 35–45. Available from: https://www.sciencedirect.com/science/journal/00852538. doi:10.1016/j.kint.2023.10.001.

Davison, S.N., Rathwell, S., 2024. Short-term and long-term survival in patients with prevalent haemodialysis—an integrated prognostic model: external validation. BMJ Support. Palliat. Care. 20454368. 14 (2), 222–229. Available from: https://spcare.bmj.com/. doi:10.1136/spcare-2022-003916.

Davison, S.N., Simpson, C., 2006. Hope and advance care planning in patients with end stage renal disease: qualitative interview study. BMJ. 0959-8138. 333 (7574), 886. doi:10.1136/bmj.38965.626250.55.

Davison, S.N., Tupala, B., Wasylynuk, B.A., Siu, V., Sinnarajah, A., Triscott, J., 2019. Recommendations for the care of patients receiving conservative kidney management focus on management of CKD and symptoms. Clin. J. Am. Soc. Nephrol. 1555905X. 14 (4), 626–634. Available from: https://cjasn.asnjournals.org/content/clinjasn/14/4/626.full.pdf. doi:10.2215/CJN.10510917.

Elliott, B.A., Gessert, C.E., Larson, P., Russ, T.E., 2012. Religious beliefs and practices in end-stage renal disease: implications for clinicians. J. Pain Symptom Manage. 18736513. 44 (3), 400–409. doi:10.1016/j.jpainsymman.2011.09.019.

Fletcher, B.R., Damery, S., Aiyegbusi, O.L., Anderson, N., Calvert, M., Cockwell, P., Ferguson, J., Horton, M., Paap, M.C.S., Sidey-Gibbons, C., Slade, A., Turner, N., Kyte, D., 2022. Symptom burden and health-related quality of life in chronic kidney disease: a global systematic review and meta-analysis. PLoS Med. 15491676. 19 (4). Available from: https://journals.plos.org/plosmedicine/article/file?id=10.1371/journal.pmed.1003954&type=printable. doi:10.1371/journal.pmed.1003954.

Fox, R.C., Swazey, J.P., 1991. The Courage to Fail: A Social View of Organ Transplants and Dialysis, University of Chicago Press. 145.

Frazier, R., Levine, S., Porteny, T., Tighiouart, H., Wong, J.B., Isakova, T., Koch-Weser, S., Gordon, E.J., Weiner, D.E., Ladin, K., 2022. Shared decision making among older adults with advanced CKD. Am. J. Kidney Dis. 15236838. 80 (5), 599–609. Available from: http://www.elsevier.com/inca/publications/store/6/2/3/2/7/6/index.htt. doi:10.1053/j.ajkd.2022.02.017.

Grubbs, V., Tuot, D.S., Powe, N.R., O'Donoghue, D., Chesla, C.A., 2017. System-level barriers and facilitators for foregoing or withdrawing dialysis: a qualitative study of nephrologists in the United States and England. Am. J. Kidney Dis. 15236838. 70 (5), 602–610. Available from: http://www.elsevier.com/inca/publications/store/6/2/3/2/7/6/index.htt. doi:10.1053/j.ajkd.2016.12.015.

Hamroun, A., Speyer, E., Ayav, C., Combe, C., Fouque, D., Jacquelinet, C., Laville, M., Liabeuf, S., Massy, Z.A., Pecoits-Filho, R., Robinson, B.M., Glowacki, F., Stengel, B., Frimat, L., 2022. Barriers to conservative care from patients' and nephrologists' perspectives: the CKD-REIN study. Nephrol. Dial. Transplant. 14602385. 37 (12), 2438–2448. Available from: http://ndt.oxfordjournals.org/. doi:10.1093/ndt/gfac009.

Harris, D.C.H., Davies, S.J., Finkelstein, F.O., Jha, V., Bello, A.K., Brown, M., Caskey, F.J., Donner, J.A., Liew, A., Muller, E., Naicker, S., O'Connell, P.J., Filho, R.P., Vachharajani, T., Alfa, A.K.A., Ashuntantang, G., Brown, E., Cullis, B., Dreyer, G., Eke, F.U., Garcia, G.G., Goh, B.L., Hemmelgarn, B., Hou, F.F., Iyengar, A., Johnson, D.W., Levin, N.W., Luyckx, V.A., Martin, D.E., McCulloch, M.I., Mengistu, Y.T., Moosa, M.R., Morton, R.L., Niang, A., Obrador, G.T., Okpechi, I.G., Ossareh, S., Shah, K.D., Sola, L., Swanepoel, C., Tchokhonelidze, I., Tonelli, M., Trask, M., Kazancioglu, R.T., Twahir, A., Walker, R., Were, A.J.O., Yang, C.W., Yeates, K., Zakharova, E., Zuniga, C., 2020. Strategic plan for integrated care of patients with kidney failure. Kidney Int. 15231755. 98 (5), S117. Available from: https://www.journals.elsevier.com/kidney-international. doi:10.1016/j.kint.2020.07.023.

Heyland, D.K., Allan, D.E., Rocker, G., Dodek, P., Pichora, D., Gafni, A., 2009. Discussing prognosis with patients and their families near the end of life: impact on satisfaction with end-of-life care. Open Med. 19112092. 3 (2), 71–80. Available from: http://www.openmedicine.ca/article/view/160/244.

Hole, B., Coast, J., Caskey, F.J., Selman, L.E., Rooshenas, L., Kimpton, G., Snead, C., Field, A., Morton, R.L., 2024. A choice experiment of older patients' preferences for kidney failure treatments. Kidney Int. doi:10.1016/j.kint.2024.08.032.

Holley, J.L., Carmody, S.S., Moss, A.H., Sullivan, A.M., Cohen, L.M., Block, S.D., Arnold, R.M., 2003. The need for end-of-life care training in nephrology: national survey results of nephrology fellows. Am. J. Kidney Dis. 42 (4), 813–820.

Holley, J.L., Schmidt, R.J., 2014. Conservative/Palliative Treatment and End-of-Life Care in Chronic Kidney Disease. Springer Science and Business Media LLC, pp. 451–461. doi:10.1007/978-3-642-54637-2_34.

House, T.R., Wightman, A., Rosenberg, A.R., Sayre, G., Abdel-Kader, K., Wong, S.P.Y., 2022. Challenges to Shared Decision Making About Treatment of Advanced CKD: a Qualitative Study of Patients and Clinicians. Am. J. Kidney Dis. 15236838. 79 (5), 657. Available from: http://www.elsevier.com/inca/publications/store/6/2/3/2/7/6/index.htt. doi:10.1053/j.ajkd.2021.08.021.

Jongejan, M., Lange, S.D., Bos, W.J.W., Pieterse, A.H., Konijn, W.S., van Buren, M., Abrahams, A.C., van Oevelen, M., 2024. Choosing conservative care in advanced chronic kidney disease: a scoping review of patients' perspectives. Nephrol. Dial. Transplant. 14602385. 39 (4), 659–668. Available from: http://ndt.oxfordjournals.org/. doi:10.1093/ndt/gfad196.

Kaufman, S.R., Shim, J.K., Russ, A.J., 2006. Old Age, Life Extension, and the Character of Medical Choice. J. Gerontol. B Psychol. Sci. Soc. Sci. 1079-5014. 61 (4), S175. doi:10.1093/geronb/61.4.S175.

Kimmel, P.L, 2002. Depression in patients with chronic renal disease: what we know and what we need to know. J. Psychosom. Res. 00223999. 53 (4), 951–956. doi:10.1016/S0022-3999(02)00310-0.

Kriston, L., Scholl, I., Hölzel, L., Simon, D., Loh, A., Härter, M., 2010. The 9-item shared decision making questionnaire (SDM-Q-9). Development and psychometric properties in a primary care sample. Patient Educ. Couns. 07383991. 80 (1), 94–99. doi:10.1016/j.pec.2009.09.034.

Kurella, M., Mapes, D.L., Port, F.K., Chertow, G.M., 2006. Correlates and outcomes of dementia among dialysis patients: the dialysis outcomes and practice patterns study. Nephrol. Dial. Transplant. 14602385. 21 (9), 2543–2548. doi:10.1093/ndt/gfl275.

Ladin, K., Lin, N., Hahn, E., Zhang, G., Koch-Weser, S., Weiner, D.E., 2017. Engagement in decision-making and patient satisfaction: a qualitative study of older patients' perceptions of dialysis initiation and modality decisions. Nephrol. Dial. Transplant. 14602385. 32 (8), 1394–1401. Available from: http://ndt.oxfordjournals.org/. doi:10.1093/ndt/gfw307.

Ladin, K., Pandya, R., Kannam, A., Loke, R., Oskoui, T., Perrone, R.D., Meyer, K.B., Weiner, D.E., Wong, J.B., 2018b. Discussing conservative management with older patients with CKD: an interview study of nephrologists. Am. J. Kidney Dis. 15236838. 71 (5), 627–635. Available from: http://www.elsevier.com/inca/publications/store/6/2/3/2/7/6/index.htt. doi:10.1053/j.ajkd.2017.11.011.

Ladin, K., Pandya, R., Perrone, R.D., Meyer, K.B., Kannam, A., Loke, R., Oskoui, T., Weiner, D.E., Wong, J.B., 2018a. Characterizing approaches to dialysis decision making with older adults: a qualitative study of nephrologists. Clin. J. Am. Soc. Nephrol. 1555905X. 13 (8), 1188–1196. Available from: http://cjasn.asnjournals.org/content/13/8/1188.full.pdf. doi:10.2215/CJN.01740218.

Ladin, K., Tighiouart, H., Bronzi, O., Koch-Weser, S., Wong, J.B., Levine, S., Agarwal, A., Ren, L., Degnan, J., Sewall, L.N., Kuramitsu, B., Fox, P., Gordon, E.J., Isakova, T., Rifkin, D., Rossi, A., Weiner, D.E., 2023. Effectiveness of an intervention to improve decision making for older patients with advanced chronic kidney disease. Ann. Intern. Med. 15393704. 176 (1), 29–38. Available from: https://www.acpjournals.org/doi/10.7326/M22-1543. doi:10.7326/M22-1543.

Lam, D.Y., Scherer, J.S., Brown, M., Grubbs, V., Schell, J.O., 2019. A conceptual framework of palliative care across the continuum of advanced kidney disease. Clin. J. Am. Soc. Nephrol. 1555905X. 14 (4), 635–641. Available from: https://cjasn.asnjournals.org/content/clinjasn/14/4/635.full.pdf. doi:10.2215/CJN.09330818.

Levy, N.B., Blumenfield, M., Beasley, C.M., Dubey, A.K., Solomon, R.J., Todd, R., Goodman, A., Bergstrom, R.R., 1996. Fluoxetine in depressed patients with renal failure and in depressed patients with normal kidney function. Gen. Hosp. Psychiatry. 01638343. 18 (1), 8–13. Available from: www.elsevier.com/locate/genhospsych.. doi:10.1016/0163-8343(95)00073-9.

Li, K.C., Brown, M.A., 2023. Conservative Kidney Management: when, Why, and For Whom? Seminars in Nephrology. 02709295. 43 (1), 151395. doi:10.1016/j.semnephrol.2023.151395.

Lopez Revuelta, K., Garcia Lopez, F.J, de Alvaro Moreno, F., Alonso, J., 2004. Perceived mental health at the start of dialysis as a predictor of morbidity and mortality in patients with end-stage renal disease (CALVIDIA Study). Nephrol. Dial. Transplant. 0931-0509. 19 (9), 2347–2353. doi:10.1093/ndt/gfh392.

Maddalena, V., O'Shea, F., Barrett, B., 2018. An exploration of palliative care needs of people with end-stage renal disease on dialysis: family caregiver's perspectives. J. Palliat. Care. 23695293. 33 (1), 19–25. Available from: https://journals.sagepub.com/home/PAL. doi:10.1177/0825859717747340.

Michel, D.M., Moss, A.H., 2005. Communicating prognosis in the dialysis consent process: a patient-centered, guideline-supported approach. Adv. Chronic Kidney Dis. 15485595. 12 (2), 196–201. Available from: http://www.elsevier.com/wps/find/journaldescription.cws_home/703170/description#description. doi:10.1053/j.ackd.2005.01.003.

Montez-Rath, M.E., Thomas, I.C., Charu, V., Odden, M.C., Seib, C.D., Arya, S., Fung, E., O'Hare, A.M., Wong, S.P.Y., Tamura, M.K., 2024. Effect of starting dialysis versus continuing medical management on survival and home time in older adults with kidney failure: a target trial emulation study. Ann. Intern. Med. 15393704. 177 (9), 1233–1243. Available from: https://www.acpjournals.org/doi/10.7326/M23-3028. doi:10.7326/M23-3028.

Morton, R.L., Snelling, P., Webster, A.C., Rose, J., Masterson, R., Johnson, D.W., Howard, K., 2012. Factors influencing patient choice of dialysis versus conservative care to treat end-stage kidney disease. CMAJ. 14882329. 184 (5), E277. Available from: http://www.cmaj.ca/content/184/5/E277full.pdf+html. doi:10.1503/cmaj.111355.

Moss, A.H., Ganjoo, J., Sharma, S., Gansor, J., Senft, S., Weaner, B., Dalton, C., MacKay, K., Pellegrino, B., Anantharaman, P., Schmidt, R., 2008. Utility of the "Surprise" question to identify dialysis patients with high mortality. Clin. J. Am. Soc. Nephrol. 1555905X. 3 (5), 1379–1384. doi:10.2215/CJN.00940208.

Murray, A.M., Tupper, D.E., Knopman, D.S., Gilbertson, D.T., Pederson, S.L., Li, S., Smith, G.E., Hochhalter, A.K., Collins, A.J., Kane, R.L., 2006. Cognitive impairment in hemodialysis patients is common. Neurology. 00283878. 67 (2), 216–223. Available from: http://www.neurology.org. doi:10.1212/01.wnl.0000225182.15532.40.

Murtagh, F.E.M., Sheerin, N.S., Addington-Hall, J., Higginson, I.J., 2011. Trajectories of illness in stage 5 chronic kidney disease: a longitudinal study of patient symptoms and concerns in the last year of life. Clin. J. Am. Soc. Nephrol. 1555905X. 6 (7), 1580–1590. Available from: http://cjasn.asnjournals.org/content/6/7/1580.full.pdf+html. doi:10.2215/CJN.09021010.

O'Hare, A.M., Hailpern, S.M., Wachterman, M., Kreuter, W., Katz, R., Hall, Y.N., Montez-Rath, M., Tamura, M.K., Daratha, K.B., 2018. Hospice use and end-of-life spending trajectories in Medicare beneficiaries on hemodialysis. Health Aff. 37 (6), 980–987.

O'Hare, A.M., Rodriguez, R.A., Hailpern, S.M., Larson, E.B., Tamura, M.K., 2010. Regional variation in health care intensity and treatment practices for end-stage renal disease in older adults. JAMA. 15383598. 304 (2), 180–186. Available from: http://jama.ama-assn.org/cgi/reprint/304/2/180. doi:10.1001/jama.2010.924.

O'Hare, A.M., Szarka, J., McFarland, L.V., Taylor, J.S., Sudore, R.L., Trivedi, R., Reinke, L.F., Vig, E.K., 2016. Provider perspectives on advance care planning for patients with kidney disease: whose job is it anyway? Clin. J. Am. Soc. Nephrol. 1555905X. 11 (5), 855–866. Available from: http://cjasn.asnjournals.org/content/11/5/855.full.pdf. doi:10.2215/CJN.11351015.

Pattison, M., Romer, A.L., 2001. Improving care through the end of life: launching a primary care clinic-based program. J. Palliat. Med. 10966218. 4 (2), 249–254. doi:10.1089/109662101750290335.

Postorino, M., Marino, C., Tripepi, G., Zoccali, C., 2007. Prognostic value of the New York Heart Association classification in end-stage renal disease. Nephrol. Dial. Transplant. 0931-0509. 22 (5), 1377–1382. doi:10.1093/ndt/gfl813.

Quill, T.E., Abernethy, A.P., 2013. Generalist plus specialist palliative care—creating a more sustainable model. N. Engl. J. Med. 15334406. 368 (13), 1173–1175. Available from: http://www.nejm.org/doi/pdf/10.1056/NEJMp1215620. doi:10.1056/NEJMp1215620.

Rakowski, D.A., Caillard, S., Agodoa, L.Y., Abbott, K.C., 2006. Dementia as a predictor of mortality in dialysis patients. Clin. J. Am. Soc. Nephrol. 1555905X. 1 (5), 1000–1005. doi:10.2215/CJN.00470705.

Ramer, S.J., McCall, N.N., Robinson-Cohen, C., Siew, E.D., Salat, H., Bian, A., Stewart, T.G., El-Sourady, M.H., Karlekar, M., Lipworth, L., Ikizler, T.A., Abdel-Kader, K., 2018. Health outcome priorities of older adults with advanced CKD and concordance with their nephrology providers' perceptions. J. Am. Soc. Nephrol. 15333450. 29 (12), 2870–2878. Available from: https://jasn.asnjournals.org/content/jnephrol/29/12/2859.full.pdf. doi:10.1681/ASN.2018060657.

Renal Physicians Association (RPA), 2010. Shared Decision-Making in the Appropriate Initiation of and Withdrawal from Dialysis, 2nd Ed. Renal Physicians Association, Rockville, MD.

Renal Physicians Association and the American Society of Nephrology, 2000. Shared Decision-Making in the Appropriate Initiation of and Withdrawal from Dialysis, Renal Physicians Association, Rockville, MD.

Rettig, R.A., Levinsky, N.G., 1991. Kidney Failure and the Federal Government, National Academies Press.

Saeed, F., Adams, H., Epstein, R.M., 2020. Matters of life and death: why do older patients choose conservative management? Am. J. Nephrol. 14219670. 51 (1), 35–42. Available from: www.karger.ch/journals/ajn/ajn_jh.htm.. doi:10.1159/000504692.

Saeed, F., Moss, A.H., Duberstein, P.R., Fiscella, K.A., 2022. Enabling patient choice: the "deciding not to decide" option for older adults facing dialysis decisions. J. Am. Soc. Nephrol. 15333450. 33 (5), 880–882. Available from: https://jasn.asnjournals.org/content/jnephrol/33/5/880.full.pdf?casa_token=HEnhHmHMJfEAAAAA%3Ay3DEk3dL5d-JR-rNHU3v1G4CreGfn7Qa6PezqYUrI3wOR2bjnsM30pdCqN7SflJ7c0aILQsYflvJh. doi:10.1681/ASN.2021081143.

Schell, J.O., Green, J.A., Tulsky, J.A., Arnold, R.M., 2013. Communication skills training for dialysis decision-making and end-of-life care in nephrology. Clin. J. Am. Soc. Nephrol. 1555905X. 8 (4), 675–680. Available from: http://cjasn.asnjournals.org/content/8/4/675.full.pdf+html. doi:10.2215/CJN.05220512.

Schmidt, R.J., Landry, D.L., Cohen, L., Moss, A.H., Dalton, C., Nathanson, B.H., Germain, M.J., 2019. Derivation and validation of a prognostic model to predict mortality in patients with advanced chronic kidney disease. Nephrol. Dial. Transplant. 14602385. 34 (9), 1517–1525. Available from: http://ndt.oxfordjournals.org/. doi:10.1093/ndt/gfy305.

Song, M.K., Lin, F.C., Gilet, C.A., Arnold, R.M., Bridgman, J.C., Ward, S.E., 2013. Patient perspectives on informed decision-making surrounding dialysis initiation. Nephrol. Dial. Transplant. 14602385. 28 (11), 2815–2823. doi:10.1093/ndt/gft238.

Speyer, E., Tu, C., Zee, J., Sesso, R., Lopes, A.A., Moutard, E., Omorou, A.Y., Stengel, B., Finkelstein, F.O., Pecoits-Filho, R., de Pinhode Pinho, N.A., Pisoni, R.L., Lopes, A., Combe, C., Jacquelinet, C., Massy, Z., Stengel, B., de Pinhode Pinho, N.A., Duttlinger, J., Fliser, D., Lonnemann, G., Reichel, H., Wada, T., Yamagata, K., Pisoni, R., Robinson, B., da Silva, V.C., Asahi, K., Hoshino, J., Narita, I., Perlman, R., Port, F., Sukul, N., Wong, M., Young, E., 2024. Symptom burden and its impact on quality of life in patients with moderate to severe CKD: the international chronic kidney disease outcomes and practice patterns study (CKDopps). Am. J. Kidney Dis. 15236838. 84 (6), 696. Available from: https://www.sciencedirect.com/science/journal/02726386. doi:10.1053/j.ajkd.2024.06.011.

Stacey, D., Lewis, K.B., Smith, M., Carley, M., Volk, R., Douglas, E.E., Pacheco-Brousseau, L., Finderup, J., Gunderson, J., Barry, M.J., Bennett, C.L., Bravo, P., Steffensen, K., Gogovor, A., Graham, I.D., Kelly, S.E., Légaré, F., Sondergaard, H., Thomson, R., Trenaman, L., Trevena, L., 2024. Decision aids for people facing health treatment or screening decisions. Cochrane Database Syst. Rev. 14651858. 2024 (1). Available from: https://www.cochranelibrary.com/cdsr/table-of-contents. doi:10.1002/14651858.CD001431.pub6.

Tam-Tham, H., King-Shier, K.M., Thomas, C.M., Quinn, R.R., Fruetel, K., Davison, S.N., Hemmelgarn, B.R., 2016. Prevalence of barriers and facilitators to enhancing conservative kidney management for older adults in the primary care setting. Clin. J. Am. Soc. Nephrol. 1555905X. 11 (11), 2012–2021. Available from: http://cjasn.asnjournals.org/content/11/11/2012.full.pdf. doi:10.2215/CJN.04510416.

Tamura, M.K., Covinsky, K.E., Chertow, G.M., Yaffe, K., Landefeld, C.S., McCulloch, C.E., 2009. Functional status of elderly adults before and after initiation of dialysis. N. Engl. J. Med. 15334406. 361 (16), 1539–1547. Available from: http://content.nejm.org/cgi/reprint/361/16/1539.pdf. doi:10.1056/NEJMoa0904655.

Tamura, M.K., Meier, D.E., 2013. Five policies to promote palliative care for patients with ESRD. Clin. J. Am. Soc. Nephrol. 8 (10), 1783–1790.

Tamura, M.K., O'Hare, A.M., Lin, E., Holdsworth, L.M., Malcolm, E., Moss, A.H., 2018. Palliative Care Disincentives in CKD: changing Policy to Improve CKD Care. Am. J. Kidney Dis. 15236838. 71 (6), 866–873. Available from: http://www.elsevier.com/inca/publications/store/6/2/3/2/7/6/index.htt. doi:10.1053/j.ajkd.2017.12.017.

United States Renal Data System, 2014. USRDS Annual Data Report: Epidemiology of Kidney Disease in the United States. National Institutes of Health, National Institute of Diabetes and Digestive and Kidney Diseases, Bethesda, MD.

Wachterman, M.W., Leveille, T., Keating, N.L., Simon, S.R., Waikar, S.S., Bokhour, B., 2019b. Nephrologists' emotional burden regarding decision-making about dialysis initiation in older adults: a qualitative study. BMC Nephrology 20 (1), 385. doi:10.1186/s12882-019-1565-x.

Wachterman, M.W., O'Hare, A.M., Rahman, O.K., Lorenz, K.A., Marcantonio, E.R., Alicante, G.K., Kelley, A.S., 2019a. One-year mortality after dialysis initiation among older adults. JAMA Intern. Med. 21686106. 179 (7), 987–990. Available from: http://archinte.jamanetwork.com/issues.aspx. doi:10.1001/jamainternmed.2019.0125.

Weisbord, S.D., Fried, L.F., Arnold, R.M., Fine, M.J., Levenson, D.J., Peterson, R.A., Switzer, G.E., 2005. Prevalence, severity, and importance of physical and emotional symptoms in chronic hemodialysis patients. J. Am. Soc. Nephrol. 10466673. 16 (8), 2487–2494. Available from: https://journals.lww.com/jasn/pages/default.aspx. doi:10.1681/ASN.2005020157.

White, N., Kupeli, N., Vickerstaff, V., Stone, P., 2017. How accurate is the 'Surprise Question' at identifying patients at the end of life? A systematic review and meta-analysis. BMC Med. 17417015. 15 (1). Available from: http://www.biomedcentral.com/bmcmed/. doi:10.1186/s12916-017-0907-4.

Wong, S.P.Y., McFarland, L.V., Liu, C.F., Laundry, R.J., Hebert, P.L., O'Hare, A.M., 2019. Care practices for patients with advanced kidney disease who forgo maintenance dialysis. JAMA Intern. Med. 21686106. 179 (3), 305–313. Available from: http://archinte.jamanetwork.com/issues.aspx. doi:10.1001/jamainternmed.2018.6197.

Wong, S.P.Y., Rubenzik, T., Zelnick, L., Davison, S.N., Louden, D., Oestreich, T., Jennerich, A.L., 2022. Long-term outcomes among patients with advanced kidney disease who forgo maintenance dialysis: a systematic review. JAMA Netw. Open. 25743805. Available from: https://jamanetwork.com/journals/jamanetworkopen. doi:10.1001/jamanetworkopen.2022.2255.

Further reading

Davison, S.N., Jhangri, G.S., Holley, J.L., Moss, A.H., 2006. Nephrologists' reported preparedness for end-of-life decision-making. Clin. J. Am. Soc. Nephrol. 1555905X. 1 (6), 1256–1262. doi:10.2215/CJN.02040606.

CHAPTER

28

Drugs to avoid with geriatric kidney disease

Stephen Z. Fadem

Department of Medicine, Section of Nephrology, Baylor College of Medicine, Houston, TX, United States

Introduction

Chronic kidney disease (CKD) is common among the elderly. It affects up to 14%–30% of individuals over 65 (Aymanns et al., 2010) with the prevalence increasing with age and in conditions like diabetes, hypertension, and heart failure. The staging of CKD relies on the estimated glomerular filtration rate (eGFR) and albuminuria. With disease progression, adverse drug reactions worsen, especially when patients are taking multiple medications. Polypharmacy is common, with most geriatric CKD patients taking between 6 and 12 medications daily, leading to potentially inappropriate medication use and adverse drug events (Chen et al., 2019; Kishi et al., 2024; Roux-Marson et al., 2020). Not only does the decrease in clearance play a role, but the impact of aging, uremic toxins, chronic inflammation, and oxidative stress also changes how medications are metabolized and how they affect older CKD patients. Altered body composition and increased sensitivity to the central nervous system and cardiovascular effects of medications further complicate treatment. The Kidney Disease: Improving Global Outcomes (KDIGO) 2024 guideline and the National Kidney Foundation Kidney Disease Outcomes Quality Initiative (KDOQI) 2025 commentary emphasize the need for individualized, patient-centered medication management with regular review and adjustment of all medications to minimize harm and optimize outcomes (Navaneethan et al., 2025).

Why aging and CKD magnify nephrotoxicity and systemic harm

Glomerular filtration and tubular secretion are the main pathways for drug elimination. CKD reduces both, resulting in drug accumulation and prolonged half-life of drugs excreted by the kidney. In addition to filtration and excretion, the renal tubules metabolize some

Aging and the Kidney
https://doi.org/10.1016/B978-0-443-34069-7.00028-8

medications, and with renal impairment, there is increased systemic exposure and, in some instances, increased renal toxicity. Well-known examples include the aminoglycosides, which cause not only kidney damage but also ototoxicity. Renal function and medication clearance are modulated by renal blood flow, tubular glomerular feedback, oncotic pressure, a variety of hormones, adipocyte health and number, protein binding, and urine pH. In health, and with low protein binding, low molecular weight drugs can be easily filtered, and tubular secretion can raise the renal clearance above the glomerular filtration rate (GFR) (KDIGO, 2024).

Aging reduces renal plasma flow and GFR and may diminish tubular transport capacity. With fewer functioning nephrons, stiffer vasculature, and attenuated repair responses, older kidneys tolerate hemodynamic stress and toxins poorly. The same drug exposure that is tolerated by younger adults can provoke injury in an older person with CKD (KDIGO, 2024). Comorbidities (e.g., heart failure, liver disease) and polypharmacy magnify these risks, raising the probability and severity of AKI and incomplete recovery (Triantafylidis et al., 2018; Roux-Marson et al., 2020). The lower total body water/lean mass and higher fat mass, with variable hepatic metabolic capacity, alter volumes of distribution and half-lives, increasing exposure to standard doses (Chen et al., 2019; Kishi et al., 2024). In practice, older adults often require lower doses or longer intervals for renally cleared and narrow-therapeutic-index drugs, with close monitoring to prevent accumulation (Triantafylidis et al., 2018; KDIGO, 2024). CKD and aging, chronic diseases, and inflammatory states often cause hypoalbuminemia, increasing the free fraction of highly protein-bound drugs and the risk of toxicity.

Polypharmacy is common in CKD, especially in the elderly, with frequent use of 6–12 medications daily, increasing the risk of drug-drug interactions and inappropriate dosing. Polypharmacy is endemic in advanced CKD and strongly associated with potentially inappropriate medication use and renally inappropriate prescriptions (Roux-Marson et al., 2020; Kurani et al., 2020). Older adults and those with CKD have increased sensitivity to drug effects, especially central nervous system and cardiovascular agents, due to altered receptor responses and homeostatic mechanisms. Sarcopenia and low albumin can distort GFR estimation and free drug fractions, respectively, heightening toxicity from highly protein-bound medicines (KDIGO, 2024; Navaneethan et al., 2025). Genetic variants sometimes influence dose needs (e.g., warfarin), but routine pharmacogenomic testing remains uncommon in CKD care (Brown et al., 2025; Singh, 2023).

Coexisting conditions, such as diabetes and heart failure, further increase vulnerability to adverse drug events and nephrotoxicity. Sarcopenia and fluid shifts in CKD and aging affect drug distribution, complicating dosing. Impaired renal elimination extends toxicity beyond the kidney. CNS effects include delirium, excessive sedation, and falls—especially with anticholinergics, benzodiazepines, opioids, and renally cleared neuromodulators (Triantafylidis et al., 2018; American Geriatrics Society 2023 updated AGS Beers Criteria® for potentially inappropriate medication use in older adults, 2023). Cardiometabolic consequences include bradyarrhythmias (e.g., with digoxin), bleeding (e.g., with renally cleared anticoagulants), dysglycemia (e.g., prolonged hypoglycemia with glyburide), and metformin-related lactic acidosis when the eGFR is low (Chen et al., 2019; Wilson et al., 2024; Kurani et al., 2020).

Many drugs lack robust safety and efficacy data in advanced CKD and older adults, increasing uncertainty in prescribing. Some have not been adequately tested (KDIGO, 2024;

Chen et al., 2019; Triantafylidis et al., 2018; Brown et al., 2025; Escribá-Martí et al., 2022; Stevens et al., 2024; Taji et al., 2020; Vondracek et al., 2021; Navaneethan et al., 2025).

Patient-specific factors that modify recommendations

Socioeconomic factors can interfere with access to care, home supervision, and the affordability of medications. Often, patients must select less costly alternatives that frequently have less desirable characteristics. Another factor to consider is the presence of chronic diseases or conditions like frailty, sarcopenia, diabetes, vascular disease, or heart failure. A low serum albumin level can raise the free fraction of protein-bound drugs, and drug dosing should be appropriately adjusted. Low muscle mass can result in an overestimation of the GFR. Patients with cognitive impairment who are still independent need home support. With chronic illness, drugs often interfere with metabolism and, in some cases, alter the risk-benefit ratio. Nephrotoxicity can be exacerbated by chronic diseases. Although less commonly considered, there is considerable genetic variation in how drugs are metabolized. Understanding the rate of metabolism will help planners provide more optimal care. Patients who have recently undergone a kidney transplant may not have regained full kidney function, and medications must often be adjusted (KDIGO, 2024; Navaneethan et al., 2025).

Use caution with these drugs (Table 28.1)

Analgesics/antiinflammatories: Systemic NSAIDs (including COX-2 inhibitors) increase the risk of hemodynamic AKI, worsen edema and blood pressure, and—especially when combined with RAAS blockade and diuretics—can precipitate acute kidney injury. This phenomenon is often referred to as the "triple whammy." In patients on a diuretic and either an angiotensin converting enzyme (ACE) inhibitor or angiogentin receptor blocker (ARB), pain relief is best achieved with topical medications. There are also several nonpharmacological approaches that can minimize pain, particularly when it is of musculoskeletal origin. Arthritis can often be alleviated through the use of topical ointments and stretching (KDIGO, 2024; Chen et al., 2019). Whenever possible, it is best to avoid or restrict the use of aminoglycosides and conventional amphotericin B, opting instead for alternatives or liposomal formulations. Patients on amphotericin should be closely monitored. Vancomycin is often toxic when infused in patients with impaired kidney function and can lead to acute kidney injury; the risk is further increased when piperacillin is used concomitantly. Sulfamethoxazole and trimethoprim are cleared by the kidneys and can also interfere with creatinine excretion and the creatinine assay, potentially leading to false-positive results for AKI. The dose should be adjusted in patients with CKD. Antiviral medication doses also need to be adjusted. Nitrofurantoin is ineffective and potentially harmful at low eGFR (Wilson et al., 2024). Many excellent drug databases, available on smartphone apps such as Epocrates, can assist clinicians in reducing drug dosing according to GFR when indicated.

In patients with cardiovascular disease, the use of RAAS blockers can interfere with kidney function, and if an NSAID is used, it can lead to acute kidney injury. If digoxin has been prescribed, the dose must be reduced, and drug levels should be obtained, as this

TABLE 28.1 Drugs requiring special consideration.

Drug	CKD Stage(s)	Recommendation	Rationale
Cisplatin, carboplatin	All, especially CKD < 50	Reduce the dose and monitor	Dose-dependent AKI Electrolyte disorders
Methotrexate	All, especially CKD < 50	Avoid if GFR < 10; reduce the dose if GFR is between 10 and 50; monitor	Renal elimination; severe toxicity risk
Calcineurin inhibitors (cyclosporine, Tacrolimus)	All	Use the lowest effective dose; monitor levels. Reduce further if oliguria occurs	Nephrotoxicity; Drug interactions
Aminoglycosides	No adjustment with liposome	Use liposomal form	Acute tubular necrosis;
Amphotericin B	All, especially CKD < 10		
Acyclovir, tenofovir disoproxyl fumarate	Reduce dose if GFR < 10		Acute tubular necrosis, proximal tubular dysfunction
Remdesivir	All		Acute tubular necrosis

These drugs require special consideration—they should only be used by experienced specialists (Table Resources: Kishi et al., 2024; Kurani et al., 2020; Wilson et al., 2024).

medication has a very narrow therapeutic margin. Direct oral anticoagulants, with the exception of reduced-dose apixaban, are generally avoided in advanced CKD patients (Wilson et al., 2024; Kan et al., 2022). Metformin is an effective antidiabetic agent but should be avoided if the eGFR is < 30 mL/min/1.73 m^2 and reduced when the eGFR is between 30 and 44, as it may result in lactic acidosis. Long-acting sulfonylureas like glyburide are associated with prolonged hypoglycemia. Gabapentinoid and insulin dosing should also be reduced according to kidney function. Avoid lithium where possible in CKD, and particularly avoid using it along with a diuretic, as it may reduce lithium excretion and result in lithium toxicity. Lithium levels should be monitored if this medication cannot be avoided. Anticholinergics, such as antihistamines and long-acting benzodiazepines, as well as nonbenzodiazepines or "Z drugs," can result in heightened CNS sensitivity. Anticholinergics have been independently associated with worsening dementia (Grossi et al., 2019; Triantafylidis et al., 2018; American Geriatrics Society 2023 updated AGS Beers Criteria® for potentially inappropriate medication use in older adults, 2023; KDIGO, 2024).

Medication risks and monitoring needs vary by context. Outpatients benefit from scheduled medication reviews and the explicit use of Beers/STOPP-START criteria to identify high-risk agents. Hospitalized older adults with CKD require intensified monitoring of kidney function, electrolytes, and drug levels for nephrotoxins and narrow-therapeutic-index agents. Perioperatively, several chronic therapies should be paused to reduce risks of hypotension, hypovolemia, and metabolic complications (Navaneethan et al., 2025; Parker et al., 2019; KDIGO, 2024; American Geriatrics Society 2023 updated AGS Beers Criteria® for potentially inappropriate medication use in older adults, 2023).

Immunosuppressants (e.g., calcineurin and mTOR inhibitors) require specialist dosing and level monitoring due to nephrotoxicity and drug–drug interactions. Chemotherapeutics like cisplatin are directly nephrotoxic, while methotrexate is excreted by the kidney and thus requires dose reduction and close surveillance to avoid systemic complications. Selected antivirals and antifungals also necessitate careful renal dosing, with preference for less nephrotoxic formulations where options exist (Navaneethan et al., 2025; Kishi et al., 2024; Kurani et al., 2020) (Table 28.2).

Strategies for reducing adverse drug effects

Medication errors are common, and efforts to reduce them must be systemic. This should start with the patient, where they bring, or photograph with their smartphones, the bottles of medications they are taking, including the labels. Looking at the date of the prescription and the number of pills in the bottle can indicate whether the medication is being used. Often, patients receive both branded medications from one doctor and a generic drug that is identical from another. Taking both is hazardous, especially in the population most vulnerable—those with declining cognitive function. The patient should also include over-the-counter medications, supplements, herbs, and "home remedies." One goal of the encounter should be centered around education and engagement—individualized and patient-centered—discussing comorbidities, life expectancy, patient goals, and expectations. Informing the patient about risks and benefits and providing tools for self-management removes many barriers to safety. The provider should be mindful of drug interactions and should also ask if the medication is really necessary or if a substitution is possible. Medications have complex actions, and involving pharmacists who have extensive experience can help reduce risks. The physician and other health providers have at their disposal a number of tools, particularly with the readiness of machine learning apps on practically every smartphone. While many artificial intelligence tools "hallucinate" when they do not have the exact answer to a question, others are designed specifically for the medical community.

Actor/Critic model

A reinforcement learning paradigm takes advantage of artificial intelligence to create a balanced decision making and implementation process. The Actor/Critic reinforcement learning model uses two neural networks. The electronic medical record encodes a patient's current clinical profile, including kidney function, comorbidities, medication exposures, laboratory values, and recent events. The Actor proposes a set of safe, guideline-constrained actions—dose adjustments, substitutions, deprescribing steps, and monitoring orders. The Critic estimates the expected value of each action bundle using a multi-objective reward that prioritizes safety and renal trajectory stabilization while preserving effectiveness and minimizing treatment burden. The policy is optimized using retrospective data and refined prospectively with clinician overrides to ensure safe learning.

Action–reward in CKD pharmacology

Key variables can be created by clinical experts and include kidney function (estimated GFR and albuminuria value), comorbidities such as diabetes, heart failure, atrial fibrillation, and atherosclerotic cardiovascular disease; frailty indicators such as a history of falls, sarcopenia, and cognitive impairment; current medications; and laboratory/vital sign features like serum potassium, bicarbonate, sodium, hemoglobin A1c, blood pressure, and weight. The action space comprises renal dose adjustments, avoidance or substitution of nephrotoxic or high-risk agents, deprescribing processes for long-term acid suppression and sedatives, initiation of disease-modifying therapies where indicated, and explicit monitoring bundles. The reward aggregates events over fixed windows (e.g., 30, 90, and 180 days), heavily weighting the absence of acute kidney injury, severe hyperkalemia, major bleeding, falls, and delirium; stability of estimated GFR slope and achievement of treatment targets; and reduced medication burden and improved adherence.

Epic or Oracle Health integration and Clinical Decision Support (CDS) Contexts

Implementing this framework into an electronic health record, such as Epic or Oracle Health, requires a layered architecture that separates feature management, inference, and workflow delivery. Data flow begins with Fast Healthcare Interoperability Resources (FHIR) to assemble a patient snapshot from the core health record elements. A feature store maintains longitudinal variables and engineered features, such as trend metrics. The Actor–Critic inference service exposes a resource known as an application programming interface, callable by CDS workflow contexts. At the point of care, best practice alerts can present top-ranked, guideline-constrained action bundles with embedded order sets. SmartSets in Epic and order panels enforce predefined safe defaults, including renal dosing and laboratory recheck intervals. Flowsheets collect structured measures, such as anticholinergic burden and sedation scores, and Synopsis tiles visualize estimated GFR and serum potassium trajectories alongside high-risk medication flags. SmartPhrases insert rationale and monitoring plans into clinical notes that can be audited.

Governance, safety, and monitoring

Safety governance is key to the system's success. The Actor is strictly limited to actions within KDIGO and Beers/STOPP–START guardrails; the Critic may only rank among these actions. Retrospective policy evaluation should use conservative offline reinforcement learning and causal adjustment to mitigate confounding. Prospective deployment begins in silent mode to establish baseline performance, followed by a pharmacist-supported pilot. Continuous dashboards should monitor alert acceptance, overrides, adverse event rates, and fairness across patient subgroups. A formal change control process should govern reward weighting, threshold tuning, and policy updates.

Clinical vignette

Case vignette: A 76-year-old lady with CKD stage G3b and an estimated GFR of 38 mL/min/1.73 m^2, hypertension, atrial fibrillation, and painful neuropathy uses apixaban 5 mg twice daily, gabapentin 600 mg three times daily, and zolpidem 10 mg nightly. The Actor flags a renal/age dose reduction for apixaban, proposes reducing gabapentin to a divided daily dose under 400 mg, and deprescribing zolpidem in favor of nonpharmacological sleep strategies. The Critic assigns the highest expected reward to the combined bundle. The Epic alert surfaces a ready-to-sign order set and an education SmartPhrase with a 2-week basic metabolic panel follow-up.

Discussion

This approach balances adherence to guidance with personalization. While randomized trials remain scarce for many geriatric CKD medication decisions, large-scale electronic health record datasets enable robust retrospective estimation of near-term safety and effectiveness signals. While not a substitute for clinical judgment, reinforcement learning creates safety options and standardizes monitoring in complex cases. This system will have limitations. Clinical users of health records often become easily fatigued by excessive clicking and alert fatigue. Data accuracy is always a challenge. The program has benefits in that it brings awareness to imminent problems centered around fundamental issues in health care. It helps keep the medication review current and fosters partnerships with pharmacists. It also focuses on deprescribing, particularly of medications deemed less safe in this patient population. Future projects can include integration of biomarkers such as cell-free deoxyribonucleic acid assays, proteomics panels such as CKD273, and pharmacogenetic markers to refine dosing and risk. A guideline-constrained Actor–Critic system operationalizes KDIGO 2024 pharmacology guidance for older adults with CKD. By structuring Action–Reward around safety-first outcomes and embedding the system within Epic, Oracle Health, or other EMR clinical decision support, healthcare teams can reduce medication-related harm while preserving therapeutic effectiveness and patient-centered goals.

Conclusion

Older adults, especially those with CKD, are vulnerable to adverse drug reactions because renal clearance, pharmacokinetics, and pharmacodynamics are altered. Many commonly used drugs, including those used without a prescription and obtained "over the counter," can be dangerous. NSAIDs and contrast agents may precipitate acute kidney injury. Polypharmacy further amplifies the likelihood of drug–drug interactions and inappropriate prescribing. Avoidance of high-risk medications, systematic deprescribing, and the use of machine learning to develop clinical decision support systems are critical strategies to reduce harm. Implementation of Beers and STOPP/START criteria, coupled with pharmacist-led medication review, can help tailor safer therapy in this vulnerable group. While current guidance is largely extrapolated from observational studies and expert consensus, future work should prioritize randomized trials focused on the geriatric CKD population. Careful prescribing and deprescribing represent effective strategies, and tools like ACTOR/CRITIC present major opportunities to improve outcomes and quality of life in older adults living with CKD.

AI disclosure

During the preparation of this work, the author(s) used Open Evidence, GPT-5, Perplexity, along with PubMed and Google Scholar to help gather information for authors to review, organize, select, and create a composition. After using this tool/service, the author(s) reviewed and edited the content as needed and take(s) full responsibility for the content of the publication.

References

American Geriatrics Society 2023 updated AGS Beers Criteria® for potentially inappropriate medication use in older adults, 2023. J. Am. Geriatr. Soc. 0002-8614. 71 (7), 2052–2081. doi:10.1111/jgs.18372.

Aymanns, C., Keller, F., Maus, S., Hartmann, B., Czock, D., 2010. Review on pharmacokinetics and pharmacodynamics and the aging kidney. Clin. J. Am. Soc. Nephrol. 1555-9041. 5 (2), 314–327. doi:10.2215/cjn.03960609.

Brown, J.C., Caesar-Gibbs, W., Delgado, C., The primary care management of chronic kidney disease (CKD). (2025).

Chen, N., Aleksa, K., Woodland, C., 2019. Pharmacokinetics in the elderly with chronic kidney disease. Clin. Pharmacokinet. 58 (2), 205–222.

Chen, T.K., Knicely, D.H., Grams, M.E., 2019. Chronic kidney disease diagnosis and management: a review. JAMA. 15383598. 322 (13), 1294–1304. Available from: http://jama.jamanetwork.com/journal.aspx. doi:10.1001/jama.2019.14745.

Escribá-Martí, G., Cámara-Ramos, I., Teresa Climent-Catalá, M., Escudero-Quesada, V., Salar-Ibáñez, L., Remuzzi, G., 2022. Pharmaceutical care program for patients with chronic kidney disease in the community pharmacy: detection of nephrotoxic drugs and dose adjustment. Viability study. PLoS One. 1932-6203. 17 (12), e0278648. doi:10.1371/journal.pone.0278648.

Grossi, C.M., Richardson, K., Fox, C., Maidment, I., Steel, N., Loke, Y.K., Arthur, A., Myint, P.K., Campbell, N., Boustani, M., Robinson, L., Brayne, C., Matthews, F.E., Savva, G.M., 2019. Anticholinergic and benzodiazepine medication use and risk of incident dementia: a UK cohort study. BMC Geriatr. 14712318. 19 (1). Available from: http://www.biomedcentral.com/bmcgeriatr/. doi:10.1186/s12877-019-1280-2.

Kan, W.C., Chen, Y.C., Wu, V.C., Shiao, C.C., 2022. Vancomycin-associated acute kidney injury: a narrative review from pathophysiology to clinical application. Int. J. Mol. Sci. 14220067. 23 (4). Available from: https://www.mdpi.com/1422-0067/23/4/2052/pdf. doi:10.3390/ijms23042052.

KDIGO, 2024. 2024 Clinical Practice Guideline for the Evaluation and Management of Chronic Kidney Disease.

Kishi, S., Kadoya, H., Kashihara, N., 2024. Treatment of chronic kidney disease in older populations. Nat. Rev. Nephrol. 1759-5061. 20 (9), 586–602. doi:10.1038/s41581-024-00854-w.

Kurani, S., Jeffery, M.M., Thorsteinsdottir, B., Hickson, L.T.J., Barreto, E.F., Haag, J., Giblon, R., Shah, N.D., McCoy, R.G., 2020. Use of potentially nephrotoxic medications by U.S. adults with chronic kidney disease: NHANES, 2011–2016. J. Gen. Intern. Med. 15251497. 35 (4), 1092–1101. Available from: http://www.springerlink.com/content/120414/. doi:10.1007/s11606-019-05557-8.

Navaneethan, S.D., Bansal, N., Cavanaugh, K.L., Chang, A., Crowley, S., Delgado, C., Estrella, M.M., Ghossein, C., Ikizler, T.A., Koncicki, H., Peter, W.S., Tuttle, K.R., William, J., 2025. KDOQI US commentary on the KDIGO 2024 clinical practice guideline for the evaluation and management of CKD. Am. J. Kidney Dis. 15236838. 85 (2), 135–176. Available from: https://www.sciencedirect.com/science/journal/02726386. doi:10.1053/j.ajkd.2024.08.003.

Parker, K., Bull-Engelstad, I., Benth, J.Š., Aasebø, W., von der Lippe, N., Reier-Nilsen, M., Os, I., Stavem, K., 2019. Effectiveness of using STOPP/START criteria to identify potentially inappropriate medication in people aged ≥ 65 years with chronic kidney disease: a randomized clinical trial. Eur. J. Clin. Pharmacol. 14321041. 75 (11), 1503–1511. Available from: https://link.springer.de/link/service/journals/00228/index.htm. doi:10.1007/s00228-019-02727-9.

Roux-Marson, C., Patel, D., Harris, K., 2020. Polypharmacy and medication-related harm in older adults with CKD. Nephrol. Dial. Transplant. 35 (11), 1908–1916.

Roux-Marson, C., Baranski, J.B., Fafin, C., Exterman, G., Vigneau, C., Couchoud, C., Moranne, O., Investigators, P.S.P.A., 2020. Medication burden and inappropriate prescription risk among elderly with advanced chronic kidney disease. BMC Geriatr. 14712318. 20 (1). Available from: http://www.biomedcentral.com/bmcgeriatr/. doi:10.1186/s12877-020-1485-4.

Singh, S., 2023. Medication safety in chronic kidney disease. Curr. Opin. Nephrol. Hypertens. 1062-4821. 32 (5), 434–438. doi:10.1097/mnh.0000000000000907.

Stevens, P.E., Ahmed, S.B., Carrero, J.J., Foster, B., Francis, A., Hall, R.K., Herrington, W.G., Hill, G., Inker, L.A., Kazancıoğlu, R., Lamb, E., Lin, P., Madero, M., McIntyre, N., Morrow, K., Roberts, G., Sabanayagam, D., Schaeffner, E., Shlipak, M., Shroff, R., Tangri, N., Thanachayanont, T., Ulasi, I., Wong, G., Yang, C.-W., Zhang, L., Levin, A., 2024. KDIGO 2024 Clinical practice guideline for the evaluation and management of chronic kidney disease. Kidney Int. 00852538. 105 (4), S117. doi:10.1016/j.kint.2023.10.018.

Taji, L., Battistella, M., Grill, A.K., Cunningham, J., Hemmelgarn, B.L., Quinn, K.M., Thomas, A., Brimble, K.S., 2020. Medications used routinely in primary care to be dose-adjusted or avoided in people with chronic kidney disease: results of a modified delphi study. Ann. Pharmacother. 15426270. 54 (7), 625–632. Available from: https://journals.sagepub.com/home/AOP. doi:10.1177/1060028019897371.

Triantafylidis, L.K., Hawley, C.E., Perry, L.P., Paik, J.M., 2018. The role of deprescribing in older adults with chronic kidney disease. Drugs Aging. 11791969. 35 (11), 973–984. Available from: http://rd.springer.com/journal/40266. doi:10.1007/s40266-018-0593-8.

Vondracek, S.F., Teitelbaum, I., Kiser, T.H., 2021. Principles of kidney pharmacotherapy for the nephrologist: core curriculum 2021. Am. J. Kidney Dis. 15236838. 78 (3), 442–458. Available from: http://www.elsevier.com/inca/publications/store/6/2/3/2/7/6/index.htt. doi:10.1053/j.ajkd.2021.02.342.

Wilson, J.A., Ratajczak, N., Halliday, K., Battistella, M., Naylor, H., Sheffield, M., Marin, J.G., Pitman, J., Kennie-Kaulbach, N., Trenaman, S., Gillis, L., 2024. Medications for community pharmacists to dose adjust or avoid to enhance prescribing safety in individuals with advanced chronic kidney disease: a scoping review and modified Delphi. BMC Nephrol. 14712369. 25 (1). Available from: https://bmcnephrol.biomedcentral.com/. doi:10.1186/s12882-024-03829-y.

CHAPTER

29

Innovations in chronic kidney disease and aging

Stephen Z. Fadem

Department of Medicine, Section of Nephrology, Baylor College of Medicine, Houston, TX, United States

Introduction

CKD remains a leading cause of morbidity and mortality in aging populations. The progressive loss of kidney function not only leads to end-stage kidney disease (ESKD) but also amplifies cardiovascular risk and frailty in older adults. Despite this burden, the management of CKD has historically been limited to controlling underlying diseases such as diabetes and hypertension and using renin–angiotensin system blockers to slow progression. Fortunately, the landscape is changing. The Kidney Disease Improving Global Outcomes (KDIGO) 2024 clinical practice guideline for CKD early management codified a new standard of care emphasizing early detection, multifaceted renoprotective therapy, risk stratification, and multidisciplinary care. This paradigm reflects the influx of new evidence-based therapies and tools that can be leveraged to improve outcomes.

This chapter provides a comprehensive review of recent and emerging innovations in CKD, with particular attention to more recent developments. The major thematic areas are: (1) therapeutic innovations, covering the expanding pipeline of CKD pharmacotherapies and regenerative treatments; (2) diagnostics and early risk stratification, highlighting novel biomarkers, imaging modalities, and screening approaches for earlier identification of high-risk CKD patients; (3) artificial intelligence (AI) applications, describing how AI and machine learning, including reinforcement learning, are being applied to CKD risk prediction and therapy optimization; (4) genomic and multiomic advances, summarizing how genetic discoveries and tissue atlas projects are enabling precision medicine in nephrology; and (5) innovations in care delivery models, examining new models of integrated care and digital health interventions improving CKD patient management.

CKD management is transitioning toward a more personalized, proactive approach. The confluence of better drugs, better diagnostics, and better care models offers hope that kidney

https://doi.org/10.1016/B978-0-443-34069-7.00031-8

function decline can be slowed, delaying the need for dialysis and transplantation, and improving the aging trajectory of patients living with CKD.

Management of CKD has entered a new era of disease-modifying therapies. Beyond conventional renin-angiotensin system inhibitors, clinical trials over the past few years have demonstrated the renal protective effects of new pharmacological agents. This section reviews both established and emerging therapeutics reshaping the treatment paradigm, and it also touches on regenerative and geroprotective strategies under investigation.

Established renoprotective therapies—best demonstrated practice

The standard therapeutic cache for CKD expanded significantly in the 2020s. Sodium–glucose cotransporter-2 inhibitors (SGLT2i) were the first breakthrough. Trials such as DAPA-CKD and EMPA-KIDNEY proved that SGLT2 inhibitors slow kidney disease progression and reduce cardiovascular events in CKD, even in patients without diabetes (Heerspink et al., 2020; Herrington et al., 2025; Theodorakopoulou and Sarafidis, 2024). These agents are now instrumental in CKD care due to consistent benefits on hard renal outcomes and mortality. Another important addition has been finerenone, a nonsteroidal mineralocorticoid receptor antagonist (Bakris et al., 2020). In patients with diabetic kidney disease (DKD) and without DKD, finerenone significantly lowers the risk of kidney and cardiac events on top of standard therapy. Pooled analyses from the FIDELITY program confirm finerenone's efficacy across a broad spectrum of CKD, with recent data indicating its benefits extend to older, frail patients as well. The incorporation of SGLT2 inhibitors and finerenone into guidelines (KDIGO 2024) reflects their role as cornerstone therapies to halt CKD progression. The CONFIDENCE trial is a study to investigate whether dual therapy with empagliflozin and finerenone together is superior to either alone in reducing proteinuria (Green et al., 2023).

New additions expanding the armamentarium

Multiple positive trials are poised to further expand CKD pharmacotherapy. This is exciting because it enables patients with significant kidney disorders to live longer lives with a higher quality of life and experience a delay in the development of serious disease until later years. One of the most notable trials is the FLOW trial of semaglutide, a glucagon-like peptide receptor agonist (GLP-1-RA). In FLOW, semaglutide, administered to 1767 patients with type 2 diabetes and CKD in a randomized controlled fashion, significantly reduced the composite of major kidney outcomes by 24% when compared with the 1766 placebo patients. It also lowered the risk of cardiovascular death (HR 0.71; 95% CI, 0.56 – 0.89) (Perkovic et al., 2024). Semaglutide is the first GLP-1 RA to demonstrate renal benefit, paving the way for regulatory approval in CKD indications beyond its glucose-lowering use. Damaged mitochondria and impaired mitophagy are hallmarks of aging. When treated with semaglutide, laboratory animals also demonstrated improved skeletal muscle mitochondrial function (Choi et al., 2025).

Another promising avenue is endothelin pathway blockade. The ZENITH-CKD trial is a Phase 2b randomized clinical trial that studied CKD patients with proteinuria. In this trial, the selective endothelin-A receptor antagonist zibotentan, when added to dapagliflozin, led to a meaningful reduction in albuminuria compared to SGLT2 inhibitor alone (Heerspink et al., 2023). This intervention targets two distinct pathways of kidney injury. A phase 3 trial is underway.

IgA nephropathy is the most common glomerulonephritis and often results in ESKD. It begins with the formation of galactose-deficient IgA that enters the systemic circulation from lymphoid tissue in the GI tract. This defective IgA leads to autoantibody formation, with resultant aggregation and immune complex deposition in the mesangium. This leads to scarring and loss of kidney function. The PROTECT trial was an international, double-blind, randomized, active-controlled study to determine if an endothelin-A combined with an angiotensin receptor antagonist (sparsentan) was effective at lowering proteinuria in patients with IgA nephropathy. There were 404 participants. By week 36, the urine protein-to-creatinine ratio in the sparsentan group was significantly lower (–49 · 8%) than in the irbesartan group (–15 · 1%), resulting in a reduction difference of 41% (least squares mean ratio = 0 · 59; 95% CI 0 · 51–0 · 69; $P < \cdot 0001$). The study was extended to 2 years with sustained results. The safety profile was similar to irbesartan's (Rovin et al., 2023).

At one time, IgA nephropathy had no successful treatment except for conservative measures and the use of omega-3 fatty acids. There are now two available drugs. The other is budesonide, a corticosteroid that specifically targets gut inflammation. It has been used in treating Crohn's disease, ulcerative colitis, and microscopic colitis. In the phase 3, randomized, double-blind, placebo-controlled, multicenter NefIgArd trial, 364 patients with IgA nephropathy were randomized. In the 182 patients who received budesonide, there was a statistically significant improvement in eGFR (5.05 mL/min/1.73m^2 difference, 95% CI 3.24–7.38, $P < .0001$). Proteinuria was also reduced (Lafayette et al., 2023). Complement activation is involved in the pathogenesis of IgA nephropathy. Iptacopan, a complement factor B inhibitor used in the treatment of paroxysmal nocturnal hemoglobinuria, was evaluated in IgA nephropathy patients in the APPLAUSE-IgAN study. This was a phase 3, double-blind, randomized, placebo-controlled trial of patients with proteinuria. Iptacopan produced a significant drop in proteinuria relative to placebo, achieving clinically meaningful reductions in albuminuria by 3–6 months. A proliferation-inducing ligand (APRIL) is a cytokine that signals IgA antibody production. Its receptor, B-cell maturation antigen, is also involved. Its elevation is associated with the overproduction of pathogenic galactose-deficient IgA. Thus, it has been targeted as a potential treatment strategy and is being evaluated in clinical trials (Mathur et al., 2024).

Trypanosomiasis is a parasitic disorder that causes African sleeping sickness. Polymorphisms in the APOL1 gene can confer immunity to trypanosomiasis, but when two copies of the variant are present, it can cause kidney disease. The presence of a viral syndrome can potentiate interferon (IFNɣ) and increase APOL1 expression. This leads to podocyte mitochondrial and lysosomal dysfunction, impaired autophagy, and cell death (Blazer et al., 2022). The discovery of APOL1's mechanism via functional genomics and CRISPR screens led to inaxaplin, which inhibits APOL1 channel function (Greensmith et al., 2024). Inaxaplin, which in preliminary studies reduced proteinuria by 47% (95% CI, – 60.0 to – 31.3), was safe and well tolerated. Phase 3 trials are underway (Egbuna et al., 2023).

Targeting aging pathways in the kidney

CKD accelerates biological aging, and conversely, aging mechanisms contribute to CKD progression. Researchers are investigating geroprotective interventions that target fundamental aging pathways, such as cellular senescence and the loss of youthful factors like Klotho. There are several antiaging therapeutics for patients with kidney disease. Senolytics clear senescent cells, and senomorphics suppress their harmful secretions. They have shown consistent renoprotective effects in preclinical models. Although paradoxical, senescent cells are more harmful than apoptotic cells because they are resistant to apoptosis but produce a catabolic factor known as the senescence-associated secretory phenotype (SASP). Dasatinib is used to treat chronic myelogenous leukemia. Quercetin is a flavonoid found in plants such as onions, green tea, apples, and berries. It has antiinflammatory and antioxidant properties but has not been investigated in any clinical trial. In aged or CKD mice, the senolytic agents dasatinib plus quercetin reduce renal fibrosis and improve function by eliminating senescent cells that drive inflammation. Senolytics, such as the combination of dasatinib and quercetin, target senescent cells and eliminate SASP (senescence-associated secretory phenotype). An early open-label clinical trial in 14 patients with idiopathic pulmonary fibrosis showed improvement in the 6 min walk test. Only 1 out of 14 patients experienced serious adverse events, with the rest of the patients having only mild discomfort. Although SASP factors were inconclusive, there were correlations with microRNAs, cytokines, and SASP-related matrix-remodeling proteins (23/48 markers, $R = 0.5$) (Justice et al., 2019; Rex et al., 2023). It is also being evaluated in intervertebral disc degeneration in mice, where it has been shown to decrease SASP as well as IL6 and other senescence markers (Novais et al., 2021). These approaches are not yet in clinical trials for CKD, although preclinical evidence supports senescence targeting as a therapeutic strategy.

α-Klotho is an antiaging protein that is abundant in the kidney; its levels decline in CKD and with age, contributing to vascular calcification, fibrosis, and frailty. Preclinical studies show that supplementation with a recombinant Klotho protein or gene therapy to boost Klotho expression protects the kidneys from injury by reducing fibrosis after acute injury and slowing CKD progression (Kanbay et al., 2024). Although, to date, there are no clinical trials in humans, low-dose subcutaneous Klotho in rhesus monkeys increases synaptic plasticity and cognition (Castner et al., 2023).

Another drug used to treat idiopathic pulmonary fibrosis is pirfenidone, a transforming growth factor beta (TGF-β) inhibitor. TGF-β binds to a receptor on the fibroblast, signaling SMAD phosphorylation, complexing of SMAD2 and SMAD3 with SMAD4, and translocation to the nucleus, where they increase profibrotic factors, extracellular matrix, and connective tissue growth factor, resulting in fibrosis, fibroblast proliferation, and myofibroblast differentiation. Thus, it leads to collagen production and fibrosis as well as fibroblast proliferation. This fibrosis is nonspecific and can affect the kidneys, liver, or eyes as well as the lungs. Pirfenidone decreases proinflammatory cytokines, inhibits oxidative stress, and blocks the activation of NF-κB. It modulates the activity of M1 and M2 macrophages, and by blocking the translocation of cytochrome C from the mitochondria to the cytosol, it can block apoptosis (Torre et al., 2024). A randomized controlled trial performed in 2011 used large doses and had a high drop out rate. The 1 year study lowered the number of patients needing dialysis and concluded that the drug was promising (Sharma et al., 2011). A Phase I bridging study

TABLE 29.1 Anti-aging therapies in Kidney Disease. Anti-aging therapies can potentially delay kidney disease progression, but in the four examples below, further clinical investigation will be necessary.

Therapy (Agent)	Target/Mechanism	Evidence
Senolytics (Dasatinib + Quercetin)	Targets senescent cells for elimination (reduces SASP inflammatory factors)	Senolytics improve pulmonary function in interstitial pulmonary fibrosis.
Metformin (as geroprotector)	Activates AMPK and mimics calorie restriction effects on metabolism	Systematic review demonstrates a mild effect of metformin on CKD
NAD + (nicotinamide riboside)	Prevents maternal-fetal malnutrition and low nephron number	Nephron number in offspring is restored when an NAD + supplement is given to rice mothers fed a low-protein diet
Anti-fibrotics (pirfenidone)	Inhibit TGF-β signaling, collagen deposition, and fibrosis	A 2011 study showed the drug had promise, but further trials are needed.

in CKD with GFR from 45–89 mL/min/1.73m^2 has shown that the drug is safe in this range and that dose adjustment is not necessary (Yu et al., 2025) (Table 29.1).

Metformin activates AMPK, mimicking calorie restriction and inducing mTOR pathway inhibition. This slows cell growth and induces autophagy. It may be associated with a reduction in both kidney and human aging. In a Cochrane review, there have been 11 studies involving either autosomal dominant polycystic kidney disease or diabetes. The review suggested only slight improvement over placebo with metformin, but little to no drug intolerance leading to drug withdrawal (El-Damanawi et al., 2024).

A factor explaining the pathogenesis of kidney disease is a low nephron number at the time of birth, induced by maternal malnutrition or premature birth. This increases the risk of later hypertension and CKD in adulthood. Animal models show that mice fed a low-protein diet give birth to offspring with reduced nephron numbers, but this is reversed with nicotinamide adenine dinucleotide (NAD +) (Pezzotta et al., 2022).

Regenerative and cell-based therapies

Regenerative medicine shows great promise. In one method, a biopsy of the patient's kidney tissue is processed to isolate and grow renal progenitor cells, which are then injected back into the patient's kidney to repair nephron segments. A Phase 2 trial indicated a potential slowdown of CKD progression in patients with diabetic kidney disease who received Rilparencel (Renal Autologous Cell Therapy [REACT]) (Stavas et al., 2024). Motivated by these results, ProKidney Corp (http://prokidney.com) has announced a Phase 3 trial (PROACT-1) in stage 3b–4 diabetic CKD patients.

Diagnostics and early risk stratification

A crucial component of improving CKD outcomes is identifying high-risk individuals early and monitoring disease activity more precisely. Traditional markers, like serum creatinine and urine albumin, have limitations in sensitivity and specificity. In response, researchers have developed novel biomarker assays and AI-driven screening tools to both detect kidney disease in early and reversible stages and track the disease course.

Biomarker-based risk prediction

KidneyIntelX (https://www.kidneyintelx.com/) has developed a diagnostic test combining three plasma biomarkers (soluble TNF receptor-1, soluble TNF receptor-2, and kidney injury molecule-1). The objective is to use machine learning algorithms and electronic health record data to predict which patients with diabetic CKD Stage 1–3 are at high risk for progressive decline and to select candidates for renoprotective therapy by creating a risk score to identify "fast progressors."

CKD273 is a panel of 273 urinary peptide fragments (mostly collagen and inflammatory proteins) whose combined pattern serves as a molecular signature of early diabetic CKD. It is able to predict CKD even when other markers, such as urine albumin, are negative. It may also be useful in tracking the course of kidney disease. In a double-blind, randomized, controlled, crossover study, type 2 diabetic patients managed with dapagliflozin, an SGLT2 inhibitor, were compared with placebo and then crossed over. Dapagliflozin significantly lowered the CKD273 score (–0.221; 95% CI – 0.356, – 0.087; P = 0.002) (Curovic et al., 2022).

Individual biomarkers are also under investigation. One of the most prominent is the soluble urokinase plasminogen activator receptor (suPAR), a circulating protein linked to focal segmental glomerulosclerosis (FSGS). In a study of over 3683 adults, those in the highest suPAR quartile had a 3.13 times greater risk of developing CKD compared to those in the lowest quartile (95% CI 2.11–4.65, P < 0.001) (Hayek et al., 2015).

Advanced imaging and liquid biopsy approaches

Renal imaging with conventional modalities has not been suitable for assessing and tracking the progression of chronic kidney disease. Using magnetic resonance imaging (MRI), T1 tissue relaxation properties appear to correlate with interstitial fibrosis and changes in tissue composition. A 2024 study of patients with CKD found that higher cortical T1 values were independently associated with a more rapid decline in glomerular filtration rate (GFR). MRI can assess water molecule diffusion in tissue, which may reflect fibrosis and inflammation in the renal parenchyma. MRI-based quantification of renal fibrosis in CKD patients is being investigated further (Shi et al., 2024).

Ultrasound with holography was developed by the late Norman S. Neidell for seismography to estimate oil reserves. Neidell also envisioned that the same techniques could be repurposed to develop holographic ultrasonography, which could noninvasively estimate cortical density and help track CKD progression. An acoustical imaging system can produce high-resolution medical images by using velocity characterizations captured by transducer arrays (USPTO 5,269,309).

Extracellular vesicles released into the extracellular space are potential markers of fibrosis, inflammation, and apoptosis. The sampling of tissues or the evaluation of urine for extracellular vesicles may help identify mRNAs, miRNAs, and proteins that provide insight into the content and specific characteristics of tubular cells and podocytes (Schnobrich and Castrop, 2025).

Artificial intelligence

An especially novel concept is harnessing routine nonrenal data (like an eye photograph) to infer kidney health via AI. The eye and kidney share many microvascular features, and subtleties in retinal images can reflect systemic microvascular disease. Recent studies have leveraged deep learning to analyze retinal fundus photographs for CKD screening with surprisingly good accuracy. The program was developed from an urban eye-screening program using a digital retinal camera. Three models were compared: the image-only model, the risk factor model, and a hybrid of the two. Risk factors included age, sex, ethnicity, duration of diabetes, HbA1C, and systolic blood pressure. The deep learning algorithm was based on a neural network architecture trained on 26,568 retinal images. The investigators used 5-fold cross-validation to evaluate model performance using two independent datasets. The area under the curve (AUC) was highest in the hybrid models in both datasets (Sabanayagam et al., 2020).

Artificial intelligence is increasingly being applied to nephrology and can augment clinical guidelines by creating a risk assessment for each individual patient. Algorithms can easily incorporate several additional variables, such as demographics, comorbidities, laboratory and imaging data, genetic testing, proteomics, and genomics, into models that can predict the risks of developing an endpoint, such as the need for renal replacement therapy, hospitalization, or even mortality. Physicians can use these scores to modify workflow to ensure the highest-risk patients are prioritized.

Reinforcement learning (RL) is an AI technique where algorithms learn optimal actions through trial-and-error feedback. In an RL framework, the agent—the entity that interacts with the environment—uses a mathematical procedure or algorithm to iteratively learn different actions by analyzing large datasets, such as dialysis sessions—to create a policy. The effect on patient outcomes is called the "reward." The policies and algorithms are applied chairside and can monitor care with the internal goal of getting rewarded.

A major problem in hemodialysis is intradialytic hypotension (IDH). Sudden drops in blood pressure are often unexpected. They usually respond to placing the patient in the Trendelenburg position, slowing the ultrafiltration rate, giving a fluid bolus, or even pausing treatment. IDH can often lead to adverse sequelae, including cardiac arrest. A reinforcement learning (RL) model was trained on historical data from 68,522 dialysis sessions at Chi Mei Medical Center. Thirty clinical, laboratory, and dialysis variables were used to create predictive models with eight algorithms. The algorithms were ranked, with the eXtreme Gradient Boosting (XGBoost) algorithm providing the best discrimination. Blood pressure, ultrafiltration rate, conductivity, and dialyzate calcium were identified as dominant determinants of hemodynamic stability. The model was implemented in a cloud-based dashboard and used for continuous risk visualization, updating every 60 min and displaying the risk of IDH up to 60 min in advance. This enabled proactive modifications in care, such as reducing ultrafiltration or elevating the patient's legs. There was a significant reduction in IDH incidences, from 26.1% to 20.6% (Yang et al., 2024).

A specific reinforcement learning architecture that is gaining attention in healthcare is the actor–critic model. In this approach, the "actor" suggests actions, and the "critic" assesses them, enabling more stable and efficient learning. Actor–critic algorithms have been used in critical care for conditions like sepsis treatment and are now being studied in nephrology for CKD-MBD management. An actor–critic AI can simultaneously recommend adjustments to both a patient's dialysis prescription and medications (e.g., fluid removal, dialyzate sodium, antihypertensives) to optimize blood pressure control without causing volume overload. The critic component evaluates each combined action based on predicted outcomes (from prior data), improving the actor's suggestions over time. While such comprehensive systems are still in the early stages, the modular actor–critic design is attractive for complex CKD management scenarios in which multiple interventions interact. It is also conducive to human-in-the-loop setups, where the AI's "actor" suggestion is reviewed by a clinician (the human is effectively an external critic).

In CKD drug management for patients not on dialysis, an actor–critic system could potentially assist with the management of chronic kidney disease mineral bone disorder, which has been developed and, although not yet validated, shows great promise (Gaweda et al., 2022; Lederer et al., 2024).

Machine learning (ML) is an aspect of artificial intelligence and refers to the ability of a machine (computer) to extract knowledge and, hence, learn from huge amounts of data using mathematical theory and algorithms to create models. These models are then validated against known datasets and subsequently tested on unseen data. Machine learning serves as both a tool in diagnostic and predictive analysis and as a means to identify latent relationships. The Nephrotic Syndrome Study Network (NEPTUNE) applies precision medicine through multilayered analysis using ML to analyze kidney biopsy images for risk analysis, influencing treatment choices and patient outcomes. Tangri has used AI to predict kidney failure from standard laboratory data derived from electronic health records. Other studies have been able to predict kidney failure timelines and transitions from decade-long blocks of data (Delrue et al., 2024). A CKD predictive model of seven variables over 5 years has resulted in a CKD classifier accurately predicting an eGFR decline of > 30%, with an area under the curve receiver-operator characteristic of 0.85 (Aoki et al., 2023).

Genomic and multiomic advances in precision nephrology

Genetic discoveries

As inaxaplin comes to market, genetic testing for APOL1 will guide its use—a clear example of precision medicine. In addition to APOL1 genetic variants, sequencing can identify a mutation in PKD1 or COL4A in a young CKD patient, altering management and allowing screening of family members. Genetic screening programs can identify nearly 385 genes responsible for monogenic kidney diseases and have been demonstrated to improve decision-making in clinical practice. In a multicenter study, 20.8% of patients had positive genetic findings that provided a new diagnosis. In the majority of circumstances, the results altered management (Dahl et al., 2023).

In addition to single-gene mutations, polygenic risk scores (PRS) for CKD are being developed. Large genome-wide association studies (GWAS) have identified common genetic variants associated with CKD risk. These include Uromodulin (UMOD) variants that interfere with tubular function and salt handling. UMOD encodes Tamm-Horsfall protein and is associated with hypertension and CKD. SHROOM3 encodes an actin-skeletal protein essential for podocyte cellular architecture and function (Khalili et al., 2016). Contemporary research has constructed PRS that aggregate dozens of such variants to estimate a person's inherited risk of developing CKD (Jefferis et al., 2024). CKD is associated with mitochondrial dysfunction. Summary-data-based Mendelian Randomization analysis of mitochondrial genes identified that increased expression of loci at glycine amidinotransferase (GATM) was associated with a decreased incidence of CKD. Loci associated with the methylation level of GATM sites were associated with an increased incidence of CKD. Decreased GATM expression was associated with diabetic nephropathy, vasculitis, IgA nephropathy, minimal change disease, FSGS, membranous GN, and hypertension. The nexus is explained by glycine amidinotransferase playing a key role in the synthesis of creatine, vital for energy release in mitochondria-rich cells. As proximal tubular cells are dependent upon mitochondria to function, GATM abnormalities are associated with Fanconi syndrome (Liu et al., 2024).

The kidney tissue atlas

A major recent multiomic project is the NIH-funded Kidney Precision Medicine Project (KPMP). KPMP is collecting research kidney biopsies from patients with CKD or acute kidney injury and analyzing them using single-cell RNA sequencing, spatial transcriptomics, proteomics, and metabolomics. The combined data are being used to build kidney-tissue atlases that will pinpoint functional pathways and druggable targets for various diseases. These include inflammatory and fibrotic pathways, as well as repair states. In addition, there are the Human Biomolecular Atlas Program and the Human Cell Atlas. Twenty-eight cellular states altered in kidney injury have been identified, defining biological pathways, repair states, and maladaptive responses that lead to kidney dysfunction (Jain et al., 2023; Lake et al., 2023).

Uremic toxins

The gut microbiome is altered in kidney disease, changing gut bacterial composition and resulting in the fermentation of uremic products into toxins (Bhargava et al., 2022). These toxins include p-cresyl sulfate (PCS) and indoxyl sulfate (IS). One theory suggests that increased urea levels promote colonization by urea-utilizing bacteria. Urea is metabolized into ammonia, raising gut pH, damaging the intestinal barrier, and allowing toxins to enter the circulation, which leads to inflammation. Uricase-containing bacteria may also increase uric acid levels, which is another toxin. There is a decrease in metabolites such as short-chain fatty acids, which benefit gut health. The uremic toxins and inflammatory cytokines result in the activation of MAP kinases and NF-κB, and they increase muscle-protein ubiquitination, contributing to sarcopenia (Zheng et al., 2024a). These toxins are strongly associated with cognitive impairment (de Oliveira Franco et al., 2019; Yu et al., 2022) cardiac disease (Wu et al., 2021), and the worsening of kidney disease (Tsuji et al., 2024). Although further investigation is needed, probiotics such as Renadyl and Lobun Forte have demonstrated improved quality-of-life scores and reduced uremic toxins, including uric acid (Borges et al., 2018).

Arginine residues, such as asymmetric dimethylarginine, are excreted by the kidney or metabolized by the liver. They are also uremic toxins, as they inhibit nitric oxide synthase (NOS), thereby reducing nitric oxide production and leading to oxidative stress, vasoconstriction, and endothelial dysfunction. This promotes hypertension and atherosclerosis, accelerates renal fibrosis, and causes mitochondrial dysfunction, inflammation, and ischemia to end organs like the brain. These negative effects are amplified by dysbiosis and the release of indoxyl sulfate and p-cresyl sulfate. Targeted therapies include RAAS inhibition, L-arginine supplements, probiotics, and lifestyle changes (exercise, dietary control, smoking cessation) (Zoccali and Kielstein, 2006; Lim et al., 2021).

Innovations in care delivery models

Scientific breakthroughs alone are not sufficient to improve patient outcomes on a broad scale—innovations in how care is delivered are equally important. In CKD, care coordination and late referrals have long been challenges, especially for older adults with multiple comorbidities. New models of care and policy initiatives are aimed at improving the management of CKD and the transition to ESRD.

Value-based and integrated care models

In the United States, the CMS Kidney Care Choices (KCC) model represents a major shift in incentivizing CKD care. Launched in 2022 and expanded through 2024, KCC is a voluntary payment program in which providers can earn performance-based payments for slowing CKD progression, increasing home dialysis and transplant rates, and improving care coordination. Participants include nephrology practices and dialysis providers who are accountable for the outcomes of their CKD and ESKD patients and share in savings if they meet targets. KCC and similar programs are driving interventions for stage 4 and 5 CKD to ensure "optimal starts," planned dialysis initiation with permanent access or preemptive transplantation. Other countries are also exploring integrated care approaches; for instance, some European health systems have implemented CKD multidisciplinary teams and seen improvements in preparation for renal replacement therapy and patient survival. Value-based care rewards keeping patients healthier longer, rather than the fee-for-service model, which unintentionally rewards acute and crisis care.

Multidisciplinary CKD clinics

Managing advanced CKD in older patients benefits from a holistic approach. Multidisciplinary CKD clinics bring together nephrologists, nurse practitioners, dietitians, pharmacists, social workers, and often cardiologists or diabetes specialists to co-manage patients. Evidence for their efficacy is growing. A prominent example is the PEAK program (Program for Education in Advanced Kidney Disease) at the Rogison Institute in New York. PEAK implemented an expanded care team plus structured care processes (including patient education on modality options, monthly team review of each case, and risk prediction tools to tailor care). Over 5 years, patients in PEAK had dramatically better transitions to ESKD. Of the patients who required dialysis, 58% achieved an "optimal" start. Fifty-four (18%) started on peritoneal dialysis, 16 (5%) on home hemodialysis, and 36 (12%) received a preemptive transplant. Patients in PEAK were more likely to start home dialysis (HR 1.34 from 2015 to 2020; 95% CI: 1.05–1.71, P = 0.018) (Shimonov et al., 2024). These outcomes underscore that comprehensive pre-ESKD care can change the trajectory. Other studies in Europe and Asia have similarly found that multidisciplinary clinics can slow eGFR decline and improve blood pressure and anemia control. Patients report higher satisfaction when they have access to diet and psychosocial support alongside medical care.

Multidisciplinary clinics also facilitate addressing the common complications in older CKD patients, such as frailty and cognitive impairment. As an example, incorporating a physical therapist can help with fall risk, mobility, flexibility, and muscle strength. Value-based programs like CMS's KCC provide a business case, as preventing dialysis, a fall-related fracture, or hospital admissions creates shared savings for providers.

Digital health and remote management

A 2024 scoping review identified 31 studies cataloging digital interventions in CKD, including smartphone apps for tracking symptoms (fatigue, itching, sleep quality), educational web platforms, and telemedicine coaching programs. The review concluded that these interventions show promise for offering patient-centric solutions, but gaps were also identified. These gaps included the fact that usability and acceptability were sometimes assumed without proper evaluation, as they did not always involve multidisciplinary stakeholders. In addition, evidence-based approaches were underused, and long-term outcomes were rarely assessed (Zheng et al., 2024b).

Conclusion summary (Table 29.2)

Novel innovations and therapeutics allow for better treatment and stabilization of a disease-complex that once had a uniformly poor prognosis. Diagnostic modalities make the detection of disease possible at an even earlier stage, offering additional opportunities to delay disease progression using existing new therapies like SGLT2 inhibitors, GLP1a, and MRA. Clinical trials are also exploring whether additive therapy is beneficial. For instance, an elderly nondiabetic patient with Stage 3B CKD might be managed not just with an SGLT2 inhibitor but also with an MRA and GLP1a. Genetic testing may help identify patients who are rapid or slow metabolizers of medications. Best demonstrated practice alerts, triggered by complex but "under the hood" AI systems that seamlessly integrate into the electronic health record, will help avoid medication errors and alert clinicians when gaps in care occur.

TABLE 29.2 Summary of advancements in aging research. Using established grouped hallmarks of aging (López-Otín et al., 2023) as a template, this table explains the relevance of each category, as well as present and emerging diagnostics and therapies.

Category(Organelle/DNA Locus)	Relevance to CKD and aging	Present diagnostics	Emerging diagnostics	Present therapies	Emerging therapies
Nuclear/Genomic/ Telomeric (Genomic instability, telomere attrition, epigenetic alterations)	CKD accelerates telomere attrition and DNA methylation drift, predicting mortality and vascular stiffness. Shared cellular aging mechanism.	Telomere length assays. DNA damage markers. DNA methylation clocks.	Multiomic biological age clocks, combining methylome, transcriptome, metabolome, and chromatin. Cell-free DNA signatures. Genome integrity mapping.	Lifestyle. Antioxidants Decrease genotoxic stress. Telomerase activators.	Partial epigenetic reprogramming, mRNA or viral telomerase therapy, and activators for DNA repair.
Mitochondrial/ Metabolic/ Nutrient-Sensing (Mitochondrial dysfunction, dysregulated nutrient sensing)	CKD involves mitochondrial fragmentation, decreases biogenesis, and impairs fatty-acid oxidation, driving sarcopenia and cognitive decline.	NAD^+/NADH ratios, mitochondrial (mt) DNA copy number, and mitochondrial respiration, as well as oxidative stress markers.	Mitochondrial metabolomics and redox flux profiling, mtDNA mutation burden, and mitochondrial imaging with PET or fluorescent probes.	Caloric restriction. Exercise. Metformin.SGLT2 inhibitors. Probiotics	NAD^+ boosters. Mitophagy activators. Mitochondrial transplants. Gene therapy. FGF-21analogs. AMPK/mTOR modulators.
Proteostasis/ Autophagy/ Lysosomal (Loss of proteostasis and impaired autophagy)	Impaired autophagy and the loss of proteostasis in tubular and podocyte cells accelerate fibrosis, which is common to renal and systemic aging.	Urinary proteomic panel (CKD273). Plasma proteostasis markers.	Proteostasis imaging (fluorescent autophagy sensors.) TFEB reporters read out mTORC1. Urinary exosomal proteostasis signatures. Serum lysosomal enzyme activity panels.	Caloric restriction. Exercise. mTOR inhibition. Pharmacologic chaperones. Statins improve lysosomal clearance.	Autophagy enhancers. TFEB agonists. Proteasome stabilizers. Lysosomal gene therapy. Senomorphic autophagy restoration.
Cellular Senescence/Stem Cell/Intercellular Communication with SASP production	Senescent tubular/ interstitial cells drive renal fibrosis. SASP amplifies systemic inflammation and frailty.	Senescence biomarkers. Stem cell biomarkers.	PET imaging of senescent cells. Plasma exosomal SASP proteome. Single-cell senescence transcriptomics.	Senolytics. Exercise. Mesenchymal stem cells.	CAR-T senolytics targeting uPAR or B2M, senomorphic JAK/STAT inhibitors, and FOXO activators, as well as exosome-based rejuvenation.

Category(Organelle/DNA Locus)	Relevance to CKD and aging	Present diagnostics	Emerging diagnostics	Present therapies	Emerging therapies
Systemic/Immune/ Microbiome (Inflammaging, Dysbiosis, Altered intercellular signaling)	Uremic dysbiosis fuels systemic inflammation, vascular calcification, and neurodegeneration—central in CKD—and accelerates aging.	hs-CRP. IL-6. TNF-α. Microbiome profiling. Kynurenine/ tryptophan ratio.	Integrated immune-microbiome "aging clocks". plasma metabolomics for uremic toxins (p-cresol, indoxyl sulfate), and multiomics inflammation risk models.	Anti-inflammatories (IL-1, IL-6 blockade), RAAS inhibitors, pro/ prebiotics, dietary modulation.	Microbiome engineering. Inflammasome inhibitors. Precision antiinflammatories. Gut–brain axis modulators.

CKD, chronic kidney disease; progressive loss of kidney function accelerated with cellular aging. *DNA,* deoxyribonucleic acid; carries genetic information—its damage or instability drives cellular senescence and CKD progression. *mtDNA,* mitochondrial DNA; encodes mitochondrial proteins—loss or mutation indicates mitochondrial dysfunction. *NAD⁺/NADH* nicotinamide adenine dinucleotide, oxidized/reduced forms; central redox cofactor regulating mitochondrial metabolism and energy balance. *mTORC1,* mechanistic target of rapamycin complex 1; nutrient-sensing kinase that suppresses autophagy when overactivated. *AMPK,* AMP-activated protein kinase; energy sensor that promotes mitochondrial biogenesis and autophagy, counteracting mTORC1. *SGLT2,* sodium-glucose cotransporter-2; renal glucose transporter—its inhibition improves metabolic and mitochondrial efficiency. *FGF-21,* fibroblast growth factor-21; hormone enhancing fatty-acid oxidation and mitochondrial health. *TFEB,* transcription factor EB; master regulator of lysosomal biogenesis and autophagy, promoting cellular clearance of waste. *mRNA,* messenger RNA; genetic transcript that carries the code from the nucleus to the ribosome—the site of protein synthesis. *PET,* positron emission tomography; imaging modality for mitochondrial or senescent-cell activity. *uPAR,* urokinase plasminogen activator receptor; marker of cellular senescence and inflammation, targeted by CAR-T senolytics. *B2M,* beta-2 microglobulin; senescence and immune activation marker, another CAR-T target. *CAR-T,* chimeric antigen receptor T-cell; engineered immune cells that selectively destroy targeted senescent or malignant cells. *SASP,* senescence-associated secretory phenotype; inflammatory cytokine and protease profile secreted by senescent cells. *JAK/STAT,* Janus kinase/signal transducer and activator of transcription; cytokine signaling pathway that promotes fibrosis—its inhibition reduces inflammation and SASP. *FOXO,* forkhead box O; transcription factors that regulate stress resistance, autophagy, and longevity. *IL-6/IL-1/TNF-α,* interleukin-6, interleukin-1, tumor necrosis factor-α; major pro-inflammatory cytokines driving systemic inflammation and "inflammaging"; *RAAS,* renin–angiotensin–aldosterone system; hormonal regulator of blood pressure and kidney perfusion—blockade limits CKD injury. *NF-κB,* nuclear factor κB; transcription factor controlling inflammatory gene expression—chronic activation drives fibrosis and aging. *CRP/ hs-CRP,* high-sensitivity C-reactive protein; circulating biomarker of systemic inflammation elevated in CKD and aging.

During dialysis, real-time learning integration can monitor and prevent drops in blood pressure.

Noninvasive diagnostics like MRI scans, holographic ultrasounds, retinal scans, AI-based risk prediction tools, and biomarkers will someday distinguish patients who require aggressive intervention from those who can be managed with standard therapy, improving both efficacy and resource allocation.

Care delivery will also be more patient-centered and proactive. Payment systems are starting to reward outcomes over volume. The adoption of multidisciplinary CKD clinics and care coordination programs enables patients to reliably interact with their care team through their smartphones. "Apps" monitor patients' home measurements, which trigger timely adjustments in care. For an aging CKD population, this could mean fewer hospital visits and a smoother transition if dialysis or transplant becomes necessary.

The new models of healthcare delivery will require interdisciplinary collaboration. The goal is to combine novel and more effective evidence-based therapy with smart diagnostic tools and AI-based decision support. The investment in hardware and software resources, training, and retooling the infrastructure is balanced by the promise of early identification and treatment, a delay in disease progression, and better kidney health.

AI Disclosure

During the preparation of this work, the author(s) used Chat GPT 5.0 Pro, Perplexity, Open Evidence, PubMed, and Google Scholar. These are valuable resources that are in the public domain and should be reviewed before composing a chapter. After using these tools/services, the author(s) reviewed and edited the content as needed and take(s) full responsibility for the content of the publication.

References

Aoki, J., Kaya, C., Khalid, O., Kothari, T., Silberman, M.A., Skordis, C., Hughes, J., Hussong, J., Salama, M.E., 2023. CKD Progression prediction in a diverse US population: a machine-learning model. Kidney Med. 25900595. 5 (9). Available from: https://www.journals.elsevier.com/kidney-medicine. doi:10.1016/j.xkme.2023.100692.

Bakris, G.L., Agarwal, R., Anker, S.D., Pitt, B., Ruilope, L.M., Rossing, P., Kolkhof, P., Nowack, C., Schloemer, P., Joseph, A., Filippatos, G., 2020. Effect of finerenone on chronic kidney disease outcomes in type 2 diabetes. N. Engl. J. Med. 15334406. 383 (23), 2219–2229. Available from: http://www.nejm.org/medical-index. doi:10.1056/NEJMoa2025845.

Bhargava, S., Merckelbach, E., Noels, H., Vohra, A., Jankowski, J., 2022. Homeostasis in the gut microbiota in chronic kidney disease. Toxins. 2072-6651. 14 (10), 648. doi:10.3390/toxins14100648.

Blazer, A., Qian, Y., Schlegel, M.P., Algasas, H., Buyon, J.P., Cadwell, K., Cammer, M., Heffron, S.P., Liang, F.X., Mehta-Lee, S., Niewold, T., Rasmussen, S.E., Clancy, R.M., 2022. APOL1 variant-expressing endothelial cells exhibit autophagic dysfunction and mitochondrial stress. Front. Genet. 16648021. 13. Available from: https://www.frontiersin.org/journals/genetics#. doi:10.3389/fgene.2022.769936.

Borges, N.A., Carmo, F.L., Stockler-Pinto, M.B., de Brito, J.S., Dolenga, C.J., Ferreira, D.C., Nakao, L.S., Rosado, A., Fouque, D., Mafra, D., 2018. Probiotic supplementation in chronic kidney disease: a double-blind, randomized, placebo-controlled trial. J. Ren. Nutr. 10512276. 28 (1), 28–36. Available from: http://www.sciencedirect.com/science/journal/10512276. doi:10.1053/j.jrn.2017.06.010.

Castner, S.A., Gupta, S., Wang, D., Moreno, A.J., Park, C., Chen, C., Poon, Y., Groen, A., Greenberg, K., David, N., Boone, T., Baxter, M.G., Williams, G.V., Dubal, D.B., 2023. Longevity factor klotho enhances cognition in aged nonhuman primates. Nat. Aging. 26628465. 3 (8), 931–937. Available from: https://www.nature.com/nataging/. doi:10.1038/s43587-023-00441-x.

Choi, R.H., Karasawa, T., Meza, C.A., Maschek, J.A., Manuel, A.M., Nikolova, L.S., Fisher-Wellman, K.H., Cox, J.E., Chaix, A., Funai, K., 2025. Semaglutide-induced weight loss improves mitochondrial energy efficiency in skeletal muscle. Obesity. 1930739X. 33 (5), 974–985. Available from: http://onlinelibrary.wiley.com/journal/10.1002/(ISSN)1930-739X. doi:10.1002/oby.24274.

Curovic, V.R., Eickhoff, M.K., Rönkkä, T., Frimodt-Møller, M., Hansen, T.W., Mischak, H., Rossing, P., Ahluwalia, T.S., Persson, F., 2022. Dapagliflozin improves the urinary proteomic kidney-risk classifier CKD273 in type 2 diabetes with albuminuria: a randomized clinical trial. Diabetes Care. 19355548. 45 (11), 2662–2668. Available from: http://care.diabetesjournals.org/content/by/year. doi:10.2337/dc22-1157.

Dahl, N.K., Bloom, M.S., Chebib, F.T., Clark, D., Westemeyer, M., Jandeska, S., Zhang, Z., Milo-Rasouly, H., Kolupaeva, V., Marasa, M., Broumand, V., Fatica, R.A., Raj, D.S., Demko, Z.P., Marshall, K., Punj, S., Tabriziani, H., Bhorade, S., Gharavi, A.G., 2023. The clinical utility of genetic testing in the diagnosis and management of adults with chronic kidney disease. J. Am. Soc. Nephrol. 15333450. 34 (12), 2039–2050. Available from: https://journals.lww.com/jasn/pages/default.aspx. doi:10.1681/ASN.0000000000000249.

de Oliveira Franco, Á., Starosta, R.T., Roriz-Cruz, M., 2019. The specific impact of uremic toxins upon cognitive domains: a review. Brazilian Journal of Nephrology. 2175-8239. 41 (1), 103–111. doi:10.1590/2175-8239-jbn-2018-0033.

Delrue, C., De Bruyne, S., Speeckaert, M.M., 2024. Application of machine learning in chronic kidney disease: current status and future prospects. Biomedicines. 22279059. 12 (3). Available from: www.mdpi.com/journal/biomedicines. doi:10.3390/biomedicines12030568.

Egbuna, O., Zimmerman, B., Manos, G., Fortier, A., Chirieac, M.C., Dakin, L.A., Friedman, D.J., Bramham, K., Campbell, K., Knebelmann, B., Barisoni, L., Falk, R.J., Gipson, D.S., Lipkowitz, M.S., Ojo, A., Bunnage, M.E., Pollak, M.R., Altshuler, D., Chertow, G.M., 2023. Inaxaplin for proteinuric kidney disease in persons with Two APOL1 variants. N. Engl. J. Med. 15334406. 388 (11), 969–979. Available from: http://www.nejm.org/medical-index. doi:10.1056/NEJMoa2202396.

El-Damanawi, R., et al., 2024. Metformin for preventing the progression of chronic kidney disease.. Cochrane Database Syst. Rev. 6 (6), CD013414. doi:10.1002/14651858.CD013414.pub2.

Gaweda, A., Lederer, E., Brier, M.E., 2022. Artificial intelligence guided precision treatment of chronic kidney disease-mineral bone disorder. CPT Pharmacometrics SYst. Pharmacol. 11, 1305-1315.

Green, J.B., Mottl, A.K., Bakris, G., Heerspink, H.J.L., Mann, J.F.E., Mcgill, J.B., Nangaku, M., Rossing, P., Scott, C., Gay, A., Agarwal, R., 2023. Design of the combination effect of finerenone and empagliflozin in participants with chronic kidney disease and type 2 diabetes using a UACR endpoint study (CONFIDENCE). Nephrol. Dial. Transplant. 14602385. 38 (4), 894–903. Available from: http://ndt.oxfordjournals.org/. doi:10.1093/ndt/gfac198.

Greensmith, R., Lape, I.T., Riella, C.V., Schubert, A.J., Metzger, J.J., Dighe, A.S., Tan, X., Hemmer, B., Rau, J., Wendlinger, S., Diederich, N., Schütz, A., Riella, L.V., Kaminski, M.M., 2024. CRISPR-enabled point-of-care genotyping for APOL1 genetic risk assessment. EMBO Mol. Med. 17574684. 16 (10), 2619–2637. Available from: https://communities.springernature.com/badges/embo-molecular-medicine. doi:10.1038/s44321-024-00126-x.

Hayek, S.S., et al., 2015. Soluble Urokinase Receptor and Chronic Kidney Disease. N. Engl. J. Med. 373 (20), 1916–1925. doi:10.1056/NEJMoa1506362.

Heerspink, H.J.L., Kiyosue, A., Wheeler, D.C., Lin, M., Wijkmark, E., Carlson, G., Mercier, A.K., Åstrand, M., Ueckert, S., Greasley, P.J., Ambery, P., 2023. Zibotentan in combination with dapagliflozin compared with dapagliflozin in patients with chronic kidney disease (ZENITH-CKD): a multicentre, randomised, active-controlled, phase 2b, clinical trial. Lancet. 1474547X. 402 (10416), 2004–2017. Available from: https://www.sciencedirect.com/science/journal/01406736. doi:10.1016/S0140-6736(23)02230-4.

Heerspink, H.J.L., Stefánsson, B.V., Correa-Rotter, R., Chertow, G.M., Greene, T., Hou, F.F., Mann, J.F.E., McMurray, J.J.V., Lindberg, M., Rossing, P., Sjöström, C.D., Toto, R.D., Langkilde, A.M., Wheeler, D.C., 2020. Dapagliflozin in patients with chronic kidney disease. N. Engl. J. Med. 15334406. 383 (15), 1436–1446. Available from: http://www.nejm.org/medical-index. doi:10.1056/NEJMoa2024816.

Herrington, W.G., Staplin, N., Agrawal, N., Wanner, C., Green, J.B., Hauske, S.J., Emberson, J.R., Preiss, D., Judge, P., Zhu, D., Dayanandan, R., Arimoto, R., Mayne, K.J., Ng, S.Y.A., Sammons, E., Hill, M., Stevens, W., Wallendszus, K., Brenner, S., Cheung, A.K., Liu, Z.H., Li, J., Hooi, L.S., Liu, W., Kadowaki, T., Nangaku, M., Levin, A., Cherney, D.Z.I., Maggioni, A.P., Pontremoli, R., Deo, R., Goto, S., Rossello, X., Tuttle, K.R., Steubl, D., Massey, D., Brueckmann, M., Landray, M.J., Baigent, C., Haynes, R., 2025. Long-term effects of empagliflozin in patients with chronic kidney disease. N. Engl. J. Med. 15334406. 392 (8), 777–787. Available from: http://www.nejm.org/medical-index. doi:10.1056/NEJMoa2409183.

Jain S., et al., 2023. Advances and prospects for the Human BioMolecular Atlas Program (HuBMAP). Nat. Cell Biol. 25 (8) 1089–1100. doi:10.1038/s41556-023-01194-w.

Jefferis, J., Hudson, R., Lacaze, P., Bakshi, A., Hawley, C., Patel, C., Mallett, A., 2024. Monogenic and polygenic concepts in chronic kidney disease (CKD). J. Nephrol. 17246059. 37 (1), 7–21. Available from: https://www.springer.com/journal/40620. doi:10.1007/s40620-023-01804-8.

Justice, J.N., Nambiar, A.M., Tchkonia, T., LeBrasseur, N.K., Pascual, R., Hashmi, S.K., Prata, L., Masternak, M.M., Kritchevsky, S.B., Musi, N., Kirkland, J.L., 2019. Senolytics in idiopathic pulmonary fibrosis: results from a first-in-human, open-label, pilot study. EBioMedicine. 23523964. 40, 554–563. Available from: http://www.journals.elsevier.com/ebiomedicine/. doi:10.1016/j.ebiom.2018.12.052.

Kanbay, M., Copur, S., Ozbek, L., Mutlu, A., Cejka, D., Ciceri, P., Cozzolino, M., Haarhaus, M.L., 2024. Klotho: a potential therapeutic target in aging and neurodegeneration beyond chronic kidney disease-a comprehensive review from the ERA CKD-MBD working group. Clin. Kidney J. 20488513. 17 (1). Available from: http://ckj.oxfordjournals.org/. doi:10.1093/ckj/sfad276.

Khalili, H., Sull, A., Sarin, S., Boivin, F.J., Halabi, R., Svajger, B., Li, A., Cui, V.W., Drysdale, T., Bridgewater, D., 2016. Developmental origins for kidney disease due to Shroom3 deficiency. J. Am. Soc. Nephrol. 15333450. 27 (10), 2965–2973. Available from: http://jasn.asnjournals.org/content/27/10/2965.full.pdf+html. doi:10.1681/ASN.2015060621.

Lafayette, R., Kristensen, J., Stone, A., Floege, J., Tesař, V., Trimarchi, H., Zhang, H., Eren, N., Paliege, A., Reich, H.N., Rovin, B.H., Barratt, J., 2023. Efficacy and safety of a targeted-release formulation of budesonide in patients with primary IgA nephropathy (NefIgArd): 2-year results from a randomised phase 3 trial. Lancet. 1474547X. 402 (10405), 859–870. Available from: http://www.journals.elsevier.com/the-lancet/. doi:10.1016/S0140-6736(23)01554-4.

Lake, B.B., et al., 2023. An atlas of healthy and injured cell states and niches in the human kidney. Nat. 619 (7970), 585–594. doi:10.1038/s41586-023-05769-3.

Lederer, E.D., Sobh, M.M., Brier, M.E., Gaweda, A.E., 2024. Application of artificial intelligence to chronic kidney disease mineral bone disorder. Clin. Kidney J. 17 (6), sfae143. doi:10.1093/ckj/sfae143.

Lim, Y.J., Sidor, N.A., Tonial, N.C., Che, A., Urquhart, B.L., 2021. Uremic toxins in the progression of chronic kidney disease and cardiovascular disease: mechanisms and therapeutic targets. Toxins. 20726651. 13 (2). Available from: https://www.mdpi.com/2072-6651/13/2/142/pdf. doi:10.3390/TOXINS13020142.

Liu, B., Gao, X., Teng, H., Zhou, H., Gao, B., Faping, L., 2024. Association between GATM gene polymorphism and progression of chronic kidney disease: a mitochondrial related genome-wide Mendelian randomization study. Sci. Rep. 2045-2322. 14 (1). doi:10.1038/s41598-024-68448-x.

López-Otín, C., Blasco, M.A., Partridge, L., Serrano, M., Kroemer, G., 2023. Hallmarks of aging: an expanding universe. Cell. 10974172. 186 (2), 243–278. Available from: https://www.sciencedirect.com/journal/cell. doi:10.1016/j.cell.2022.11.001.

Mathur, M., Barratt, J., Chacko, B., Chan, T.M., Kooienga, L., Oh, K.H., Sahay, M., Suzuki, Y., Wong, M.G., Yarbrough, J., Xia, J., Pereira, B.J.G., 2024. A phase 2 trial of sibeprenlimab in patients with IgA nephropathy. N. Engl. J. Med. 15334406. 390 (1), 20–31. Available from: http://www.nejm.org/medical-index. doi:10.1056/NEJMoa2305635.

Novais, E.J., Tran, V.A., Johnston, S.N., Darris, K.R., Roupas, A.J., Sessions, G.A., Shapiro, I.M., Diekman, B.O., Risbud, M.V., 2021. Long-term treatment with senolytic drugs Dasatinib and Quercetin ameliorates age-dependent intervertebral disc degeneration in mice. Nat. Commun. 20411723. 12 (1). Available from: http://www.nature.com/ncomms/index.html. doi:10.1038/s41467-021-25453-2.

Perkovic, V., Tuttle, K.R., Rossing, P., Mahaffey, K.W., Mann, J.F.E., Bakris, G., Baeres, F.M.M., Idorn, T., Bosch-Traberg, H., Lausvig, N.L., Pratley, R., 2024. Effects of semaglutide on chronic kidney disease in patients with type 2 diabetes. N. Engl. J. Med. 15334406. 391 (2), 109–121. Available from: http://www.nejm.org/medical-index. doi:10.1056/NEJMoa2403347.

Pezzotta, A., Perico, L., Morigi, M., Corna, D., Locatelli, M., Zoja, C., Benigni, A., Remuzzi, G., Imberti, B., 2022. Low Nephron number induced by maternal protein restriction is prevented by nicotinamide riboside supplementation depending on sirtuin 3 activation. Cells. 2073-4409. 11 (20), 3316. doi:10.3390/cells11203316.

Rex, N., Melk, A., Schmitt, R., 2023. Cellular senescence and kidney aging. Clin. Sci. 0143-5221. 137 (24), 1805–1821. doi:10.1042/cs20230140.

Rovin, B.H., Barratt, J., Heerspink, H.J.L., Alpers, C.E., Bieler, S., Chae, D.W., Diva, U.A., Floege, J., Gesualdo, L., Inrig, J.K., Kohan, D.E., Komers, R., Kooienga, L.A., Lafayette, R., Maes, B., Małecki, R., Mercer, A., Noronha, I.L., Oh, S.W., Peh, C.A., Praga, M., Preciado, P., Radhakrishnan, J., Rheault, M.N., Rote, W.E., Tang, S.C.W., Tesar, V., Trachtman, H., Trimarchi, H., Tumlin, J.A., Wong, M.G., Perkovic, V., Abbasciano, I., Abrantes, C., Accarino, S., Adler, S., Adoberg, A., Afsari, R., Ahmad, S., Ahmed, J., Ahn, W., Ajayi, B., Aksamit, D., Chalabi, S.A., Alamartine, E., Alchi, B., Ali, M., Aliotta, R., Almaani, S., Almeida, C., Almeida, E., Alvarez, F.D.L.P., Alves, P., Annese, F., Appel, G., Arduan, A.O., Arena, M., Arevalo, M.C., Arfaania, D., Arias, C., Aristoy, E.C., Asakiene, E., Ashley, S., Assefi, A., Atenza, A., Auerbach, A., Augustyniak-Bartosik, H., Avella, M., Ayling-Smith, J., Ayoub, I., Ayvazyan, C., Baccaro, R., Bailey, A., Baker, B., Balamuthusamy, S., Ballarin, J., Barata, R., Barbic, J., Barisic, D., Barreto, J.C.D.J., Barrios, C., Belingheri, M., Benesova, A., Bernabeu, A.A., Bernhardt, W., Bhadra, S., Biancone, L., Blanchard, A., Boaglio, E., Bolignano, D., Bomback, A., Bonilla, G.A.U., Bordoli, M., Bose, B., Boudville, N., Brandon, D., Brown, K., Broyet, C., Bucknall, T., Buffet, A., Bumblyte', I.A., Burdese, M., Burgos, N.A., Burguet, L., Burtey, S., Busch, M., Cakiroglu, F., Campbell, V., Canetta, P., Capaccio, F., Carbonell, J., Cardoso, F., Carro, C.G., Carroll, R., Carron, P.L., Carullo, N., Cassia, M., Caster, D., Castillo, B.V., Catucci, D., Cavalli, A., Chakera, A., Chan, D., Chan, G.C.W., Chan, A.T.P., Chan, L.W., Chang, J.H., Chang, M.S., Chapman, F., Charytan, C., Chaudhry, A., Cheetham, M., Chen, C.H., Chen, H.Y., Chen, C.L., Chen, H.Y., Chen, H.C., Chenine, L., Cheung, S.F., Cheung, C.K., Chiche-Jourde, N., Chiu, H.F., Chiu, Y.L., Chiu, Y.W., Chiu, I., Choi, H.Y., Chou, K.J., Chowdhury, P., Chowdhury, P., Chrysochou, C., Chukwu, C., Chun, K.Y., Chung, W., Cieniawski, D., Claisse, G., Clayton, P., Cleary, C.M., Clement, N., Coates, T., Cogno, C., Colla, L., Collins, M., Colucci, M., Combe, C., Comi, N., Comunale, R., Contreras, G., Cooper, B., Coppock, G., Costa, A.C., Costanzi, S., Cozzolino, M.,

Crail, S., Cunha, L., Curry, E., Dai, T., Daina, E., Daneshvari, S., Dasgupta, I., DaSilva, L., Davidson, R., De Bhailis, A.M., de Précigout, V., Decupere, M., Delmas, Y., Deodato, F., Dhaun, N., Dhaygude, A., Dhelaria, R., Di Maio, F., Diezhandino, M.A.G., Dika, Z., Dinic, M., Dittmer, I., Dobre, M., Doctor, G., Donati, G., Doubel, P., Douthit, N., Draganova, D., Drexler, Y., Drinkovic, M., Drinovska, K., Dudreuilh, C., Dumond, C., Durlen, I., Dussol, B., Encarnacion, M.D., Endre, Z., Enrique, J., Eqbal, Y., Erlich, J., Esposito, V., Esposito, C., Fakih, F., Fang, H.C., Farinha, A., Fearday, A., Felgueiras, J.D.S.S., Felicjanczuk, E., Fernandes, J.C., Fernandes, S., Fernandes, A., Fernandez, J.L., Fernandez, V., Fernando, M., Figueiredo, A.C., Firre, E., Flossmann, O., Floyd, L., Fonseca, N., Fonseca, J.N.D.A.A., Foote, C., Forbes, S., Forcen, A., Fornoni, A., Fouassier, D., Fraser, I., Fung, K.S.S., Furlano, M., Furtado, T., Gadh, R., Gaisset, R., Gallagher, M., Gameiro, J., Gangadharan, M., Garcia, F.A., Garcia, O.G., Garg, G., Garrouste, C., Gautam, A., Geara, A., Geddes, C., Gellineo, L., Germain, M., Ghalli, F., Giaroni, F., Giles, H., Gillies, A., Gimeno, A.V., Girardet, A., Glaze, J., Goh, T., Gois, M., Goldsmith, C., Goma, E., Gomes, A.M., Goncalves, L.P.F., Goncalves, S., Gontarek-Kacprzak, J., Gonzalez, C., Gopu, A., Gowda, N., Gray, N., Greco, B., Green, H., Greze, C., Griffin, S., Guldris, S.C., Guzman, U.V., Ha, J.T.K., Hall, A., Hamilton, P., Han, S.H., Haws, R., Hayat, A., Heath, L., Heinrichs, S., Henderson, A., Henderson, A., Hendren, E., Heng, A.E., Heres, S.V.P., Herfurth, J.K., Herrero, E.M., Ho, T.Y., Hogan, J., Hohenstein, B., Hollett, P., Horvatic, I., Hsu, B.G., Hsu, C.T., Hsu, C.Y., Hsu, S.P., Huang, C.W., Hudson, A., Hung, C.C., Hwang, S.J., Hwang, D.Y., Hyun, Y.Y., Ilmoja, M., Irish, G., Jacob, R., Jahan, S., Jain, A., Jamar, S., Jander, A., Jang, H.R., Janko, C., Jardine, M., Jaskowski, P., Jeantet, G., Jelakovic, B., Jeon, J., Jeong, J.C., Jesudason, S., Jittirat, A., Jo, S.K., Jones, R., Joo, N., Jorge, S., Julian, B., Jung, J.Y., Jyothinagaram, P., Kadakia, J., Kamal, F., Kanigicherla, D., Karanovic, S., Karras, A., Kasimatis, T., Kassem, M., Kattamanchi, S., Keller, C., Kentric, D.T., Kettner, C., Khalil, K., Kim, D., Kim, S.J., Kim, Y.H., Kim, Y., Kim, H.W., Kim, S., Kim, J.K., Kim, A., Kim, M.G., Kimber, C., Klamm, K., Koch, A., Koester, E., Kolvald, K., Kon, S., Kotwal, S., Krajewska, M., Kratka, K., Krishnan, A., Krishnasamy, R., Krueger, T., Kruljac, I., Kulka, S., Kunzendorf, U., Kuo, M.C., Kuo, H.T., Kuo, S., Kwan, L.P.Y., Kwella, N., Kwella, B., Kyaw, K., Labat, A., Lagatta, M., Lam, C.K.D., Lambie, M., Lanaret, C., Latif, F., Laute, M., Law, W.P., Lawman, S., Lazo, M.S., Lee, H., Lee, M.H., Lee, K.B., Lee, H.S., Lee, J.E., Lee, H.H., Lee, P.T., Leis, L., Lemahieu, W., Leung, J., Li, Y., Lie, D.N.W., Lifland, H., Lilienthal, K., Lim, W., Limardo, M., Livrozet, M., Longhi, S., Lopes, D., Lopes, J.A., Lorde, N., Luxton, G., Ma, M., Madhrira, M., Madonia, P., Mahadevan, K., Mahdi, A., Mahdi, E., Maillard, N., Maixnerova, D., Barac, K.M., Malecki, R., Malfait, T., Malvica, S., Mandayam, S., Manley, P., Mansfield, N., Marcantoni, C., Mariat, C., Marin, T.M., Marin, L.M.R., Mark, P., Marques, J., Martinez, E.G., Martinez, S., Masset, C., Masson, I., Mather, A., Maung Myint, T.M., Mayet, V., McCafferty, K., McCarthy, E., McDonald, S., McGreal, K., McMahon, K., McNally, A., McQuarrie, E., Medina, A., Meeus, G., Mehta, K., Mendoza, E., Menezes, M., Meng, J., Messa, P., Messias, A., Miarka, P., Miglinas, M., Mikacic, I., Mikhail, A., Milicevic, M., Minasian, R., Moeller, M., Mohey, H., Mojarrab, J., Mok, M.M.Y., Moncasi, E.P., Moonen, M., Morales, W.A.A., Moreno, E.V., Moreno, A., Morris, A., Moutzouris, D., Moya, M.G., Mucha, S., Musolino, M., Napodano, P., Natario, A., Negrea, L., Nelson, B., Neuen, B., Newsome, B., Ng, K.C.J., Nguyen, T., Nguyen, V., Nicolo, C., Nitschke, M., Noble, E., Nolasco, F., O'Lone, E., Ochoa, A.S., Oh, K.H., Oh, S.W., Okoh, P., Ombelet, S., O'Shaughnessy, M., Ou, S.H., Packham, D., Padiyar, A., Pai, M.F., Pamplona, I.A., Pan, S.Y., Pandya, B., Papadia, F., Pardinhas, C., Parikh, N., Parikh, S., Park, H.C., Park, J.T., Parreira, L., Passerini, P., Patak, R., Patecki, M., Patel, R., Patel, J., Patel Suthar, M., Patella, G., Patrikyan, A., Pavlovic, D., Paxton, W., Peh, C., Peleg, Y., Pelicano, J.M.B., Peng, Y.S., Pereira de Vicente, M., Perez, J.P., Perez, E., Perez de Jose, A., Pérez Gómez, M.V., Perez Lluna, L., Peri, U., Perico, N., Philipponnet, C., Phua, E., Piel, J., Pillai, U., Pilmore, H., Plavljanic, D., Plaza, M.V., Pollock, C., Ponnusamy, A., Ponti, S., Powell, T., Pradhan, N., Prado, R.F., Prkacin, I., Pruthi, R., Pugh, D., Quinn, S., Quintana, L.F., Raakesh, L., Rabindranath, K., Radermacher, L., Ragy, O.S.I., Raichoudhury, R., Raimundo, M., Randone, P., Razavian, M., Reichel, H., Reis, M., Remuzzi, G., Reynolds, A., Ricchiuto, A., Rico, I.M.B., Rigothier, C., Ritchie, A., Rivero, M.A.A., Rizk, D., Ro, H., Rodriguez, A., Garcia, E.R., Roger, S., Rony, M., Rosenberg, M., Roueff, S., Rovin, B., Roxburgh, S., Ruiz, M., Rusinol, H.M., Rychlik, I., Sá, H., Salehi, T., Sánchez de la Nieta, M.D., Sanden, S., Santockiene, L., Santos, P.V., Santos, I.D.S., Sargsyan, M., Sarnow, F., Sat, S., Satora, E., Savuk, A., Sayer, M., Schlieper, G., Schlosser, M., Schmidt-Guertler, H., Schockaert, O., Schulte, K., Schulz, L., Selvaskandan, H., Semple, D., Sen, S., Seppet, E., Serrano, A.G., Serre, J.E., Sevillano, A., Shah, S., Shen, Y., Sheridan, B., Shu, K.H., Sightler, F., Silva, S., Silva, A., Sinha, S., Siriwardana, A., Sitas, Z., Sivo, C., Sizeland, P., Sly, C., Smith, P., Snow, B., Soares, E.S.Q., Solazzo, A., Solis, E.G., Solomon, L., Song, Y.R., Sousa, H., Spinowitz, B., Stallworthy, E., Stamellou, E., Stanczyk, M., Stangenberg, S., Stankovic, M., Stankuviene, A., Stea, E.D., Stompor, T., Storrar, J., Sullivan, J., Sulowicz, W., Suyumova, I., Szeto, C.C., Tamarit, E., Tan, E., Tan, M., Tang, H., Teixeira, C., Telling, K., Terrades, N.R., Tez, D., Thervet, E., Thibaudin, D., Thomas, M., Thyagarajan, N., Tkaczyk, M., Torreggiani, M., Trillini, M., Tsai, S.F., Tsai, W.C., Tsai, J.C., Tseng, P.Y.,

Tumlin, J., Tung, K.T., Turnbull, A., Udani, S., Uhlinova, J., Unt, K., Urciuolo, F., Vanacker, A., Vandewiele, B., Vaz, A., Veermae, K., Viaene, L., Vickiene, A., Vigano, S., Vila, M.A.M., Vilayur, E., Villanueva, C.M., Villarroya, C.M., Villen, A.S., Viramontes, V., Vita, C., Vujcic, D., Wahba, M., Wan, S., Wang, C.H., Warling, X., Waters, G., Waugh, J., Weiland, L., Weiner, S., Weinreich, T., Werth, S.C., Wickens, O., Wijeratne, V., Wilder, K., Willcocks, L., Williams, A., Winiarska, A., Wirtz, N., Wolf, L., Wolf, G., Wong, Y.H., Wong, S.H.S., Workeneh, B., Wu, M.J., Wu, H.Y., Wyndham, R., Yang, J., Yang, J.Y., Yeap, C., Yim, K.F., Yong, K., Yoo, T.H., Yoon, S., Yu, T.M., Yue, T.T.A., Zakari, M., Zakauskiene, U., Zaoui, P., Zbrzezniak, J., Zielinska, D., Zizzi, C.F., 2023. Efficacy and safety of sparsentan versus irbesartan in patients with IgA nephropathy (PROTECT): 2-year results from a randomised, active-controlled, phase 3 trial. Lancet. 1474547X. 402 (10417), 2077–2090. Available from: https://www.sciencedirect.com/science/journal/01406736. doi:10.1016/S0140-6736(23)02302-4.

Sabanayagam, C., Xu, D., Ting, D.S.W., Nusinovici, S., Banu, R., Hamzah, H., Lim, C., Tham, Y.C., Cheung, C.Y., Tai, E.S., Wang, Y.X., Jonas, J.B., Cheng, C.Y., Lee, M.L., Hsu, W., Wong, T.Y., 2020. A deep learning algorithm to detect chronic kidney disease from retinal photographs in community-based populations. Lancet Digit. Health. 25897500. 2 (6), e295. Available from: https://www.sciencedirect.com/journal/the-lancet-digital-health. doi:10.1016/S2589-7500(20)30063-7.

Schnobrich, L., Castrop, H., 2025. Urinary microvesicles: a window into the kidney. Clin. Kidney J. 2048-8505. 18 (7). doi:10.1093/ckj/sfaf189.

Sharma, K., Ix, J.H., Mathew, A.V., Cho, M., Pflueger, A., Dunn, S.R., Francos, B., Sharma, S., Falkner, B., McGowan, T.A., Donohue, M., RamachandraRao, S., Xu, R., Fervenza, F.C., Kopp, J.B., 2011. Pirfenidone for diabetic nephropathy. J. Am. Soc. Nephrol. 15333450. 22 (6), 1144–1151. Available from: http://jasn.asnjournals.org/content/22/6/1144.full.pdf+html. doi:10.1681/ASN.2010101049.

Shi, Z., Sun, C., Zhou, F., Yuan, J., Chen, M., Wang, X., Wang, X., Zhang, Y., Pylypenko, D., Yuan, L., 2024. Native T1-mapping as a predictor of progressive renal function decline in chronic kidney disease patients. BMC Nephrol. 1471-2369. 25 (1). doi:10.1186/s12882-024-03559-1.

Shimonov, D., Tummalapalli, S.L., Donahue, S., Narayana, V., Wu, S., Walters, L.S., Billman, R., Desiderio, B., Pressman, S., Fielding, O., Sweeney, K., Cukor, D., Levine, D.M., Parker, T.S., Srivatana, V., Silberzweig, J., Liu, F., Bohmart, A., 2024. Clinical outcomes of a novel multidisciplinary care program in advanced kidney disease (PEAK). Kidney Int. Rep. 24680249. 9 (10), 2904–2914. Available from: https://www.sciencedirect.com/science/journal/24680249. doi:10.1016/j.ekir.2024.07.018.

Stavas, J., Silva, A.L., Wooldridge, T.D., Aqeel, A., Saad, T., Prakash, R., Bakris, G., 2024. Rilparencel (Renal autologous cell therapy-REACT®) for chronic kidney disease and type 1 and type 2 diabetes: phase 2 trial design evaluating bilateral kidney dosing and redosing triggers. Am. J. Nephrol. 14219670. 55 (3), 389–398. Available from: www.karger.ch/journals/ajn/ajn_jh.htm.. doi:10.1159/000537942.

Theodorakopoulou, M.P., Sarafidis, P., 2024. SGLT2 inhibitors and finerenone in non-diabetic CKD: a step into the (near) future? Clin. Kidney J. 20488513. 17 (1). Available from: http://ckj.oxfordjournals.org/. doi:10.1093/ckj/sfad272.

Torre, A., Martínez-Sánchez, F.D., Narvaez-Chávez, S.M., Herrera-Islas, M.A., Aguilar-Salinas, C.A., Córdova-Gallardo, J., 2024. Pirfenidone use in fibrotic diseases: what do we know so far? Immun. Inflamm. Dis. 20504527. 12 (7). Available from: http://onlinelibrary.wiley.com/journal/10.1002/(ISSN)2050-4527. doi:10.1002/iid3.1335.

Tsuji, U., Nakanoh, F., Haraguchi, K., Wada J., 2024. The gut-kidney axis in chronic kidney diseases. Diagnostics 15 (21).

Wu, P.H., Lin, Y.T., Chiu, Y.W., Baldanzi, G., Huang, J.C., Liang, S.S., Lee, S.C., Chen, S.C., Hsu, Y.L., Kuo, M.C., Hwang, S.J., 2021. The relationship of indoxyl sulfate and p-cresyl sulfate with target cardiovascular proteins in hemodialysis patients. Sci. Rep. 20452322. 11 (1). Available from: www.nature.com/srep/index.html.. doi:10.1038/s41598-021-83383-x.

Yang, I.N., Liu, C.F., Chien, C.C., Wang, H.Y., Wang, J.J., Shen, Y.T., Chen, C.C., 2024. Personalized prediction of intradialytic hypotension in clinical practice: development and evaluation of a novel AI dashboard incorporating risk factors from previous and current dialysis sessions. Int. J. Med. Inform. 18728243. 190. Available from: https://www.sciencedirect.com/science/journal/13865056. doi:10.1016/j.ijmedinf.2024.105538.

Yu, D., Zhang, R., Zhou, J., Guo, P., Li, P., Ye, M., Liu, Y., Shi, S., 2025. Pharmacokinetics and safety of pirfenidone in individuals with chronic kidney disease stage G2 and G3a: a single-dose, Phase I, bridging study. J. Pharm. Sci. 15206017. 114 (2), 1087–1094. Available from: https://www.sciencedirect.com/science/journal/00223549. doi:10.1016/j.xphs.2024.11.020.

Yu, Y.H., Kim, S.W., Im, H., Oh, S.W., Cho, N.J., Park, S., Park, D.K., Kim, D.S., Gil, H.W., 2022. Cognitive sequelae and hippocampal dysfunction in chronic kidney disease following 5/6 nephrectomy. Brain Sci. 20763425. 12 (7). Available from: http://www.mdpi.com/journal/brainsci. doi:10.3390/brainsci12070905.

Zheng, G., Cao, J., Wang, X.H., He, W., Wang, B., 2024a. The gut microbiome, chronic kidney disease, and sarcopenia. Cell Commun. Signal. 1478811X. 22 (1). Available from: https://biosignaling.biomedcentral.com/. doi:10.1186/s12964-024-01922-1.

Zheng, X., Yang, Z., Liu, S., Yuqian, L., Wang, A., 2024b. Digital symptom management interventions for people with chronic kidney disease: a scoping review based on the UK Medical Research Council Framework. BMC Public Health. 1471-2458. 24 (1). doi:10.1186/s12889-024-20871-5.

Zoccali, C., Kielstein, J.T., 2006. Asymmetric dimethylarginine: a new player in the pathogenesis of renal disease? Curr. Opin. Nephrol. Hypertens. 10624821. 15 (3), 314–320. doi:10.1097/01.mnh.0000222701.22583.e8.

Index

Note: Page numbers followed by "*f*" indicate figures, "*t*" indicate tables.

I

K

L

Q

R

Printed and bound by CPI Group (UK) Ltd, Croydon, CR0 4YY
26/08/2026
02204302-0016